Clinical Laboratory Tests

Values and Implications

THIRD EDITION

CONTENTS

Margaret E. Barnes, *RN, MSN*
Staff Development Educator
Sisters of Charity Hospital
Buffalo, N.Y.

Thomas A. Brabson, *DO, FACOEP, FACEP*
Emergency Physician
Albert Einstein Medical Center
Philadelphia

Barbara S. Buckner, *RN, BSN*
Staff Nurse
Harton Regional Medical Center
Tullahoma, Tenn.

Christine S. Clayton, *RN, MSN*
Nurse Practitioner/Clinical Nurse Specialist
Sioux Valley Hospital and University Medical Center
Sioux Falls, S. Dak.

Ellen P. Digan, *MA, MT(ASCP)*
Professor of Biology/Coordinator, MLT Program
Manchester (Conn.) Community College

Diane Dixon, *PA-C, MA, MMSC*
Assistant Professor, Dept. of PA Studies
University of South Alabama
Mobile

Kathleen Ellstrom, *RN, CS, PhD, CNS*
Pulmonary Clinical Nurse Specialist
UCLA Medical Enterprise

Peggi Guenter, *RN, PhD*
Editor-in-Chief, Nutrition in Clinical Practice
American Society for Parenteral and Enteral Nutrition
Silver Spring, Md.

Victoria Hackett, *HT(ASCP)*
Histotechnology Specialist
Health Network Labs
Allentown, Pa.

Connie S. Heflin, *RN, MSN*
Professor
Paducah (Ky.) Community College

Marianne Hoy, *RN, MSN*
Director of Nursing
Cumberland County College
Vineland, N.J.

Elaine G. Lange, *RN, MSN, CCRN, ANP-C*
Adult Nurse Practitioner
Deerfield Valley Health Center
Wilmington, Vt.

Hal S. Larsen, *PhD, MT(ASCP), CLS(NCA)*
Associate Dean, School of Allied Health
Texas Tech University Health Sciences Center
Lubbock

Michel E. Lloyd, *MT(ASCP), SBB*
Technical Coordinator, Blood Bank
St. Luke's Hospital
Bethlehem, Pa.

Julia A. McAvoy, *RN, MSN, CCRN*
Clinical Nurse Specialist, Critical Care
The Washington (Pa.) Hospital

Cathy D. McNew, *CRNP, MS*
Adult Epilepsy Nurse Practitioner
Penn State Geisinger Health System
Hershey, Pa.

Teresa A. Richardson, *MT, BS*
Medical Technologist—Generalist
St. Luke's Quakertown (Pa.) Hospital

Mary Jean Rutherford, *MEd, MT(ASCP), SC*
Associate Professor and CLS Programs Director
Arkansas State University
Jonesboro

Bruce Austin Scott, *RN,CS, MSN*
Nursing Instructor, San Joaquin Delta College
Staff Nurse, St. Joseph's Behavioral Health Center
Stockton, Calif.

Sylvia J. Smith, *RN, CRNP*
OB/GYN Nurse Practitioner
Rosedale Women's Care, P.C.
Pottstown, Pa.

Patricia D. Weiskittel, RN, MSN, CNN, CS
Renal Clinical Nurse Specialist
University Hospital
Cincinnati, Ohio

Jay W. Wilborn, MEd, MT(ASCP)
Program Director
Garland County Community College
Hot Springs, Ark.

Denise Zacher, RN, MSN, CCRN
Administrative Supervisor
Taylor Hospital
Ridley Park, Pa.

Special thanks to the following, who served as contributors for previous editions:

Lolita M. Adrien, RN, MS, ET
Bonnie L. Anderson, MD
G. David Ball, PhD
Wendy L. Baker, RN, BSN, MS
Carol K. Barker, RN, MSN, Med
Deborah M. Berkowitz, RN, MSN, FNP
Barbara Gross Braverman, RN, MSN, DS
Debra C. Broadwell, RN, PhD, ET
Frank Lowell Brown, CUT
Mary Buritt, PhD
Judith Byrne, BS, MT(ASCP)
Ricardo L. Camponovo, MD
Donald C. Cannon, MD, PhD
Raynell J. Clark, BA, MT
Deborah L. Dalrymple, RN, MSN
Gordon DeWald, PhD
William M. Dougherty, BS
Mahmoud A. ElSohly, PhD
John J. Fenton, PhD, DABcc, FNACB
Sr. Rebecca Fidler, MT(ASCP), PhD
Katherine L. Fulton, RN
Shirley Given, HTR(ASCP)
Thad C. Hagen, MD
Patrice M. Harman, RN
Annette L. Harmon, RN, MSN
Lenora R. Haston, RN, MSN
Kathy A. Hausman, RN, MS, CNRN
Tobie Virginia Hittle, RN, BSN, CCRN·
Henry A. Hornburger, MD
Richard Edward Honigman, MD
Jerry A. Katzmann, PhD

Alicia Beth Kavka, MD

Susan A. Kayes, BS, MT(ASCP)

Sr. Mary Brian Kelber, RN, DNS

Sherry L. Keramidas, PhD

Catherine E. Kirby, RN, BSN

George Klee, MD, PhD

William E. Kline, MS, MT(ASCP), SBB

Jeananne Krejci, RN, BS

Clarke Lambe, MD

Laurel Kareus Lambe, MS, RD

George Lawson, PhD

Dennis E. Leavelle, MD

Vanda A. Lennon, MD, PhD

Claire B. Mailhot, RN, MS

Elizabeth Anne Mallon, BS, MT(ASCP)

Harry G. McCoy, PharmD

Marylou K. McHugh, RN, EdD

Joan C. McManus, RN, MA

Malinda Mitchell, RN, MS

S. Breanndan Moore, MD, DCH, FCAP

Susan F. Morrow, RN

John O'Brien, PhD

Whyte G. Owen, PhD

Lynda Palmer, RN, BSN

Deborah S. Parziale, RN, MS

Dale Rabe, MLT(ASCP)

Frank C. Riggall, MD

Carolyn Robertson, RN, MSN

Suzanne G. Rotzell, RN, BSN

Janice Selekman, RN, MSN, DNSc

Ellen Shipes, RN, MN, MEd, ET

Thomas F. Smith, PhD

Mary C. Smolenski, MSN, RN, C, ARNP

Barbara L. Solomon, RN, DNSc, CCNS

Harvey Spector, MD

Howard F. Taswell, MD

Barry L. Tonkonow, MD

Ronald J. Wapner, MD

Beverly A. Zenk Wheat, RN, MA

Elaine Gilligan Whelan, RN, MSN, MA

FOREWORD

Health care consumers are becoming more demanding and informed as a result of recent legislation, a change in attitudes and expectations, and an increase in available information. The availability of home diagnostic tests has also increased, and it appears that this will only expand in the future.

Most clients want to take an active part in their own health care. Informed clients tend to be more compliant and to become participants in the diagnostic, treatment, and healing process. However, the availability of information from television, magazines, and the Internet is a two-edged sword. A little knowledge, or information misunderstood, can be confusing to the client and a detriment to the process.

The health care provider is faced with two significant tasks. The first, of course, is to provide care to the client. The second is to provide accurate and meaningful information to the client that will assist that person in participating in, and understanding, health care decisions.

Clinical Laboratory Tests: Values and Implications, Third Edition, aids the provider in both respects. It's a practical reference that serves as a guide by extending the provider's knowledge base. Its value lies in explaining the more technical aspects of the diagnostic tests as well as providing background for dealing with client questions. This is especially true of the appendix entitled, "Illustrated guide to home tests," which details instructions for performing a number of commonly performed laboratory tests such as cholesterol and glucose. Practitioners will find this section helpful when teaching clients.

This practical reference includes concise descriptions of more than 350 clinical laboratory tests. Each entry begins with a brief description of the test. *Purpose* lists the specific diagnostic indications for performing the test. *Patient preparation* includes specific instructions that must be given the client to ensure a meaningful result. *Procedure* describes the protocol for specimen collection. The normal and abnormal values of each test are listed in *Reference values* or *Normal findings*. *Impli-*

cations of results provides interpretive information in relation to the various disease states that a particular laboratory test is used to evaluate. *Posttest care* describes appropriate client management that is indicated by test results. *Interfering factors* lists the known factors that may interfere with the test and possibly yield misleading results.

Especially helpful for quick reference are the appendices that offer quick-scan charts on crisis or "panic" values and a guide to common abbreviations. Selected references provide opportunity for more detailed reading when necessary. The index is detailed and allows the reader to find important topics quickly and easily.

Clinical Laboratory Tests: Values and Implications, Third Edition, serves as a valuable reference to practicing professionals as well as students. It is a very practical reference that provides important information that will contribute to the quality of client management and appropriate treatment.

Hal S. Larsen, PhD, MT(ASCP), CLS(NCA)
Associate Dean, School of Allied Health
Texas Tech University Health Sciences Center
Lubbock

COLLECTION TECHNIQUES FOR BLOOD AND URINE SAMPLES

Blood

The nature of the test and the patient's age and condition determine the appropriate blood sample, collection site, and technique. *Whole blood*—containing all blood elements—is the sample of choice for blood gas analysis, determination of hemoglobin derivatives, and measurement of red blood cell (RBC) constituents. In addition, most routine hematologic studies, such as complete blood count, erythrocyte sedimentation rate, reticulocyte and platelet counts, and the osmotic fragility test, require whole blood samples.

Plasma is the liquid part of whole blood, which contains all the blood proteins; *serum* is the liquid that remains after whole blood clots. Plasma and serum samples, which contain most of the physiologically and clinically significant substances found in blood, are used for most biochemical, immunologic, and coagulation studies as well as electrolyte evaluation, enzyme analysis, glucose concentration, protein determination, and bilirubin level.

Venous, arterial, and capillary blood

Venous blood returns to the heart through the veins. It carries a high concentration of carbon dioxide (CO_2) from the cells back to the lungs, where it is excreted in exhaled air. Because the biochemical content of venous blood represents physiologic conditions throughout the body and is relatively easy to obtain, it's used for most laboratory procedures.

Arterial blood, replenished with oxygen from the lungs, leaves the heart through the arteries to distribute nutrients throughout the capillary network. Arterial blood samples are necessary for determining pH, partial pressure of arterial oxygen, partial pressure of carbon dioxide, and oxygen saturation, although an arterial puncture increases the risks of hematoma and arterial spasm.

Capillary, or peripheral, blood does the real work of the circulatory system—exchanging fluids, nutrients, and wastes between blood and tissues. Capillary blood samples are most useful for such studies as hemoglobin and hematocrit determinations; blood smears; microtechniques for clinical chemistry; and platelet, RBC, and white blood cell counts requiring only small amounts of blood.

Quantities and containers

The most recent guidelines from the Centers for Disease Control and Prevention mandate that gloves always be worn when obtaining and handling blood and urine specimens as well as any other body fluid. (See *Precautions.*)

Sample quantities needed for diagnostic studies depend on the laboratory, available equipment, and the type of test. Some laboratories, for example, use automated analyzer systems that require a serum sample of 100 µl or less; others use manual systems that require a larger amount. The desired sample quantity determines the collection procedure and the type and size of the container. A single venipuncture with a conventional glass or disposable plastic syringe can provide 10 ml of blood—sufficient for many hematologic, immunologic, chemical, and coagulation tests but hardly enough for a series of tests.

To avoid doing multiple venipunctures when tests require a large blood sample, use an evacuated tube system (Vacutainer, Corvac) with interchangeable glass tubes, optional draw capacities, and a selection of additives. Evacuated tubes are commercially prepared with or without additives (indicated by their color-coded stoppers) and with enough vacuum to draw a predetermined blood volume (2 to 20 ml per tube).

Microanalysis of minute amounts of capillary blood collected with micropipettes or glass capillary tubes allows numerous hematologic and routine laboratory studies to be performed on infants, children, and patients with severe burns or poor veins. Micropipettes are color-coded by sample capacity and hold 30 to 50 µl of whole blood; glass capillary tubes hold 80 to 130 µl of serum or plasma.

Venipuncture

Most tests require venous blood. Although a relatively simple procedure, venipuncture must be performed carefully to avoid hemolysis or hemoconcentration of the sample, hematoma formation, and damage to the patient's veins.

EQUIPMENT

Gloves ▪ tourniquet ▪ 70% alcohol or povidone-iodine solution ▪ sterile syringes or evacuated tubes ▪ sterile

PRECAUTIONS

The Centers for Disease Control and Prevention and the Hospital Infection Control Practices Advisory Committee have developed two
categories of guidelines for preventing the transmission of nosocomial infections. These latest guidelines—*standard precautions*
and *transmission-based precautions*—replace the previous universal precautions and category-specific guidelines.

Standard precautions

Standard precautions are designed to decrease the risk of transmitting organisms from recognized and unrecognized sources of infection in hospitals. They should be followed at all times, with every
patient.

Standard precautions combine the major features of the former
universal precautions, which were developed in response to the increasing incidence of human immunodeficiency virus (HIV), hepatitis B virus (HBV), and other blood-borne diseases, and the former
body-substance isolation precautions, which were developed to
reduce the risk of pathogen transmission from moist body surfaces.
Because standard precautions reduce the risk of transmitting
blood-borne and other pathogens, many patients with diseases that
previously required category- or disease-specific isolation precautions now require only standard precautions.

The specific substances covered by standard precautions include
blood and all other body excretions, except sweat, even if blood is
not visible. Standard precautions should also be followed in the
presence of nonintact skin or exposed mucous membranes.

EQUIPMENT

Gloves ■ masks, goggles, or face shields ■ gowns or aprons ■ resuscitation masks ■ bags for specimens ■ 1:10 dilution of bleach to
water (mixed daily) or hospital-strength disinfectant certified effective against HIV and HBV

IMPLEMENTATION

■ Wash your hands immediately if they become contaminated with
blood or body fluids; also wash them before and after patient care
and after removing gloves. Hand washing retards the growth of organisms on your skin.

■ Wear a gown and face shield (or goggles and a mask) during
procedures that are likely to generate droplets of blood or body fluid, such as surgery, endoscopic procedures, and dialysis.

■ Wear gloves if you will, or could, come in contact with blood,
specimens, tissue, body fluids, or excretions as well as contaminated surfaces or objects. Change your gloves between patient con-
tacts to prevent cross-contamination.

■ Handle used needles and other sharp implements carefully. Do
no bend or break them, reinsert them into their original sheaths, or
handle them unnecessarily. Discard them intact immediately after
use in a sharps biohazard container. These measures reduce the risk
of accidental injury or infection.

■ Notify your employee health provider immediately about all
needlestick injuries, mucosal splashes, and contamination of open
wounds with blood or body fluids to allow investigation of the accident and appropriate care and documentation.

(continued)

PRECAUTIONS (continued)

- Properly label all specimens collected from patients, and place them in plastic biohazard bags at the collection site.
- Promptly clean all blood and body fluids with a 1:10 dilution of bleach to water (mixed daily) or with an approved hospital-strength disinfectant that's effective against HIV and HBV.
- Disposable food trays and dishes are not necessary.
- If you have an exudative lesion, avoid all direct patient contact until the condition has resolved and you've been cleared by your employee health provider. Intact skin is your best defense against infection.

SPECIAL CONSIDERATIONS

Standard precautions are intended to supplement—not replace—recommendations for routine infection control, such as hand washing and wearing gloves.

Keep mouthpieces, resuscitation bags, and other ventilation devices nearby to minimize the need for emergency mouth-to-mouth resuscitation, thus reducing the risk of exposure to body fluids.

Because precautions can't be specified for every clinical situation, you must use your judgment in individual cases. If your job requires exposure to blood, make sure you receive an HBV vaccine.

COMPLICATIONS

Failure to follow standard precautions may lead to exposure to blood-borne diseases and all the complications they may incur.

Transmission-based precautions

Transmission-based precautions are divided into three types, based on the mode of transmission: *airborne precautions, droplet precautions,* and *contact precautions.* These precautions should be followed—in addition to standard precautions—whenever a patient is known or suspected to be infected with a highly contagious and epidemiologically important pathogen that is transmitted by air, by droplets, or by contact with dry skin or other contaminated surfaces. Examples include the pathogens that cause measles (transmitted by air), influenza (transmitted by droplets), and GI, respiratory, skin, and wound infections (transmitted by contact).

Transmission-based precautions replace all previous categories of isolation precautions, including strict isolation, contact isolation, respiratory isolation, enteric precautions, and drainage and secretion precautions as well as other disease-specific precautions. One or more transmission-based precautions may be combined when a patient has a disease with multiple modes of transmission.

needle (20G or 21G for forearm; 25G for wrist, hand, or ankle and for children) ■ color-coded tubes with appropriate additives ■ identification labels ■ small adhesive bandage ■ sterile 2″ × 2″ gauze pads.

TECHNIQUE

Label all test tubes clearly with the patient's name, date, and collection time.

When drawing the sample at bedside, instruct the patient to lie on his back, with his head slightly elevated

SAFEGUARDS FOR VENIPUNCTURE

When performing venipuncture:
- Make sure the patient is well supported in case of syncope.
- To avoid injecting air into a vein when using a syringe to withdraw a sample, first make sure that the plunger is fully depressed.
- Avoid drawing blood from an arm or leg used for I.V. infusion of blood, dextrose, or electrolyte solutions because this dilutes the blood sample. If you must collect blood near an I.V. site, choose a location below it.
- For easier identification of veins in patients with tortuous or sclerosed veins or veins damaged by repeated venipuncture, antimicrobial therapy, or chemotherapy, apply warm, wet compresses 15 minutes before attempting venipuncture.
- If you are not successful after two attempts, ask another phlebotomist to do the venipuncture.
- When you can't find a vein quickly, release the tourniquet temporarily to avoid tissue necrosis and circulation problems.
- Be sure to insert the needle at the correct angle to reduce the risk of puncturing the opposite wall of the vein and causing a hematoma.
- Always release the tourniquet before withdrawing the needle to prevent a hematoma. When drawing multiple samples, release the tourniquet within 1 minute after beginning to draw blood to prevent hemoconcentration.

and his arms resting at his sides. Have an ambulatory patient sit in a chair, with his arm supported on an armrest or a table. Restrain small children if necessary.

Select a venipuncture site. The most common site is the antecubital fossa area; other sites are the wrist and the dorsum of the hand or foot. Do the venipuncture below all I.V. sites or in the opposite arm.

Always wash your hands and put on gloves before drawing a blood sample. When using an evacuated tube, attach the needle to the holder before applying the tourniquet.

Unless cautioned otherwise, apply a soft rubber tourniquet above the puncture site to increase venous pressure, which makes the veins more prominent. Make sure the tourniquet is snug but not constrictive. If the patient's veins appear distinct, you may not need to apply a tourniquet. Using a tourniquet for a patient with large, distended, and highly visible veins increases the risk of hematoma. Instruct the patient to make a fist several times to enlarge the veins.

Select a vein by palpation and inspection. If you can't feel a vein distinctly, *don't* attempt the venipuncture. (See *Safeguards for venipuncture*.)

Working in a circular motion from the center outward, clean the puncture site with alcohol or povidone-iodine solution, and dry it with a gauze pad. If you must touch the cleaned puncture site again to relocate the vein, palpate with an antiseptically clean, gloved finger, and wipe the area again with an alcohol pad.

Draw the skin tautly over the vein by pressing just below the puncture site with your thumb to keep the vein from moving.

Hold the syringe or tube with the needle bevel up and the shaft parallel to the path of the vein at a 15-degree angle to the arm. Enter the vein with a single direct puncture of the skin and vein wall.

If you use a syringe, venous blood flows into the hub. Withdraw the blood slowly, gently pulling on the syringe to create steady suction until you obtain the desired amount.

If you're using an evacuated tube, a drop of blood appears just inside the needle holder. Grasp the needle holder securely and push down on the collection tube until the needle punctures the rubber stopper; blood then flows into the tube automatically. When the tube is filled, remove it; if you're drawing multiple samples, repeat the procedure with additional tubes.

To prevent stasis, release the tourniquet as soon as you establish adequate blood flow. If the flow is sluggish, you may want to leave the tourniquet in place longer. However, always remove the tourniquet before withdrawing the needle.

After drawing the sample, ask the patient to open his fist as soon as you collect the desired amount. Release the tourniquet if you haven't already done that. Place a gauze pad over the puncture site; then withdraw the needle slowly and gently. Apply gentle pressure to the puncture site. If the patient is alert and cooperative, tell him to hold the gauze pad in place for several minutes until the bleeding stops to prevent hematoma. If the patient is not alert or cooperative, hold the pad in place or apply a small adhesive bandage.

After collection with a syringe, remove the needle and carefully empty the sample into the appropriate test tube without delay. To prevent foaming and hemolysis, don't eject the blood through the needle or force it out of the syringe. Place the appropriate color-coded stoppers on the tubes. Gently invert a tube containing an anticoagulant several times to mix the sample thoroughly. Examine the sample for clots or clumps; if none appear, send the sample to the laboratory. Don't shake the tube.

Before leaving the patient, check his condition. If a hematoma develops at the puncture site, apply warm soaks. If the patient has lingering discomfort or excessive bleeding, instruct him to lie down. Watch for anxiety or signs of shock, such as hypotension and tachycardia. Send the sample to the laboratory immediately.

Many laboratories use automated electronic systems that can perform multiple tests on a blood sample.

Arterial sample

Arterial blood is rarely required for routine studies. Because arterial puncture carries risks, a doctor or a specially trained nurse or physician assistant usually collects these samples.

Before drawing a blood sample for arterial blood gas (ABG) analysis, carefully check the patient's oxygen therapy. If ABG levels are being measured to monitor his response to withdrawal of oxygen but the patient continues to receive it, results will be misleading. For the same reason, wait 15 to 30 minutes before drawing an arterial sample after suctioning the patient or placing him on a ventilator to allow circulating blood levels to reflect mechanical ventilation. Blood gases should not be drawn during dialysis.

EQUIPMENT

If available, use an ABG kit, which contains all the necessary equipment, including a heparinized syringe. Gloves ■ 10-ml luer-lock glass syringe ■ 1-ml ampule heparin ■ 20G 1½" short-bevel needle ■ 23G 1" short-bevel needle ■ rubber stopper or cork ■ antiseptic swabs ■ 70% alcohol or povidone-iodine solution ■ sterile 2" × 2" gauze pads ■ tape or adhesive bandage ■ iced specimen container ■ labels (for syringe and specimen bag) for patient's name, doctor's name, hospital number, date, collection time, and details of oxygen therapy.

TECHNIQUE

Before drawing an arterial blood sample, administer a local anesthetic at the puncture site, if necessary. Perform Allen's test to assess radial artery circulation. (See *Performing Allen's test*, page 8.) Try to obtain the specimen from the radial artery; use the brachial artery only when necessary. Don't draw arterial blood from an arm that had a vascular graft or has an atrioventricular fistula in situ.

Next, using a circular motion, clean the puncture site with povidone-iodine solution. Then wipe the site with alcohol to remove the povidone-iodine solution, which is sticky and may hinder palpation.

Palpate the artery with the forefinger and middle finger of one hand while holding the syringe over the puncture site with the other hand. With the needle bevel up, puncture the skin at a 45-degree angle for the radial

PERFORMING ALLEN'S TEST

Before obtaining a specimen from an arterial site, assess the blood supply to your patient's hand. If the radial artery is blocked by a blood clot — a common complication — the ulnar artery alone must supply blood to the hand. The Allen's test is a simple, reliable procedure that quickly assesses arterial function.

Just follow these steps:

1. Have the patient rest his arm on the bedside table. Support his wrist with a rolled towel. Ask him to clench his fist. Use your index and middle fingers to exert pressure over both the radial and the ulnar arteries.

2. Without removing your fingers, ask the patient to unclench his fist. You'll notice his palm is blanched because you've impaired the normal blood flow with your fingers. *Tip:* If your patient is unconscious or unable to clench his fist for some other reason, you can encourage his palm to blanch by occluding both arteries, elevating his hand, and massaging his palm.

3. Release the pressure on the ulnar artery, and ask the patient to open his fist. If the ulnar artery is functioning well, his palm will turn pink in about 5 seconds, even though the radial artery is still occluded. But if blood return is slow and his fingers begin to contract, blood supply from the ulnar artery may not be adequate. In that case, try Allen's test on his other wrist; you may get better results. *Note:* Slow blood return may indicate poor cardiac output or poor capillary refill due to shock.

---

artery and at a 60-degree angle for the brachial artery. For a femoral arterial puncture, insert the needle at a 90-degree angle.

Advance the needle, but don't pull the plunger back. When you've punctured the artery, blood will pulsate into the syringe. Allow 5 to 10 ml to fill the syringe.

If the syringe doesn't fill immediately, you may have pushed the needle through the artery. If so, pull the needle back slightly, but don't pull the plunger back. If the syringe still doesn't fill, withdraw the needle and start over with a fresh heparinized needle. Never make more than two attempts to draw blood from one site.

After drawing the sample, remove the needle and apply firm pressure to the puncture site with a gauze pad for at least 5 minutes to prevent hematoma (a significant risk after arterial puncture). If the patient is receiving an anticoagulant or has a bleeding disorder, apply pressure for at least 15 minutes. Do not ask the patient to apply pressure to the site; he may not apply the continuous, firm pressure that's needed.

Rotate the syringe to mix the heparin with the sample. Try to remove air bubbles by holding the syringe upright and tapping it lightly with your finger. If the bubbles don't disappear, hold the syringe upright and pierce a 2" × 2" gauze pad or alcohol pad with the needle. Slowly forcing some of the blood out of the syringe eliminates the bubbles, and the gauze pad catches the ejected blood. After removing air bubbles, plunge the needle into a rubber stopper to seal it, or remove the needle and apply the syringe stopper from the ABG kit, if available. Transfer the sample to the iced specimen container.

Note on the laboratory request the type and amount of oxygen the patient is receiving. In certain instances (such as hypothermia), you may also be asked to provide the patient's temperature and hemoglobin count. Send the sample to the laboratory immediately.

After releasing pressure on the puncture site, tape a bandage firmly over it. (Don't tape the entire wrist.)

After arterial puncture, observe the patient closely for signs of circulatory impairment distal to the puncture site, such as swelling or discoloration. Ask if he feels pain, numbness, or tingling in the extremity.

Capillary sample

Collection of a capillary blood sample requires puncturing the fingertip or earlobe of adults or the great toe or heel of neonates.

EQUIPMENT

Gloves ■ sterile, disposable blood lancet ■ sterile 2" × 2" gauze pads ■ 70% alcohol or povidone-iodine solution ■ glass slides, heparinized capillary tubes, or pipettes ■ appropriate solutions.

TECHNIQUE

To facilitate collection of a capillary sample, first dilate the vessels by applying warm, moist compresses to the area for about 10 minutes. Avoid cold, cyanotic, or swollen sites.

Select the puncture site, wipe it with gauze and alcohol pads, and dry it thoroughly with another gauze pad so the blood will well up. To draw a sample from the fingertip, use an automatic lancing device and make the puncture perpendicular to the lines of the patient's fingerprints.

After drawing the sample, wipe away the first drop of blood and avoid squeezing the puncture site to reduce the risk of diluting the sample with tissue fluid. After collecting the sample, apply pressure to the puncture site briefly to prevent painful extravasation of blood into the subcutaneous tissues. Ask the adult patient to hold a sterile gauze pad over the puncture site until bleeding has stopped. Then apply a small adhesive bandage.

Interfering factors

Because food and medications can interfere with test methods, be sure to check the patient's diet and medication history before tests, and try to schedule blood collection after an overnight fast of 12 to 14 hours. Although the concentration of most blood constituents doesn't change significantly after a meal, fasting is customary because blood collected shortly after eating often appears cloudy (turbid) from a temporary increase in triglyceride levels, which can interfere with many chemical reactions. Transient, food-related lipemia usually disappears 4 to 6 hours after a meal, making such short fasts acceptable before blood collection. Baseline studies often depend on the patient's diet. For example, valid glucose tolerance test results require an adequate daily carbohydrate intake (250 mg) for 3 days before testing. Similarly, recent protein and fat consumption influences uric acid, urea, and lipid levels.

Numerous drugs and their metabolites can affect test results by pharmacologic or chemical interference. Pharmacologic interference results from temporary or permanent drug-induced physiologic changes in a blood component. For example, long-term administration of aminoglycosides can damage the kidneys and alter the results of renal function studies.

Chemical interference results from a drug's physical characteristic that alters the test reaction. For example, high doses of ascorbic acid may raise blood glucose levels. To identify such interference with test results, all unexpected changes in blood values require a meticulous review of the patient's drug and dietary history and of his clinical status.

Urine

The type of urine specimen required—random, second-voided, first morning, fasting, clean-catch midstream, or timed—depends on the patient's condition and the purpose of the test.

Collection by patients

Random, second-voided, and clean-catch midstream specimens can be collected at any time; first morning, fasting, and timed specimens require collection at specific times.

RANDOM, SECOND-VOIDED, FIRST MORNING, OR FASTING COLLECTION

A *random urine specimen*, usually collected as part of a physical examination or at various times during hospitalization, permits laboratory screening for urinary and systemic disorders as well as for drug screening. A *second-voided* (or *double-voided*) *specimen* rinses the urethra and produces a truer specimen of urine from the bladder. It's used in diabetic patients to obtain a true determination of the amount of sugar and ketones spilled at any particular time. *First morning* and *fasting specimens* produce a more accurate urine-values list because values aren't influenced or tainted by ingestion of food or chemicals.

Equipment Clean, dry bedpan or urinal (for nonambulatory patients) ■ gloves ■ specimen container ■ specimen labels ■ laboratory request slip.

Random specimen To collect a *random specimen* (for such routine tests as urinalysis), the patient simply collects urine by voiding into a specimen container. Although this method provides quick laboratory results, the information it supplies is less reliable than that from a controlled specimen.

For random collection, tell the ambulatory patient to urinate directly into a clean, dry specimen container. Tell the nonambulatory patient to void into a clean bedpan or urinal to minimize bacterial or chemical contamination and then put on gloves, transfer about 30 ml of urine to the specimen container, and secure the cap.

Second-voided specimen To collect a *second-voided specimen*, the patient voids, discards the urine, and then voids again 30 minutes later into a specimen container.

For second-voided collection, instruct the patient to void and discard the urine. Then offer him at least one glass of water to stimulate urine production. Collect urine 30 minutes later, using the random collection technique.

Label the specimen container with the patient's name and room number, and send the labeled container to the laboratory immediately. On the chart, record the procedure and the time the specimen was sent.

First morning and fasting specimens These must be collected when the patient awakens. Because the first morning specimen is the most concentrated of the day, it's the specimen of choice for nitrate, protein, and urinary sediment analyses. To obtain this specimen, the patient voids and discards the urine just before going to bed, then collects the urine from the first voiding of the morning. For the fasting specimen, which is used for glucose testing, the patient maintains an overnight fast and collects a first morning specimen.

Unless the patient is an infant or is catheterized or unable to urinate, use the following collection techniques:

For fasting specimen collection, instruct the patient to restrict food and fluids after midnight before the test. For both collection procedures, instruct the patient to void and discard the urine before retiring for the night and then collect the first voiding of the next day in a clean, dry specimen container. (If the patient must void during the night, note it on the specimen label, for example, "Urine specimen, 2:15 a.m. to 8:00 a.m.")

Label the container with the patient's name and room number (if applicable), doctor's name, date, and collection time. Send the specimen and a completed request to the laboratory immediately. On the chart, record the procedure and the time the specimen was sent.

CLEAN-CATCH SPECIMEN

The patient begins voiding into either a bedpan or toilet and then collects a sample in midstream. Originally used mainly to test for bacteriuria and pyuria, this type of specimen is now replacing the random specimen because it's aseptic, producing a virtually uncontaminated specimen without the need for catheterization.

Equipment Commercially prepared kit containing necessary equipment and directions for the patient in several languages (English, Spanish, and French), or antiseptic solution (green soap or povidone-iodine solution) ■ water ■ cotton balls ■ sterile gloves ■ specimen labels ■ laboratory request slip.

Technique This aseptic technique for obtaining a clean-catch midstream urine specimen has become the acceptable procedure for collecting a random urine specimen. It's especially valuable for collecting urine specimens from women because it provides a specimen that's virtually free of bacterial contamination.

Teach the patient how to obtain a clean-catch midstream specimen. Send the specimen to the laboratory immediately or refrigerate it to prevent proliferation of bacteria. On the chart, record the procedure and the time the specimen was sent.

TIMED SPECIMENS

A *timed specimen* determines the urinary concentration of such substances as hormones, proteins, creatinine, and electrolytes over a specified period—usually 2, 12, or 24 hours. The 24-hour collection, the most common duration, provides a measure of average excretion for substances eliminated in variable amounts during the day, such as hormones. A timed specimen may also be collected after administration of a challenge dose of a chemical to measure physiologic efficiency — for example, ingestion of glucose to test for incipient diabetes mellitus or hypoglycemia. This type of specimen is also preferred for quantitative analysis of urobilinogen, amylase, or dye excretion.

Equipment Clean, dry gallon containers or commercial urine collection containers ■ preservative, as ordered ■ labels for collection container ■ display signs.

Technique All timed specimens — 2-, 12-, and 24-hour specimens — are collected in virtually the same way. This procedure is used for uncatheterized adults and continent children.

Explain the procedure to the patient, and instruct him to collect all urine during the test period, to notify you after each voiding, and to avoid contaminating the specimen with toilet tissue or stool. Also, provide him with written instructions for home collection. Explain any necessary dietary, drug, or activity restrictions.

Obtain the proper preservative from the laboratory. Write down the test requirements on the nursing-care Kardex. Label a gallon jug or a commercial urine collection container with the patient's name and room number (if applicable), the doctor's name, the date and time the collection begins and ends, a "Do Not Discard" warning, and instructions to keep the container refrigerated. Prominently display signs indicating that a 24-hour urine collection is in progress: one at the head of the patient's bed, a second over the toilet bowl in his bathroom, and a third over the utility room bedpan hopper.

Tell the patient to void and discard the urine; then begin a 24-hour collection with the next voiding. After placing the urine from the first voiding in the container, add the preservative. Add each subsequent urine specimen to the container immediately. If any urine is lost, restart the test, but remember that the test should end at a time that the laboratory is open. Just before the end of the collection period, instruct the patient to void, and add the urine to the gallon jug.

Send the labeled container to the laboratory as soon as the collection period has ended. On the chart, record the time that urine collection ended and when the specimen was sent to the laboratory.

Special timed collections Some tests require specimen collection at specified times — for example, the glucose tolerance test requires collection of urine at 30 minutes,

1 hour, 2 hours, 3 hours and, occasionally, 4 and 5 hours after a test meal. To ensure that the patient can void at the specified times, have him drink water at least every hour.

Other tests, including urea clearance, require only 2-hour collection periods. For these tests, give the patient at least 20 oz (600 ml) of water 30 minutes before the test, and instruct him to drink at least one full glass each hour during the test.

Collection from infants

Use this technique to obtain a random, second-voided, first morning, fasting, or timed specimen from infants.

EQUIPMENT

Gloves ■ disposable plastic collection bags ■ specimen containers ■ laboratory request slip ■ cotton swabs ■ soap and water ■ diapers.

TECHNIQUE

Position the infant on his back, with his hips externally rotated and abducted, and knees flexed. Put on gloves. Clean the perineal area with cotton swabs, soap, and water. Rinse the area with warm water and dry it thoroughly.

Males: Apply the collection device over the penis and scrotum with gloved hands, and closely press the flaps of the bag against the perineum to secure it.

Females: Tape the pediatric collection device to the perineum, starting between the anus and the vagina and working anteriorly.

Place a diaper over the collection bag to discourage the child from tampering with it. Elevate the head of the bed to facilitate drainage.

Remove the bag immediately after collection is complete to prevent skin excoriation. Transfer the urine to a clean, dry specimen container. Label the container with the patient's name and room number (if applicable), doctor's name, date, and collection time. Send the specimen and the completed request to the laboratory immediately, and note the collection time on the chart.

Collection by catheter

Although use of a catheter increases the risk of bacterial infection in the lower genitourinary tract, it may be necessary to obtain a random, second-voided, first morning, fasting, or timed specimen in a patient who can't void voluntarily.

EQUIPMENT

Sterile catheterization set (sterile gloves, sterile catheter [#16F for adults, #8F for children]) ▪ sterile forceps ▪ soap, water, towelette ▪ sterile water-soluble lubricant ▪ sterile cotton balls ▪ antiseptic solution ▪ sterile drapes ▪ sterile specimen container ▪ labels for specimen container.

TECHNIQUE

Tell the patient you'll collect a urine specimen by inserting a small tube into the bladder through the urethra and that, although this procedure may cause some discomfort, it takes only a few minutes.

Males: Put on gloves and wash the perineal area with soap and water. Place a sterile drape under the patient's buttocks and around the penis, making sure that you don't contaminate the drape. Remove the contaminated gloves, and put on sterile gloves. Place the antiseptic solution on the cotton balls.

Arrange all sterile articles within easy reach on a sterile wrapper.

Open the sterile specimen container, and lubricate the sterile catheter.

Grasp the shaft of the penis in one hand and elevate it about 90 degrees to the upright position; hold it in this position until the procedure is completed.

Retract the foreskin and, with the forceps, grasp an antiseptic-moistened cotton ball.

Clean the urethral meatus, wiping with a circular motion away from the urethral opening toward the glans. Repeat twice, each time with a clean cotton ball.

Gently insert the lubricated catheter until urine flows. Allow a few milliliters to drain into the basin; then collect 10 to 60 ml in a sterile plastic container, depending on test requirements.

After gently removing the catheter, clean and dry the periurethral area.

Send the specimen and the laboratory request to the laboratory within 10 minutes, or refrigerate the specimen. On the chart, record the procedure and the time the specimen is sent.

Females: Put on gloves, and wash the perineal area with soap and water.

Place the patient in the supine position, with knees flexed and feet on the bed.

Place a sterile drape under her buttocks and around the perineal area, making sure that you don't contaminate the drape.

Remove the contaminated gloves, and put on sterile gloves.

Place the antiseptic solution on the cotton balls, and lubricate the sterile catheter.

Arrange all sterile articles within easy reach on a sterile wrapper, and open the sterile specimen container.

Separate the labia majora and keep them open with one hand. With the forceps, grasp an antiseptic-moistened cotton ball and make two vertical swipes on the labia minora. (Use a new cotton ball for each swipe, cleaning from the urethral meatus toward the anus.)

Position the sterile tray with the lubricated catheter on the sterile field between the patient's legs.

Gently insert the catheter into the urethra until urine flows. Allow a few milliliters of urine to flow into a basin; then collect 10 to 60 ml in a sterile plastic container, depending on the test requirements.

After gently removing the catheter, clean and dry the urethral area.

Send the specimen and a laboratory request to the laboratory within 10 minutes after collection, or refrigerate the specimen. On the chart, record the procedure and the time that the specimen was sent.

Collection from an indwelling catheter

You can minimize the risk of bacterial contamination by aspirating a urine specimen from an indwelling urinary catheter made of self-sealing rubber or from a collection tube with a special sampling port. (However, *don't* aspirate a Silastic, silicone, or plastic catheter.) This technique can provide a random, second-voided, first morning, fasting, or timed specimen.

EQUIPMENT

Gloves ▪ sterile syringe (10 to 20 ml) ▪ sterile needle (21G to 25G) ▪ alcohol sponge ▪ sterile specimen container ▪ specimen labels ▪ laboratory request slip.

TECHNIQUE

About 30 minutes before collecting the specimen, clamp the collection tube unless the patient has just undergone genitourinary surgery.

Never insert the needle into the shaft of the catheter because this may puncture the lumen leading to the balloon.

If the collection tube has a sampling port, put on gloves and wipe the port with an alcohol sponge. Insert the needle at a 90-degree angle and aspirate the urine into the syringe.

If the collection tube has a rubber catheter but not a port, obtain the specimen from the catheter.

Put on gloves, and wipe the catheter with alcohol just above the connection of the collection tube to the catheter.

Insert the needle at a 45-degree angle into the catheter, and withdraw the urine specimen.

If you can't draw any urine, lift the tube a little, but make sure urine doesn't return to the bladder.

Aspirate urine and unclamp the tube after collecting the specimen. Failure to do so can cause bladder distention and may predispose the patient to a bladder infection.

Transfer the specimen to a sterile container, and cap the container securely. Send it to the laboratory in a plastic bag.

Interfering factors

A common interfering factor in urine collection, especially in timed collections, is the patient's failure to follow the correct collection procedure. Inaccurate test results may be due to *overcollection*, failing to discard the last voiding before the test period; *undercollection*, failing to include all urine voided during the test; *contamination*, including toilet tissue or stool in the specimen; or, for procedures requiring collection at specified times or for the second-voided collection, the patient's *inability to urinate on demand*.

In urine specimens collected from females, vaginal drainage (such as menses, which elevates the RBC count) can alter the results of a urinalysis.

Improper collection or handling of the specimen can also produce unreliable results. For instance, failure to thoroughly clean the urethral meatus and glans before collection can contaminate a clean-catch midstream specimen. Similarly, failure to send a urine specimen to the laboratory immediately allows bacterial proliferation and thus invalidates the colony count on bacterial culture.

Foods and drugs can affect test results by changing the composition of the urine. For example, ingestion of sugar increases urine glucose levels. Drugs can cause chemical or pharmacologic interference with the laboratory analysis. For example, corticosteroids tend to elevate glucose levels.

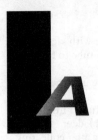

ABO blood type test

This test classifies blood according to the presence of major antigens A and B on red blood cell (RBC) surfaces and of serum antibodies anti-A and anti-B. ABO blood typing is required before transfusions to prevent a lethal reaction — even if the patient is carrying an ABO blood group identification card.

In forward typing, the patient's RBCs are mixed with anti-A serum and then with anti-B serum; the presence or absence of agglutination determines the blood group. In reverse typing, the results of the forward method are verified by mixing the patient's serum with known group A and group B cells. Blood group determination is confirmed when the results of forward and reverse typing match perfectly. (See *ABO blood types*.)

Purpose

■ To establish blood group according to the ABO system
■ To check compatibility of donor and recipient blood before a transfusion.

Patient preparation

Tell the patient that this test determines blood type. If he is scheduled for a transfusion, explain that determining his blood type makes it possible to match his blood with the correct donor blood. Inform the patient that fasting isn't necessary. Explain that the test requires a blood sample, tell him who will perform the venipuncture and when, and note that the needle puncture and the pressure of the tourniquet may cause transient discomfort. Check the patient's history for recent administration of blood, dextran, or I.V. contrast media, which may affect test results.

Procedure

Perform the venipuncture, and collect the sample in a 10-ml tube without additives.

Precautions

■ Before the transfusion, compare current and past ABO typing and cross-matching to detect mistaken identification and prevent transfusion reaction.

ABO BLOOD TYPES

ABO RECIPIENT-DONOR COMPATIBILITY

Recipient's blood type	Compatible donor type
A	A, O
B	B, O
AB	A, B, AB, O
O	O

ABO BLOOD TYPES IN U.S. POPULATION

Blood type	Percent	Blood type	Percent
O+	38%	B+	9%
O-	7%	B-	2%
A+	34%	AB+	3%
A-	6%	AB-	1%

Note: Distribution may differ for specific ethnic and racial groups.

Source: American Association of Blood Banks, September 1999.

- Label the sample with the patient's name, the hospital or blood bank number, the date, and the initials of the phlebotomist.
- Handle the sample gently, and send it to the laboratory immediately with a properly completed laboratory request.

Normal findings and implications of results

In forward typing, agglutination when the patient's RBCs are mixed with anti-A serum means the A antigen is present, and the blood is typed A. Agglutination when the patient's RBCs are mixed with anti-B serum means the B antigen is present, and the blood is typed B. If agglutination occurs in both mixes, both A and B antigens are present, and the blood is typed AB. If it doesn't occur in either mix, no antigens are present, and the blood is typed O.

In reverse typing, agglutination when B cells are mixed with the patient's serum means that anti-B is present, and the blood is typed A. Agglutination when A cells are mixed with the patient's serum means that anti-A is present, and the blood is typed B. If agglutination occurs when both A and B cells are mixed, anti-A and anti-B are present, and the blood is typed O. If agglutination doesn't occur when both A and B cells are mixed, neither anti-A nor anti-B is present, and the blood is typed AB.

Posttest care

If a hematoma develops at the venipuncture site, apply warm soaks.

Interfering factors

■ Recent administration of dextran or I.V. contrast media causes cellular aggregation that resembles agglutination.

■ Hemolysis caused by rough handling of the sample may affect test results.

■ New antibodies may interfere with compatibility testing if the patient has received blood or been pregnant in the past 3 months.

Acetylcholine receptor antibody test

The acetylcholine receptor (AChR) antibodies test is the most useful way to confirm myasthenia gravis (MG), a disorder of neuromuscular transmission. In normal muscle contraction, acetylcholine (ACh) is released from the terminal end of the nerve and binds to AChR sites on the muscle motor end plate. In MG, antibodies block and destroy AChR sites, causing muscle weakness that can be either generalized or localized to the ocular muscles.

Two test methods—a binding assay and a blocking assay—are available to determine the relative concentration of AChR antibodies in serum. In the binding assay, purified AChRs are complexed with ^{125}I-labeled alpha-bungarotoxin, a molecule that binds specifically to AChRs and blocks them. A serum sample is added to this complex; after incubation, antihuman immunoglobulin is added. Antibodies bind to AChR–^{125}I-labeled alpha-bungarotoxin complexes, which coprecipitate with the total human immunoglobulin. The amount of radioactivity is then measured to assay the available AChR sites. AChR-binding antibodies are found in about 90% of patients with generalized MG and in about 50% of those with localized MG.

When the AChR-binding assay is negative in a patient with symptoms of MG, the AChR-blocking assay may be performed. In this test, the patient's serum is incubated with purified AChRs before ^{125}I-labeled alpha-bungarotoxin is added to detect antibodies whose antigenic sites would otherwise be blocked. Although the blocking assay is relatively new and its clinical significance isn't yet fully known, it's specific for autoimmune MG and is useful for research. Determination of AChR antibodies by either method also helps monitor immunosuppressive therapy for MG, although antibody levels don't usually parallel the severity of disease.

Purpose

- To confirm a diagnosis of MG
- To monitor the effectiveness of immunosuppressive therapy for MG.

Patient preparation

Explain to the patient that this test helps confirm MG or, when indicated, that it assesses the effectiveness of treatment for MG. Tell the patient that fasting isn't necessary. Explain that the test requires a blood sample, tell him who will perform the venipuncture and when, and note that the needle puncture and the pressure of the tourniquet may cause transient discomfort. Check the patient's medication history for immunosuppressive drugs that may affect test results, and note their use on the laboratory request.

Procedure

Perform a venipuncture, and collect the sample in a 7-ml tube without additives.

Precautions

Keep the sample at room temperature, and send it to the laboratory immediately.

Reference values

Normal serum contains 0 to 0.03 nmol/L AChR-binding antibodies and is negative for AChR-blocking antibodies.

Implications of results

Positive AChR antibodies in symptomatic adults confirm the diagnosis of MG. Patients with only ocular symptoms tend to have lower antibody titers than those with generalized symptoms.

Posttest care

- Check the venipuncture site for infection, and promptly report any change because patients with autoimmune disease have compromised immune systems. Keep a clean, dry bandage over the site for at least 24 hours.
- If a hematoma develops at the venipuncture site, apply warm soaks.

Interfering factors

- Patients undergoing thymectomy, thoracic duct drainage, immunosuppressive therapy, or plasmapheresis may show reduced AChR-antibody levels.
- Failure to maintain the sample at room temperature and send it to the laboratory immediately may affect the accuracy of test results.

■ Patients with amyotrophic lateral sclerosis may show false-positive test results.

Acid mucopolysaccharide test, urine

This quantitative test measures the urine level of acid mucopolysaccharides (AMPs), a group of polysaccharides or carbohydrates, in infants who have a family history of one of the group of rare diseases called mucopolysaccharidosis. These inborn errors of metabolism cause enzyme deficiencies and accumulation of AMPs—especially dermatan sulfate and heparitin sulfate. The most severe form, Hurler's syndrome (gargoylism), results from deposition of these macromolecular complexes in several organs, particularly the heart and kidneys, and excretion of large amounts of mucopolysaccharides in the urine.

AMPs are precipitated out of a 24-hour urine specimen with cetyltrimethylammonium bromide and are then extracted with ethanol. The glucuronic acid in the now-isolated AMPs is measured by the Dische carbazole reaction, and the AMP value is expressed as milligrams of glucuronic acid. Dividing this number by the amount of creatinine (which reflects the glomerular filtration rate) in the same specimen yields a ratio that overcomes irregularities in the 24-hour urine collection.

Purpose

To diagnose mucopolysaccharidosis.

Patient preparation

Explain to the parents of the infant that this test helps determine the efficiency of carbohydrate metabolism. Inform them that they don't need to restrict the child's food or fluids. Tell them that the test requires urine collection for 24 hours, and teach them the proper way to collect the specimen at home.

CLINICAL ALERT If the child is receiving therapy with heparin and must continue it, note this on the laboratory request.

Procedure

Obtain a 24-hour urine specimen. Add 20 ml of toluene as a preservative at the start of the collection period. Indicate the patient's age on the laboratory request, and send the specimen to the laboratory as soon as the 24-hour collection period is over.

Precautions

During the collection period, refrigerate the specimen or place it on ice.

Reference values

The normal AMP value for adults is less than 13.3 μg glucuronic acid/mg creatinine/24 hours. For children, values vary with age.

Implications of results

Elevated AMP levels reliably indicate mucopolysaccharidosis. Supplementary quantitative analysis and detailed blood studies can identify the specific enzyme that is defective.

Posttest care

Be sure to remove all adhesive from the infant's perineum after removing the urine collector. Wash the area gently with soap and water, and watch for irritation.

Interfering factors

- Heparin elevates urine AMP levels.
- Failure to collect all urine during the test period or to store the specimen properly may alter test results.

Acid perfusion test

The lower esophageal sphincter normally prevents gastric reflux. However, if this sphincter is incompetent, the recurrent backflow of acidic juices (and of bile salts, if the pyloric sphincter is also incompetent) into the esophagus inflames the esophageal mucosa. The inflammation, esophagitis, manifests in burning epigastric or retrosternal pain that may radiate to the back or arms.

The acid perfusion test, also known as the Bernstein test, distinguishes such pain from that caused by angina pectoris or other disorders. In this test, normal saline and acidic solutions are perfused separately into the esophagus through a nasogastric (NG) tube.

Purpose

To distinguish heartburn-like pains caused by esophagitis from those caused by cardiac disorders.

Patient preparation

Explain to the patient that this test helps determine the cause of heartburn. Instruct the patient to observe the following pretest restrictions: no antacids for 24 hours, no food for 12 hours, and no fluids or smoking for 8 hours. Tell the patient who will perform the test and where it will be performed, and advise that the test will take about 1 hour.

Inform the patient that the test requires passage of a tube through his nose into the esophagus and that he may experience some discomfort, coughing, or gagging during tube passage. Explain that during the test, liquid is slowly perfused through the tube into the esophagus and that he should immediately report any pain or burning during perfusion.

Immediately before the test, check the patient's pulse rate and blood pressure, ask the patient if he's experiencing any heartburn and, if he is, ask him to describe it.

Procedure

- After seating the patient, insert into the patient's stomach an NG tube that has been marked at 12″ (30 cm) from the tip.
- Attach a 20-ml syringe to the tube, and aspirate the stomach contents. Then withdraw the tube into the esophagus (to the 12″ mark).
- Hang labeled containers of normal saline solution and 0.1 N HCl solution on an I.V. pole behind the patient; then connect the NG tube to I.V. tubing.
- Open the line from the normal saline solution, and begin a drip at a rate of 60 to 120 drops/minute.
- Continue to perfuse this solution for 5 to 10 minutes; then ask the patient if he's experiencing any discomfort, and record his response.
- Without the patient's knowledge, close the line from the saline solution and open the line from the acidic solution. Begin a drip into the esophagus at the same rate as for the saline solution, and continue the perfusion for 30 minutes or until the patient indicates that he's experiencing discomfort.
- If the patient experiences discomfort, immediately close the line from the acidic solution and open the line from the saline solution. Continue to perfuse saline solution until the discomfort subsides.
- If ordered, repeat perfusion of the acidic solution to verify the patient's response. If this isn't required, or if the patient experiences no discomfort after perfusion of the acidic solution for 30 minutes, stop the drip and withdraw the NG tube.
- If the patient continues to experience pain or burning, administer an antacid. If the patient reports a sore throat, provide soothing lozenges or obtain an order for an ice collar.

Precautions

- The acid perfusion test is contraindicated in patients with esophageal varices, heart failure, acute myocardial infarction, or other cardiac disorders.
- During intubation, make sure the tube enters the esophagus, not the trachea. Withdraw the tube immediately if the patient develops cyanosis or paroxysmal coughing.

■ Observe the patient closely for arrhythmias.
■ Clamp the tube before removing it to prevent aspiration of fluid into the lungs.

Normal findings

Absence of pain or burning during perfusion of either solution indicates a healthy esophageal mucosa.

Implications of results

In patients with esophagitis, the acidic solution causes pain or burning, whereas the normal saline solution usually produces no adverse reactions. Occasionally, both solutions cause pain in patients with esophagitis; they may cause no pain in patients with asymptomatic esophagitis.

Posttest care

The patient may resume usual diet and medications withheld before the test.

Interfering factors

■ Failure to adhere to pretest restrictions may interfere with the accuracy of test results.
■ Drugs that may affect test results include adrenergic blockers, anticholinergics, reserpine, corticosteroids, histamine-2 blockers, and acid pump inhibitors. Note the use of any of these drugs on the laboratory request.

Acid phosphatase test

Acid phosphatases are a group of enzymes most active at a pH of about 5.0. They are present in the prostate gland and semen and, to a lesser extent, in the liver, spleen, red blood cells, bone marrow, and platelets. Each of these variants is called an isoenzyme.

This test measures total acid phosphatase and the prostatic fraction in serum by radioimmunoassay or biochemical enzyme assay. The more widespread the cancer, the more likely that serum acid phosphatase levels will be increased.

Purpose

■ To detect prostate cancer
■ To monitor response to therapy for prostate cancer (successful treatment decreases acid phosphatase levels).

Patient preparation

Explain to the patient that this test helps evaluate prostate function. Inform him that restriction of food or fluids before the test isn't necessary. Tell him that the test requires a blood sample, explain who will perform the venipuncture and when, and tell him he may experience discomfort from the needle puncture and the tourniquet.

Withhold fluorides, phosphates, and clofibrate before the test, if ordered. If any of these drugs must be continued, be sure to note this on the laboratory request.

Procedure

Perform a venipuncture, and collect the sample in a 7-ml tube without additives; some laboratories ask for a heparinized tube so they won't have to wait for the sample to clot. Put the tube in ice for immediate delivery to the laboratory. If the sample can't be analyzed in less than 30 minutes, it should be frozen.

Precautions

■ Don't draw the sample within 48 hours of prostate manipulation (rectal examination).
■ Handle the collection tube gently.
■ Send the sample to the laboratory immediately. Acid phosphatase levels drop by 50% within 1 hour if the sample remains at room temperature without a preservative or if it isn't packed in ice.

Reference values

Total serum acid phosphatase levels vary with the assay method; they generally range from 0.5 to 1.9 U/L.

Implications of results

High levels of prostatic acid phosphatase usually indicate that a tumor has spread beyond the prostatic capsule. If the tumor has metastasized to bone, alkaline phosphatase (ALP) levels are also high, reflecting increased osteoblastic activity.

Misleading results may occur if ALP levels are high because acid phosphatase and ALP enzymes are chemically similar and differ mainly in the optimum pH ranges. Some ALP isoenzymes may react at a lower pH and thus be detected as acid phosphatase. Increased levels may reflect the presence of prostatic carcinoma, multiple myeloma, Paget's disease, Gaucher's disease, cancer of breast or bone or metastases to bone, cirrhosis, thrombocytosis, hyperparathryoidism, or renal impairment.

Acid phosphatase levels rise moderately in patients with prostatic infarction or Gaucher's disease, in some patients with Paget's disease, and occasionally in patients with other conditions such as multiple myeloma.

Posttest care

■ If a hematoma develops at the venipuncture site, apply warm soaks to ease discomfort.

■ Resume administration of any medications discontinued before the test.

Interfering factors

■ Fluorides, phosphates, and oxalates can cause false-negative test results; clofibrate can cause false-positive results.

■ Prostate massage, catheterization, or rectal examination within 48 hours of the test may interfere with interpretation of the test results.

■ Hemolysis caused by rough handling of the sample or improper sample storage may interfere with test results.

■ Delayed delivery of the specimen to the laboratory may cause false-low results or results in the reference range.

ACTH test, plasma

This test measures the plasma levels of adrenocorticotropic hormone (ACTH)—also known as corticotropin—by radioimmunoassay. ACTH, a polypeptide hormone released by the basophilic cells of the anterior pituitary, stimulates the adrenal cortex to secrete cortisol and, to a lesser degree, androgens and aldosterone. ACTH also has some melanocyte-stimulating activity and increases the uptake of amino acids by muscle cells, promotes lipolysis by fat cells, stimulates pancreatic beta cells to secrete insulin, and may contribute to the release of growth hormone. ACTH levels vary diurnally, peaking between 6 a.m. and 8 a.m. and ebbing between 6 p.m. and 11 p.m.

Through a negative feedback mechanism, plasma cortisol levels control ACTH secretion; for example, high cortisol levels suppress ACTH secretion. Emotional and physical stress, such as pain, surgery, or insulin-induced hypoglycemia, stimulate secretion and can override the effects of plasma cortisol levels.

The plasma ACTH test may be ordered for patients with signs of adrenal hypofunction (insufficiency) or hyperfunction (Cushing's syndrome). However, ACTH suppression or stimulation (see "ACTH test, rapid," page 29) testing is usually necessary to confirm diagnosis. The instability and unavailability of plasma ACTH greatly limit its diagnostic significance and reliability of the stimulation test, and the ACTH rapid test is gradually replacing it.

Purpose

■ To facilitate differential diagnosis of primary and secondary adrenal hypofunction

■ To aid differential diagnosis of Cushing's syndrome.

Patient preparation

Explain to the patient that this test helps to determine if his hormonal secretion is normal. Advise him to fast and limit physical activity for 10 to 12 hours before the test. Tell the patient that the test requires a blood sample, explain who will perform the venipuncture and when, and note that he may feel transient discomfort from the needle puncture and the pressure of the tourniquet. Advise the patient that the laboratory may take up to 4 days to complete the analysis.

Check the patient's drug history for the use of any medications that may affect accurate determination of test results, such as corticosteroids and drugs that affect cortisol levels, including estrogens, amphetamines, spironolactone, calcium gluconate, and alcohol (ethanol). Withhold these drugs for 48 hours or more before the test; if they must be continued, note this on the laboratory request. Arrange for the patient to have a low-carbohydrate diet for 2 days before the test. This requirement may vary, depending on the laboratory.

Procedure

■ For a patient with suspected adrenal hypofunction, draw the sample between 6 a.m. and 8 a.m. (peak secretion); for a patient with suspected Cushing's syndrome, draw the sample between 6 p.m. and 11 p.m. (low secretion).

■ Collect the sample in a *plastic* tube, because ACTH may adhere to glass, or in an ethylenediaminetetraacetic acid (EDTA) tube. The tube must be full because excess anticoagulant will affect results. Pack the sample in ice, and send it to the laboratory immediately. The collection technique may vary, depending on the laboratory.

Precautions

Because proteolytic enzymes in the plasma degrade ACTH, maintaining a temperature of 39.2° F (4° C) is necessary to retard enzyme activity. Immediately transfer the sample, packed in ice, to the laboratory for reliable test results.

Reference values

Normal baseline values are usually less than 60 pg/ml, but they may vary, depending on the laboratory.

Implications of results

A higher-than-normal plasma ACTH level suggests primary adrenal hypofunction (Addison's disease), in which the pituitary gland attempts to compensate for the unresponsiveness of the target organ by releasing excessive ACTH. The underlying cause of adrenocortical hypofunction may be idiopathic atrophy of the adrenal cortex or partial destruction of the gland by granuloma, neoplasm, amyloidosis, or inflammatory necrosis.

CLINICAL ALERT A low-normal plasma ACTH level suggests adrenal hypofunction secondary to pituitary or hypothalamic dysfunction. The primary determinant may be panhypopituitarism, absence of corticotropin-releasing hormone in the hypothalamus, or chronic blunting of ACTH levels by long-term corticosteroid therapy.

In suspected Cushing's syndrome, an elevated plasma ACTH level suggests Cushing's *disease*, a related disorder in which pituitary dysfunction (associated with adenoma) causes continuous hypersecretion of ACTH and, consequently, continuously elevated plasma cortisol levels without diurnal variations. Moderately elevated ACTH levels suggest pituitary-dependent adrenal hyperplasia or nonadrenal tumors, such as oat cell carcinoma of the lungs.

A low-normal ACTH level implies adrenal hyperfunction resulting from adrenocortical tumor or hyperplasia; ACTH levels are low-normal or undetectable because the high plasma cortisol levels suppress ACTH secretion through negative feedback.

Posttest care

■ If a hematoma develops at the puncture site, apply warm soaks.
■ Resume diet and administration of medications that were discontinued before the test.

Interfering factors

■ Failure to observe restrictions of diet, medications, or physical activity may interfere with accurate determination of test results. ACTH levels are depressed by corticosteroids, including cortisone and its analogues, and by drugs that increase endogenous cortisol secretion, including estrogens, calcium gluconate, amphetamines, spironolactone, and ethanol. Lithium carbonate decreases cortisol levels and may interfere with ACTH secretion. ACTH levels are also affected by the menstrual cycle and pregnancy.
■ Any radioactive scan performed within 1 week before the test may influence test results.

ACTH test, rapid

The rapid adrenocorticotropic hormone (ACTH) test, also known as the cosyntropin test, is gradually replacing the 8-hour ACTH stimulation test as the most effective test for evaluating adrenal hypofunction (insufficiency). Using cosyntropin, a synthetic analogue of the biologically active part of ACTH, the rapid ACTH test provides faster results and causes fewer allergic reactions than the 8-hour test, which uses natural ACTH from animal sources. This test requires prior determination of baseline plasma cortisol levels to evaluate the effect of cosyntropin administration on cortisol secretion. An unequivocally high morning cortisol level rules out adrenal hypofunction and makes further testing unnecessary.

Purpose

To aid in identification of primary and secondary adrenal hypofunction.

Patient preparation

Explain to the patient that this test helps determine if his condition is caused by a hormonal deficiency. Inform him that he may be required to fast for 10 to 12 hours before the test and that he must be relaxed and rest quietly for 30 minutes before the test. Tell him the test, which takes at least 1 hour to perform, requires three venipunctures and an injection.

This test may be given on an outpatient basis. If so, instruct the patient to withhold ACTH and all corticosteroid medications for as long as instructed, generally 24 to 48 hours, before the test. If the patient is hospitalized, withhold these medications. If they must be continued, note this on the laboratory request.

Procedure

■ Draw 5 ml of blood for a baseline value. Collect the sample in a 5-ml heparinized tube. Label this sample "preinjection," and send it to the laboratory. Inject v 250 µg (0.25 mg) of cosyntropin I.V. (preferably) or I.M.; I.V. administration yields more accurate test results because ineffective absorption after I.M. administration may cause wide variations in response. Direct I.V. injection should take 2 minutes.

■ Draw another 5 ml of blood at 30 minutes and again at 60 minutes after the cosyntropin injection. Collect the samples in 5-ml heparinized tubes. Label the samples "30 minutes postinjection" and "60 minutes postinjection," and send them to the laboratory. Include the actual collection times on the laboratory request.

CLINICAL ALERT Observe the patient for signs of an allergic reaction to cosyntropin, which is rare; symptoms include hives, itching, or tachycardia.

Precautions

Handle the samples gently to prevent hemolysis.

Reference values

Normally, plasma cortisol levels rise 7 µg/dl or more above the baseline value to a peak of 18 µg/dl (or more) 60 minutes after the cosyntropin injection. Generally, a doubling of the baseline value indicates a normal response.

Implications of results

A normal result excludes adrenal hypofunction. In patients with primary adrenal hypofunction (Addison's disease), cortisol levels remain low. Thus, the rapid ACTH test provides an effective method of screening for adrenal hypofunction. However, if test results show subnormal increases in plasma cortisol levels, prolonged stimulation of the adrenal cortex may be required to differentiate between primary and secondary adrenal hypofunction.

Posttest care

■ If a hematoma develops at the venipuncture sites, apply warm soaks.
■ Resume diet and administration of medications that were discontinued before the test.

Interfering factors

■ Failure to observe restrictions of diet and physical activity may hinder accurate determination of test results.
■ Drugs that increase plasma cortisol levels, including estrogens (which increase plasma cortisol-binding proteins) and amphetamines, may interfere with test results. Smoking and obesity may also increase plasma cortisol levels.
■ Lithium carbonate decreases plasma cortisol levels.
■ A radioactive scan performed within 1 week before the test may influence test results because plasma cortisol levels are determined by radioimmunoassay.
■ Hemolysis caused by rough handling of the sample may interfere with accurate determination of test results.

Activated clotting time test

Activated clotting time, or automated coagulation time (ACT), measures whole-blood clotting time. This test is commonly performed during procedures that require extracorporeal circulation, such as cardiopulmonary bypass, ultrafiltration, hemodialysis, and extracorporeal membrane oxygenation (ECMO).

Purpose

■ To monitor the effect of heparin

■ To monitor the effect of protamine sulfate in heparin neutralization

■ To detect severe deficiencies in clotting factors (except factor VII).

Patient preparation

Explain to the patient or parents that this test is used to monitor the effect of heparin on the blood's ability to coagulate. Tell him that the test requires a blood sample, which is usually drawn from an existing vascular access site, so venipuncture won't be needed. Explain who will perform the test and that the test is usually done at the bedside. Explain that two blood samples will be drawn; the first one will be discarded so that any heparin in the tubing doesn't interfere with the results. If the sample is drawn from a line with a continuous infusion, stop the infusion before drawing the sample.

Procedure

■ Withdraw 5 to 10 ml of blood from the line and discard it.

■ Withdraw a clean sample of blood into the special tube containing celite (purified inert silica) provided with the ACT unit.

■ Activate the ACT unit and wait for the signal to insert the tube.

■ If the specimen must be sent to the laboratory (if the ACT machine is not in the room) the specimen should be placed in ice for transport.

Precautions

Guard against contamination with heparin if drawn from an access site containing heparin.

Reference values and implications of results

In the patient who is not receiving an anticoagulant, normal ACT is 107 ± 13 seconds. During cardiopulmonary bypass, heparin is titrated to maintain ACT between 400 and 600 seconds. During ECMO, heparin is titrated to maintain ACT between 220 and 260 seconds.

Posttest care

Flush the vascular access site according to your facility's protocol.

Interfering factors

■ Failure to fill the collection tube completely, to use the proper anticoagulant, to adequately mix the sample and the anticoagulant, or to send the sample to the laboratory immediately or place it on ice may alter test results.

■ Hemolysis caused by rough handling of the sample may affect test results.

■ Failure to draw and discard at least 5 ml of waste when drawing sample from a venous access device that is used for heparin infusion may contaminate the sample.

Activated partial thromboplastin time test

The activated partial thromboplastin time (APTT) test evaluates all the clotting factors of the intrinsic pathway — except platelets — by measuring the time required for formation of a fibrin clot after the addition of calcium and phospholipid emulsion to a plasma sample. Because most congenital coagulation deficiencies occur in the intrinsic pathway, the APTT test is valuable in preoperative screening for bleeding tendencies. This is also the test of choice for monitoring heparin therapy.

Purpose

■ To screen for deficiencies of the clotting factors in the intrinsic pathways
■ To monitor response to heparin therapy. (For information about another test used to monitor heparin therapy, see *Heparin neutralization assay*, page 34.)

Patient preparation

Explain to the patient that this test helps determine if his blood clots normally. Explain that fasting isn't necessary and that the test requires a blood sample. Tell him who will perform the venipuncture and when, and note that he may feel transient discomfort from the needle puncture and the pressure of the tourniquet.

When appropriate, tell the patient receiving heparin therapy that this test may be repeated at regular intervals to assess his response to treatment.

Procedure

Perform a venipuncture, and collect the sample in a 7-ml tube containing sodium citrate.

Precautions

■ To prevent hemolysis, avoid excessive probing at the venipuncture site and handle the sample gently.
■ Completely fill the collection tube, invert it gently several times, and send it to the laboratory on ice.
■ For a patient on anticoagulant therapy, additional pressure may be needed at the venipuncture site to control bleeding.

HEPARIN NEUTRALIZATION ASSAY

This complex, quantitative test is sometimes used to monitor heparin therapy. It can also help determine if prolonged thrombin time results from effective heparin therapy or from the presence of other circulating anticoagulants such as fibrin split products.

To perform this test, a specimen is divided into small plasma samples. Thrombin time is determined on one sample; the other samples are added to various dilutions of protamine sulfate. After a brief incubation, equal amounts of thrombin are added to each solution and thrombin time is measured. Because protamine sulfate neutralizes heparin, reduced thrombin time in the protamine-treated samples indicates the presence of heparin.

A fibrometer is used to select the sample with the thrombin time closest to the control value. Then, a chart or formula is used to convert the sample's protamine concentration to units of heparin per milliliter, providing an accurate measurement of heparin blood levels. If none of the samples show a reduced thrombin time, no heparin is present, indicating that prolonged thrombin time is associated with other anticoagulants, such as fibrin split products.

Reference values

Normally, a fibrin clot forms 21 to 35 seconds after addition of reagents. For a patient on anticoagulant therapy, values will differ with the type of anticoagulant being used.

Implications of results

Prolonged APTT may indicate a deficiency of certain plasma clotting factors, the presence of heparin, or the presence of fibrin split products, fibrinolysins, or circulating anticoagulants that are antibodies to specific clotting factors.

Posttest care

If a hematoma develops at the venipuncture site, apply warm soaks.

Interfering factors

■ Failure to use the proper anticoagulant, fill the collection tube completely, or mix the sample and the anticoagulant adequately may affect the accuracy of test results.

■ Hemolysis caused by rough handling of the sample or excessive probing at the venipuncture site may alter test results.

■ Failure to send the sample to the laboratory immediately or place it on ice may cause spurious test results.

Alanine aminotransferase test, serum

Alanine aminotransferase (ALT) is one of two enzymes that catalyze a reversible amino-group transfer reaction in the Krebs cycle, also called the citric acid or tricarboxylic acid cycle. This enzyme is necessary for energy production. Unlike aspartate aminotransferase (AST), the other aminotransferase, ALT is primarily present in hepatocellular cytoplasm—with lesser amounts in the kidneys, heart, and skeletal muscles—and is a relatively specific indicator of acute hepatocellular damage. When such damage occurs, ALT is released from the cytoplasm into the bloodstream, often before jaundice appears. The consequent abnormally high serum levels may not return to normal for days or weeks. This test measures serum ALT levels by spectrophotometry.

Purpose

■ To help detect and evaluate treatment of acute hepatic disease—especially hepatitis and cirrhosis without jaundice

■ To help distinguish between myocardial and hepatic tissue damage (used with AST)

■ To assess hepatotoxicity of some drugs.

Patient preparation

Explain to the patient that this test helps assess liver function. Inform the patient that fasting isn't necessary. Tell the patient that the test requires a blood sample, discuss who will perform the venipuncture and when, and note that transient discomfort may be felt from the needle puncture and the pressure of the tourniquet.

Withhold hepatotoxic or cholestatic drugs, such as methotrexate, chlorpromazine, salicylates, and narcotics, before the test. If they must be continued, note this on the laboratory request.

Procedure

Perform a venipuncture, and collect the sample in a 7-ml tube without additives.

Precautions

Handle the sample gently to prevent hemolysis. ALT activity is stable in serum for up to 3 days at room temperature.

Reference values

Normal serum ALT levels are 0 to 35 U/L in males and 9 to 24 U/L in females.

Implications of results

Very high ALT levels (up to 50 times normal) suggest viral or severe drug-induced hepatitis or another hepatic disease with extensive necrosis. In these cases, AST levels are also elevated but usually to a lesser degree. Moderate to high levels may indicate infectious mononucleosis, chronic hepatitis, intrahepatic cholestasis or cholecystitis, early or improving acute viral hepatitis, or severe hepatic congestion associated with heart failure.

Slight to moderate ALT elevations, usually with higher increases in AST levels, may reflect the presence of any condition that causes acute hepatocellular injury, such as active cirrhosis or drug-induced or alcoholic hepatitis. Marginal elevations occasionally occur in association with acute myocardial infarction, reflecting secondary hepatic congestion or the release of small amounts of ALT from myocardial tissue.

Posttest care

■ Unless otherwise directed, resume administration of drugs that were withheld before the test.
■ If a hematoma develops at the venipuncture site, apply warm soaks.

Interfering factors

■ Many medications produce hepatic injury by competitively interfering with cellular metabolism. Falsely elevated ALT levels can follow use of barbiturates, griseofulvin, isoniazid, nitrofurantoin, methyldopa, phenothiazines, phenytoin, salicylates, tetracycline, chlorpromazine, para-aminosalicylic acid, and other drugs that affect the liver.
■ Narcotic analgesics, such as morphine, codeine, and meperidine, may falsely elevate ALT levels by increasing intrabiliary pressure.
■ Ingestion of lead or exposure to carbon tetrachloride causes direct injury to hepatic cells and sharp elevations of ALT.
■ Hemolysis caused by rough handling of the sample may affect test results.

Aldosterone test, serum

This test measures serum aldosterone levels by quantitative analysis and radioimmunoassay. Aldosterone, the principal mineralocorticoid secreted by the zona glomerulosa of the adrenal cortex, regulates ion transport across cell membranes in the renal tubules to promote reabsorption of sodium and chloride in exchange for potassium and hydrogen ions. Consequently, aldosterone helps to maintain blood pressure and blood volume and to regulate fluid and electrolyte balance.

Aldosterone secretion is controlled primarily by the renin-angiotensin system and by the circulating serum levels of potassium. Thus, high serum potassium levels elicit secretion of aldosterone through a potent feedback system; similarly, hyponatremia, hypovolemia, and other disorders that provoke the release of renin stimulate aldosterone secretion.

This test identifies aldosteronism and, when supported by plasma renin levels, distinguishes between its primary and secondary forms. Thus, it's helpful in identifying adrenal adenoma and adrenal hyperplasia, causes of primary aldosteronism. Secondary aldosteronism is commonly associated with salt depletion, potassium excess, congestive heart failure with ascites, or other conditions that increase activity of the renin-angiotensin system.

Purpose

To aid diagnosis of primary and secondary aldosteronism, adrenal hyperplasia, hypoaldosteronism, and salt-losing syndrome.

Patient preparation

Explain to the patient that this test helps determine whether his symptoms are caused by improper hormonal secretion. Instruct the patient to maintain a low-carbohydrate, normal-sodium diet for at least 2 weeks or, preferably, 30 days before the test. Explain that the test requires a blood sample and that the needle puncture may cause some discomfort. Advise the patient that the laboratory may take up to 5 days to complete the multistage analysis.

Withhold all drugs that alter fluid, sodium, and potassium balance, especially diuretics, antihypertensives, corticosteroids, cyclic progestational agents, and estrogens, for at least 2 weeks or, preferably, 30 days before the test. Also withhold all renin inhibitors (such as propranolol) for 1 week before the test. If these medications must be continued, note this on the laboratory request. Warn the patient that licorice produces an aldosterone-like effect and should be avoided for at least 2 weeks before the test.

Procedure

■ While the patient is still supine after a night's rest, perform a venipuncture. Collect the sample in a 7-ml clot-activator collection tube, and send it to the laboratory.

■ To evaluate the effect of postural change, draw another sample 4 hours later, with the patient in a standing position after he has been up and moving around. Collect the second sample in a 7-ml clot-activator collection tube, and send it to the laboratory.

Precautions

■ Handle the sample gently to prevent hemolysis.
■ Record on the laboratory request whether the patient was supine or standing during the venipuncture.
■ If the patient is a premenopausal female, specify the phase of her menstrual cycle because aldosterone levels may fluctuate during the menstrual cycle.
■ Send the specimen to the laboratory immediately.

Reference values

Normal serum aldosterone levels vary with age, as follows:

■ *0 to 3 weeks:* 16.5 to 154 ng/dl
■ *1 to 11 months:* 6.5 to 86 ng/dl
■ *1 to 10 years:* 3 to 39.5 ng/dl (supine); 3.5 to 124 ng/dl (upright)
■ *11 years and older:* 1 to 21 ng/dl.

Implications of results

Excessive aldosterone secretion may indicate a primary or secondary disease. Primary aldosteronism (Conn's syndrome) may result from adrenocortical adenoma or carcinoma or from bilateral adrenal hyperplasia. Secondary aldosteronism can result from renovascular hypertension, congestive heart failure, cirrhosis of the liver, nephrotic syndrome, idiopathic cyclic edema, or the third trimester of pregnancy.

Depressed serum aldosterone levels may indicate primary hypoaldosteronism, salt-losing syndrome, toxemia of pregnancy, or Addison's disease.

Posttest care

■ Resume diet and medications discontinued before the test.
■ If a hematoma develops at the venipuncture site, apply warm soaks.

Interfering factors

■ Serum aldosterone levels are affected by positional changes. Urine aldosterone levels are more reliable, in part because they aren't affected by position changes. (See "Aldosterone, urine," page 39.)
■ Failure to observe restrictions of diet, medications, or posture may interfere with accurate determination of test results.

■ Some antihypertensives such as methyldopa promote sodium and water retention and therefore may reduce aldosterone levels.

■ Diuretics promote sodium excretion and may raise aldosterone levels.

■ Some corticosteroids such as fludrocortisone mimic mineralocorticoid activity and therefore may lower aldosterone levels.

■ Hemolysis caused by rough handling of the sample may interfere with accurate determination of test results.

■ A radioactive scan performed within 1 week before the test may affect results.

Aldosterone test, urine

This test measures urine levels of aldosterone, the principal mineralocorticoid secreted by the zona glomerulosa of the adrenal cortex. Aldosterone promotes retention of sodium and excretion of potassium by the renal tubules, thereby helping regulate blood pressure and fluid and electrolyte balance.

Aldosterone secretion is controlled by the renin–angiotensin system. Renin, an enzyme released in the kidneys in response to low plasma volume, stimulates production of angiotensin I, which is converted to angiotensin II, a powerful vasopressor that stimulates the adrenal cortex to secrete aldosterone. Potassium levels also affect aldosterone secretion: Increased potassium stimulates the adrenal cortex, triggering substantial increase in aldosterone secretion to promote potassium excretion. This feedback mechanism is vital to maintaining fluid and electrolyte balance.

Urine aldosterone levels, measured by radioimmunoassay, are usually evaluated after measurement of serum electrolyte and renin levels.

Serum aldosterone levels are affected by positional changes. Urine aldosterone levels are more reliable, in part because they aren't affected by position changes.

Purpose

To aid diagnosis of primary and secondary aldosteronism.

Patient preparation

Explain to the patient that this test evaluates hormonal balance. Instruct him to maintain a normal sodium diet (3 g/day) before the test; to avoid sodium-rich foods, such as bacon, barbecue sauce, corned beef, bouillon cubes or powder, and olives; and to avoid strenuous physical exercise and stressful situations during the collection period. Tell the patient the test requires collection of a 24-hour urine specimen, and provide instruction on the proper collection technique.

Check the patient's medication history for drugs that may affect aldosterone levels.

Procedure

Collect a 24-hour specimen in a bottle containing a preservative such as boric acid to keep the specimen at a pH of 4.0 to 4.5.

Precautions

Refrigerate the specimen or place it on ice during the collection period. Send the specimen to the laboratory as soon as the collection is completed.

Reference values

Normally, urine aldosterone levels range from 2 to 20 µg/24 hours.

Implications of results

Increased urine aldosterone levels suggest primary or secondary aldosteronism. The primary form usually arises from an aldosterone-secreting adenoma of the adrenal cortex but may also result from adrenocortical hyperplasia. Patients with primary aldosteronism have increased aldosterone and decreased renin levels.

Secondary aldosteronism, the more common form, results from external stimulation of the adrenal cortex, such as that produced when hypertensive and edematous disorders activate the renin-angiotensin system. The major systemic disorders that result in secondary aldosteronism are malignant hypertension, congestive heart failure, cirrhosis of the liver, nephrotic syndrome, and idiopathic cyclic edema.

Low urine aldosterone levels may result from Addison's disease, hypernatremia, overhydration, and toxemia of pregnancy. Aldosterone levels normally rise during pregnancy but rapidly decline after parturition.

Posttest care

■ After collection, resume administration of any medications that were discontinued before the test.
■ Tell the patient that normal physical activity can be resumed.

Interfering factors

■ Patient's failure to avoid strenuous physical exercise and emotional stress before the test can stimulate adrenocortical secretions and thus increase aldosterone levels.

■ Patient's failure to maintain normal dietary intake of sodium and to avoid excess intake of licorice or glucose can influence test results.

■ Antihypertensive drugs promote sodium and water retention and may suppress urine aldosterone levels.

■ Diuretics and most corticosteroids promote sodium excretion and may raise aldosterone levels.

■ Some corticosteroids such as fludrocortisone mimic mineralocorticoid activity and consequently may lower aldosterone levels.

■ Failure to collect *all* urine during the 24-hour specimen collection period or to store the urine specimen properly can affect the accuracy of test results.

■ A radioactive scan performed within 1 week before the test may affect the accuracy of test results.

Alkaline phosphatase test

An enzyme that is most active at about pH 10.0, alkaline phosphatase (ALP) influences bone calcification and lipid and metabolite transport. Total serum levels reflect the combined activity of several ALP isoenzymes found in the liver, bones, kidneys, intestinal lining, and placenta. (See *ALP isoenzymes*, page 42.) Bone and liver ALP are always present in adult serum; liver ALP is most prominent—except during the third trimester of pregnancy, when about half of all ALP originates from the placenta. The intestinal isoenzyme is a genetically controlled characteristic found almost exclusively in the sera of patients with blood groups B or O. It may be a normal component—occurring in fewer than 10% of patients with otherwise normal patterns, or it may be an abnormal finding associated with hepatic disease.

The ALP test is particularly sensitive to mild biliary obstruction and is a primary indicator of space-occupying hepatic lesions. Although both skeletal and hepatic diseases can raise ALP levels, this test is most useful for diagnosing metabolic bone disease. Additional liver function studies are usually required to identify hepatobiliary disorders.

Purpose

■ To detect and identify skeletal diseases, primarily those characterized by marked osteoblastic activity

■ To detect focal hepatic lesions causing biliary obstruction, such as tumor or abscess

■ To supplement information from other liver function studies and GI enzyme tests

■ To assess response to vitamin D treatment of deficiency-induced rickets.

ALP ISOENZYMES

Separation of alkaline phosphatase (ALP) isoenzymes in the laboratory, using heat inactivation, electrophoresis, or chemical means, is sometimes used in place of serum gamma-glutamyl transferase, leucine aminopeptidase, or 5'-nucleotidase to differentiate between hepatic and skeletal disease.

Sixteen molecularly distinct isoenzyme fractions have been identified electrophoretically in human serum, stimulating continuing controversy about the origins, proportions, and methods of isoenzyme determination. Although the number and concentration of ALP isoenzymes in total serum levels vary with the laboratory separation method used, the five isoenzymes of greatest clinical significance originate in the liver (includes kidney and bile fractions), bone (may also include bile fraction), intestine, and placenta.

Reference values

On electrophoresis, liver isoenzyme levels usually range from 20 to 130 U/L; bone isoenzyme levels, from 20 to 120 U/L; and intestinal isoenzyme levels (which occur almost exclusively in individuals with blood group B or O and are markedly elevated 8 hours after a fatty meal), from undetectable to 18 U/L.

The placental isoenzyme first appears in the second trimester of pregnancy, accounts for roughly half of all ALP during the third trimester, and drops to normal levels the first month postpartum. Another isoenzyme, Regan, resembles the placental isoenzyme and appears in a small percentage of patients with cancer; it may be used as a tumor marker.

Patient preparation

Explain to the patient that this test assesses liver or bone function. Instruct the patient to fast for at least 8 hours before the test because fat intake stimulates intestinal ALP secretion. Explain that this test requires a blood sample, discuss who will perform the venipuncture and when, and note that discomfort may be felt from the needle puncture and the pressure of the tourniquet.

Procedure

Perform a venipuncture, and collect the sample in a 7-ml clot-activator tube.

Precautions

Handle the collection tube gently to prevent hemolysis, and send the sample to the laboratory immediately because ALP activity increases at room temperature in association with a rise in pH.

Reference values

When measured by chemical inhibition, total ALP levels normally range from 98 to 251 U/L for males and from 81 to 312 U/L for females, depending on age.

Implications of results

Although significant ALP elevations may occur in association with diseases that affect many organs, they usually indicate skeletal disease or extrahepatic or intrahepatic biliary obstruction. In many acute hepatic diseases, ALP elevations precede any change in serum bilirubin levels. A moderate rise in ALP levels may reflect acute biliary obstruction from hepatocellular inflammation, inactive cirrhosis, mononucleosis, or viral hepatitis. Moderate increases are also seen in osteomalacia and deficiency-induced rickets.

Sharp elevations of ALP levels may result from complete biliary obstruction by malignant or infectious infiltration or fibrosis. Such markedly high levels are most common in Paget's disease and, occasionally, in biliary obstruction, extensive bone metastases, or hyperparathyroidism. Metastatic bone tumors resulting from pancreatic cancer raise ALP levels without a concomitant rise in serum alanine aminotransferase levels.

Isoenzyme fractionation and additional enzyme tests (gamma-glutamyl transferase, lactate dehydrogenase, 5'-nucleotidase, and leucine aminopeptidase) are sometimes performed when the cause of ALP elevations (skeletal or hepatic disease) is in doubt. However, hepatic scans are replacing these tests as a diagnostic tool and sometimes are used to follow disease progression. In rare cases, low ALP levels are associated with hypophosphatasia or with protein or magnesium deficiency.

Posttest care

■ Tell the patient that a normal diet may be resumed.
■ If a hematoma develops at the venipuncture site, apply warm soaks.

Interfering factors

■ Recent ingestion of vitamin D may increase ALP levels through its effect on osteoblastic activity.
■ Recent infusion of albumin prepared from placental venous blood causes a marked increase in serum ALP levels.
■ Drugs that influence liver function or cause cholestasis, such as barbiturates, chlorpropamide, oral contraceptives, isoniazid, methyldopa, phenothiazines, phenytoin, and rifampin, can cause a mild increase in ALP levels.

■ In patients with halothane sensitivity, use of that anesthetic may increase levels drastically.
■ Clofibrate decreases ALP levels.
■ Healing long-bone fractures and pregnancy (third trimester) can increase ALP levels. Levels are also typically elevated in infants, children, adolescents, and individuals over 45 years old.
■ Hemolysis caused by rough handling of the sample may alter test results.
■ The specimen should be analyzed within 4 hours.

Alpha₁-antitrypsin test

A protein produced by the liver, alpha₁-antitrypsin (also known as AAT or alpha₁-AT) is believed to inhibit the release of protease into body fluids by dying cells and is a major component of alpha₁-globulin. AAT is measured by radioimmunoassay or isoelectric focusing. Congenital absence or deficiency of AAT has been linked to high susceptibility to emphysema.

Purpose

■ To screen for high-risk emphysema patients
■ As a nonspecific method of detecting inflammation, severe infection, and necrosis
■ To test for congenital AAT deficiency.

Patient preparation

Explain to the patient that this test is used to diagnose respiratory or liver disease as well as inflammation, infection, or necrosis. Tell the patient to avoid smoking because irritants in tobacco stimulate leukocytes in the lungs to release protease. Tell the patient who is taking oral contraceptives or corticosteroids to discontinue them 24 hours before the test. Instruct the patient to fast for at least 8 hours before the test. Tell the patient that collecting the sample usually takes less than 3 minutes.

Procedure

Perform a venipuncture, and collect the sample in a 7-ml tube without additives.

Precautions

■ Handle the sample gently to avoid hemolysis, and send the sample to the laboratory promptly.
■ If clinically indicated, patients with AAT levels lower than 125 mg/dl should be phenotyped to confirm homozygous and heterozygous deficiencies; only homozygous patients seem to be at increased risk for early emphysema.

Reference values
AAT levels vary by age, but the normal range is 110 to 200 mg/dl.

Implications of results
AAT levels may be decreased in patients with early-onset emphysema as well as in those with cirrhosis, nephrotic syndrome, malnutrition, or congenital alpha$_1$-globulin deficiency or, transiently, in the normal neonate.

Increased AAT levels can occur in patients with chronic inflammatory disorders, necrosis, pregnancy, acute pulmonary infections, hyaline membrane disease in infants, hepatitis, systemic lupus erythematosus, and rheumatoid arthritis.

Posttest care
If a hematoma develops at the venipuncture site, apply warm soaks.

Interfering factors
■ Failure to fast for 8 hours before the test may cause false-high test results.
■ Oral contraceptives and corticosteroids may cause false-high test results.
■ Smoking may cause false-high test results.

Alpha-fetoprotein test
Alpha-fetoprotein (AFP) is a glycoprotein produced by fetal tissue and tumors that differentiate from midline embryonic structures. During fetal development, AFP levels in serum and amniotic fluid rise; because this protein crosses the placenta, it appears in maternal serum. In late stages of pregnancy, AFP levels in fetal and maternal serum and in amniotic fluid begin to diminish. During the first year of life, serum AFP levels continue to decline and usually remain low thereafter.

Elevated maternal serum AFP levels at 14 to 22 weeks' gestation may suggest fetal neural tube defects, such as spina bifida or anencephaly, but positive confirmation requires amniocentesis or ultrasonography. Other congenital anomalies may also be associated with high maternal serum AFP concentrations; evaluation for Down syndrome can be performed on serum samples at 15 to 20 weeks' gestation. Elevated AFP levels in persons who aren't pregnant may occur in malignancy such as hepatocellular carcinoma or in certain nonmalignant conditions such as ataxia-telangiectasia; in these conditions, AFP assays are more useful for monitoring response to therapy than for diagnosis. AFP levels are best determined by enzyme immunoassay of amniotic fluid or serum and should be used only as a tumor marker.

Purpose

■ To monitor the effectiveness of therapy in malignant diseases, such as hepatomas and germ cell tumors, and in certain nonmalignant disorders such as ataxia-telangiectasia

■ To screen for the need for amniocentesis or high-resolution ultrasound in a pregnant woman.

Patient preparation

Explain to the patient that this test monitors response to therapy or helps detect possible congenital defects in a fetus by measuring a specific blood protein. Advise the patient that she may need further testing. Tell her that food, fluids, and medications don't need to be restricted before the test.

Procedure

■ Perform a venipuncture, and collect the sample in a 7-ml clot-activator tube.

■ Record the patient's age, race, weight, and gestational period on the laboratory request.

Precautions

Handle the sample gently.

Reference values

When testing by immunoassay, AFP values are less than 15 ng/ml in males and nonpregnant females. For values in pregnant women, see *Alpha-fetoprotein values in pregnant women*. Values in maternal serum are less than 2.5 multiples of median for fetal gestational age.

Implications of results

Elevated maternal serum AFP levels may suggest a neural tube defect or other neural tube anomaly after 14 weeks' gestation. AFP levels rise sharply in approximately 90% of fetuses with anencephaly and in 50% of those with spina bifida. Definitive diagnosis requires ultrasonography and amniocentesis. High AFP levels may reflect the presence of intrauterine death or such anomalies as duodenal atresia, omphalocele, tetralogy of Fallot, or Turner's syndrome.

Serum AFP levels are elevated in 70% of pregnant women; in nonpregnant persons elevations may indicate hepatocellular carcinoma (although low AFP levels don't rule it out) or germ cell tumor of gonadal, retroperitoneal, or mediastinal origin. Serum AFP level rises in patients with ataxia-telangiectasia or cancer of the pan-

ALPHA-FETOPROTEIN VALUES IN PREGNANT WOMEN

Gestational age (weeks)	Median value in white women (IU/ml)	Median value in black women (IU/ml)
14	19.9	23.2
15	23.2	26.9
16	27.0	31.1
17	31.5	35.9
18	36.7	41.6
19	42.7	48.0
20	49.8	55.6
21	58.1	64.2
22	67.8	74.2

creas, stomach, or biliary system. Transient modest elevations can occur in nonneoplastic hepatocellular disease, such as alcoholic cirrhosis and acute or chronic hepatitis. Elevation of AFP levels after remission suggests tumor recurrence.

In patients with hepatocellular carcinoma, a gradual decrease in serum AFP levels indicates a favorable response to therapy. In patients with germ cell tumors, serum AFP and human chorionic gonadotropin levels should be measured concurrently.

Posttest care

If a hematoma develops at the venipuncture site, apply warm soaks.

Interfering factors

■ Hemolysis may alter test results.
■ Multiple pregnancy may cause false-positive test results.

Amino acid test, plasma

This is a qualitative but effective test performed on neonates to detect inborn errors of amino acid metabolism. The test uses thin-layer chromatography, which can profile many amino acids simultaneously.

Amino acids are the chief components of all proteins and polypeptides. The body contains at least 20 amino acids; 10 are considered "essential" — that is, they must be acquired through diet because the body doesn't form them. Certain congenital enzymatic deficiencies interfere with normal metabolism of one or more amino acids, causing them to accumulate or become deficient.

Excessive accumulation of amino acids typically produces overflow aminoacidurias. Congenital abnormalities of the amino acid transport system in the kidneys produce a second group of disorders called renal aminoacidurias.

Purpose

To screen for inborn errors of amino acid metabolism.

Patient preparation

Explain to the parents that this test determines how well their infant metabolizes amino acids. Tell the parents the infant must fast for 4 hours before the test and that a small amount of blood will be drawn from the infant's heel.

Procedure

Perform a heelstick, and collect 0.1 ml of blood in a heparinized capillary tube.

Precautions

Handle the sample gently.

Normal findings

Chromatography shows a normal plasma amino acid pattern.

Implications of results

The plasma amino acid pattern is normal in renal aminoacidurias and abnormal in overflow aminoacidurias. Comparisons of blood and urine chromatography can help distinguish between the two types of aminoacidurias.

Posttest care

The infant can resume feeding.

Interfering factors

■ Failure to observe dietary restrictions may influence amino acid levels.
■ Hemolysis may alter test results.

Amino acid screening test, urine

This test screens for aminoaciduria—elevated urine amino acid levels—a condition that may result from inborn errors of metabolism caused by the absence of specific enzymatic activities. Normally, up to 200 mg of amino acids may be excreted in the urine in 24 hours. Abnormal metabolism causes an excess of one or more amino acids in plasma and, as the renal threshold is exceeded, in urine.

Aminoacidurias may be classified as primary (overflow) aminoacidopathies or secondary (renal) aminoacidopathies. The latter type is associated with conditions marked by defective tubular reabsorption from congenital disorders. A more specific defect such as cystinuria may cause one or more amino acids to appear in urine.

To screen neonates, children, and adults for congenital aminoacidurias, plasma or urine specimens may be used. The plasma test is the better indicator of overflow aminoaciduria; urine testing is used to confirm or monitor certain amino acid disorders and to screen for renal aminoacidurias.

Various laboratory techniques are available to screen for aminoacidurias, but chromatography is the preferred method. Positive findings on chromatography can be elaborated by fractionation, which shows specific amino acid levels. Testing for specific amino acid levels is also necessary for infants or young children with acidosis, severe vomiting and diarrhea, and abnormal urine odor. Such testing is especially important in newborns because early diagnosis and prompt treatment of certain aminoacidurias may prevent mental retardation.

Purpose

- To screen for renal aminoacidurias
- To follow up plasma test findings when results of these tests suggest certain overflow aminoacidurias.

Patient preparation

Explain to the patient (or to the parents if the patient is an infant or a child) that this test helps detect amino acid disorders and that additional tests may be necessary. Tell the patient that food and fluids don't need to be restricted before the test. Tell the patient that the test requires a urine specimen.

Check the patient's medication history for drugs that may interfere with test results. If such drugs must be continued, note this on the laboratory request. If the patient is a breast-fed infant, record any drugs that the mother is taking.

Procedure

- If the patient is an infant, clean and dry the genital area, attach the collection device, and observe for voiding. Transfer at least 20 ml of urine to a specimen container.
- If the patient is an adult or a child, collect a fresh random specimen.

Precautions

- For infants, remove the collection device carefully to prevent skin irritation.
- For an infant, apply adhesive flanges of the collection device securely to the skin to prevent leakage.
- Send the specimen to the laboratory immediately.

Reference values

Reported values are age-dependent and are indicated as normal or abnormal.

Implications of results

If thin-layer chromatography shows gross changes or abnormal patterns, blood and 24-hour urine quantitative column chromatography will identify specific amino acid abnormalities and differentiate overflow from renal aminoaciduria.

Posttest care

Be sure to remove all adhesive residue after removing the collection device.

Interfering factors

■ Failure to send the urine specimen to the laboratory immediately may affect the accuracy of test results.
■ Results are invalid in a neonate who hasn't ingested dietary protein in the 48 hours preceding the test.

Ammonia test, plasma

This test measures plasma levels of ammonia, a nonprotein nitrogen compound that helps maintain acid–base balance. Most ammonia is absorbed from the intestinal tract, where it's produced by bacterial action on protein; a smaller amount is produced in the kidneys from hydrolysis of glutamine. Normally, the body uses the nitrogen fraction of ammonia to rebuild amino acids and then converts the ammonia to urea in the liver for excretion by the kidneys. In diseases such as cirrhosis of the liver, ammonia can bypass the liver and accumulate in the blood. Therefore, measurement of plasma ammonia levels may help indicate the severity of hepatocellular damage.

Purpose

■ To help monitor the progression of severe hepatic disease and the effectiveness of therapy
■ To recognize impending or established hepatic coma.

Patient preparation

Explain to the patient that this test evaluates liver function. If the patient is comatose, explain the procedure to a family member. Inform the patient who's conscious that he must observe an overnight fast before the test because plasma ammonia levels may vary with protein intake. Check the patient's medication history for drugs that may influence plasma ammonia levels.

Procedure

Perform a venipuncture, and collect the sample in a 10-ml heparinized tube.

Precautions

■ Notify the laboratory before performing the venipuncture so that preliminary preparations can begin.
■ Handle the sample gently, pack it in ice, and send it to the laboratory immediately. *Don't* use a chilled container.

Reference values

Normally, plasma ammonia levels are less than 50 µg/dl.

Implications of results

Elevated plasma ammonia levels are common in patients with severe hepatic disease, such as cirrhosis and acute hepatic necrosis, and may lead to hepatic coma. Elevated levels are also possible in patients with Reye's syndrome, severe congestive heart failure, GI hemorrhage, and erythroblastosis fetalis.

Posttest care

■ Make sure bleeding has stopped before removing pressure from the venipuncture site. If a hematoma develops, apply warm soaks.
■ Watch for signs of impending or established hepatic coma if plasma ammonia levels are high.

Interfering factors

■ Acetazolamide, thiazides, ammonium salts, and furosemide raise ammonia levels, as can total parenteral nutrition or a portacaval shunt.
■ Lactulose, neomycin, and kanamycin depress ammonia levels.
■ Hemolysis caused by rough handling of the sample may alter test results.
■ Smoking, poor venipuncture technique, and exposure to ammonia-based cleaners in the laboratory may elevate results.
■ Delay in testing may alter results.

Amniotic fluid analysis

Amniocentesis is the transabdominal needle aspiration of 10 to 20 ml of amniotic fluid for laboratory analysis. This test can be performed only when the amniotic fluid level reaches 150 ml, usually after the 16th week of pregnancy. Such analysis can detect several birth defects (especially Down syndrome and spina bifida), detect hemolytic disease of the newborn, detect gender and chromosomal abnormalities (through karyotyping), and determine fetal maturity (especially pulmonary maturity).

Amniotic fluid reflects important metabolic changes in the fetus, the placenta, and the mother. It protects the fetus from external trauma, allows the fetus to move, allows the fetus to have an even body temperature, and provides a limited source of protein (10% to 15%). Although the origin of amniotic fluid is uncertain, its original composition is essentially the same as that of interstitial fluid. As the fetus matures, the amniotic fluid becomes progressively more diluted with hypotonic fetal urine.

One of the chief differences between amniotic fluid and maternal plasma during intrauterine development is the amniotic fluid's relatively high levels of uric acid, urea, and creatinine. The volume of amniotic fluid steadily rises from 50 ml at the end of the first trimester to an average of 1000 ml near term; at 40 weeks' gestation, the volume decreases to 700 to 800 ml.

Amniocentesis is indicated when a pregnant woman is over age 35; has a family history of genetic, chromosomal, or neural tube defects; or has had a previous miscarriage. Complications from this test are rare but may include spontaneous abortion, trauma to the fetus or placenta, bleeding, premature labor, infection, and Rh sensitization from fetal bleeding into the maternal circulation. For these reasons, amniocentesis is contraindicated as a general screening test. Abnormal test results or failure of the tissue cultures to grow may necessitate repetition of the test.

Purpose

- To detect fetal abnormalities, particularly chromosomal and neural tube defects
- To detect hemolytic disease of the newborn
- To diagnose metabolic disorders, amino acid disorders, and mucopolysaccharidoses
- To determine fetal age and maturity, especially pulmonary maturity
- To assess fetal health by detecting the presence of meconium or blood or by measuring amniotic levels of estriol and fetal thyroid hormone
- To identify the fetus's gender when one or both parents are carriers of a sex-linked disorder.

Patient preparation

Describe the procedure to the patient, and explain that this test detects fetal abnormalities. Assess her understanding of the test, and answer any questions she may have. Inform her that she doesn't need to restrict food or fluids. Explain that the test requires a specimen of amniotic fluid, and tell her who will perform the test. Advise her that normal test results can't guarantee a normal fetus because some fetal disorders are undetectable.

Make sure the patient has signed a consent form. Explain that she'll feel a stinging sensation and pressure when the local anesthetic is injected. Provide emotional support before and during the test, and reassure her that complications are rare.

Just before the test, ask her to urinate to minimize the risk of puncturing the bladder and aspirating urine instead of amniotic fluid.

Equipment

70% alcohol or povidone-iodine solution ∎ sponge forceps ∎ 2″ × 2″ gauze pads ∎ local anesthetic (1% lidocaine) ∎ sterile 25G needle ∎ 3-ml glass syringe ∎ sterile 20G to 22G spinal needle with stylet ∎ 10-ml glass syringe ∎ sterile amber or foil-covered 10-ml glass test tube.

Procedure

∎ After determining fetal and placental position, usually through palpation and ultrasonography, the doctor locates a pool of amniotic fluid. After preparing the skin with an antiseptic and alcohol, he injects 1 ml of 1% lidocaine with a 25G needle, first intradermally and then subcutaneously. Then he inserts the 20G to 22G spinal needle with a stylet into the amniotic cavity and withdraws the stylet. After attaching a 10-ml syringe to the needle, he aspirates the fluid and places it in an amber or foil-covered test tube. Approximately 20 to 30 ml of fluid is drawn when cells from amniotic fluid are needed for culturing. After the needle is withdrawn, an adhesive bandage is placed over the needle insertion site.

∎ Monitor fetal heart rate and maternal vital signs every 15 minutes for at least 30 minutes.

∎ If the patient feels faint or nauseated or perspires profusely, position her on the left side to counteract uterine pressure on the vena cava.

∎ Before discharge, instruct the patient to notify the doctor immediately of any abdominal pain or cramping, chills, fever, vaginal bleeding or leakage of serous vaginal fluid, or fetal hyperactivity or unusual fetal lethargy.

Precautions

∎ Instruct the patient to fold her hands behind her head to prevent her from accidentally touching the sterile field and causing contamination.

∎ Send the specimen to the laboratory immediately.

Normal findings

Amniotic fluid should be clear but may contain white flecks of vernix caseosa when the fetus is near term. (See *Amniotic fluid analysis findings*.)

Implications of results

Blood in amniotic fluid is usually of maternal origin and doesn't indicate a fetal abnormality. However, it does inhibit cell growth and changes the level of other amniotic fluid constituents.

Large amounts of *bilirubin*, a breakdown product of red blood cells, may indicate hemolytic disease of the newborn. Normally, the bilirubin level increases from the 14th to the 24th week of pregnancy and then declines as the fetus matures, essentially reaching zero at term. Testing for bilirubin usually isn't performed until the 26th week, the earliest time that successful therapy for Rh sensitization can begin.

Meconium, a semisolid viscous material found in the fetal GI tract, consists of mucopolysaccharides, desquamated cells, vernix, hair, and cholesterol. Meconium passes into the amniotic fluid when hypoxia causes fetal distress and relaxation of the anal sphincter; it's a normal finding in breech presentation. Meconium in the amniotic fluid produces a peak of 410 mµ on the spectrophotometric analysis. However, serial amniocentesis may show a clearing of meconium over 2 to 3 weeks.

If meconium is present during labor, the newborn's nose and throat require thorough cleaning to prevent meconium aspiration.

Creatinine, a product of fetal urine, increases in the amniotic fluid as the fetus's kidneys mature. The creatinine level usually exceeds 2 mg/dl in a mature fetus.

Alpha-fetoprotein (AFP) is a fetal alpha globulin produced first in the yolk sac and later in the parenchymal cells of the liver and GI tract. Fetal serum levels of AFP are about 150 times greater than amniotic fluid levels; maternal serum levels are far less than amniotic fluid levels. High amniotic fluid levels indicate neural tube defects, but levels may remain normal if the defect is small and closed. Elevated AFP levels may occur in multiple pregnancy; in disorders such as omphalocele, congenital nephrosis, esophageal or duodenal atresia, cystic fibrosis, exomphalos, Turner's syndrome, and obstruction of the fetal bladder neck with hydronephrosis; and in impending fetal death.

The amount of *uric acid* in the amniotic fluid increases as the fetus matures, but these levels fluctuate widely and can't accurately predict fetal maturity. Laboratory studies indicate that severe erythroblastosis fetalis, fa-

AMNIOTIC FLUID ANALYSIS FINDINGS

Test	Normal findings	Fetal implications of abnormal findings
Color	Clear, with white flecks of vernix caseosa in a mature fetus	Blood of maternal origin is usually harmless. "Port wine" fluid may indicate abruptio placentae. Fetal blood may indicate damage to the fetal, placental, or umbilical cord vessels.
Bilirubin	Absent at term	High levels indicate hemolytic disease of the newborn in isoimmunized pregnancy.
Meconium	Absent (except in breach presentation)	Presence indicates fetal hypotension or distress.
Creatinine	More than 2 mg/dl in a mature fetus	Decrease may indicate immature fetus (less than 37 weeks).
Lecithin-sphingomyelin ratio	More than 2 generally indicates fetal pulmonary maturity	Less than 2 indicates pulmonary immaturity and subsequent respiratory distress syndrome.
Phosphatidylglycerol	Present	Absence indicates pulmonary immaturity.
Glucose	Less than 45 mg/dl	Excessive increases at term or near term indicate hypertrophied fetal pancreas and subsequent neonatal hypoglycemia.
Alpha-fetoprotein	Variable, depending on gestation age and laboratory technique; highest concentration (about 18.5 µg/ml) occurs at 13 to 14 weeks	Inappropriate increases indicate neural tube defects, such as spina bifida or anencephaly, impending fetal death, congenital nephrosis, or contamination of fetal blood.
Bacteria	Absent	Presence indicates chorioamnionitis.
Chromosome	Normal karyotype	Abnormal karyotype may indicate fetal sex and chromosome disorders.
Acetylcholinesterase	Absent	Presence may indicate neural tube defects, exomphalos, or other serious malformations.

milial hyperuricemia, and Lesch-Nyhan syndrome tend to increase the level of uric acid.

Estrone, estradiol, estriol, and *estriol conjugates* appear in amniotic fluid in varying amounts. Estriol, the most prevalent form of estrogen, increases from 25.7 ng/ml during the 16th to 20th weeks to almost 1000 ng/ml at term. Severe erythroblastosis fetalis decreases the estriol level.

THE APT TEST

Blood in the amniotic fluid can be of maternal or fetal origin. The APT test, based on the premise that fetal hemoglobin is alkali-resistant and adult hemoglobin changes to alkaline hematin after the addition of alkali, can differentiate between the two. This test may be performed on all bloody amniotic fluid samples.

To perform this test, dilute 1 ml of amniotic fluid with water until it turns pink. Centrifuge for 10 minutes, and decant the supernatant. Add five parts supernatant to one part 0.25 N (1%) sodium hydroxide, and observe for 1 to 2 minutes. Fetal blood appears red; maternal blood, yellow-brown. To confirm results, repeat the test with known maternal blood.

Blood in the amniotic fluid, which occurs in about 10% of amniocenteses, results from a faulty tap. If the origin is maternal, the blood generally has no special significance; however, "port wine" fluid may be a sign of premature separation of the placenta, and blood of fetal origin may indicate damage to the fetal, placental, or umbilical cord vessels by the amniocentesis needle. (See *The APT test.*)

The type 2 cells lining the fetal lung alveoli produce *lecithin* slowly in early pregnancy and then markedly increase production around the 35th week.

The *sphingomyelin* level parallels that of lecithin until the 35th week, when it gradually decreases. Measuring the lecithin-sphingomyelin (L/S) ratio confirms fetal pulmonary maturity (L/S ratio above 2) or suggests a risk of respiratory distress (L/S ratio below 2). However, fetal respiratory distress may develop in the fetus of a diabetic patient or in a fetus with sepsis even if the L/S ratio is greater than 2.

As the pulmonary system matures, *phosphatidylglycerol* (indicating that respiratory distress is unlikely) replaces *phosphatidylinositol.* Measuring *glucose* levels in the fluid can aid in assessing glucose control in a diabetic patient, but it isn't done routinely. A level greater than 45 mg/dl indicates poor maternal and fetal control. Insulin levels normally increase slightly from the 27th to the 40th week but increase sharply (up to 27 times the normal level) in a patient with poorly controlled diabetes.

Laboratory analysis can identify at least 25 different enzymes (usually in low concentrations) in amniotic fluid. The enzymes have few known clinical implications, although elevated *acetylcholinesterase* levels may be associated with neural tube defects, exomphalos, and other serious malformations.

When the mother carries an X-linked disorder, determining the fetus's sex is important: A male fetus has a 50% chance of being affected; a female fetus won't be affected but has a 50% chance of being a carrier.

Posttest care
■ Make sure bleeding has stopped before removing pressure from the venipuncture site.
■ If a hematoma develops, apply warm soaks.

Interfering factors
■ Failure to place the fluid specimen in an appropriate amber or foil-covered tube may result in abnormally low bilirubin levels.
■ Blood or meconium in the fluid adversely affects the L/S ratio.
■ Maternal blood in the fluid may lower creatinine levels.
■ Fetal blood in the fluid specimen invalidates the AFP results because even small amounts of fetal blood can double AFP concentrations.
■ Several disorders that aren't associated with pregnancy (including infectious mononucleosis, cirrhosis, hepatic cancer, teratoma, endodermal sinus tumor, gastric carcinoma, pancreatic carcinoma, and subacute hereditary tyrosinemia) can cause increased AFP levels.
■ Plastic disposable syringes can be toxic to amniotic fluid cells.

Amylase test, serum
Alpha-amylase (amylase or AML) is synthesized primarily in the pancreas and the salivary glands and secreted into the GI tract. This enzyme helps digest starch and glycogen in the mouth, stomach, and intestine. In cases of suspected acute pancreatic disease, measurement of serum or urine amylase is the most important laboratory test.

More than 20 methods of measuring serum amylase exist, with different ranges of normal values. Unfortunately, test values can't always be converted to a standard measurement.

Purpose
■ To diagnose acute pancreatitis
■ To distinguish between acute pancreatitis and other causes of abdominal pain that require immediate surgery

■ To evaluate possible pancreatic injury caused by abdominal trauma or surgery.

Patient preparation

Explain to the patient that this test helps assess pancreatic function. Inform the patient that fasting isn't necessary before the test but abstaining from alcohol is required.

Withhold drugs that may elevate serum amylase levels. These drugs include aminosalicylic acid asparaginase, azathioprine, bethanechol, chloride salts, cholinergics, corticosteroids, cyproheptadine hydrochloride, ethacrynic acid, ethyl alcohol, fluoride salts, furosemide, indomethacin, mercaptopurine, methacholine, narcotic analgesics, pancreozymin, rifampin, sulfasalazine, and thiazide diuretics. Citrates and oxalates may cause false low results. If these drugs must be continued, note this on the laboratory request.

Procedure

Perform a venipuncture, and collect the sample in a 7-ml clot-activator tube.

Precautions

■ If the patient has severe abdominal pain, draw the sample before diagnostic or therapeutic intervention. For accurate results, obtaining an early sample is important.

■ Handle the sample gently to prevent hemolysis.

Reference values

Serum amylase levels for adults age 18 and older normally range from 25 to 125 U/L.

Implications of results

After the onset of acute pancreatitis, serum amylase levels begin to rise within 2 hours, peak at 12 to 48 hours, and return to normal in 3 to 4 days. Determination of urine levels should follow normal serum amylase results to rule out pancreatitis.

Moderate serum elevations may accompany pancreatic injury from perforated peptic ulcer, pancreatic cancer, acute salivary gland disease, impaired renal function, or obstruction of the common bile duct, the pancreatic duct, or the ampulla of Vater. Levels may be slightly elevated in a patient who's asymptomatic or who has an unusual response to therapy.

Depressed amylase levels can occur in patients with chronic pancreatitis, pancreatic cancer, cirrhosis, hepatitis, or toxemia of pregnancy.

MACROAMYLASEMIA

An uncommon, benign condition, macroamylasemia doesn't cause any symptoms, but it occasionally causes elevated serum amylase levels. This condition occurs when macroamylase—a complex of amylase and an immunoglobulin or other protein—is present in a patient's serum.

A typical patient with macroamylasemia has an elevated serum amylase level and a normal or slightly decreased urine amylase level. This characteristic pattern helps differentiate macroamylasemia from conditions in which both serum and urine amylase levels rise, such as pancreatitis. But it doesn't differentiate macroamylasemia from hyperamylasemia associated with impaired renal function, which may raise serum amylase levels and lower urine amylase levels. Chromatographic, ultracentrifugation, or precipitation tests are necessary to detect macroamylase in serum and definitively confirm macroamylasemia.

Posttest care

- Resume administration of drugs discontinued before the test.
- If a hematoma develops at the venipuncture site, apply warm soaks.

Interfering factors

- Conditions that may produce false-positive test results include ingestion of ethyl alcohol in large amounts and use of certain drugs, such as aminosalicylic acid, asparaginase, azathioprine, corticosteroids, cyproheptadine, narcotic analgesics, oral contraceptives, rifampin, sulfasalazine, and thiazide or loop diuretics.
- Hemolysis may alter test results.
- Conditions that may produce false-positive test results include recent peripancreatic surgery, perforated ulcer or intestine, or abscess; spasm of the sphincter of Oddi; and, in rare cases, macroamylasemia. (See *Macroamylasemia.*)

Amylase test, urine

Amylase is a starch-splitting enzyme produced primarily in the pancreas and salivary glands, usually secreted into the alimentary tract, and absorbed into the blood; small amounts of amylase are also absorbed into the blood directly from the pancreas and salivary glands. After glomerular filtration, amylase is excreted in the urine. If renal function is adequate, serum and urine levels usually rise in tandem. However, within 2 to 3 days after the onset of acute pancreatitis, serum amylase levels fall to normal, but urine amylase levels remain elevated for

7 to 10 days. One method of determining urine amylase levels is the dye-coupled starch method.

Purpose

■ To diagnose acute pancreatitis when serum amylase levels are normal or borderline

■ To aid diagnosis of chronic pancreatitis and salivary gland disorders.

Patient preparation

Explain to the patient that this test evaluates the function of the pancreas and the salivary glands. Inform the patient that restricting food or fluids isn't necessary. Explain that the test requires urine collection for 2, 6, 8, or 24 hours, and provide instruction on how to collect a timed specimen. If a female patient is menstruating, the test may have to be rescheduled.

Withhold morphine, meperidine, codeine, pentazocine, bethanechol, thiazide diuretics, indomethacin, and ethyl alcohol for 24 hours before the test. If any of the medications must be continued, note this on the laboratory request.

Procedure

Collect a 2-, 6-, 8-, or 24-hour specimen.

Precautions

■ Cover and refrigerate the specimen during the collection period. If the patient is catheterized, keep the collection bag on ice.

■ Instruct the patient not to contaminate the specimen with toilet tissue or stool.

■ Send the specimens to the laboratory as soon as the test is completed.

Reference values

Values differ from laboratory to laboratory, but urinary excretion of 10 to 80 amylase units/hour is generally considered normal.

Implications of results

Elevated amylase levels occur in association with acute pancreatitis; obstruction of the pancreatic duct, intestines, or salivary duct; carcinoma of the head of the pancreas; mumps; acute injury to the spleen; renal disease with impaired absorption; perforated peptic or duodenal ulcers; and gallbladder disease.

Depressed levels occur in association with chronic pancreatitis, cachexia, alcoholism, cancer of the liver, cirrhosis, hepatitis, and hepatic abscess. (See *Serum and urine amylase values in acute pancreatitis.*)

SERUM AND URINE AMYLASE VALUES IN ACUTE PANCREATITIS

	Serum	Urine
Normal	■ 138 to 404 amylase units/L	■ 10 to 80 amylase units/hour
Elevation	■ Rises rapidly within 3 to 6 hours after onset of attack ■ May rise to 40 times normal value ■ Increase isn't proportional to severity of attack	■ Reflects rise in serum level but lags 6 to 10 hours
Duration	■ Peaks 20 to 30 hours after onset ■ Returns to normal level within 2 or 3 days, although active inflammation of pancreas may persist ■ Persistent elevation suggests pseudocyst, necrosis, or renal disease that inhibits amylase formation	■ Elevation persists for 7 to 10 days ■ Allows retrospective diagnosis of acute or relapsing pancreatitis when serum level registers in normal range ■ Persistent elevation in the absence of renal disease suggests pseudocyst formation

Interfering factors

■ Ingestion of morphine, meperidine, codeine, pentazocine, bethanechol, thiazide diuretics, indomethacin, or alcohol within 24 hours of the test may raise urine amylase levels.

■ Fluoride may lower urine amylase levels.

■ High levels of bacterial contamination of the specimen or blood in the urine may affect test results.

■ Salivary amylase in the urine resulting from coughing or talking over the sample may raise urine amylase levels.

■ Failure to collect all urine during the test period or store the specimen properly may alter test results.

Androstenedione test

This test identifies the causes of disorders related to abnormal estrogen levels. Androstenedione, secreted by the adrenal cortex and the gonads, is converted to estrone (an estrogen of relatively low biological activity) by adipose tissue and the liver. In premenopausal women, the amount of estrogen derived from androstenedione is relatively small compared with the amount of estradiol, a more potent estrogen secreted by the ovaries. Usually, estrogen derived from androstenedione doesn't interfere with gonadotropin feedback during the menstrual cycle. In obese patients, increased levels of estrone may interfere with normal feedback, causing menstrual irregularities.

In children and postmenopausal women, estrone is a major source of estrogen. Increased androstenedione production may induce premature sexual development in children. It may produce renewed ovarian stimulation, endometriosis, bleeding, and polycystic ovaries in postmenopausal women. In men, overproduction of androstenedione may cause feminization such as gynecomastia.

Purpose

To aid in determining the cause of gonadal dysfunction, menstrual or menopausal irregularities, and premature sexual development.

Patient preparation

Explain that this test determines the cause of symptoms. Tell the patient that the test requires a blood sample. If appropriate, explain that the test should be done 1 week before or after her menstrual period and that it may be repeated. Withhold corticosteroid and pituitary-based hormones before the test. If they must be continued, note this on the laboratory request.

Procedure

Perform a venipuncture, and collect a serum sample in a 17-ml clot-activator tube. Collect a plasma sample in a separate heparinized tube. Label each tube appropriately, and send them to the laboratory immediately.

Precautions

■ Handle the sample gently to prevent hemolysis. Refrigerate plasma samples or place them on ice.
■ Record the patient's age, sex, and (if appropriate) phase of menstrual cycle on the laboratory request.

Reference values

Normal values by radioimmunoassay in females age 18 and older are 0.2 to 3.1 ng/ml; in males age 18 and older, 0.3 to 3.1 ng/ml. Values for children vary by age.

Implications of results

Elevated androstenedione levels are associated with Stein-Leventhal syndrome, Cushing's syndrome, ectopic tumors that produce adrenocorticotropic hormone, late-onset congenital adrenal hyperplasia, ovarian stromal hyperplasia, and ovarian, testicular, or adrenocortical tumors. Elevated levels result in increased estrone levels, causing premature sexual development in children; menstrual irregularities in premenopausal women; bleeding, endometriosis, or polycystic ovaries in postmenopausal women; and feminization such as gynecomastia in men. Decreased levels occur in hypogonadism.

Posttest care

- If a hematoma develops at the venipuncture site, apply warm soaks.
- Resume medications discontinued before the test.

Interfering factors

- Ingestion of corticosteroids or pituitary hormones may alter test results.
- Hemolysis caused by rough handling of the sample may interfere with accurate determination of test results.

Angiotensin-converting enzyme test

This test measures serum levels of angiotensin-converting enzyme (ACE), an enzyme found in high concentrations in lung capillaries and in lesser concentrations in blood vessels and kidney tissue. Its primary function is to help regulate arterial pressure by converting angiotensin I to angiotensin II, a powerful vasoconstrictor.

Despite the role of ACE in blood pressure regulation, this test is of little use in diagnosing hypertension. Instead, it's primarily used to diagnose sarcoidosis because of the high correlation between elevated serum ACE levels and this disease. Presumably, elevated serum levels reflect macrophage activity. This test also monitors response to treatment in sarcoidosis and helps confirm a diagnosis of Gaucher's disease or Hansen's disease.

Purpose

- To aid diagnosis of sarcoidosis, especially pulmonary sarcoidosis
- To monitor response to therapy in sarcoidosis
- To help confirm Gaucher's disease or Hansen's disease.

Patient preparation

Explain to the patient that this test helps diagnose sarcoidosis, Gaucher's disease, or Hansen's disease or, if appropriate, that it checks the response to treatment for sarcoidosis. Inform the patient that a 12-hour fast is necessary before the test. Explain that the test requires a blood sample, discuss who will perform the venipuncture and when, and note that slight discomfort may be felt from the needle puncture and the pressure of the tourniquet.

Note the patient's age on the laboratory request. If the patient is younger than age 20, ask the doctor about postponing the test because ACE levels vary in patients younger than age 20.

Procedure

Perform a venipuncture, and collect the sample in a 7-ml clot-activator tube.

Precautions

- Avoid using a collection tube with ethylenediamine-tetraacetic acid because this can decrease ACE levels, altering test results.
- Handle the collection tube gently to prevent hemolysis, which may interfere with determination of ACE levels.
- Send the sample to the laboratory immediately, or freeze it and place it on dry ice until the test can be done.

Reference values

In the colorimetric assay, normal serum ACE values for patients age 20 and older range from 6.1 to 21.1 U/L.

Implications of results

Elevated serum ACE levels may indicate sarcoidosis, Gaucher's disease, or Hansen's disease, but results must be correlated with the patient's clinical condition. In some patients, elevated ACE levels may result from hyperthyroidism, diabetic retinopathy, or liver disease.

Serum ACE levels decline as the patient responds to steroid or prednisone therapy for sarcoidosis.

Posttest care

If a hematoma develops at the venipuncture site, apply warm soaks.

Interfering factors

- Failure to fast before the test may cause significant lipemia of the sample, interfering with accurate test results.
- Use of a collection tube with ethylenediaminetetraacetic acid can falsely lower ACE levels.
- Hemolysis caused by excessive agitation of the sample may alter test results.
- Failure to send the sample to the laboratory immediately or to freeze it and place it on dry ice may cause enzyme degradation and artificially low ACE levels.

Anion gap test

The anion gap reflects anion–cation balance in the serum and helps distinguish types of metabolic acidosis without expensive, time-consuming measurement of all serum electrolytes. This test uses serum levels of routinely measured electrolytes — sodium (Na^+), chloride (Cl^-), and bicarbonate (HCO^{3-}) — for a quick calculation based on a simple physical principle: Total concentrations of cations and anions are normally equal, thereby maintaining electrical neutrality in serum.

Because sodium accounts for more than 90% of circulating cations, whereas chloride and bicarbonate together account for 85% of the counterbalancing anions, the gap between measured cation and anion levels represents those anions not routinely measured, including sulfate, phosphates, proteins, and organic acids, such as ketone bodies and lactic acid.

An increased anion gap indicates an increase in one or more of these unmeasured anions, which may occur with acidosis characterized by excessive organic or inorganic acids, such as lactic acidosis or ketoacidosis.

A normal anion gap occurs in hyperchloremic acidoses, renal tubular acidosis, and severe bicarbonate-wasting conditions, such as biliary or pancreatic fistulas and poorly functioning ileal loops.

Purpose

- To distinguish types of metabolic acidosis
- To monitor renal function and total parenteral nutrition.

Patient preparation

Explain to the patient that this test helps determine the cause of metabolic acidosis. Explain that food or fluids don't need to be restricted before the test. Tell the patient that the test requires a blood sample, discuss who will perform the venipuncture and when, and note that transient discomfort may be felt from the needle puncture and the pressure of the tourniquet.

Check the patient history for use of drugs that may influence sodium, chloride, or bicarbonate blood levels, such as diuretics, corticosteroids, and antihypertensives. If these drugs must be continued, note this on the laboratory request.

Procedure

Perform a venipuncture, and collect the sample in a 7-ml clot-activator tube.

Precautions

Handle the sample gently to prevent hemolysis, which can interfere with accurate determination of test results.

Reference values

Normally, the anion gap ranges from 8 to 14 mEq/L.

Implications of results

A normal anion gap doesn't rule out metabolic acidosis. When acidosis results from loss of bicarbonate in the urine or other body fluids, renal reabsorption of sodium promotes retention of chloride and the anion gap remains unchanged. Thus, metabolic acidosis associated with excessive chloride levels is known as *normal anion gap acidosis.*

When acidosis results from accumulation of metabolic acids, as with lactic acidosis, the anion gap increases above 14 mEq/L, with the increase being in unmeasured anions. Metabolic acidosis caused by such accumulation is known as a *high anion gap acidosis.* (See *Anion gap and metabolic acidosis.*)

Because the anion gap only determines total anion–cation balance, it doesn't necessarily reflect abnormal values for individual electrolytes. Further investigation and diagnostic tests are usually necessary to determine the specific cause of metabolic acidosis.

A decreased anion gap (less than 8 mEq/L) is rare but may occur in hypermagnesemia and in paraproteinemic states, such as multiple myeloma and Waldenström's macroglobulinemia.

Posttest care

- If a hematoma develops at the venipuncture site, ease discomfort by applying warm soaks.
- Instruct the patient to resume use of any drugs discontinued before the test.

Interfering factors

- Diuretics, lithium, chlorpropamide, and vasopressin suppress serum sodium levels, possibly decreasing the anion gap; corticosteroids and antihypertensives elevate serum sodium levels, possibly increasing the anion gap.
- Salicylates, paraldehyde, methicillin, dimercaprol, ammonium chloride, acetazolamide, ethylene glycol, and methyl alcohol decrease serum bicarbonate levels, which may increase the anion gap; adrenocorticotropic hormone, cortisone, mercurial or chlorothiazide diuretics, and excessive ingestion of alkalis or licorice elevate serum bicarbonate levels, which may decrease the anion gap.
- Ammonium chloride, cholestyramine, boric acid, oxyphenbutazone, phenylbutazone, and excessive I.V. infusion of sodium chloride may elevate serum chloride levels, possibly decreasing the anion gap.
- Thiazide diuretics, ethacrynic acid, furosemide, bicarbonates, and prolonged I.V. infusion of dextrose 5% in

ANION GAP AND METABOLIC ACIDOSIS

Metabolic acidosis with a *normal anion gap* (8 to 14 mEq/L) occurs in conditions characterized by loss of bicarbonate, such as:
■ hypokalemic acidosis associated with renal tubular acidosis, diarrhea, or ureteral diversions
■ hyperkalemic acidosis caused by acidifying agents (e.g., ammonium chloride or hydrochloric acid), hydronephrosis, or sickle cell nephropathy.
　　Metabolic acidosis with an *increased anion gap* (>14 mEq/L) occurs in conditions characterized by accumulation of organic acids, sulfates, or phosphates, such as:
■ renal failure
■ ketoacidosis associated with starvation, diabetes mellitus, or alcohol abuse
■ lactic acidosis
■ ingestion of toxins, such as salicylates, methanol, ethylene glycol (antifreeze), and paraldehyde.

water can lower serum chloride levels, possibly increasing the anion gap.
■ Iodine absorption from wounds packed with povidone-iodine or excessive use of magnesium-containing antacids (especially by patients with renal failure) may cause a falsely low anion gap.
■ Hemolysis caused by rough handling of the sample may interfere with accurate determination of test results.

Antibody screening test

This test, also known as the indirect Coombs' test and the indirect antiglobulin test, detects unexpected circulating antibodies in the patient's serum. After incubating the serum with group O red blood cells (RBCs), which are unaffected by anti-A or anti-B antibodies, an antiglobulin (Coombs') serum is added. Agglutination occurs if the patient's serum contains an antibody to one or more antigens on the RBCs.

The antibody screening test detects 95% to 99% of the circulating antibodies. After this screening procedure detects them, the antibody identification test can determine the specific identity of the antibodies present. (See *Antibody identification test*, page 68.)

Purpose

■ To detect unexpected circulating antibodies to RBC antigens in the recipient's or donor's serum before a transfusion
■ To determine the presence of anti-$Rh_0(D)$ (Rh-positive) antibody in maternal blood

> ### ANTIBODY IDENTIFICATION TEST
>
> This test identifies unexpected circulating antibodies detected by the antibody screening test (indirect Coombs' test). In this test, group O red blood cells (RBCs) — at least three with and three without a specific antigen — are combined with serum containing unknown antibodies and are observed for agglutination. If the serum contains the corresponding antibody to the RBC antigen, a positive reaction occurs with RBCs that have the antigen but not with those that lack the antigen. For example, serum that reacts with Rh-positive cells but not Rh-negative cells probably contains the anti-Rh_o(D) antibody.
>
> At least three RBCs containing the antigen and three without it are used in each test to reduce error. Serum that contains rare or multiple antibodies requires more complicated procedures.

■ To evaluate the need for administration of Rh_o(D) immune globulin
■ To aid diagnosis of acquired hemolytic anemia.

Patient preparation

Explain to the prospective blood recipient that the antibody screening test helps evaluate the possibility of a transfusion reaction. If the test is being performed because the patient is anemic, explain that it helps identify the specific type of anemia.

Inform the patient that fasting before the test isn't necessary. Explain that this test requires a blood sample, discuss who will perform the venipuncture and when, and note that transient discomfort may be felt from the needle puncture and the pressure of the tourniquet.

Check the patient history for recent administration of blood, dextran, or I.V. contrast media. Be sure to note any such administration on the laboratory request to prevent spurious interpretation of test results.

Procedure

Perform a venipuncture, and collect the sample in two 10-ml tubes. If the antibody screen is positive, antibody identification is performed on the blood.

Precautions

■ Handle the sample gently to prevent hemolysis.
■ Label the sample with the patient's name, the hospital or blood bank number, the date, and the initials of the phlebotomist. Be sure to include the patient's diagnosis and any history of transfusions, pregnancy, or drug therapy on the laboratory request.

■ Send the sample to the laboratory immediately. The antibody screening must be done within 72 hours after the sample is drawn.

Normal findings

A negative test result is normal. That is, agglutination doesn't occur, indicating that the patient's serum contains no circulating antibodies (other than anti-A and anti-B).

Implications of results

A positive result indicates the presence of unexpected circulating antibodies to RBC antigens. Such a reaction demonstrates donor and recipient incompatibility.

A positive result in a pregnant patient with Rh-negative blood may indicate the presence of antibodies to the Rh factor from previous a transfusion with incompatible blood or from a previous pregnancy with an Rh-positive fetus.

A positive result above a titer of 1:8 indicates that the fetus may develop hemolytic disease of the newborn. As a result, repeated testing throughout the patient's pregnancy is necessary to evaluate progressive development of circulating antibody levels.

Posttest care

If a hematoma develops at the venipuncture site, apply warm soaks.

Interfering factors

■ Previous administration of blood, dextran, or I.V. contrast media causes aggregation that resembles agglutination.

■ Hemolysis caused by rough handling of the sample may affect the accuracy of test results.

■ The administration of certain drugs can produce antibodies that may alter test results.

■ If the patient has received a transfusion or has been pregnant within the past 3 months, antibodies may develop and linger, thereby interfering with the patient's compatibility testing.

Antideoxyribonucleic acid antibody test

This test measures antinative deoxyribonucleic acid (DNA) antibody levels in a serum sample, using radioimmunoassay or a less sensitive technique, such as agglutination, complement fixation, or immunoelectrophoresis. For radioimmunoassay, the sample is mixed with radiolabeled native DNA. If antinative DNA antibodies are in the serum sample, they combine with the native DNA, forming complexes that are too large to pass through a membrane filter. If such antibodies aren't present, the radiolabeled DNA is able to pass through the filter. The DNA that doesn't pass through the membrane filter is then counted.

In autoimmune diseases such as systemic lupus erythematosus (SLE), native DNA is thought to be the antigen that complexes with antibody and complement, causing local tissue damage where these complexes are deposited. Serum antinative DNA levels are directly related to the extent of renal or vascular damage caused by the disease.

Two different types of anti-DNA antibodies are present in patients with SLE: anti–single-stranded (denatured) DNA and anti–double-stranded (native) DNA. Antibodies to native DNA, however, are more specific for SLE. Determination of these antibodies, with serum complement, is also useful in monitoring immunosuppressive therapy.

Purpose

■ To confirm SLE after a positive antinuclear antibody test

■ To monitor response to therapy.

Patient preparation

Explain to the patient that this test detects certain antibodies and that test results help determine the diagnosis and appropriate therapy. Or, when indicated, tell the patient that the test assesses the effectiveness of present treatment. Tell the patient that food and fluids don't need to be restricted before the test. Explain that the test requires a blood sample, discuss who will perform the venipuncture and when, and note that transient discomfort may be felt from the needle puncture and the pressure of the tourniquet.

If the patient is scheduled for a radionuclide scan, make sure the sample is collected before the scan.

Procedure

Perform a venipuncture, and collect the sample in a 7-ml tube with no additives. Some laboratories may specify a tube with either ethylenediaminetetraacetic acid or sodium fluoride and potassium oxalate added.

Precautions

Handle the sample gently.

Reference values

Normal values are less than 7 IU of native DNA bound per milliliter of serum.

Implications of results

Elevated antinative DNA levels may indicate SLE. A value of 1 to 2.5 mg/ml suggests a remission phase of SLE or the presence of other autoimmune disorders. A value of 10 to 15 mg/ml indicates active SLE. Depressed levels following immunosuppressive therapy demonstrate effective treatment of SLE.

Posttest care

If a hematoma develops at the venipuncture site, apply warm soaks.

Interfering factors

■ Penicillin, procainamide, and hydralazine may cause a false-positive reaction.
■ Hemolysis caused by rough handling of the sample may alter test results.
■ A radioactive scan performed within 1 week of collecting the sample may alter test results.

Antidiuretic hormone test, serum

Antidiuretic hormone (ADH), also known as vasopressin, is a polypeptide produced by the hypothalamus and released from storage sites in the posterior pituitary on neural stimulation. The primary function of ADH is to promote water reabsorption in response to increased osmolality (water deficiency with high concentration of sodium and other solutes). In response to decreased osmolality (water excess), reduced secretion of ADH allows increased excretion of water to maintain fluid balance. (See *ADH release and regulation*, page 72.) In an interlocking feedback mechanism with aldosterone, ADH helps regulate sodium, potassium, and fluid balance. It also stimulates vascular smooth-muscle contraction, causing an increase in arterial blood pressure.

This relatively rare test, a quantitative analysis of serum ADH level, may identify diabetes insipidus and other causes of severe homeostatic imbalance. It may be ordered as part of dehydration or hypertonic saline infusion testing, which determines the body's response to states of hyperosmolality.

Purpose

To aid in the differential diagnosis of pituitary diabetes insipidus, nephrogenic diabetes insipidus (congenital or familial), and syndrome of inappropriate antidiuretic hormone (SIADH).

Patient preparation

Explain to the patient that this test to measure hormonal secretion may aid in identifying the cause of his

ADH RELEASE AND REGULATION

Neural impulses signal the supraoptic nuclei of the hypothalamus to produce antidiuretic hormone (ADH). After it's formed, ADH moves along the hypothalamicohypophysial tract to the posterior pituitary, where it's stored until needed by the kidneys to maintain fluid balance. In the kidneys, ADH acts on the collecting tubules to retain water.

Homeostasis is maintained by a negative feedback mechanism: Ample water or excess water inhibits further ADH secretion by the supraoptic nuclei of the hypothalamus or by ADH release from the posterior pituitary. A similar negative feedback mechanism that is vital to hormonal homeostasis prevents oversecretion of other hormones.

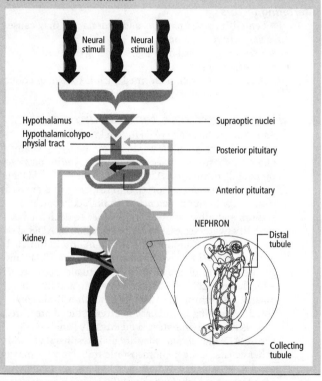

symptoms. Instruct the patient to fast and limit physical activity for 10 to 12 hours before the test. Explain that a blood sample will be drawn and that discomfort may be felt from the needle puncture. Tell the patient that the laboratory requires at least 5 days to complete the analysis.

As ordered, withhold conjugated estrogens, morphine, tranquilizers, hypnotics, oxytocin, anesthetics (such as ether), lithium carbonate, vincristine, carbamazepine, cyclophosphamide, and chlorothiazide before the test;

these drugs and others may cause SIADH. If these medications must be continued, note this on the laboratory request.

Make sure the patient is relaxed and recumbent for 30 minutes before the test.

Procedure

Perform a venipuncture, and collect the sample in a plastic collection tube without additives or a chilled ethylenediaminetetraacetic acid tube. Immediately send the sample to the laboratory, where serum or plasma must be separated from the red blood cells within 10 minutes. Perform a serum osmolality test at the same time to facilitate interpretation of results.

Precautions

The syringe and the collection tube *must* be plastic because the fragile ADH degrades on contact with glass.

Reference values

ADH values range from 1 to 5 pg/ml, but they can be evaluated in light of serum osmolality. If serum osmolality is less than 285 mOsm/kg, ADH is normally less than 2 pg/ml. If it's greater than 290 mOsm/kg, ADH may range from 2 to 12 pg/ml.

Implications of results

Absent or below-normal ADH levels indicate pituitary diabetes insipidus resulting from a neurohypophysial or hypothalamic tumor, a viral infection, metastatic disease, sarcoidosis, tuberculosis, Hand-Schüller-Christian disease, syphilis, neurosurgical procedures, or head trauma.

Normal ADH levels in the presence of signs of diabetes insipidus, such as polydipsia, polyuria, and hypotonic urine, may indicate the nephrogenic form of the disease, which is marked by renal tubular resistance to ADH; however, levels may rise if the pituitary tries to compensate.

Elevated ADH levels may also indicate SIADH, possibly as a result of bronchogenic carcinoma, acute porphyria, hypothyroidism, Addison's disease, cirrhosis of the liver, infectious hepatitis, severe hemorrhage, or circulatory shock.

Posttest care

■ If a hematoma develops at the venipuncture site, apply warm soaks.
■ Resume diet and medications discontinued before the test.

Interfering factors

- Failure to restrict diet, medications, or activity may affect test results. Morphine, anesthetics, estrogen, oxytocin, chlorpropamide, vincristine, carbamazepine, cyclophosphamide, and chlorothiazide elevate ADH levels, as do stress, pain, and positive-pressure ventilation. Alcohol and negative-pressure ventilation inhibit ADH secretion.
- A radioactive scan performed within 1 week before the test may influence test results.

Anti–double-stranded DNA antibody test

About two-thirds of patients with active systemic lupus erythematosus (SLE) have measurable levels of autoantibodies to double-stranded (native) deoxyribonucleic acid (known as anti-ds-DNA). These antibodies are rarely detected in patients with other connective tissue diseases.

The anti-ds-DNA antibody test measures and differentiates these antibody levels in a serum sample, using radioimmunoassay, agglutination, complement fixation, or immunoelectrophoresis. If anti-ds-DNA antibodies are present, they combine with native DNA and form complexes that are too large to pass through a membrane filter. The test counts these oversized complexes.

Purpose

- To confirm a diagnosis of SLE
- To monitor the SLE patient's response to therapy and determine prognosis.

Patient preparation

Explain to the patient that this test helps diagnose and determine the appropriate therapy for SLE. Tell the patient that restricting food or fluids isn't necessary before the test. Explain that the test requires a blood sample, discuss who will perform the venipuncture and when, and explain that transient discomfort may be felt from the needle puncture and the tourniquet but collecting the sample usually takes less than 3 minutes. If the patient has had a recent radioactive test, note this on the laboratory request.

Procedure

Perform a venipuncture, and collect the sample in a 7-ml tube with no additives. Some laboratories may specify a tube with either ethylenediaminetetraacetic acid or sodium fluoride and potassium oxalate added.

Precautions

Handle the sample gently to prevent hemolysis.

Reference values

An anti-ds-DNA antibody level less than 25 IU is considered negative for SLE.

Implications of results

Elevated anti-ds-DNA antibody levels may indicate SLE. Values of 25 to 30 IU are considered borderline positive. Values of 31 to 200 IU are positive, and those greater than 200 IU are strongly positive.

Depressed anti-ds-DNA antibody levels may follow immunosuppressive therapy, demonstrating effective treatment of SLE.

Posttest care

If a hematoma develops at the venipuncture site, apply warm soaks.

Interfering factors

- A radioactive scan performed within 1 week before collection of a sample.
- Hemolysis caused by rough handling of the sample.

Anti-insulin antibody test

Some diabetic patients form antibodies to the insulin they take. These antibodies bind with some of the insulin, making less insulin available for glucose metabolism and necessitating increased insulin dosages. This phenomenon is known as insulin resistance.

Performed on the blood of a diabetic patient receiving insulin, the anti-insulin antibody test detects insulin antibodies. Insulin antibodies are immunoglobulins, called anti-insulin Ab. The most common type of anti-insulin Ab is immunoglobulin G (IgG), but anti-insulin Ab is also found in the other four classes of immunoglobulins—IgA, IgD, IgE, and IgM. IgM may cause insulin resistance, and IgE has been associated with allergic reactions.

Purpose

- To determine insulin allergy
- To confirm insulin resistance
- To determine if hypoglycemia is caused by insulin overuse.

Patient preparation

Tell the patient that this test is used to determine the most appropriate treatment for his diabetes and to determine the presence of insulin resistance or an allergy to insulin. Explain that the test requires a blood sample and discuss who will perform the venipuncture and when. Tell the patient that transient discomfort may be felt from the needle puncture and the tourniquet but collecting the sample takes only a few minutes. Tell the patient that fasting before the test isn't necessary. If the patient has recently had a radioactive test, note this on the laboratory request.

Procedure

Perform a venipuncture, and collect the sample in a 7-ml tube with no additives.

Precautions

Handle the sample gently to prevent hemolysis.

Reference values

Less than 3% of the patient's serum should bind with labeled beef, human, and pork insulin.

Implications of results

Elevated levels may occur in insulin allergy or resistance and in factitious hypoglycemia.

Posttest care

If a hematoma develops at the venipuncture site, apply warm soaks.

Interfering factors

A radioactive test performed within 1 week before the test may interfere with test results.

Antimitochondrial antibody test

Usually performed with the test for anti–smooth-muscle antibodies, this test detects antimitochondrial antibodies in serum by indirect immunofluorescence. Antimitochondrial antibodies react with mitochondria in the renal tubules, gastric mucosa, and other organs in which cells expend large amounts of energy.

These autoantibodies are present in several hepatic diseases, although their etiology is unknown and there's no evidence that they cause hepatic damage. They are most commonly associated with primary biliary cirrhosis and sometimes with chronic active hepatitis and drug-induced jaundice. Antimitochondrial antibodies are also associated with autoimmune diseases, such as systemic lupus erythematosus, rheumatoid arthritis, pernicious anemia, and idiopathic Addison's disease. (See *Incidence of serum antibodies in various disorders*.)

Purpose

■ To aid diagnosis of primary biliary cirrhosis
■ To distinguish between extrahepatic jaundice and biliary cirrhosis.

INCIDENCE OF SERUM ANTIBODIES IN VARIOUS DISORDERS

The chart below shows the percentage of patients with certain disorders who have antimitochondrial or anti–smooth-muscle antibodies in the serum. The presence of these antibodies requires further testing to confirm the diagnosis. Up to 1% of healthy people also show antimitochondrial antibodies.

Disorder	Antimitochondrial antibodies	Anti–smooth-muscle antibodies
Primary biliary cirrhosis	75% to 95%	0% to 50% [a]
Chronic active hepatitis	0% to 30%	50% to 80%
Extrahepatic biliary obstruction	0% to 5%	0%
Cryptogenic cirrhosis	0% to 25%	0% to 1%
Viral (infectious) hepatitis	0%	1% to 2% [b]
Drug-induced jaundice	50% to 80%	0%
Intrinsic asthma	0%	20%
Rheumatoid arthritis and other collagen diseases	1% to 2%	0%
Systemic lupus erythematosus	3% to 5% [c]	0%

a In chronic disease, values fall at upper end of range.
b Much higher incidence occurs with hepatic damage.
c Much higher incidence occurs with renal involvement.

Patient preparation

Explain that this test evaluates liver function. Advise the patient that restriction of food or fluids isn't necessary. Explain that this test requires a blood sample, discuss who will perform the venipuncture and when, and note that discomfort may be felt from the needle puncture and the pressure of the tourniquet.

Check the patient's medication history for oxyphenisatin use, and report such use to the laboratory because this drug may produce antimitochondrial antibodies.

Procedure

■ Perform a venipuncture, and collect the sample in a 7-ml tube with no additives.
■ Apply pressure to the venipuncture site until bleeding stops because patients with hepatic disease may bleed excessively.

Reference values

Serum is negative for antimitochondrial antibodies at a titer less than 20.

Implications of results

Although antimitochondrial antibodies appear in 75% to 95% of patients with primary biliary cirrhosis, this test alone doesn't confirm the diagnosis. Further tests, such as serum alkaline phosphatase, serum bilirubin, alanine aminotransferase, aspartate aminotransferase and, possibly, liver biopsy or cholangiography may also be necessary.

Antimitochondrial autoantibodies also appear in some patients with chronic active hepatitis, drug-induced jaundice, or cryptogenic cirrhosis. However, they rarely appear in patients with extrahepatic biliary obstruction, and a positive test helps rule out this condition.

Posttest care

If a hematoma develops at the venipuncture site, apply warm soaks.

Interfering factors

■ Confusion of antimitochondrial antibodies with heterophil antibodies, cardiolipin antibodies to syphilis, ribosomal antibodies, or microsomal hepatic or renal autoantibodies may affect the accuracy of test results.
■ Oxyphenisatin can produce antimitochondrial antibodies in patients taking this drug.

Antinuclear antibody test

In conditions such as systemic lupus erythematosus (SLE), scleroderma, and certain infections, the body's immune system may perceive portions of its own cell nuclei as foreign and may produce antinuclear antibodies (ANAs). Specific types of ANA include antibodies to deoxyribonucleic acid (DNA), nucleoprotein, histones, nuclear ribonucleoprotein, and other nuclear constituents. Although ANAs are harmless on their own because they don't penetrate living cells, they sometimes form antigen-antibody complexes that cause damage, as in SLE. Because of multi-organ involvement, test results aren't diagnostic and can only partially confirm clinical evidence.

This test measures the relative level of ANA in a serum sample through indirect immunofluorescence. Serial dilutions of serum are mixed with either Hep-2 or mouse kidney substrate. If the serum contains ANA, it forms antigen-antibody complexes with the substrate. After the preparation is mixed with fluorescein-labeled antihuman serum, it's examined under an ultraviolet microscope. If ANAs are present, the complex fluoresces. Titer is taken as the greatest dilution that shows the reaction.

About 99% of patients with SLE exhibit ANA; a large percentage of these patients do so at high titers. (See *Incidence of antinuclear antibodies in various disorders.*) Although this test isn't specific for SLE, it's a useful

INCIDENCE OF ANTINUCLEAR ANTIBODIES IN VARIOUS DISORDERS

The chart below indicates the percentage of patients with certain disorders whose serum contains antinuclear antibodies (ANAs). About 40% of elderly people and 5% of the general population also have positive ANA findings.

Disorder	Positive ANA
Systemic lupus erythematosus (SLE)	95% to 100%
Lupoid hepatitis	95% to 100%
Felty's syndrome	95% to 100%
Progressive systemic sclerosis (scleroderma)	75% to 80%
Drug-associated SLE-like syndrome (hydralazine, procainamide, isoniazid)	Approximately 50%
Sjögren's syndrome	40% to 75%
Rheumatoid arthritis	25% to 60%
Healthy family member of SLE patient	Approximately 25%
Chronic discoid lupus erythematosus	15% to 50%
Juvenile arthritis	15% to 30%
Polyarteritis nodosa	15% to 25%
Miscellaneous diseases	10% to 50%
Dermatomyositis, polymyositis	10% to 30%
Rheumatic fever	Approximately 5%

screening tool. Failure to detect ANA essentially rules out active SLE.

Purpose

■ To screen for SLE (failure to detect ANAs essentially rules out active SLE)
■ To monitor the effectiveness of immunosuppressive therapy for SLE.

Patient preparation

Explain that this test evaluates the immune system and that further testing is usually required for diagnosis. If appropriate, inform the patient that the test will be repeated to monitor response to therapy. Explain that restricting food or fluids isn't necessary. Tell the patient that this test requires a blood sample, discuss who will perform the venipuncture and when, and note that discomfort may be felt from the needle puncture and the pressure of the tourniquet.

Check the patient's history for drugs that may affect test results, such as isoniazid, hydralazine, and procainamide. Note such drug use on the laboratory request.

Procedure

Perform a venipuncture, and collect the sample in a 7-ml tube with no additives.

Reference values

Using Hep-2 cells, the test for ANA is negative at a titer of 1:40 or below. If mouse kidney substrate is being used, the test is negative at a titer of less than 1:20. Results are reported as positive, with pattern and serum titer noted, or negative.

Implications of results

Although this test is a sensitive indicator of ANA, it isn't specific for SLE. Low titers may occur in patients with viral diseases, chronic hepatic disease, collagen vascular disease, or autoimmune diseases as well as in some healthy adults; incidence increases with age. The higher the titer, the more specific the test is for SLE, for which the titer often exceeds 1:256.

The pattern of nuclear fluorescence helps identify the type of immune disease present. A peripheral pattern is almost exclusively associated with SLE because it indicates the presence of anti-DNA antibodies; anti-DNA antibodies are sometimes measured by radioimmunoassay if ANA titers are high or a peripheral pattern is observed. A homogeneous, or diffuse, pattern is also associated with SLE as well as with related connective tissue disorders; a nucleolar pattern, with scleroderma; and a speckled, irregular pattern, with infectious mononucleosis and mixed connective tissue disorders (such as SLE and scleroderma).

A single serum sample, especially one collected from a patient with collagen vascular disease, may contain antibodies to several parts of the cell's nucleus. In addition, as serum dilution increases, the fluorescent pattern may change because different antibodies are reactive at different titers.

Posttest care

CLINICAL ALERT Observe the venipuncture site for signs of infection, and report any changes to the doctor immediately because patients with autoimmune disease have a compromised immune system. Keep a clean, dry bandage over the site for at least 24 hours.

■ If a hematoma develops at the venipuncture site, apply warm soaks.

Interfering factors

Certain drugs, most commonly isoniazid, hydralazine, and procainamide, can produce a syndrome resembling

SLE; other such drugs include para-aminosalicylic acid, chlorpromazine, clofibrate, phenytoin, griseofulvin, ethosuximide, gold salts, methyldopa, oral contraceptives, penicillin, propylthiouracil, phenylbutazone, methysergide, streptomycin, sulfonamides, tetracyclines, mephenytoin, quinidine, primidone, reserpine, and trimethadione.

Anti–smooth-muscle antibody test

Using indirect immunofluorescence, this test measures the relative concentration of anti–smooth-muscle antibodies in serum and is usually performed with the test for antimitochondrial antibodies. The serum sample is exposed to a thin section of smooth muscle and incubated; then a fluorescent-labeled antiglobulin is added. This antiglobulin binds only to antibodies that have complexed with smooth muscle and appears fluorescent when viewed through the microscope under ultraviolet light.

Anti–smooth-muscle antibodies appear in several hepatic diseases, especially chronic active hepatitis and, less often, primary biliary cirrhosis. Although these antibodies are most commonly associated with hepatic diseases, their etiology is unknown, and they aren't considered a cause of hepatic damage.

Purpose

To aid diagnosis of chronic active hepatitis and primary biliary cirrhosis.

Patient preparation

Explain to the patient that this test helps evaluate liver function. Inform the patient that restricting food or fluids isn't necessary. Explain that the test requires a blood sample, discuss who will perform the venipuncture and when, and note that transient discomfort may be felt from the needle puncture and the pressure of the tourniquet.

Procedure

■ Perform a venipuncture, and collect the sample in a 7-ml tube without additives.
■ Apply pressure to the venipuncture site until bleeding stops because patients with hepatic disease may bleed excessively.

Reference values

Normal titer of anti–smooth-muscle antibodies is less than 1:20. Results are reported as positive or negative.

Implications of results

The test for anti–smooth-muscle antibodies isn't very specific; these antibodies appear in about 66% of patients with chronic active hepatitis and 30% to 40% of patients with primary biliary cirrhosis. Anti–smooth-muscle antibodies may also be present in patients with infectious mononucleosis, acute viral hepatitis, malignant tumor of the liver, and intrinsic asthma. (See *Incidence of serum antibodies in various disorders*, page 77.)

Posttest care

If a hematoma develops at the site, apply warm soaks.

Interfering factors

None reported.

Antistreptolysin-O test

Because streptococcal infections are often overlooked, serologic testing is valuable in patients with glomerulonephritis or acute rheumatic fever to confirm antecedent infection by showing a serologic response to streptococcal antigen. The antistreptolysin-O (ASO) test measures the relative serum levels of the antibody to streptolysin O, an oxygen-labile enzyme produced by group A beta-hemolytic streptococci.

In this test, also known as the streptococcal antibody test, a serum sample is diluted with commercially prepared streptolysin O and incubated. After the addition of rabbit or human red blood cells (RBCs), the tube is reincubated and examined visually. If hemolysis fails to develop, ASO has complexed with the antigen, inactivated it, and prevented RBC destruction, indicating recent beta-hemolytic streptococcal infection. The end point is read in Todd units, the reciprocal of the highest dilution (titer) that inhibits hemolysis.

Very high ASO titers occur in poststreptococcal diseases, such as rheumatic fever or glomerulonephritis. High titers may also occur in patients with uncomplicated streptococcal disease, but the incidence is lower and the titers are lower than in poststreptococcal diseases. Microscopic methods for detecting ASO, such as the Rapi/tex ASO latex agglutination test, currently screen for beta-hemolytic streptococcal infection.

Purpose

■ To confirm recent or ongoing infection with beta-hemolytic streptococci
■ To help diagnose rheumatic fever and poststreptococcal glomerulonephritis in the presence of clinical symp-

---

TEST FOR ANTI-DNASE B

The antideoxyribonuclease B (anti-DNase B) test, a process similar to the antistreptolysin-O (ASO) test, detects antibodies to DNase B, a potent antigen produced by all group A streptococci.

For adults and preschool-age children, normal anti-DNase B titer is ≥ 85 Todd units/ml; for school-age children, less than 170 Todd units/ml. Elevated anti-DNase B titers appear in 80% of patients with acute rheumatic fever, in 75% of those with poststreptococcal glomerulonephritis (following streptococcal pharyngitis), and in 60% of those with glomerulonephritis (following group A streptococcal pyoderma). This is a much higher percentage than those with ASO titer elevations (25%), making the test for anti-DNase B especially valuable in detecting a reaction to group A streptococcal pyoderma.

Other streptococcal antigens are of limited diagnostic value, or their use is controversial.

---

toms (See *Test for anti-DNase B*, for information about another method of diagnosing these two diseases.)

■ To distinguish between rheumatic fever and rheumatoid arthritis when joint pain is present.

Patient preparation

Explain to the patient that this test detects an immune response to certain bacteria. Tell the patient that food or fluids don't need to be restricted. Explain that this test requires a blood sample, discuss who will perform the venipuncture and when, and note that transient discomfort may be felt from the needle puncture and the pressure of the tourniquet.

If the test is to be repeated at regular intervals to identify active and inactive states of rheumatic fever or to confirm acute glomerulonephritis, tell the patient that measuring changes in antibody levels helps determine the effectiveness of therapy.

Check the patient's medication history for drugs that may suppress the streptococcal antibody response. If such drugs must be continued, note this on the laboratory request.

Procedure

Perform a venipuncture, and collect the sample in a 7-ml tube with no additives.

Precautions

Handle the sample gently to prevent hemolysis.

Reference values

Even healthy people have some detectable ASO titer from previous minor streptococcal infections. For preschool-age children and adults, the normal ASO titer is up to 85 Todd units/ml and, for school-age children, less than 170 Todd units/ml.

Implications of results

High ASO titers usually occur only after prolonged or recurrent infections, but 15% to 20% of patients with poststreptococcal disease don't have high titers. Generally, a titer greater than 166 Todd units is considered a definite elevation. A low titer is good evidence for the absence of rheumatic fever. Titers of 500 to 5000 Todd units suggest acute rheumatic fever or acute poststreptococcal glomerulonephritis. Serial titers, determined at 10- to 14-day intervals, provide more reliable information than a single titer. An increase in titer 2 to 5 weeks after the acute infection, which peaks 4 to 6 weeks after the initial increase, confirms poststreptococcal disease.

CLINICAL ALERT False-negative results are likely in patients with streptococcal skin infections, who rarely have abnormal ASO titers even with poststreptococcal disease.

Posttest care

If a hematoma develops at the venipuncture site, apply warm soaks.

Interfering factors

■ Antibiotic or corticosteroid therapy may suppress the streptococcal antibody response and thus alter test results.
■ Hemolysis caused by rough handling of the sample may affect test results.

Antithyroid antibody test

In autoimmune disorders such as Hashimoto's thyroiditis and Graves' disease (hyperthyroidism), thyroglobulin, the major colloidal storage compound, is released into blood. Because thyroxine usually separates from thyroglobulin before its release into blood, thyroglobulin doesn't normally enter the circulation. When it does, antithyroglobulin antibodies are formed to attack this foreign substance; the ensuing autoimmune response damages the thyroid gland. The serum of a patient whose autoimmune system produces antithyroglobulin antibodies usually contains antimicrosomal antibodies, which react with the microsomes of the thyroid epithelial cells.

The tanned red cell hemagglutination test detects antithyroglobulin and antimicrosomal antibodies. In this assay, sheep red blood cells that have been pretreated with tannic acid and coated with thyroglobulin or microsomal fragments are mixed with a serum sample. The mixture agglutinates in the presence of these specific antibodies, and serial dilutions can quantify the antibody concentration. Another laboratory technique, indirect immunofluorescence, can detect antimicrosomal antibodies.

Purpose

To detect circulating antithyroglobulin antibodies when clinical evidence indicates Hashimoto's thyroiditis, Graves' disease, or another thyroid disorder.

Patient preparation

Explain to the patient that this test evaluates thyroid function. Tell the patient that food or fluids don't need to be restricted. Explain that this test requires a blood sample, discuss who will perform the venipuncture and when, and note that transient discomfort may be felt from the needle puncture and the pressure of the tourniquet.

Procedure

Perform a venipuncture, and collect the sample in a 7-ml tube with no additives.

Reference values

The normal titer is less than 1:100 for both antithyroglobulin and antimicrosomal antibodies. Low levels of these antibodies are normal in 10% of the general population and in 20% or more of people age 70 and older.

Implications of results

The presence of antithyroglobulin or antimicrosomal antibodies in serum can indicate subclinical autoimmune thyroid disease, Graves' disease, or idiopathic myxedema. High titers (1:400 or more) strongly suggest Hashimoto's thyroiditis. (See *Incidence of thyroid autoantibodies in various disorders*, page 86.) These antibodies may also occur in patients with other autoimmune disorders, such as systemic lupus erythematosus, rheumatoid arthritis, or autoimmune hemolytic anemia.

Posttest care

If a hematoma develops at the venipuncture site, apply warm soaks.

Interfering factors

None reported.

INCIDENCE OF THYROID AUTOANTIBODIES IN VARIOUS DISORDERS

The chart below indicates the percentage of people with thyroid disorders who have antithyroglobulin or antimicrosomal antibodies in the serum.

Disorder	Antithyroglobulin antibodies	Antimicrosomal antibodies
Hashimoto's thyroiditis	60% to 95%	70% to 90%
Idiopathic myxedema	75%	65%
Thyroid carcinoma	40%	15%
Graves' disease	30% to 40%	50% to 85%
Adenomatous goiter	20% to 30%	20%
Pernicious anemia	25%	10%

Arginine test

This test, also known as the growth hormone stimulation test, measures plasma growth hormone (hGH) levels after I.V. administration of arginine, an amino acid that normally stimulates hGH secretion. It's commonly used to identify pituitary dysfunction in infants and children with growth retardation and to confirm hGH deficiency. This test may be performed concomitantly with an insulin tolerance test or after administration of other hGH stimulants, such as glucagon, vasopressin, and levodopa.

Purpose

- To aid diagnosis of pituitary tumors
- To confirm hGH deficiency in infants and children with low baseline levels.

Patient preparation

Explain to the patient or his parents that this test identifies hGH deficiency. Explain that the patient must fast and limit physical activity for 10 to 12 hours before the test. Explain that this test requires venous infusion of a drug and collection of several blood samples. The test takes at least 2 hours to perform; results are available in 2 days.

Before the test, withhold all corticosteroid medications, including pituitary-based hormones. If these medications must be continued, record this on the laboratory request. Because hGH levels may rise after exercise or excitement, make sure the patient is relaxed and recumbent for at least 90 minutes before the test.

Procedure

■ Between 6 a.m. and 8 a.m., draw 6 ml of venous blood (basal sample) into a clot-activator tube. Start an I.V. infusion of arginine (0.5 g/kg of body weight) in normal saline solution, and continue for 30 minutes. Use an indwelling venous catheter to avoid repeated venipunctures and minimize stress and anxiety. After discontinuing the I.V. infusion, draw a 6-ml sample three times at 30-minute intervals. Collect each sample in a clot-activator tube, and label appropriately.

Precautions

■ Draw each sample at the scheduled time, and specify the collection time on the laboratory request.
■ Send each sample to the laboratory immediately because hGH has a half-life of 20 to 25 minutes.
■ Handle the samples gently to prevent hemolysis.

Reference values

Arginine should raise hGH levels to more than 10 ng/ml in men, to more than 15 ng/ml in women, and to 48 ng/ml in children. Such an increase may appear in the first sample drawn 30 minutes after arginine infusion is discontinued or in the samples drawn 60 and 90 minutes afterward.

Implications of results

Elevated fasting levels and increases during sleep help to rule out hGH deficiency. Failure of hGH levels to rise after arginine infusion indicates decreased anterior pituitary hGH reserve. In children, this deficiency causes dwarfism; in adults, it can indicate panhypopituitarism. When hGH levels fail to reach 10 ng/ml, retesting is required at the same time of day as the original test.

Posttest care

■ If a hematoma develops at the venipuncture site, apply warm soaks.
■ Resume diet and medications discontinued before the test.

Interfering factors

■ Failure to observe restrictions of diet, medications, and physical activity may affect test results.
■ A radioactive scan performed within 1 week before the test may affect results.
■ Hemolysis caused by rough handling of the sample may affect test results.

Arterial blood gas analysis

Arterial blood gas (ABG) analysis evaluates gas exchange in the lungs by measuring the partial pressures of oxygen (PaO_2) and carbon dioxide ($PaCO_2$) as well as the pH of an arterial sample. PaO_2 measures the amount of oxygen crossing the alveolar capillary membrane and dissolving in the blood. $PaCO_2$ measures the adequacy of alveolar ventilation and respiratory response to acid–base balance. The pH measures the hydrogen ion (H^+) concentration, indicating acidity of alkalinity of the blood. An increase in H^+ causes an increase in pH. Bicarbonate (HCO_3^-) is a measure of the metabolic component of acid–base balance. Oxygen saturation (SaO_2) is the ratio of the amount of oxygen in the blood combined with hemoglobin to the total amount of oxygen that the hemoglobin can carry. Oxygen content (O_2CT) measures the amount of oxygen combined with hemoglobin and isn't frequently used in blood gas evaluation. (See *Balancing pH*.)

Purpose

- To evaluate the efficiency of pulmonary gas exchange
- To assess integrity of the ventilatory control system
- To determine the acid–base level of the blood
- To monitor respiratory therapy.

Patient preparation

Explain to the patient that this test evaluates how well the lungs are delivering oxygen to blood and eliminating carbon dioxide. Tell the patient that restricting food or fluids isn't necessary. Explain that the test requires a blood sample, discuss who will perform the arterial puncture and when, and tell the patient which site — radial, brachial, or femoral artery — has been selected for the puncture. Instruct the patient to breathe normally during the test, and warn him that brief cramping or throbbing pain may be felt at the puncture site.

Procedure

- Perform a cutaneous arterial puncture, or draw blood from an arterial line. Use a heparinized blood gas syringe to draw the sample, eliminate all air from the sample, place it on ice immediately, and transport it for analysis.
- After applying pressure for 3 to 5 minutes to the puncture site, tape a gauze pad firmly over it. If the puncture site is on the arm, don't tape the entire circumference because this may restrict circulation. If the patient is receiving anticoagulants or has a coagulopathy, hold the puncture site longer than 5 minutes if necessary.

BALANCING pH

To measure the acidity or alkalinity of a solution, chemists use a pH scale of 1 to 15 that measures hydrogen ion concentrations. As hydrogen ions and acidity increase, pH falls below 7.0, which is neutral. Conversely, when hydrogen ions decrease, pH and alkalinity increase. Acid–base balance, or homeostasis of hydrogen ions, is necessary if the body's enzyme systems are to work properly.

The slightest change in ionic hydrogen concentration alters the rate of cellular chemical reactions; a sufficiently severe change can be fatal. To maintain a normal blood pH — generally between 7.35 and 7.45 — the body relies on the following three mechanisms.

Buffers
Chemically composed of two substances, buffers prevent radical pH changes by replacing strong acids added to a solution (such as blood) with weaker ones. For example, strong acids capable of yielding many hydrogen ions are replaced by weaker ones that yield fewer hydrogen ions. Because of the principal buffer coupling of bicarbonate and carbonic acid — normally in a ratio of 20:1 — the plasma acid–base level rarely fluctuates. Increased bicarbonate, however, indicates alkalosis, whereas decreased bicarbonate points to acidosis. Increased carbonic acid indicates acidosis, and decreased carbonic acid indicates alkalosis.

Respiration
Respiration is important in maintaining blood pH. The lungs convert carbonic acid to carbon dioxide and water. With every expiration, carbon dioxide and water leave the body, decreasing the carbonic acid content of the blood. Consequently, fewer hydrogen ions are formed, and blood pH increases. When the blood's hydrogen ion or carbonic acid content increases, neurons in the respiratory center stimulate respiration.

Hyperventilation eliminates carbon dioxide and hence carbonic acid from the body, reduces hydrogen ion formation, and increases pH. Conversely, increased blood pH from alkalosis — decreased hydrogen ion concentration — causes hypoventilation, which restores blood pH to its normal level by retaining carbon dioxide and thus increasing hydrogen ion formation.

Urine excretion
The third factor in acid–base balance is urine excretion. Because the kidneys excrete varying amounts of acids and bases, they control urine pH, which in turn affects blood pH. For example, when blood pH is decreased, the distal and collecting tubules remove excessive hydrogen ions (carbonic acid forms in the tubular cells and dissociates into hydrogen and bicarbonate) and displaces them in urine, thereby eliminating hydrogen from the body. In exchange, basic ions in the urine — most often sodium — diffuse into the tubular cells, where they combine with bicarbonate. This sodium bicarbonate is then reabsorbed in the blood, resulting in decreased urine pH and, more importantly, increased blood pH.

Precautions

■ Wait at least 20 minutes before drawing ABG in the following situations:
– after initiating, changing, or discontinuing oxygen therapy
– after initiating or changing settings of mechanical ventilation
– after extubation.
■ Include the following information on the laboratory request:
– room air or amount of oxygen and method of delivery (e.g., 40% aerosol face mask)
– ventilator settings if on mechanical ventilation (FIO_2, tidal volume, mode, respiratory rate, positive-end respiratory pressure [PEEP])
– the patient's temperature.

Reference values

Normal ABG values fall within the following ranges:
■ PO_2: 75 to 100 mm Hg
■ $PaCO_2$: 35 to 45 mm Hg
■ *pH*: 7.35 to 7.45
■ O_2CT: 15% to 23%
■ SaO_2: 94% to 100%
■ HCO_3^-: 22 to 26 mEq/L.

Implications of results

Low PaO_2, O_2CT, and SaO_2 levels in combination with a high $PaCO_2$ may be associated with conditions that impair respiratory function, such as respiratory muscle weakness or paralysis (as in Guillain-Barré syndrome or myasthenia gravis), respiratory center inhibition (from head injury, brain tumor, or drug abuse), and airway obstruction (possibly from mucus plugs or a tumor). Low readings also may result from bronchiole obstruction associated with asthma or emphysema, from an abnormal ventilation-perfusion ratio resulting from partially blocked alveoli or pulmonary capillaries, or from alveoli that are damaged or filled with fluid because of disease, hemorrhage, or near-drowning.

When inspired air contains insufficient oxygen, PaO_2, O_2CT, and SaO_2 also decrease, but $PaCO_2$ may be normal. Such findings are common in pneumothorax, impaired diffusion between alveoli and blood (such as that caused by interstitial fibrosis), or in an arteriovenous shunt that permits blood to bypass the lungs.

Low O_2CT with normal PaO_2, SaO_2, and possibly $PaCO_2$ may result from severe anemia, decreased blood volume, and reduced oxygen-carrying capacity of hemoglobin.

ACID–BASE DISORDERS

This chart lists the arterial blood gas (ABG) values, possible causes, and clinical effects associated with acid–base disorders.

Disorders and ABG findings	Possible causes	Signs and symptoms
Respiratory acidosis (excess CO_2 retention) pH < 7.35 HCO_3^- > 26 mEq/L (if compensating) $Paco_2$ > 45 mm Hg	■ Central nervous system depression from drugs, injury, or disease ■ Asphyxia ■ Hypoventilation associated with pulmonary, cardiac, musculoskeletal, or neuromuscular disease ■ Obesity ■ Postoperative pain ■ Abdominal distention	■ Diaphoresis, headache, tachycardia, confusion, restlessness, apprehension
Respiratory alkalosis (excess CO_2 excretion) pH > 7.42 HCO_3^- < 22 mEq/L (if compensating) $Paco_2$ < 35 mm Hg	■ Hyperventilation associated with anxiety, pain, or improper ventilator settings ■ Respiratory stimulation due to drugs, disease, hypoxia, fever, or high room temperature ■ Gram-negative bacteremia	■ Rapid, deep respirations; paresthesias; lightheadedness; twitching; anxiety; fear
Metabolic acidosis (HCO_3^- loss, acid retention) pH < 7.35 HCO_3^- < 22 mEq/L $Paco_2$ < 35 mm Hg (if compensating)	■ HCO_3^- depletion caused by renal disease, diarrhea, or small-bowel fistulas ■ Excessive production of organic acids associated with hepatic disease, endocrine disorders (including diabetes mellitus), hypoxia, shock, or drug intoxication ■ Inadequate excretion of acids resulting from renal disease	■ Rapid, deep breathing; fruity breath; fatigue; headache; lethargy; drowsiness; nausea; vomiting; coma (if severe)
Metabolic alkalosis (HCO_3^- retention, acid loss) pH > 7.45 HCO_3^- > 26 mEq/L $Paco_2$ > 45 mm Hg (if compensating)	■ Loss of hydrochloric acid from prolonged vomiting or gastric suctioning ■ Loss of potassium caused by increased renal excretion (as in diuretic therapy) or corticosteroid overdose ■ Excessive alkali ingestion	■ Slow, shallow breathing; hypertonic muscle; restlessness; twitching; confusion; irritability; apathy; tetany; seizures; coma (if severe)

In addition to clarifying blood oxygen disorders, ABG values can provide considerable information about acid–base disorders. (See *Acid–base disorders.*)

Because ABG results represent ventilatory status, abnormal values must be addressed immediately. The patient may require changes in oxygen therapy or mechanical ventilation based on these values.

Posttest care

CLINICAL ALERT Monitor vital signs and observe for signs of circulatory impairment, such as swelling, discoloration, pain, numbness, or tingling in the bandaged arm or leg.

■ Watch for bleeding or hematoma formation at the puncture site.

Interfering factors

■ Bicarbonate, ethacrynic acid, hydrocortisone, metolazone, prednisone, and thiazides may elevate $PaCO_2$. Acetazolamide, methicillin, nitrofurantoin, and tetracycline may decrease $PaCO_2$.

■ Exposing the sample to air affects PaO_2 and $PaCO_2$ and interferes with accurate determination of results.

■ Failure to comply with correct specimen-handling procedures (heparinize the syringe, place the sample in an iced bag, and transport the sample to the laboratory immediately) will adversely affect the test results.

■ Venous blood in the sample may lower PaO_2 and elevate $PaCO_2$.

Arylsulfatase A test, urine

Arylsulfatase A (ARS A), a lysosomal enzyme found in every cell except the mature erythrocyte, is principally active in the liver, the pancreas, and the kidneys, where exogenous substances are detoxified into ester sulfates. When ARS A is present in large amounts, it reverses this process by catalyzing the release of free phenylsulfates, such as benzidine and naphthaline, from the ester sulfates.

Although urine ARS A levels rise in transitional bladder cancer, colorectal cancer, and leukemia, research hasn't resolved whether elevated ARS A levels provoke malignant growths or are simply an enzymatic response to them. This test measures urine ARS A levels by colorimetric or kinetic techniques.

Purpose

To aid diagnosis of bladder, colon, or rectal cancer; myeloid (granulocytic) leukemia; and metachromatic leukodystrophy (an inherited lipid storage disease).

Patient preparation

Explain to the patient that this test measures an enzyme that is present throughout the body. Tell the patient restriction of food or fluids isn't necessary before the test. Explain that the test requires 24-hour urine collection, and provide instruction on how to collect a timed specimen. Test results are generally available in 2 or 3 days.

If a female patient is menstruating, the test may have to be rescheduled because increased numbers of epithelial cells in the urine raise ARS A levels.

Procedure

Collect a 24-hour urine specimen.

Precautions

■ Tell the patient not to contaminate the urine specimen with toilet tissue or stool.

■ Keep the collection container refrigerated or on ice during the collection period, and send the specimen to the laboratory as soon as the collection period is over. If the patient has an indwelling urinary catheter in place, keep the collection bag on ice for the duration of the test; the continuous urinary drainage apparatus should be changed before beginning the test.

Reference values

ARS A values normally range from 1.4 to 19.3 U/L in men, from 1.4 to 11 U/L in women, and over 1 U/L in children.

Implications of results

Elevated ARS A levels may result from bladder, colon, or rectal cancer or from myeloid leukemia. Decreased ARS A levels can result from metachromatic leukodystrophy. In these patients, urine studies show metachromatic granules in the urinary sediment.

Interfering factors

■ Failure to collect all urine during the test period may alter test results.

■ Contamination of the urine specimen by stool or menstrual blood or by improper storage may alter test results.

■ Surgery performed within 1 week before the test may raise ARS A levels.

Aspartate aminotransferase (AST) test, serum

Aspartate aminotransferase (AST) is one of two enzymes that catalyze the conversion of the nitrogenous portion of an amino acid to an amino acid residue. This enzyme is essential to energy production in the Krebs cycle (tricarboxylic acid or citric acid cycle). AST is found in the cytoplasm and mitochondria of many cells, primarily in the liver, heart, skeletal muscles, kidneys, and pancreas and, to a lesser extent, in red blood cells. It's released into serum in proportion to cellular damage.

Although a high correlation exists between myocardial infarction (MI) and elevated AST levels, this test is sometimes considered superfluous for diagnosing MI because of its relatively low organ specificity; it doesn't allow differentiation between acute MI and the effects of hepatic congestion associated with heart failure.

Purpose

■ To aid detection and differential diagnosis of acute hepatic disease
■ To monitor patient progress and prognosis in cardiac and hepatic diseases
■ To aid in diagnosing MI in correlation with creatine kinase and lactate dehydrogenase levels.

Patient preparation

Explain to the patient that this test helps assess heart and liver function. Tell the patient that restriction of food or fluids isn't necessary. Explain that the test usually requires three venipunctures—one at admission and one each day for the next 2 days. Provide reassurance that any discomfort from the needle and the tourniquet will be temporary.

Before the test, withhold morphine, codeine, meperidine, chlorpropamide, methyldopa, phenazopyridine, and antituberculosis drugs (e.g., isoniazid, para-aminosalicylic acid, and pyrazinamide). If any of these medications must be continued, note this on the laboratory request.

Procedure

Perform a venipuncture, and collect the sample in a 7-ml clot-activator tube.

Precautions

■ To avoid missing peak AST levels, draw serum samples at the same time each day.
■ Handle the collection tube gently to prevent hemolysis, and send the sample to the laboratory immediately.

Reference values

AST levels range from 8 to 20 U/L in males and from 5 to 40 U/L in females. Values for children are typically higher.

Implications of results

AST levels fluctuate in response to the extent of cellular necrosis and therefore may be transiently and minimally elevated early in the disease process and extremely elevated during the most acute phase. Depending on when during the course of the disease the initial sample was drawn, AST levels can rise, indicating increasing disease severity and tissue damage, or fall, indicating disease resolution and tissue repair. Thus, the relative change in AST values serves as a reliable monitoring mechanism.

Very high AST levels (more than 20 times normal) may indicate acute viral hepatitis, severe skeletal muscle trauma, extensive surgery, drug-induced hepatic injury, or severe passive liver congestion. Notify the doctor for further investigation of these results.

High levels (ranging from 10 to 20 times normal) may indicate severe MI, severe infectious mononucleosis, or alcoholic cirrhosis. They also occur during the prodromal or resolving stages of conditions listed above that cause very high elevations.

Moderate to high levels (ranging from 5 to 10 times normal) may indicate Duchenne muscular dystrophy, dermatomyositis, or chronic hepatitis. They also occur during prodromal and resolving stages of diseases that cause high elevations.

Low to moderate levels (ranging from two to five times normal) may indicate hemolytic anemia, metastatic hepatic tumors, acute pancreatitis, pulmonary emboli, delirium tremens, or fatty liver. AST levels also rise slightly after the first few days of biliary duct obstruction.

Posttest care

- If a hematoma develops at the venipuncture site, apply warm soaks.
- Resume medications discontinued before the test.

Interfering factors

- Chlorpropamide, opiates, methyldopa, erythromycin, sulfonamides, pyridoxine, dicumarol, and antituberculosis agents; large doses of acetaminophen, salicylates, or vitamin A; and many other drugs known to affect the liver cause elevated AST levels.
- Strenuous exercise and muscle trauma associated with I.M. injections raise AST levels.
- Hemolysis caused by rough handling of the sample may affect test results.
- Failure to draw the sample as scheduled, thus missing peak AST levels, may interfere with accurate determination of test results.

Atrial natriuretic factor test, plasma

This radioimmunoassay measures the plasma level of atrial natriuretic factor (ANF), a vasoactive and natriuretic hormone that is secreted from the heart when expansion of blood volume stretches atrial tissue. An extremely potent natriuretic agent and vasodilator, ANF (also known as atrial natriuretic hormone, atrionatriuretic peptide, and atriopeptin) rapidly produces diuresis and increases the glomerular filtration rate.

The role of ANF in regulating extracellular fluid volume, blood pressure, and sodium metabolism appears critical. It promotes sodium excretion, inhibits the renin-angiotensin system's effect on aldosterone secretion, and decreases atrial pressure by decreasing venous return, thereby reducing blood pressure and volume.

Researchers have found that patients with overt heart failure (HF) have highly elevated ANF levels. Patients with cardiovascular disease and elevated cardiac filling pressure, but without HF, also have markedly elevated ANF levels. Recent findings support ANF as a possible marker for early asymptomatic left ventricular dysfunction and increased cardiac volume.

Purpose

- To confirm HF
- To identify asymptomatic cardiac volume overload.

Patient preparation

As appropriate, explain the purpose of the test to the patient. Inform him that he must fast before the test. Explain that this test requires a blood sample, discuss who will perform the venipuncture and when, and note that transient discomfort may be felt from the needle puncture. Tell the patient that the laboratory may take up to 4 days for analysis.

Check the patient history for use of medications that can influence test results. Withhold beta blockers, calcium antagonists, diuretics, vasodilators, and digitalis glycosides for 24 hours before sample collection.

Procedure

Perform a venipuncture, and collect the sample in a prechilled potassium–ethylenediaminetetraacetic acid (EDTA) tube. After chilled centrifugation, the EDTA plasma should be promptly frozen and sent to the laboratory to be analyzed.

Precautions

- Handle the specimen gently to prevent hemolysis.
- Place the specimen on ice, and send it to the laboratory immediately.

Reference values

ANF levels normally range from 20 to 77 pg/ml.

Implications of results

Markedly elevated ANF levels are found in patients with frank HF and significantly elevated cardiac filling pressure. Notify the doctor for further investigation of these results.

Posttest care

- If a hematoma develops at the venipuncture site, apply warm soaks.
- The patient may resume his normal diet and any medications discontinued before the test.

Interfering factors

Cardiovascular drugs, including beta blockers, calcium antagonists, diuretics, vasodilators, and cardiac glycosides, interfere with test results.

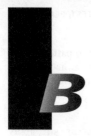

Bacterial meningitis antigen test

This test, usually performed by latex agglutination, can detect specific antigens of *Streptococcus pneumoniae*, *Neisseria meningitidis*, and *Haemophilus influenzae* type b, the principal etiologic agents in meningitis. This test can be performed on samples of serum, cerebrospinal fluid (CSF), urine, pleural fluid, or joint fluid; however, the preferred specimen is CSF or urine.

Purpose

- To identify the etiologic agent in meningitis
- To aid diagnosis of bacterial meningitis
- To aid diagnosis of meningitis when the Gram-stained smear and culture are negative.

Patient preparation

Explain the purpose of the test, and inform the patient that a urine or CSF specimen is required. If a CSF specimen is needed, describe how it will be obtained. Explain who will perform the procedure and when and that transient discomfort may be felt from the needle puncture. Advise the patient that a headache is the most common adverse effect of lumbar puncture but that cooperation during the test minimizes this effect. Make sure the patient or a family member has signed a consent form.

Procedure

As required, a 10-ml urine specimen or a 1-ml CSF specimen is collected in a sterile container.

Precautions

- Maintain specimen sterility during collection.
- Wear gloves when obtaining or handling all specimens.
- Make sure all caps are tightly fastened on specimen containers.
- Promptly send the specimen to the laboratory on a refrigerated coolant.

Normal findings

Results should be negative for bacterial antigens.

Implications of results

Positive results identify the specific bacterial antigen: *S. pneumoniae, N. meningitidis, H. influenzae* type b, or group B streptococci in infants younger than 3 months.

Interfering factors

■ Results may be influenced by previous antimicrobial therapy.

■ Failure to maintain sterility during collection of the specimen can interfere with accurate test results.

Bence Jones protein test, urine

Bence Jones proteins are abnormal light-chain immunoglobulins of low molecular weight that are derived from the clone of a single plasma cell (monoclonal). This globulin appears in the urine of 50% to 80% of patients with multiple myeloma and in most patients with Waldenström's macroglobulinemia. It can also be seen in amyloidosis and adult Fanconi's syndrome.

In most cases, these proteins—thought to be synthesized by malignant plasma cells in the bone marrow— are rapidly cleared from the plasma and don't usually appear in serum. When these proteins exceed renal tubular capacity to break down and reabsorb them, they overflow and are excreted in the urine (overflow proteinuria). Eventually, the renal tubular cells degenerate from the effort of reabsorbing excess amounts of protein. Consequently, protein precipitates and inclusions occur in the renal tubular cells. If renal failure results from such precipitation or from hypercalcemia, increased uric acid, or infiltration by abnormal plasma cells, more Bence Jones proteins and other proteins then appear in the urine because the dysfunctional nephrons no longer control protein excretion.

Urine screening tests, such as thermal coagulation and Bradshaw's test, can detect Bence Jones proteins, but urine immunoelectrophoresis is usually the method of choice for quantitative studies. Serum immunoelectrophoresis, which is sometimes used, is less sensitive than the urine tests. Nevertheless, both urine and serum studies are frequently used for patients suspected of having multiple myeloma.

Purpose

To confirm the presence of multiple myeloma in patients with characteristic clinical signs, such as bone pain (especially in the back and thorax) and persistent anemia and fatigue.

Patient preparation

Explain to the patient that this test can detect an abnormal protein in the urine. Explain that the test requires an early-morning urine specimen, and provide instruction on how to collect a clean-catch specimen.

Procedure

Collect an early-morning urine specimen of at least 50 ml.

Precautions

■ Tell the patient not to contaminate the urine specimen with toilet tissue or stool.
■ Send the specimen to the laboratory immediately. If transport is delayed, refrigerate the specimen.

Normal findings

Urine should contain no Bence Jones proteins.

Implications of results

The presence of Bence Jones proteins in urine suggests multiple myeloma or Waldenström's macroglobulinemia. Very low levels in the absence of other symptoms may result from benign monoclonal gammopathy. However, clinical evidence figures prominently in diagnosis of multiple myeloma.

Interfering factors

■ False-positive results may occur in connective tissue disease, renal insufficiency, and certain cancers.
■ Contamination of the specimen with menstrual blood, prostatic secretions, or semen may cause false-positive results.
■ Failure to send the specimen to the laboratory immediately or to keep the specimen refrigerated may produce a false-positive result because heat-coagulable protein denatures or decomposes at room temperature.

Beta-hydroxybutyrate test, serum

A quantitative colorimetric assay, this test measures levels of beta-hydroxybutyrate, which is one of three ketone bodies; the other two are acetoacetate and acetone. At 78%, the relative proportion in the blood is greater than acetoacetate (20%) or acetone (2%).

A small amount of acetoacetate and beta-hydroxybutyrate is formed during the normal hepatic metabolism of free fatty acids and is then metabolized in the peripheral tissues. In some conditions, increased acetoacetate production may exceed the metabolic capacity of the peripheral tissues. As acetoacetate accumulates in the blood, a small portion is converted to acetone by sponta-

---

VON GIERKE'S DISEASE

Glycogen storage diseases, such as Von Gierke's disease, alter the synthesis or degradation of glycogen, the form in which glucose is stored in the body.

Von Gierke's disease, a type I glycogen storage disease, is caused by a deficiency of glucose-6-phosphate dehydrogenase. It affects the liver and kidneys, causing hepatomegaly, hypoglycemia, hyperuricemia, xanthomas, bleeding, and adiposity.

This type I glycogen storage disease is transmitted as an autosomal recessive trait. Two types, types Ia and Ib, exist. Type Ib (pseudo type I) is similar to but more severe than type Ia, although patients with this disease may live well into adulthood.

Laboratory studies of plasma demonstrate low glucose levels but high levels of free fatty acids, triglycerides, cholesterol, and uric acid in type Ia disease. Serum analysis reveals elevated pyruvic acid and lactic acid levels.

---

neous decarboxylation. The remaining and greater portion of acetoacetate is converted to beta-hydroxybutyrate. This accumulation of all three ketone bodies is referred to as ketosis: Excessive formation of ketone bodies in the blood is called ketonemia.

Purpose

- To diagnose carbohydrate deprivation, which may result from starvation, digestive disturbances, dietary imbalances, or frequent vomiting
- To aid diagnosis of diabetes mellitus resulting from decreased use of carbohydrates
- To aid diagnosis of glycogen storage diseases, specifically Von Gierke's disease (See *Von Gierke's disease.*)
- To diagnose or monitor the treatment of metabolic acidosis, such as diabetic ketoacidosis or lactic acidosis.

Patient preparation

Explain to the patient that this test evaluates ketones in the blood and fasting isn't necessary. Explain that the test requires a blood sample, discuss who will perform the venipuncture and when, and tell the patient that transient discomfort may be felt from the needle puncture and the pressure of the tourniquet.

Procedure

Perform a venipuncture, and collect the sample in a 5-ml clot-activator tube. Centrifuge and remove the serum. If an acetone level is requested, have this analysis performed first. Serum beta-hydroxybutyrate remains stable for at least 1 week at 25.6° F to 46.4° F (2° C to 8° C). Plasma may also be used for analysis of beta-hydroxybutyrate.

Precautions

Send the specimen to the laboratory immediately.

Reference values

The normal value for serum or plasma beta-hydroxybutyrate levels is less than 0.4 mmol/L.

Implications of results

The determination of ketone bodies in the blood, more so than in the urine, is extremely helpful in treating ketosis associated with diabetes and other conditions. Because it possesses greater concentration and stability than acetoacetate and acetone, beta-hydroxybutyrate has become an extremely reliable guide in monitoring the effect of insulin therapy during treatment of diabetic ketoacidosis. This test is also helpful during emergency management of hypoglycemia, acidosis, alcohol ingestion, or an unexplained increase in the anion gap.

Notify the patient's doctor immediately if values exceed 2 mmol/L.

Posttest care

If a hematoma develops at the venipuncture site, apply warm soaks.

Interfering factors

- If the patient has fasted, values will increase with increased fasting time.
- Heparin doesn't appear to interfere with the reaction.
- The presence of both lactate dehydrogenase (at high concentrations) and lactic acid (at concentrations greater than 10 mmol/L) may elevate beta-hydroxybutyrate levels by at least 0.2 mmol/L, thereby altering test results.
- Sodium fluoride at concentrations greater than 2.5 nmol/L appears to lower the levels of beta-hydroxybutyrate by at least 0.1 mmol/L.
- Hemolysis, jaundice, or lipemia has little or no effect on results.

Bilirubin test, serum

This test measures serum levels of bilirubin, the main pigment in bile. Bilirubin is the major product of hemoglobin catabolism. After being formed in the reticuloendothelial cells, bilirubin is bound to albumin and transported to the liver, where it's conjugated with glucuronide by the enzymatic action of glucuronyl transferase. The resulting compound, bilirubin diglucuronide, is then excreted in bile.

The conjugated bilirubin is transported to the small intestine, where it's converted to urobilinogen. Part of the urobilinogen is excreted in the feces, and the remainder is returned to the liver where it's removed from the blood. Traces of urobilinogen that aren't removed from the blood by the liver are carried to the kidneys and excreted in the urine.

Effective bilirubin conjugation and excretion depend on a properly functioning hepatobiliary system and a normal red blood cell (RBC) turnover rate. Therefore, measurement of unconjugated (indirect or prehepatic) bilirubin and conjugated (direct or posthepatic) bilirubin can help evaluate hepatobiliary and erythropoietic function. Serum bilirubin values are especially significant in neonates because excessive unconjugated bilirubin can accumulate in the brain, causing irreparable damage.

Purpose

- To evaluate liver function
- To aid differential diagnosis of jaundice and to monitor its progression
- To aid diagnosis of biliary obstruction and hemolytic anemia
- To determine whether a neonate requires an exchange transfusion or phototherapy because of dangerously high unconjugated bilirubin levels.

Patient preparation

Explain that this test evaluates liver function and the condition of RBCs. If the patient is a neonate, tell the parents why the test is important. Inform the adult patient that restriction of fluids isn't necessary but that he should fast at least 4 hours before the test. Fasting isn't necessary for neonates. Tell the patient that this test requires a blood sample, discuss who will perform the venipuncture and when, and note that discomfort may be felt from the needle puncture and the tourniquet. Tell the parents of an infant that a small amount of blood will be drawn from the infant's heel, and tell them who will perform the heelstick and when. Check the patient's medication history for use of drugs that are known to interfere with serum bilirubin levels.

Procedure

- If the patient is an adult, perform a venipuncture, and collect the sample in a 7-ml clot-activator tube.
- If the patient is an infant, perform a heelstick and fill the microcapillary tube to the designated level with blood.
- If a hematoma develops at the venipuncture or heelstick site, apply warm soaks.

Precautions

- Protect the sample from strong sunlight and ultraviolet light because bilirubin breaks down when exposed to light.
- Handle the sample gently, and send it to the laboratory immediately.

Reference values

In adults, indirect serum bilirubin measures 1.1 mg/dl or less; direct serum bilirubin, less than 0.5 mg/dl. In neonates, total serum bilirubin measures 1 to 12 mg/dl.

Implications of results

Elevated indirect serum bilirubin levels often indicate hepatic damage in which the parenchymal cells can no longer conjugate bilirubin with glucuronide. Consequently, indirect bilirubin re-enters the bloodstream. High levels of indirect bilirubin are also common in patients with severe hemolytic anemia, when excessive indirect bilirubin overwhelms the liver's conjugating mechanism. If hemolysis continues, both direct and indirect bilirubin may rise. Other causes of elevated indirect bilirubin levels include congenital enzyme deficiency, such as Gilbert's disease and Crigler-Najjar syndrome.

Elevated direct serum bilirubin levels usually indicate biliary obstruction, in which direct bilirubin, blocked from its normal pathway from the liver into the biliary tree, overflows into the bloodstream. If the obstruction continues, both direct and indirect bilirubin eventually may be elevated because of hepatic damage. In severe chronic hepatic damage, direct bilirubin concentrations may return to normal or near-normal levels, but elevated indirect bilirubin levels persist.

Elevated blood bilirubin levels result in a condition known as jaundice, or icterus, characterized by a yellow discoloration of the skin, sclera, and mucous membranes; dry, itchy skin; dark urine; and light- or clay-colored stools. Jaundice is classified as hemolytic (prehepatic), hepatocellular (hepatic), or obstructive (intrahepatic or extrahepatic). In neonates, physiologic jaundice is caused by a combination of the breakdown of fetal red blood cells and the limited conjugation and excretion of bilirubin by the liver. This condition is common, especially in preterm infants. Serum levels can rise to 5 mg/dl/24 hours, peaking between the 2nd and 4th day of life and decreasing thereafter.

In neonates, total bilirubin levels that reach or exceed 18 mg/dl indicate the need for an exchange transfusion.

Notify the doctor immediately of the results so prompt action can be taken.

Posttest care

If a hematoma develops at the venipuncture site, apply warm soaks.

Interfering factors

■ Exposure of the sample to direct sunlight or ultraviolet light may depress bilirubin levels.
■ Hemolysis caused by rough handling of the sample may alter test results.

Bilirubin test, urine

This screening test, based on a color reaction with a specific reagent, detects abnormally high urine levels of direct (conjugated) bilirubin. The reticuloendothelial system produces the pigment bilirubin from hemoglobin breakdown. Bilirubin then combines with albumin, a plasma protein, and is transported to the liver as indirect (unconjugated) bilirubin.

In the liver, most indirect bilirubin joins with glucuronic acid to form bilirubin glucuronide and bilirubin diglucuronide — water-soluble compounds almost totally excreted into the bile. In the intestine, bacterial action converts direct bilirubin to urobilinogen. Normally, only a small amount of direct bilirubin — unbound or bound to albumin — returns to plasma. The kidneys filter the unbound portion, which may appear in trace amounts in the urine. Fat-soluble indirect bilirubin can't be filtered by the glomeruli and is never present in urine. Bilirubin in the urine may indicate liver disease caused by infections, biliary disease, or hepatotoxicity.

When combined with urobilinogen measurements, this test helps identify disorders that can cause jaundice. The analysis can be performed at bedside, using a bilirubin reagent strip, or in the laboratory. Highly sensitive spectrophotometric assays may be needed to detect trace amounts of urine bilirubin. This screening test doesn't detect such minute amounts.

Purpose

To help identify the cause of jaundice.

Patient preparation

Explain to the patient that this test helps determine the cause of jaundice. Explain that restriction of food or fluids isn't necessary before the test. Explain that the test requires a random urine specimen, and tell the patient whether the specimen will be tested at bedside or in the laboratory. Bedside analysis can be performed immediately; laboratory analysis is completed in 1 day.

Procedure

Collect a random urine specimen in the container provided. For bedside analysis, use one of the following procedures:

■ *Dipstrip*: Dip the reagent strip into the specimen, and remove it immediately. After 20 seconds, compare the strip color with the color standards. Record the test results on the patient's chart.

■ *Ictotest*: This test is easier to read and more sensitive than the dipstrip method. Place five drops of urine on the asbestos-cellulose test mat. If bilirubin is present, it will be absorbed into the mat. Next, put a reagent tablet on the wet area of the mat, and place two drops of water on the tablet. If bilirubin is present, a blue to purple coloration will develop on the mat. Pink or red indicates that no bilirubin is present — a negative test.

Precautions

■ Use only a freshly voided specimen. Bilirubin disintegrates after 30 minutes of exposure to room temperature or light.

■ If the specimen is to be analyzed in the laboratory, send it to the laboratory immediately. Record the time of collection on the patient's chart.

■ If the specimen is tested at bedside, make sure 20 seconds elapse before interpreting the color change on the dipstrip. Also make sure lighting is adequate when determining the color.

Normal findings

Normally, bilirubin isn't found in urine in a routine screening test.

Implications of results

High levels of direct bilirubin in urine may be evident from the specimen's appearance (dark, with a yellow foam). To diagnose jaundice, however, the presence or absence of direct bilirubin in urine must be correlated with serum test results and with urine and fecal urobilinogen levels. (See *Comparing bilirubin and urobilinogen values.*)

Interfering factors

■ Phenazopyridine and phenothiazine derivatives, such as chlorpromazine and acetophenazine maleate, can cause false-positive results.

■ Dipstrip testing, such as with Chemstrip or N-Multistix, is affected by large amounts of ascorbic acid and ni-

COMPARING BILIRUBIN AND UROBILINOGEN VALUES

Two types of hyperbilirubinemia, unconjugated (indirect) and conjugated (direct), are associated with jaundice. Patients with unconjugated hyperbilirubinemia have an excess of unconjugated serum bilirubin, which normally makes up more than 80% of total serum bilirubin. Because unconjugated bilirubin is bound to albumin, it isn't water-soluble and is thus absent from urine. Conversely, patients with conjugated hyperbilirubinemia have an excess of conjugated serum bilirubin. Because conjugated bilirubin is protein-free, it can be filtered by the glomeruli and appears in urine.

To aid differential diagnosis of jaundice, urobilinogen assays are used to further distinguish the various hyperbilirubinemias. Normally, only trace amounts (1 to 4 mg daily) of this colorless compound, which is converted from conjugated bilirubin by intestinal bacteria, are reabsorbed into the bloodstream and excreted in urine. The rest (50 to 250 mg daily) is eliminated in feces. Because fecal urobilinogen measurements vary, an increase generally refers to levels above 250 mg daily; a decrease refers to levels below 5 mg daily.

This chart shows the changes in bilirubin and urobilinogen levels associated with both types of hyperbilirubinemia.

Causes of jaundice	Serum		Urine		Feces
	Indirect bilirubin	Direct bilirubin	Bilirubin	Urobilinogen	Urobilinogen
Unconjugated hyperbilirubinemia					
Hemolytic disorders (hemolytic anemia, erythroblastosis fetalis)	Increased	Normal	Absent	May be increased	Increased
Gilbert's disease (constitutional hepatic dysfunction)	Moderately increased	Normal	Absent	Normal or decreased	Normal or decreased
Crigler-Najjar syndrome (congenital hyperbilirubinemia)	Markedly increased	Normal	Absent	Normal or decreased	Normal or decreased
Conjugated hyperbilirubinemia					
Extrahepatic obstruction (calculi, tumor, scar tissue in common bile duct or hepatic excretory duct)	Normal	Increased	Present	Decreased or absent	Decreased or absent
Hepatocellular disorders (viral, toxic, alcoholic hepatitis; cirrhosis; parenchymal injury)	Increased	Increased	Present	Variable	Normal or decreased
Hepatocanalicular disorders or intrahepatic obstruction (drug-induced cholestasis; some familial defects, such as Dubin-Johnson and Rotor's syndromes; viral hepatitis; primary biliary cirrhosis)	Increased	Increased	Present	Variable	Normal or decreased

trite, which may lower bilirubin levels and cause false-negative test results.

■ Exposure of the specimen to room temperature or light can lower bilirubin levels because of bilirubin degradation.

Bleeding time test

This test measures the duration of bleeding after a standardized skin incision. Bleeding time depends on the elasticity of the blood vessel wall and on the number and functional capacity of platelets. Although this test is usually performed on patients with a personal or family history of bleeding disorders, it's also useful for preoperative screening, along with a platelet count.

Bleeding time may be measured by one of three methods: Duke, Ivy, or template. The template method is used most frequently and is the most accurate because it standardizes the incision size, making test results reproducible.

This test usually isn't recommended for a patient whose platelet count is less than 75,000/µl. However, some patients with altered platelet morphology may have normal bleeding times despite low platelet counts.

Purpose

■ To assess overall hemostatic function (platelet response to injury and functional capacity of vasoconstriction)
■ To detect congenital and acquired platelet function disorders.

Patient preparation

Explain to the patient that this test measures the time required to form a clot and stop bleeding. Tell the patient who will perform the test and when. Inform the patient that restriction of food or fluids isn't necessary before the test. Tell the patient that some discomfort may be felt from the incisions, the antiseptic, and the tightness of the blood pressure cuff. Also inform the patient that, depending on the method used, incisions or punctures may leave tiny scars that should be barely visible when healed.

Check the patient history for recent ingestion of drugs that prolong bleeding time. If the patient has taken such drugs, check with the laboratory for special instructions. If the test is being used to identify a suspected bleeding disorder, it should be postponed and the drugs discontinued; if it's being used preoperatively to assess hemostatic function, it should proceed as scheduled.

Equipment

Blood pressure cuff ■ disposable lancet ■ template with 9-mm slits (template method) ■ 70% alcohol or povidone-iodine solution ■ filter paper ■ small pressure bandage ■ stopwatch.

Procedure

■ Template method: Wrap the pressure cuff around the upper arm, and inflate the cuff to 40 mm Hg. Select an area on the forearm free of superficial veins, and clean it with antiseptic. Allow the skin to dry completely before making the incision. Apply the appropriate template lengthwise to the forearm. Use the lancet to make two incisions, each being 1 mm deep and 9 mm long. Start the stopwatch. Without touching the cuts, gently blot the drops of blood with filter paper every 30 seconds until the bleeding stops in both cuts. Average the time of the two cuts, and record the results.

■ Ivy method: After applying the pressure cuff and preparing the test site, make three small punctures with a disposable lancet. Start the stopwatch immediately. Taking care not to touch the punctures, blot each site with filter paper every 30 seconds until the bleeding stops. Average the bleeding time of the three punctures, and record the result.

■ Duke method: Drape the patient's shoulder with a towel. Clean the earlobe, and let the skin air-dry. Then make a puncture wound 2 to 4 mm deep on the earlobe with a disposable lancet. Start the stopwatch. Being careful not to touch the ear, blot the site with filter paper every 30 seconds until bleeding stops. Record bleeding time.

■ For a patient with a bleeding tendency (such as hemophilia), maintain a pressure bandage over the incision for 24 to 48 hours to prevent further bleeding. If the template method was used, keep the edges of the cuts aligned to minimize scarring. Otherwise, a piece of gauze held in place by an adhesive bandage is sufficient. Check the test area frequently.

Precautions

■ Maintain a pressure of 40 mm Hg throughout the test.
■ If the bleeding doesn't diminish after 15 minutes, discontinue the test.

Reference values

The normal bleeding time is 3 to 6 minutes for the template method, 3 to 6 minutes for the Ivy method, and 1 to 3 minutes for the Duke method.

Implications of results

Prolonged bleeding time may indicate the presence of many disorders associated with thrombocytopenia, such as Hodgkin's disease, acute leukemia, disseminated intravascular coagulation, hemolytic disease of the newborn, Schönlein-Henoch purpura, severe hepatic disease (such as cirrhosis), or severe deficiency of factors I, II, V, VII, VIII, IX, or XI. Prolonged bleeding time in a person with a normal platelet count suggests a platelet function disorder (thrombasthenia or thrombocytopathia) and requires further investigation with clot retraction, prothrombin consumption, and platelet aggregation tests.

Posttest care

Resume administration of medications discontinued before the test.

Interfering factors

Sulfonamides, thiazide diuretics, antineoplastics, anticoagulants, nonsteroidal anti-inflammatory drugs, aspirin and aspirin compounds, and some nonnarcotic analgesics may prolong bleeding times.

Blood culture

A blood culture is performed by inoculating a culture medium with a blood sample and incubating it for isolation and identification of the causative pathogens in bacteremia (bacterial invasion of the bloodstream) and septicemia (systemic spread of such infection). Blood culture can identify about 67% of pathogens within 24 hours and up to 90% within 72 hours.

Bacteria from local tissue infection usually invade the bloodstream through the lymphatic system by way of the thoracic duct. Occasionally, they enter the bloodstream directly through infusion lines or thrombophlebitis or as bacterial endocarditis from prosthetic heart valve replacements.

Bacteremia may be transient, intermittent, or continuous. The timing of specimen collection for blood cultures varies; it usually depends on the type of bacteremia (intermittent or continuous) suspected and on whether drug therapy needs to be started regardless of test results.

Purpose

■ To confirm bacteremia
■ To identify the causative organism in bacteremia and septicemia.

Patient preparation

Explain to the patient that this procedure may identify the organism causing his symptoms. Inform the patient that restriction of food or fluids isn't necessary before the test. Tell the patient how many samples the test will require, explain who will perform the venipunctures and when, and note that transient discomfort may be felt from the needle punctures and the pressure of the tourniquet.

Equipment

Gloves ■ tourniquet ■ small adhesive bandages ■ alcohol swabs ■ povidone-iodine swabs ■ 10- to 20-ml syringe for an adult, 6-ml syringe for a child ■ three or four sterile needles ■ two blood culture bottles, one vented (aerobic) and one unvented (anaerobic), with nutritionally enriched broths and sodium polyethanol sulfonate added, or bottles with resin, or a lysis-centrifugation tube.

Procedure

■ Put on gloves. After cleaning the venipuncture site with an alcohol swab, clean it again with a povidone-iodine swab, starting at the site and working outward in a circular motion. Wait at least 1 minute for the skin to dry; then remove the residual iodine with an alcohol swab. Alternatively, iodine can be removed after the venipuncture. Apply the tourniquet.

■ Perform a venipuncture; draw 10 to 20 ml of blood for an adult or 2 to 6 ml for a child. Clean the diaphragm tops of the culture bottles with alcohol or iodine, and change the needle on the syringe. If broth is being used, add blood to each bottle until a 1:5 or 1:10 dilution is achieved. For example, add 10 ml of blood to a 100-ml bottle. Note that the size of the bottle may vary depending on hospital protocol. If a special resin is being used, such as Bactec resin medium or Antimicrobial Removal Device, add blood to the resin in the bottles and invert gently to mix. Draw the blood directly into a special collection-processing tube if the lysis-centrifugation technique (Isolator) is being used. Next, indicate the tentative diagnosis on the laboratory request, and note any current or recent antimicrobial therapy. Whenever possible, blood cultures should be collected prior to administration of antimicrobial agents.

Precautions

■ Use gloves when performing the procedure and handling the specimens.

■ Send each sample to the laboratory immediately after collection.

Normal findings

Blood cultures normally contain no pathogens.

Implications of results

Positive blood cultures don't necessarily confirm pathologic septicemia. Mild, transient bacteremia may occur during the course of many infectious diseases or may complicate other disorders. Persistent, continuous, or recurrent bacteremia reliably confirms the presence of serious infection. To detect most causative agents, blood cultures are ideally performed on 2 consecutive days.

Isolation of most organisms takes about 72 hours; however, for negative specimens, reports should be made at 24 hours, 48 hours, and 1 week of incubation. Negative reports for some suspected infections, such as Brucella infection, are held for about 4 weeks.

Common blood pathogens include *Neisseria meningitidis*, *Streptococcus pneumoniae* and other *Streptococcus* species, *Haemophilus influenzae*, *Staphylococcus aureus*, *Pseudomonas aeruginosa*, *Brucella*, and organisms classified as Bacteroidaceae and Enterobacteriaceae. Although 2% to 3% of cultured blood samples are contaminated by skin bacteria, such as *S. epidermidis*, diphtheroids, and *Propionibacterium*, these organisms may be clinically significant when isolated from multiple cultures or from immunocompromised patients.

Debilitated or immunocompromised patients may have isolates of *Candida albicans*. In patients with human immunodeficiency virus infection, *Mycobacterium tuberculosis* and *M. avium* complex may be isolated as well as other *Mycobacterium* species on a less frequent basis.

Posttest care

If a hematoma develops at the venipuncture site, apply warm soaks.

Interfering factors

■ Previous or current antimicrobial therapy may give false-negative results.

■ Improper collection technique may contaminate the sample.

■ Removal of culture bottle caps at bedside may prevent anaerobic growth; use of incorrect bottle and media may prevent aerobic growth.

Blood urea nitrogen (BUN) test

This test measures the nitrogen fraction of urea, the chief end product of protein metabolism. Formed in the liver from ammonia and excreted by the kidneys, urea constitutes 40% to 50% of the blood's nonprotein nitrogen. Because the level of reabsorption of urea in the renal tubules is directly related to the rate of urine flow through the kidneys, the blood urea nitrogen (BUN) is a less reliable indicator of uremia than the serum creatine level. Photometry is a commonly used test method.

Purpose

■ To evaluate renal function and aid diagnosis of renal disease
■ To aid assessment of hydration.

Patient preparation

Tell the patient that this test evaluates kidney function. Inform the patient that restriction of food or fluids isn't necessary but a diet high in meat should be avoided. Explain that the test requires a blood sample, tell the patient who will perform the venipuncture and when, and explain that some discomfort may be felt from the needle puncture and the pressure of the tourniquet. Check the patient's medication history for drugs that may influence BUN levels.

Procedure

■ Perform a venipuncture, and collect the sample in a 7-ml clot-activator tube.
■ If a hematoma develops at the venipuncture site, apply warm soaks.

Precautions

Handle the sample gently to prevent hemolysis.

Reference values

BUN values normally range from 8 to 20 mg/dl, with slightly higher values in elderly patients.

Implications of results

Elevated BUN levels occur in renal disease, reduced renal blood flow (as with dehydration), urinary tract obstruction, and increased protein catabolism (as occurs in burns).

Depressed BUN levels occur in severe hepatic damage, malnutrition, and overhydration.

Posttest care

If a hematoma develops at the venipuncture site, apply warm soaks.

Interfering factors

■ Chloramphenicol can depress BUN levels.
■ Nephrotoxic drugs, such as aminoglycosides, amphotericin B, and methicillin, can elevate BUN levels.

■ Hemolysis caused by rough handling of the sample may affect test results.

Bone biopsy

Bone biopsy is the removal of a piece or a core of bone for histologic examination. It's performed either by using a special drill needle under local anesthesia or by surgical excision under general anesthesia. Bone biopsy is indicated in patients with bone pain and tenderness after a bone scan, a computed tomography scan, radiographs, or arteriography reveals a mass or deformity. Excision provides a larger specimen than drill biopsy and permits immediate surgical treatment if rapid histologic analysis of the specimen reveals a malignant tumor. In the presence of tumors, bone bows slightly, thickens, and sometimes fractures — the result of increased osteoblastic or osteoclastic activity, or both.

Possible complications of bone biopsy include bone fracture, damage to surrounding tissue, and infection (osteomyelitis).

Purpose

To distinguish between benign and malignant bone tumors.

Patient preparation

Describe the procedure to the patient, and answer any questions. Explain that this test permits microscopic examination of a bone specimen. If the patient is to have a drill biopsy, inform him that restriction of food or fluids isn't necessary. If the patient is to have an open biopsy, instruct him to fast overnight before the test. Explain who will perform the biopsy, where it will be done, and that it should take no longer than 30 minutes.

Tell the patient that he'll receive a local anesthetic but will still experience discomfort and pressure when the biopsy needle enters the bone. Explain that a special drill forces the needle into the bone; if possible, show him a photograph of the bone drill to make the biopsy seem less ominous. Stress the importance of his cooperation during the biopsy.

Make sure the patient has signed a consent form; if the patient is a minor, ask a responsible parent or guardian to do so. Check the patient history for hypersensitivity to the local anesthetic.

Procedure

■ *Drill biopsy*: Position the patient properly, and shave and prepare the biopsy site. After the local anesthetic is injected, the doctor makes a small incision (usually about 3 mm) and pushes the biopsy needle with pointed trocar into the bone, using firm, even pressure. After the needle is engaged in the bone, it's rotated about 180 degrees while steady pressure is maintained. When the bone core is obtained, the trocar is withdrawn by reversing the drilling motion, and the specimen is placed in a properly labeled bottle containing 10% formalin solution. Apply pressure to the site with a sterile gauze pad. When bleeding stops, remove the gauze and apply a topical antiseptic (povidone-iodine ointment) and an adhesive bandage or other sterile covering to close the wound and prevent infection.

■ *Open biopsy*: After the patient is anesthetized, shave the biopsy site, clean it with surgical soap, and then disinfect it with an iodine wash and alcohol. The doctor makes an incision, removes a piece of bone, and sends it to the histology laboratory immediately for analysis. Further surgery can then be performed, depending on bone specimen findings.

■ Check vital signs and the dressing at the biopsy site. Ask the doctor how much drainage is expected, and notify him if drainage is excessive.

■ If the patient experiences pain at the biopsy site, administer an analgesic.

Precautions

■ Bone biopsy should be performed cautiously in patients with coagulopathy.

■ Send the specimen to the laboratory immediately.

Normal findings

Bone tissue consists of fibers of collagen, osteocytes, and osteoblasts. It can be classified as one of two histologic types: compact or cancellous. Compact bone has dense, concentric layers of mineral deposits, or lamellae. Cancellous bone has widely spaced lamellae, with osteocytes and red and yellow marrow lying between them.

Implications of results

Histologic examination of a bone specimen can reveal benign or malignant tumors. Benign tumors, generally well circumscribed and nonmetastasizing, include osteoid osteoma, osteoblastoma, osteochondroma, unicameral bone cyst, benign giant cell tumor, and fibroma.

Malignant tumors spread irregularly and rapidly. The most common types are multiple myeloma and osteosarcoma; the most lethal is Ewing's sarcoma. Most malignant tumors metastasize to bone through the blood and lymph systems from the breast, lungs, prostate, thyroid, or kidneys.

Posttest care

CLINICAL ALERT For several days after the biopsy, watch for indications of bone infection: fever, headache, pain on movement, and tissue redness or abscess at or near the biopsy site. Notify the doctor if these symptoms develop.

■ Advise the patient that a usual diet may be resumed.

Interfering factors

Failure to obtain a representative bone specimen, to use the proper fixative, or to send the specimen to the laboratory immediately may alter test results.

Bone marrow aspiration and biopsy

Bone marrow, the soft tissue contained in the medullary canals of long bone and in the interstices of cancellous bone, may be removed by aspiration or needle biopsy under local anesthesia. In aspiration biopsy, a fluid specimen in which pustulae of marrow are suspended is removed from the bone marrow. In needle biopsy, a core of marrow — cells, not fluid — is removed. These methods are often used concurrently to obtain the best possible marrow specimens.

Because bone marrow is the major site of hematopoiesis, the histologic and hematologic examination of its contents provides reliable diagnostic information about blood disorders. Marrow removed from the bone may be red or yellow. Red marrow, which constitutes about 50% of an adult's marrow, actively produces red blood cells; yellow marrow contains fat cells and connective tissue and is inactive. Because yellow marrow can become active in response to the body's needs, an adult has a large hematopoietic capacity. An infant's marrow is mainly red and, consequently, reflects a small hematopoietic capacity.

Bleeding and infection may result from bone marrow biopsy at any site, but the most serious complications occur at the sternum. Such complications are rare but include puncture of the heart and major vessels, which causes severe hemorrhage, and puncture of the mediastinum, which causes mediastinitis or pneumomediastinum.

Purpose

■ To diagnose thrombocytopenia, leukemias, granulomas, and aplastic, hypoplastic, and pernicious anemias
■ To diagnose primary and metastatic tumors
■ To determine the cause of infection
■ To aid staging of disease, such as Hodgkin's disease

■ To evaluate the effectiveness of chemotherapy and help monitor myelosuppression.

Patient preparation

Describe the procedure to the patient, and answer any questions. Explain that the test permits microscopic examination of a bone marrow specimen. Inform the patient that restriction of food or fluids isn't necessary before the test. Explain who will perform the biopsy, where it will be done, and that it usually takes only 5 to 10 minutes. Inform the patient that more than one bone marrow specimen may be required and that a blood sample will be collected before the biopsy for laboratory testing.

Make sure the patient has signed a consent form; if the patient is a minor, ask a responsible parent or guardian to do so. Check the patient history for hypersensitivity to the local anesthetic. After checking with the doctor, tell the patient which bone—sternum, anterior or posterior iliac crest, vertebral spinous process, rib, or tibia—will be used as the biopsy site. Inform the patient that a local anesthetic will be given but pressure on insertion of the biopsy needle and a brief, pulling pain on removal of the marrow will be felt. Administer a mild sedative 1 hour before the test.

Procedure

■ After positioning the patient, instruct him to remain as still as possible. Offer emotional support during the biopsy by talking to him quietly, describing what is being done, and answering any questions.

■ *Aspiration biopsy*: After the skin over the biopsy site is prepared and the area is draped, the local anesthetic is injected. With a twisting motion, the marrow aspiration needle is inserted through the skin, the subcutaneous tissue, and the cortex of the bone. The stylet is removed from the needle, and a 10- to 20-ml syringe is attached. The examiner aspirates 0.2 to 0.5 ml of marrow and then withdraws the needle. Pressure is applied to the site for 5 minutes while the marrow slides are being prepared. If the patient has thrombocytopenia, pressure is applied for 10 to 15 minutes. The biopsy site is cleaned again, and a sterile adhesive bandage is applied. If an adequate marrow specimen hasn't been obtained on the first attempt, the needle may be repositioned within the marrow cavity or may be removed and reinserted in another site within the anesthetized area. If the second attempt fails, a needle biopsy may be necessary.

■ *Needle biopsy*: After preparing the biopsy site and draping the area, the examiner marks the skin at the site

BONE MARROW: NORMAL VALUES AND IMPLICATIONS OF ABNORMAL FINDINGS

Cell types	Normal mean values		
	Adults	Children	Infants
Normoblasts, total	25.6%	23.1%	8.0%
Pronormoblasts	0.2% to 1.3%	0.5%	0.1%
Basophilic	0.5% to 2.4%	1.7%	0.34%
Polychromatic	17.9% to 29.2%	18.2%	6.9%
Orthochromatic	0.4% to 4.6%	2.7%	0.54%
Neutrophils, total	56.5%	57.1%	32.4%
Myeloblasts	0.2% to 1.5%	1.2%	0.62%
Promyelocytes	2.1% to 4.1%	1.4%	0.76%
Myelocytes	8.2% to 15.7%	18.3%	2.5%
Metamyelocytes	9.6% to 24.6%	23.3%	11.3%
Bands	9.5% to 15.3%	0	14.1%
Segmented	6.0% to 12.0%	12.9%	3.6%
Eosinophils	3.1%	3.6%	2.6%
Basophils	0.01%	0.06%	0.07%
Lymphocytes	16.2%	16.0%	49.0%
Plasma cells	1.3%	0.4%	0.02%
Megakaryocytes	0.1%	0.1%	0.05%
Myeloid-erythroid ratio	2.3%	2.9%	4.4%

with an indelible pencil or marking pen. A local anesthetic is then injected intradermally, subcutaneously, and at the surface of the bone. The biopsy needle is inserted into the periosteum, and the needle guard is set as indicated.

■ The needle is advanced with a steady boring motion until the outer needle passes through the cortex of the bone. The inner needle with trephine tip is inserted into the outer needle, and the stylet is removed. By alternately rotating the inner needle clockwise and counterclockwise, the examiner directs the needle into the marrow cavity and then removes a tissue plug. The needle assembly is withdrawn, and the marrow is expelled into a

Implications of abnormal findings

Elevated values	Depressed values
Polycythemia vera	Vitamin B_{12} or folic acid deficiency; hypoplastic or aplastic anemia
Acute myeloblastic or chronic myeloid leukemia	Lymphoblastic or acute monocytic leukemia; aplastic anemia
Bone marrow carcinoma, lymphadenoma, myeloid leukemia, eosinophilic leukemia, pernicious anemia (in relapse)	
No relationship between basophil count and symptoms	No relationship between basophil count and symptoms
B- and T-cell chronic lymphocytic leukemia, other lymphatic leukemias, lymphoma, mononucleosis, aplastic anemia, macroglobulinemia	
Myeloma, collagen disease, infection, antigen sensitivity, malignancy	
Old age, chronic myeloid leukemia, polycythemia vera, megakaryocytic myelosis, infection, idiopathic thrombocytopenic purpura, thrombocytopenia	Pernicious anemia
Myeloid leukemia, infection, leukemoid reactions, depressed hematopoiesis	Agranulocytosis, hematopoiesis after hemorrhage or hemolysis, iron-deficiency anemia, polycythemia vera

labeled bottle containing a special fixative such as Zenker's or bovine solution. After the biopsy site is cleaned, a sterile adhesive bandage or a pressure dressing is applied.

Precautions

■ Bone marrow biopsy is contraindicated in patients with severe bleeding disorders.
■ Send the tissue specimen or slides to the laboratory immediately.

Normal findings

Yellow marrow contains fat cells and connective tissue; red marrow contains hematopoietic cells, fat cells, and connective tissue. In addition, special stains that detect hematologic disorders produce these normal findings: the iron stain, which measures hemosiderin (storage iron), has a +2 level; the Sudan black B (SBB) stain, which shows granulocytes, is negative; and the periodic acid-Schiff (PAS) stain, which detects glycogen reactions, is negative.

Implications of results

Histologic examination of a bone marrow specimen can help detect myelofibrosis, granulomas, lymphomas, or cancer. Hematologic analysis, including the differential count and the myeloid-erythroid ratio, can implicate a wide range of disorders. (See *Bone marrow: Normal values and implications of abnormal findings*, pages 118 and 119.)

In an iron stain, decreased hemosiderin levels may indicate a true iron deficiency. Increased levels may accompany other types of anemias or blood disorders. A positive SBB stain can differentiate acute myelogenous leukemia from acute lymphoblastic leukemia (negative SBB), or it may indicate granulation in myeloblasts. A positive PAS stain may indicate acute or chronic lymphocytic leukemia, amyloidosis, thalassemia, lymphoma, infectious mononucleosis, iron-deficiency anemia, or sideroblastic anemia.

Posttest care

■ Check the biopsy site for bleeding and inflammation.
■ Observe the patient for signs of hemorrhage and infection, such as rapid pulse rate, low blood pressure, and fever.

Interfering factors

Failure to obtain a representative specimen, to use a fixative (for histologic analysis), or to send the specimen to the laboratory immediately may alter test results.

Breast biopsy

Although mammography, thermography, and ultrasonography aid diagnosis of breast masses, only histologic examination of breast tissue obtained by biopsy can confirm or rule out cancer. Needle biopsy or fine-needle biopsy can provide a core of tissue or a fluid aspirate, but needle biopsy should be restricted to fluid-filled cysts and advanced malignant lesions. Both methods have limited diagnostic value because of the small and perhaps unrepresentative specimens they provide. Open biopsy provides a complete tissue specimen, which can be sectioned to allow more accurate evaluation. All three techniques require only a local anesthetic and can often be performed on outpatients; however, open biopsy may require a general anesthetic if the patient is fearful or uncooperative.

A new advance in stereotactic biopsy has recently become available in some medical centers. (See *Advances in breast biopsy*, page 122.)

Breast biopsy is indicated for patients with palpable masses, suspicious areas in mammography, bloody discharge from the nipples, or persistently encrusted, inflamed, or eczematoid breast lesions. During mammography and before biopsy, a probe may be placed to help identify the precise site of the biopsy.

Breast tissue analysis often includes an estrogen and progesterone receptor assay to help select therapy if the mass proves malignant. This assay measures quickfrozen tumor tissue to determine binding capacity of its estrogen and progesterone receptors.

Purpose

To differentiate between benign and malignant breast tumors.

Patient preparation

Obtain a complete medical history, including when the patient first noticed the lesion, the presence or absence of pain or nipple discharge, a change in the lesion's size, association with the patient's menstrual cycle, and nipple or skin changes such as the characteristic "orangepeel" skin that may indicate an underlying inflammatory carcinoma.

Describe the procedure to the patient, and explain that this test permits microscopic examination of a breast tissue specimen. Offer her emotional support, and assure her that breast masses don't always indicate cancer.

If the patient is to receive a local anesthetic, tell her that restriction of food, fluids, or medication isn't needed prior to the biopsy. If she's to receive a general anesthetic, advise her to fast from midnight the night before the test until after the biopsy. Tell her who will perform the biopsy, where it will be done, and that it will take 15 to 30 minutes. Explain that pretest studies, such as blood tests, urine tests, and radiographs of the chest, may be required.

Make sure the patient has signed a consent form. Check the patient history for hypersensitivity to anesthetics.

ADVANCES IN BREAST BIOPSY

A diagnostic procedure that improves the accuracy of breast biopsies is available in a number of medical centers in the United States. The Advanced Breast Biopsy Instrument procedure, which involves computers linked to radiographs, offers patients less pain and a lower risk of deformity than conventional biopsies, requires only local anesthesia, and can be completed in about an hour.

In the new procedure, doctors use the computer to pinpoint the exact location of the area to be biopsied. Using computer coordinates, a probing tube is then inserted into the breast to remove a tissue specimen. Test results usually take less than 2 days.

In the past, doctors had to rely on two-dimensional radiographs to locate the calcium deposits they wanted to biopsy and couldn't be absolutely sure if they were cutting into the correct area.

The method provides 100% accuracy, according to surgeons who've used it, allowing determination of the exact three-dimensional location of the calcium deposits while the patient lies face down on a raised operating table. A rotating camera under the table takes radiographs of the breast from every angle. Doctors can then match up the coordinates to make sure they extract a specimen from the correct area.

Procedure

■ *Needle biopsy*: Instruct the patient to undress to the waist. After guiding her to a sitting or recumbent position with her hands at her sides, tell her to remain still. The biopsy site is prepared, a local anesthetic is administered, and the syringe (luer-lock syringe for aspiration, Vim-Silverman needle for tissue specimen) is introduced into the lesion. Fluid aspirated from the breast is expelled into a properly labeled, heparinized tube; the tissue specimen is placed in a labeled specimen bottle containing normal saline solution or formalin. With fine-needle aspiration, a slide is made for cytology and viewed immediately under a microscope. Pressure is exerted on the biopsy site and, after bleeding stops, an adhesive bandage is applied. Because breast fluid aspiration isn't considered diagnostically accurate, some doctors aspirate fluid only from cysts. If such fluid is clear yellow and the mass disappears, the aspiration procedure is both diagnostic and therapeutic, and the aspirate is discarded. If aspiration yields no fluid or if the lesion recurs two or three times, an open biopsy is then considered appropriate.

■ *Open biopsy*: After the patient receives a general or local anesthetic, an incision is made in the breast to expose the mass. The examiner may then incise a portion of tissue or excise the entire mass. If the mass is smaller than ¾" (2 cm) in diameter and appears benign, it's usually excised; if it's larger or appears malignant, a specimen is usually incised before the mass is excised. Incisional biopsy generally provides an adequate specimen for histologic analysis. The specimen is placed in a properly labeled specimen bottle containing 10% formalin solution. Tissue that appears malignant is sent for frozen section and receptor assays. Receptor assay specimens mustn't be placed in the formalin solution. The wound is sutured, and an adhesive bandage is applied.

Precautions

■ Open breast biopsy is contraindicated in patients with conditions that preclude surgery.

■ Send the specimen to the laboratory immediately.

Normal findings

Breast tissue normally consists of cellular and noncellular connective tissue, fat lobules, and various lactiferous ducts. It's normally pink, more fatty than fibrous, and shows no abnormal development of cells or tissue elements.

Implications of results

Abnormal breast tissue may exhibit a wide range of malignant or benign pathology. Breast tumors are common in women and account for 32% of female cancers; they're rare in men, accounting for only 0.2% of male cancers. Benign conditions include fibrocystic disease, adenofibroma, intraductal papilloma, mammary fat necrosis, and plasma cell mastitis (mammary duct ectasia). Malignant tumors include adenocarcinoma, cystosarcoma, intraductal carcinoma, infiltrating carcinoma, inflammatory carcinoma, medullary or circumscribed carcinoma, colloid carcinoma, lobular carcinoma, sarcoma, and Paget's disease.

The receptor assays evaluate tumors for estrogen and progesterone protein and assign a positive or negative value to the estrogen and progesterone receptors. This positive or negative value assists in the prognosis and treatment of breast cancer.

Posttest care

■ If the patient has received a local anesthetic during needle or open biopsy, check vital signs and provide medication for pain. Watch for and report bleeding, tenderness, or redness at the biopsy site.

■ If the patient has received a general anesthetic, check vital signs every 30 minutes for the first 4 hours, every hour for the next 4 hours, and then every 4 hours. Administer an analgesic. Watch for and report bleeding, tenderness, or redness at the biopsy site.

■ An ice bag applied to the biopsy site may provide comfort. Instruct the patient to wear a support bra at all times until healing is complete.

■ Provide emotional support to the patient who's awaiting diagnosis.

If the biopsy confirms cancer, the patient will require follow-up tests, including radiographic tests, blood studies, bone scans, and urinalysis, to determine appropriate treatment.

Interfering factors

Failure to obtain an adequate tissue specimen or to place the specimen in the proper solution container may interfere with test results.

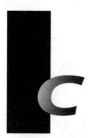

Calcitonin test, plasma

This radioimmunoassay measures plasma levels of calcitonin (also known as thyrocalcitonin), a polypeptide hormone. Interstitial or parafollicular cells (specialized C cells) of the thyroid gland secrete it in response to rising plasma calcium levels. Although the exact role of calcitonin in normal human physiology hasn't been fully determined, calcitonin is known to inhibit bone resorption by osteoclasts and osteocytes and to increase calcium excretion by the kidneys. Therefore, calcitonin acts as an antagonist to parathyroid hormone and lowers serum calcium levels.

The usual clinical indication for this test is suspected medullary carcinoma of the thyroid, which causes hypersecretion of calcitonin without associated hypocalcemia. Equivocal results require provocative testing with I.V. pentagastrin or calcium to rule out this disease. (See *Calcitonin stimulation tests*, page 126.)

Purpose

To aid diagnosis of thyroid medullary carcinoma or ectopic calcitonin-producing tumors (rare).

Patient preparation

Explain to the patient that this test helps evaluate thyroid function. Instruct the patient to observe an overnight fast because eating may interfere with calcium homeostasis and, subsequently, calcitonin levels. Explain that this test requires a blood sample, discuss who will perform the venipuncture and when, and note that transient discomfort may be felt from the needle puncture. Advise the patient that the laboratory requires several days to complete the analysis.

Procedure

Draw venous blood into a 7-ml heparinized tube.

Precautions

Handle the sample gently to prevent hemolysis and send it to the laboratory immediately.

CALCITONIN STIMULATION TESTS

Stimulation testing is often necessary in patients with medullary thyroid carcinoma when baseline calcitonin levels don't rise high enough to confirm the diagnosis.

The most common test is a 4-hour I.V. calcium infusion (15 mg/kg) to provoke calcitonin secretion. Samples are taken just before the infusion and at 3 and 4 hours afterward. Calcitonin levels rise rapidly after the infusion in patients with medullary thyroid carcinoma.

Another test involves I.V. infusion of pentagastrin (0.5 μg/kg over 5 to 10 seconds). A blood sample is drawn just before the I.V. infusion and at 90 seconds, 5 minutes, and 10 minutes afterward. In patients with medullary thyroid carcinoma, calcitonin levels rise markedly over the baseline reading.

Reference values

Normal basal plasma calcitonin levels:
- males: 40 pg/ml or less
- females: 20 pg/ml or less.

After provocative testing with 4-hour calcium infusion:
- males: 190 pg/ml or less
- females: 130 pg/ml or less.

After provocative testing with pentagastrin infusion:
- males: [less than or equal to] 110 pg/ml
- females: [less than or equal to] 30 pg/ml.

Implications of results

Elevated plasma calcitonin levels in the absence of hypocalcemia usually indicate medullary carcinoma of the thyroid. Transmitted as an autosomal dominant trait, this disease may occur as part of multiple endocrine neoplasia. Occasionally, increased calcitonin levels may be associated with ectopic calcitonin production resulting from oat cell carcinoma of the lung or from breast carcinoma.

Posttest care

If a hematoma develops, apply warm soaks.

Interfering factors

- Failure to fast overnight before the test may interfere with accurate determination of test results.
- Hemolysis resulting from rough handling of the sample may interfere with test results.

Calcium test, serum

Serum calcium is needed for the proper function of many metabolic processes, muscle contraction, cardiac function, transmission of nerve impulses, blood clotting, and stability of plasma membrane permeability.

Measurement of total calcium is the most frequently performed test for evaluation of serum calcium levels. Approximately 99% of the total calcium in the body is stored in the bones and teeth; the remaining 1% circulates in the blood. Of this, about 50% is bound to plasma proteins and 40% is ionized, or free, and is the most physiologically active form of serum calcium.

Many laboratories don't have the equipment to measure ionized calcium levels. If ionized calcium assays are not available, measuring serum albumin at the same time as serum calcium provides a way to estimate the level of ionized calcium. Because of protein binding, the serum calcium level falls by 8 mg/dl for every 1-g decrease in the serum albumin level. The measured serum calcium is then adjusted upward by the amount of decrease in serum albumin. Ionized calcium is estimated to be approximately half of the adjusted calcium value.

Parathyroid hormone (PTH), vitamin D, and calcitonin are the three substances that regulate calcium balance. PTH is secreted in response to low calcium levels and promotes movement from bone to plasma. PTH also activates vitamin D in the liver and kidney. The activated vitamin D circulates in the blood and promotes the absorption of dietary calcium from the small intestine. Calcitonin, produced by the thyroid gland, is secreted in response to high serum calcium levels and promotes movement of calcium from the blood to the bones.

Purpose

■ To evaluate endocrine function, calcium metabolism, and acid-base balance
■ To guide therapy in patients with renal failure, renal transplant, endocrine disorders, malignancies, cardiac disease, and skeletal disorders.

Patient preparation

Explain to the patient that this test determines blood calcium level. Inform the patient that restriction of food or fluids is not necessary. Explain that the test requires a blood sample, discuss who will perform the venipuncture and when, and note that some discomfort may be felt at the puncture site.

Procedure

Perform a venipuncture without using a tourniquet if possible, and collect the sample in a 7-ml clot-activator tube.

Reference values

- Total calcium: 8.9 to 10.1 mg/dl in adults; 8.9 to 10.6 mg/dl in children
- Ionized calcium: 4 to 5 mg/dl.

Implications of results

HYPERCALCEMIA

- Abnormally high serum calcium levels, or hypercalcemia, may occur in patients with hyperparathyroidism and parathyroid tumors (because of oversecretion of PTH), Paget's disease of the bone, multiple myeloma, metastatic carcinoma, multiple fractures, or prolonged immobilization. Elevated serum calcium levels may also result from inadequate excretion of calcium, as in adrenal insufficiency and renal disease; from excessive calcium ingestion; or from overuse of antacids such as calcium carbonate.

CLINICAL ALERT Observe the patient with hypercalcemia for deep bone pain, flank pain (caused by renal calculi), and muscle hypotonicity. Hypercalcemic crisis begins with nausea, vomiting, and dehydration and may lead to stupor, coma, and possibly cardiac arrest.

CLINICAL ALERT Monitor the electrocardiogram (ECG) for cardiac arrhythmias and shortened QT interval.

- Increasing mobility whenever possible decreases the risk for hypercalcemia.
- Encourage adequate fluid intake, if not contraindicated, to decrease the incidence of renal calculi and promote calcium excretion. In patients with severe hypercalcemia and adequate renal function, hydration with normal saline solution is indicated to promote calcium excretion. Loop diuretics are also administered. Certain drugs, including calcitonin, mithramycin, phosphates, and diphosphates, may also be used.

HYPOCALCEMIA

- Low calcium levels, or hypocalcemia, may result from hypoparathyroidism, total parathyroidectomy, or malabsorption. Decreased serum levels of calcium may follow calcium loss in patients with Cushing's syndrome, renal failure, acute pancreatitis, or peritonitis.

CLINICAL ALERT In a patient with hypocalcemia, be alert for circumoral and peripheral numbness and tingling, muscle twitching, Chvostek's sign (facial muscle spasm), tetany, muscle cramping, Trousseau's sign (carpopedal spasm), seizure activity, laryngeal spasm, arrhythmias, and prolongation of the QT interval.

CLINICAL ALERT Monitor and maintain a patent airway to prevent respiratory distress related to laryngeal spasm. Symptomatic hypocalcemia is treated with I.V. calcium chloride. Administration that is too rapid can cause severe bradycardia and subsequent cardiac arrest. Diluting the ordered dose in 50 ml of normal saline solution and infusing it over 20 to 30 minutes is the safest method of administration.

■ Educate patients at risk for hypocalcemia and related disease processes such as osteoporosis.

Posttest care

If a hematoma develops, apply warm soaks.

Interfering factors

■ Excessive ingestion of vitamin D or its derivatives (dihydrotachysterol, calcitriol) or the use of androgens, calciferol-activated calcium salts, progestins-estrogens, or thiazide diuretics can elevate serum calcium levels.

■ Chronic laxative use, excessive transfusions of citrated blood, and administration of acetazolamide, corticosteroids, or mithramycin can alter test results.

■ Prolonged application of a tourniquet causes venous stasis and may falsely increase calcium results.

Calcium and phosphate test, urine

This test measures the urine levels of calcium and phosphates, elements essential for the formation and resorption of bone. Urine calcium and phosphate levels generally parallel serum levels.

Normally absorbed in the upper intestine and excreted in feces and urine, calcium and phosphates help maintain tissue and fluid pH, electrolyte balance in cells and extracellular fluids, and permeability of cell membranes. Calcium promotes enzymatic processes, aids blood coagulation, and lowers neuromuscular irritability; phosphates aid carbohydrate metabolism. Factors that affect the calcium level and, indirectly, the phosphate level, include parathyroid hormone and calcitonin levels and plasma proteins.

Purpose

■ To evaluate calcium and phosphate metabolism and excretion

■ To monitor treatment of calcium or phosphate deficiency.

Patient preparation

Explain to the patient that this test measures the amount of calcium and phosphates in the urine. Encourage the patient to be as active as possible before the test. Explain that the test requires 24-hour urine specimen collection. If the specimen is to be collected at home, teach the correct collection technique.

Provide the Albright-Reifenstein diet (which contains about 130 mg of calcium/24 hours) for 3 days before the test, or provide a copy of the diet for the patient to follow at home. Note recent use of thiazide diuretics, sodium phosphate, or glucocorticoids on the laboratory request.

Procedure

Collect a 24-hour urine specimen.

Precautions

Tell the patient not to contaminate the specimen with toilet tissue or stool.

Reference values

Normal values depend on dietary intake. Males excrete less than 275 mg of calcium/24 hours; females, less than 250 mg/24 hours. Hypercalciuria is excretion of more than 350 mg of calcium/24 hours. Normal excretion of phosphates is less than 1,000 mg/24 hours.

Implications of results

Many disorders can affect urine calcium and phosphate levels. (See *Disorders that affect urine calcium and phosphate levels.*)

Posttest care

CLINICAL ALERT In patients with low urine calcium levels, observe for tetany.

Interfering factors

■ Thiazide diuretics decrease excretion of calcium. Prolonged inactivity and ingestion of corticosteroids, sodium phosphate, or calcitonin increase excretion. Vitamin D increases phosphate absorption and excretion.
■ Parathyroid hormone increases urinary excretion of phosphates and decreases urinary excretion of calcium.
■ Failure to collect all urine during the test period may affect the accuracy of test results.

Candida *antibody test*

Commonly present in the body, *Candida albicans* is a saprophytic yeast that can become pathogenic when the environment favors proliferation or the host's defenses have been significantly weakened.

Candidiasis is usually limited to the skin and mucous membranes but may cause life-threatening systemic infection. Susceptibility to candidiasis is associated with antibacterial, antimetabolic, and corticosteroid therapy as well as with immunologic defects, pregnancy, obesity, diabetes, and debilitating diseases. Oral candidiasis is

DISORDERS THAT AFFECT URINE CALCIUM AND PHOSPHATE LEVELS

The following disorders can cause changes in urine calcium or phosphate levels:

Disorder	Urine calcium level	Urine phosphate level
Acute nephritis	Suppressed	Suppressed
Acute nephrosis	Suppressed	Suppressed or normal
Chronic nephrosis	Suppressed	Suppressed
Hyperparathyroidism	Elevated	Elevated
Hypoparathyroidism	Suppressed	Suppressed
Metastatic carcinoma	Elevated	Normal
Milk-alkali syndrome	Suppressed or normal	Suppressed or normal
Multiple myeloma	Elevated or normal	Elevated or normal
Osteomalacia	Suppressed	Suppressed
Paget's disease	Normal	Normal
Renal insufficiency	Suppressed	Suppressed
Renal tubular acidosis	Elevated	Elevated
Sarcoidosis	Elevated	Suppressed
Steatorrhea	Suppressed	Suppressed
Vitamin D intoxication	Elevated	Suppressed

common and benign in children; in adults, it may be an early indication of acquired immunodeficiency syndrome.

Diagnosis of candidiasis is usually made by culture or histologic study. When such diagnosis can't be made, identifying *Candida* antibodies may be helpful in diagnosing systemic candidiasis. Be aware that serologic testing to detect antibodies in candidiasis is not reliable, and investigators continue to disagree about its usefulness.

Purpose

To aid diagnosis of candidiasis when culture or histologic study can't confirm the diagnosis.

Patient preparation

As appropriate, explain the purpose of the test to the patient. Inform the patient that restriction of food or fluids isn't necessary. Explain that the test requires a blood sample and discuss who will perform the venipuncture and when. Explain that the needle puncture and the tourniquet may cause transient discomfort, but collecting the sample takes less than 3 minutes.

Procedure

Perform a venipuncture, and collect the sample in a 5-ml sterile collection tube without additives.

Precautions

- Handle the sample gently to prevent hemolysis.
- Send the sample to the laboratory promptly.
- Note any recent antimicrobial therapy on the laboratory request form.

Normal findings

A normal test result is negative for *Candida* antibodies.

Implications of results

A positive test for *C. albicans* antibodies is common in patients with disseminated candidiasis, although this test yields a significant percentage of false-positive results.

Posttest care

If a hematoma develops, apply warm soaks.

Interfering factor

Rough handling of the sample can cause hemolysis.

Capillary fragility test

A nonspecific method of evaluating bleeding tendencies, the capillary fragility test (also known as the positive-pressure test, tourniquet test, and Rumpel-Leede test) measures the ability of capillaries to remain intact under increased intracapillary pressure. In this test, a blood pressure cuff is placed around the patient's upper arm. The cuff is inflated to 70 to 90 mm Hg or midway between the diastolic and systolic pressures. Pressure is maintained for 5 minutes. This temporary increase in pressure may cause rhexis bleeding of the capillaries and formation of petechiae on the arm, wrist, or hand. The number of petechiae within a given circular space is recorded as the test result.

Purpose

- To assess the fragility of capillary walls
- To identify platelet deficiency (thrombocytopenia).

Patient preparation

Explain to the patient that this test helps identify abnormal bleeding tendencies. Inform the patient that restriction of food or fluids isn't necessary. Explain who will perform the procedure and when and that the compression of the blood pressure cuff may cause discomfort.

Procedure

■ Select and mark a 2-inch (5-cm) space on the patient's forearm. Ideally, the site should be free of petechiae; if not, record the number of petechiae present on the site before starting the test. The patient's skin temperature and the room temperature should be normal to ensure accurate results.

■ Fasten the cuff around the arm and raise the pressure to a point midway between the systolic and diastolic blood pressures. Maintain this pressure for 5 minutes, then release the cuff. Count the number of petechiae that appear in the 2-inch space and record the results.

Precautions

■ Don't repeat this test on the same arm within 1 week.

■ This test is contraindicated in patients with disseminated intravascular coagulation (DIC) or other bleeding disorders and in those who already have significant petechiae.

Reference values

A few petechiae may normally be present before the test. Fewer than 10 petechiae on the forearm 5 minutes after the test is considered normal, or negative; more than 10 petechiae is considered a positive result. The following scale may also be used to report test results:

Number of petechiae/5 cm	Score
0 to 10	1+
10 to 20	2+
20 to 50	3+
50	4+

Implications of results

A positive finding (more than 10 petechiae present or a score of 2+ to 4+) indicates weakness of the capillary walls (vascular purpura) or a platelet defect. This occurs in conditions such as thrombocytopenia, thrombasthenia, purpura senilis, scurvy, DIC, von Willebrand's disease, vitamin K deficiency, dysproteinemia, and polycythemia vera as well as in severe deficiencies of factor VII, fibrinogen, or prothrombin.

Conditions unrelated to bleeding defects, such as scarlet fever, measles, influenza, chronic renal disease, hypertension, and diabetes with coexistent vascular disease, may also increase capillary fragility. An abnormal number of petechiae sometimes appears before onset of menstruation and at other times in some healthy persons, especially in women over age 40.

Posttest care

Encourage the patient to open and close the hand on the affected arm a few times to hasten return of blood to the forearm.

Interfering factors

■ Glucocorticoids may increase capillary resistance, even in a patient with thrombocytopenia.
■ Decreased estrogen levels in postmenopausal women may increase capillary fragility.
■ Repeating the test on the same arm within 1 week may yield inaccurate results by causing errors in counting the number of petechiae.

Carbon dioxide content test, total

Carbon dioxide (CO_2) is present in the body as an end product of metabolic processes as well as being present in small amounts in the air. When the pressure of CO_2 in the red blood cells exceeds 40 mm Hg, CO_2 flows out of the cells and dissolves in plasma. There it combines with water to form carbonic acid, which in turn dissociates into hydrogen and bicarbonate ions.

This test measures the total concentration of all forms of CO_2 in serum, plasma, or whole blood samples. Because about 90% of CO_2 in serum is in the form of bicarbonate, this test provides a close approximation of bicarbonate levels. Total CO_2 content reflects the efficiency of the carbonic acid-bicarbonate buffer system, which maintains acid-base balance and normal pH. Consequently, this test is commonly ordered to assess electrolyte balance. It is not highly accurate in measuring acid-base balance because exposure to air affects the CO_2 level in the specimen. For maximum clinical significance, test results must be considered with both pH and arterial blood gas values.

Purpose

To help evaluate acid-base balance.

Patient preparation

Explain to the patient that this test measures the amount of CO_2 in the blood. Inform the patient that restriction of food or fluids isn't necessary. Explain that this test requires a blood sample, discuss who will perform the venipuncture and when, and note that the needle puncture and pressure of the tourniquet may cause transient discomfort. Check the patient history for use of medications that may influence CO_2 blood levels.

Procedure

Perform a venipuncture. Because CO_2 content is usually measured along with electrolytes, a 7-ml clot-activator tube may be used. When this test is performed alone, a heparinized tube is appropriate.

Precautions

Fill the tube completely to prevent diffusion of CO_2 into the vacuum.

Reference values

Normally, total CO_2 levels range from 22 to 34 mEq/L.

Implications of results

High CO_2 levels may occur in metabolic alkalosis (due to excessive ingestion or retention of base bicarbonate), respiratory acidosis (from hypoventilation, for example, as in emphysema or pneumonia), primary aldosteronism, and Cushing's syndrome. CO_2 levels may also be elevated after excessive loss of acids, as in severe vomiting and continuous gastric drainage.

Decreased CO_2 levels are common in metabolic acidosis (such as diabetic acidosis or renal tube acidosis caused by renal failure). Decreased total CO_2 levels in metabolic acidosis also result from loss of bicarbonate (as in severe diarrhea or intestinal drainage). Levels also may fall below normal in respiratory alkalosis (for example, from hyperventilation after trauma).

Posttest care

If a hematoma develops, apply warm soaks.

Interfering factors

■ CO_2 levels rise with excessive use of corticotropin, cortisone, or thiazide diuretics or with excessive ingestion of alkalis or licorice.
■ CO_2 levels decrease with use of salicylates, paraldehyde, methicillin, dimercaprol, ammonium chloride, or acetazolamide and after ingestion of ethylene glycol or methyl alcohol.
■ Underfilling the collection tube allows CO_2 to escape, resulting in inaccurate levels.

Carcinoembryonic antigen test

Carcinoembryonic antigen (CEA), a glycoprotein secreted onto the glycocalyx surface of cells lining the GI tract, appears during the first or second trimester of fetal life. Production of CEA usually stops before birth but may begin again later if a neoplasm develops.

Because CEA levels are raised by biliary obstruction, alcoholic hepatitis, chronic heavy smoking, and other

USING CEA TO MONITOR CANCER TREATMENT

Because many patients in the early stages of colorectal cancer have normal or low levels of carcinoembryonic antigen (CEA), the CEA test doesn't screen successfully for early malignancy. However, it is a good tool for monitoring response to cancer therapy.

After a patient's serum CEA level has decreased following surgery, chemotherapy, or other treatment, any increase suggests recurrence of cancer or diminished effectiveness of treatment.

The charts below illustrate CEA response in two patients during and after treatment for colorectal cancer.

PATIENT #1

Initial results of chemotherapy show the usual dramatic drop in CEA levels. The subsequent rise indicates a diminishing response to treatment.

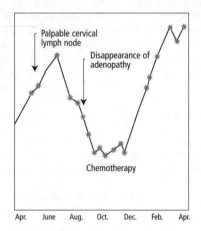

PATIENT #2

The progressive rise in CEA levels after surgery signals a recurrence of cancer months before radiologic evidence or clinical signs.

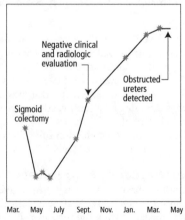

TWO CANCER TESTS

These two tests are used to diagnose certain cancers.

CA19-9 antigen test
The CA19-9 carbohydrate antigen test has proven to be a valuable tool in the early detection of pancreatic cancer. Found in the blood, the antigen is a tumor marker that helps in differentiating benign pancreatic tumors from malignant tumors. High blood levels of the antigen may indicate cancer of the pancreas or other GI sites, such as the liver or colon.

Hercep test
The Hercep test is used to detect breast cancer. This immunohistochemical assay detects breast tumors that produce excessive amounts of the HER2 protein. It may also be helpful in diagnosing a relapse of breast cancer.

---

conditions as well as by benign or malignant neoplasms, this test can't be used as a general indicator of cancer. Measuring CEA levels is useful for staging colorectal cancer, assessing the adequacy of surgical resection, and monitoring the effectiveness of colorectal cancer therapy because serum CEA levels, measured by enzyme immunoassay, usually return to normal within 6 weeks if cancer treatment is successful. (See *Using CEA to monitor cancer treatment.*) Other tests are used to diagnose certain types of cancer. (See *Two cancer tests.*)

Purpose
- To monitor the effectiveness of cancer therapy
- To help stage colorectal cancer preoperatively and to test for its recurrence.

Patient preparation
Explain to the patient that this test detects and measures a special protein in the blood. If appropriate, inform the patient that the test will be repeated to monitor the effectiveness of therapy. Advise the patient that restriction of food, fluids, or medications isn't necessary. Explain that the test requires a blood sample, discuss who will perform the venipuncture and when, and note that the needle puncture and the pressure of the tourniquet may cause transient discomfort.

Procedure
Perform a venipuncture, and collect the sample in a 7-ml tube without additives.

Precautions
Handle the sample gently to prevent hemolysis and send it to the laboratory immediately.

Reference values

Normal serum CEA values are less than 5 ng/ml in healthy nonsmokers. Approximately 5% of the population has above-normal CEA levels.

Implications of results

If serum CEA levels are above normal before surgical resection, chemotherapy, or radiation therapy, a return to normal within 6 weeks after therapy suggests successful treatment. Persistent elevation of CEA levels, however, suggests residual or recurrent tumor.

High CEA levels are characteristic in various malignant conditions, particularly endodermally derived neoplasms of the GI organs and the lungs and in certain nonmalignant conditions, such as benign hepatic disease, hepatic cirrhosis, alcoholic pancreatitis, and inflammatory bowel disease. Elevated CEA levels may also result from nonendodermal cancers, such as breast cancer and ovarian cancer.

Posttest care

If a hematoma develops, apply warm soaks.

Interfering factors

■ Chronic cigarette smoking may elevate serum CEA levels, altering test results.
■ Hemolysis caused by rough handling may alter test results.

Cardiolipin antibody test

This test measures serum concentrations of IgG or IgM antibodies in relation to the phospholipid cardiolipin. These antibodies appear in some patients with lupus erythematosus (LE) whose serum also contains a coagulation inhibitor (lupus anticoagulant). They also appear in some patients who don't fulfill all the diagnostic criteria for LE but who experience recurrent episodes of spontaneous thrombosis, fetal loss, or thrombocytopenia. Cardiolipin antibodies are measured by enzyme-linked immunosorbent assay.

Purpose

To aid diagnosis of cardiolipin antibody syndrome in patients with or without LE who experience recurrent episodes of spontaneous thrombosis, thrombocytopenia, or fetal loss.

Patient preparation

Explain the purpose of the test. Tell the patient that restriction of food or fluids before the test is not necessary. Inform the patient that the test requires a blood sample, discuss who will perform the venipuncture and when, and note that the needle puncture and pressure of the tourniquet may cause transient discomfort.

Procedure

Perform a venipuncture, and collect the sample in a 5-ml tube without additives.

Precautions

Handle the sample gently to prevent hemolysis and send it to the laboratory immediately.

Reference values

Cardiolipin antibody results are reported as dilution titers obtained by making 1:2 serial dilutions of serum. The highest dilution is reported. A 1:4 titer is a borderline result. A lower titer (1:2) is negative; a higher titer (1:8, 1:16), positive.

Implications of results

A positive result along with a history of recurrent spontaneous thrombosis, thrombocytopenia, or fetal loss suggests cardiolipin antibody syndrome. Treatment may involve anticoagulant or platelet-inhibitor therapy.

Posttest care

If a hematoma develops, apply warm soaks.

Interfering factors

Hemolysis will affect results.

Catecholamine test, plasma

This test, a quantitative (total or fractionated) analysis of plasma catecholamines, is clinically significant in patients with hypertension and signs of adrenal medullary tumor and in patients with neural tumors that affect endocrine function. Elevated plasma catecholamine levels necessitate supportive confirmation by urinalysis that shows catecholamine degradation products, such as metanephrine.

Major catecholamines include the hormones epinephrine, norepinephrine, and dopamine, which are produced almost entirely in the brain, sympathetic nerve endings, and adrenal medulla. When secreted into the bloodstream, adrenal medullary catecholamines prepare the body for the fight-or-flight reaction: They increase heart rate and contractility, constrict blood vessels, redistribute circulating blood toward the skeletal and coronary muscles, mobilize carbohydrate and lipid reserves, and sharpen alertness. These effects resemble those produced by direct stimulation of the sympathetic nervous system, but they are intensified and prolonged. Excessive catecholamine secretion by tumors causes hypertension, weight loss, episodic sweating, headache, palpitations, and anxiety.

Plasma levels commonly fluctuate in response to temperature, stress, postural change, diet, smoking, anoxia, volume depletion, renal failure, obesity, and use of certain drugs.

Purpose

■ To rule out pheochromocytoma (adrenal medullary or extra-adrenal) in patients with hypertension
■ To identify neuroblastoma, ganglioneuroblastoma, and ganglioneuroma
■ To aid diagnosis of autonomic nervous system dysfunction such as idiopathic orthostatic hypotension
■ To distinguish between adrenal medullary tumors and other catecholamine-producing tumors through fractional analysis; in these cases, urinalysis for catecholamine degradation products is recommended to support the diagnosis.

Patient preparation

Explain that this test helps determine if hypertension or other symptoms are related to improper hormonal secretion. Advise the patient to strictly follow pretest instructions to ensure a reliable test result. Instruct him to refrain from using self-prescribed medications, especially cold or allergy remedies that may contain sympathomimetics, for 2 weeks; to exclude amine-rich foods and beverages, such as bananas, avocados, cheese, coffee, tea, cocoa, beer, and Chianti wine from his diet for 48 hours; to maintain vitamin C intake, which is necessary for formation of catecholamines; to abstain from smoking for 24 hours; and to fast for 10 to 12 hours. Tell the patient that this test requires one or two blood samples, explain who will perform the venipunctures and when, and note that the needle punctures may cause some discomfort. Advise the patient that the laboratory requires up to 1 week to complete the analysis.

If the patient is hospitalized, withhold medications that affect catecholamine levels, such as amphetamines, phenothiazines, sympathomimetics, and tricyclic antidepressants.

Insert an indwelling venous catheter (heparin lock) 24 hours before the test. This may be needed because the stress of the venipuncture itself may significantly raise catecholamine levels. Make sure the patient is relaxed and recumbent for 45 to 60 minutes before the test. If necessary, provide blankets to keep him warm as low temperatures stimulate catecholamine secretion.

Procedure

■ Perform a venipuncture between 6 a.m. and 8 a.m. Collect the sample in a 10-ml chilled tube containing EDTA (sodium metabisulfite solution), which can be obtained from the laboratory on request.

■ If a second sample is requested, have the patient stand for 10 minutes, and draw the sample into another tube exactly like the first.

■ If a heparin lock is used, you may need to discard the first 1 or 2 ml of blood. Check with the laboratory for the preferred procedure.

Precautions

■ After collecting each sample, roll the tube slowly between your palms to distribute the EDTA without agitating the blood.

■ Pack the tube in crushed ice to minimize deactivation of catecholamines, and send it to the laboratory immediately. Indicate on the laboratory request whether the patient was supine or standing and the time the sample was drawn.

Reference values

In fractional analysis, catecholamine levels range as follows:

■ *supine*: epinephrine, undetectable to 110 pg/ml; norepinephrine, 70 to 750 pg/ml; dopamine, undetectable to 30 pg/ml

■ *standing*: epinephrine, undetectable to 140 pg/ml; norepinephrine, 200 to 1,700 pg/ml; dopamine, undetectable to 30 pg/ml.

Implications of results

High catecholamine levels may indicate pheochromocytoma, neuroblastoma, ganglioneuroblastoma, or ganglioneuroma. (See *Clonidine suppression test*, page 142.) Elevations suggest but don't directly confirm thyroid disorders, hypoglycemia, or cardiac disease. Electroconvulsive therapy or shock resulting from hemorrhage, endotoxins, or anaphylaxis also raises catecholamine levels.

In the patient with normal or low baseline catecholamine levels, absence of an increase in the sample taken after standing suggests autonomic nervous system dysfunction.

Fractional analysis helps identify the cause of elevated catecholamine levels. For example, adrenal medullary tumors secrete epinephrine, whereas ganglioneuromas,

---

CLONIDINE SUPPRESSION TEST

This test uses clonidine as an aid in the differential diagnosis of pheochromocytoma and essential hypertension.
To perform the test:
- Place the patient in the supine position.
- Collect a blood sample to obtain baseline catecholamine levels, and then administer 0.3 mg of oral clonidine.
- Collect a blood sample after 3 hours to measure catecholamine levels again and allow for comparison of findings.
  Patients with pheochromocytoma show no decrease in catecholamine levels after clonidine administration. In contrast, patients with essential hypertension have catecholamine levels in the normal range.

---

ganglioneuroblastomas, and neuroblastomas secrete norepinephrine.

Posttest care
- If a hematoma develops, apply warm soaks.
- Resume normal diet and any medications discontinued before the test.

Interfering factors
- Failure to observe pretest restrictions may interfere with test results.
- Epinephrine, levodopa, amphetamines, phenothiazines, sympathomimetics, decongestants, and tricyclic antidepressants raise plasma catecholamine levels. Reserpine lowers them.
- A radioactive scan performed within 1 week before the test may affect results.

Catecholamine test, urine
This test uses spectrophotofluorometry to measure urine levels of the major catecholamines — dopamine, epinephrine, and norepinephrine. Dopamine is secreted by the central nervous system; epinephrine by the adrenal medulla; and norepinephrine by both. Catecholamines help regulate metabolism and prepare the body for the fight-or-flight response to stress. Certain tumors can also secrete catecholamines. One of the most common of these is a pheochromocytoma, which causes intermittent or persistent hypertension.

A 24-hour urine specimen is preferred for this test because catecholamine secretion fluctuates diurnally and in response to pain, heat, cold, emotional stress, physical exercise, hypoglycemia, injury, hemorrhage, asphyxia, and drugs. A random specimen may be useful for evaluating catecholamine levels after a hypertensive episode.

For a complete diagnostic workup of catecholamine secretion, urine levels of the catecholamine metabolites are measured concurrently. These metabolites — metanephrine, normetanephrine, homovanillic acid (HVA), and vanillylmandelic acid (VMA) — normally appear in the urine in greater quantities than the catecholamines.

Purpose

■ To aid diagnosis of pheochromocytoma in a patient with unexplained hypertension
■ To aid diagnosis of neuroblastoma, ganglioneuroma, and dysautonomia.

Patient preparation

Explain to the patient that this test evaluates adrenal function. Inform the patient that restriction of food or fluids isn't necessary before the test but stressful situations and excessive physical activity should be avoided during the collection period. Explain whether a 24-hour or a random specimen is required and explain the collection procedure.

Check the patient's drug history for medications that may affect catecholamine levels (such as those listed under "Interfering factors"). Review your findings with the laboratory, then notify the doctor, who may want to restrict such medications before the test.

Procedure

24-hour urine specimen: collect it in a bottle containing a preservative to keep the specimen acidified to a pH of 3.0 or less.

CLINICAL ALERT *Random specimen:* collect it immediately after a hypertensive episode.

Precautions

Refrigerate a 24-hour specimen or place it on ice during the collection period. At the end of the collection period, send the specimen to the laboratory immediately.

Reference values

Normally, urine epinephrine values range from undetectable to 20 μg/24 hours; urine norepinephrine values, from undetectable to 80 μg/24 hours; and urine dopamine values, from undetectable to 400 μg/24 hours.

Implications of results

In a patient with undiagnosed hypertension, elevated urine catecholamine levels following a hypertensive episode usually indicate a pheochromocytoma. With the exception of HVA, a metabolite of dopamine, catecholamine metabolites may also be elevated. Abnormally high HVA levels rule out a pheochromocytoma because this tumor mainly secretes epinephrine, whose primary metabolite is VMA, not HVA. If tests indicate a pheochromocytoma, the patient may also be tested for multiple endocrine neoplasia.

Elevated catecholamine levels without marked hypertension may be caused by a neuroblastoma or a ganglioneuroma, although HVA levels reflect these conditions more accurately. Neuroblastomas and ganglioneuromas primarily composed of immature cells secrete large quantities of dopamine and HVA. Elevated catecholamine levels may also be seen in severe systemic situations (such as burns, peritonitis, shock, and septicemia), cor pulmonale, manic depressive disorders, or in depressive neurosis.

Myasthenia gravis and progressive muscular dystrophy commonly cause urine catecholamine levels to rise above normal, but this test is rarely performed to diagnose these disorders.

Consistently low-normal catecholamine levels may indicate dysautonomia, marked by orthostatic hypotension.

Posttest care

- Tell the patient that he may resume activity restricted during the test.
- Resume administration of medications withheld before the test.

Interfering factors

- Excessive physical exercise or emotional stress raises catecholamine levels.
- Caffeine, insulin, nitroglycerin, aminophylline, ethanol, sympathomimetics, methyldopa, tricyclic antidepressants, chloral hydrate, quinidine, quinine, tetracycline, B-complex vitamins, isoproterenol, levodopa, and monoamine oxidase inhibitors may raise urine catecholamine levels.
- Clonidine, guanethidine, reserpine, and iodine-containing contrast media may lower urine catecholamine levels.
- Phenothiazines, erythromycin, and methenamine compounds may raise or suppress catecholamine levels.
- Failure to comply with drug restrictions, to collect all urine during the test period, or to store the specimen properly may affect test results.

Cerebrospinal fluid analysis

Cerebrospinal fluid (CSF), a clear substance that circulates in the subarachnoid space, has many vital functions. It protects the brain and spinal cord from injury and transports products of neurosecretion, cellular biosynthesis, and cellular metabolism through the central nervous system (CNS). For qualitative analysis, CSF is most commonly obtained by lumbar puncture (usually between the third and fourth lumbar vertebrae); in rare instances, by cisternal or ventricular puncture. (See *Alternative methods of obtaining CSF*, page 146.) Specimens of CSF for laboratory analysis are commonly obtained during other neurologic tests such as myelography.

Purpose

■ To measure CSF pressure as an aid in detecting obstruction of CSF circulation
■ To aid diagnosis of viral or bacterial meningitis, subarachnoid or intracranial hemorrhage, tumors, and brain abscesses
■ To aid diagnosis of neurosyphilis and chronic CNS infections

Two tests use CSF specimens to check for Alzheimer's disease. (See *Two tests for Alzheimer's disease*, page 147.)

Patient preparation

Describe the procedure to the patient and explain that this test analyzes the fluid surrounding the spinal cord. Inform the patient that restriction of food or fluids isn't necessary. Tell the patient who will perform the procedure and where and that it usually takes at least 15 minutes.

Advise the patient that a headache is the most common adverse effect of lumbar puncture, but reassure him that his cooperation during the test helps minimize this reaction. Make sure the patient or a responsible family member has signed a consent form if required. If the patient is unusually anxious, assess his vital signs and notify the doctor.

Equipment

Lumbar puncture tray ■ sterile gloves ■ local anesthetic (usually 1% lidocaine) ■ povidone-iodine ■ small adhesive bandage.

Procedure

■ Position the patient on his side at the edge of the bed with his knees drawn up to his abdomen and his chin tucked against his chest (the fetal position). Provide pil-

ALTERNATIVE METHODS OF OBTAINING CSF

Cisternal puncture

When lumbar puncture is contraindicated by infection at the puncture site, lumbar deformity, or some other problem, the doctor may perform a cisternal puncture to obtain cerebrospinal fluid (CSF). A short-beveled, hollow needle is inserted into the cisterna cerebellomedullaris posterior, below the occipital bone, between the first cervical vertebra and the trim of the foramen magnum. Adverse reactions are minimal; the severe headaches that often occur after lumbar puncture are uncommon with this procedure. Cisternal puncture is hazardous because the needle is positioned close to the brain stem.

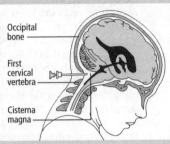

Contraindications are the same as for lumbar puncture — infection or deformity at the puncture site; increased intracranial pressure; or a history of thrombocytopenia or anticoagulant therapy, which may increase the potential for hemorrhage into the posterior fossa or cerebellar–brain stem area.

Prepare the patient as for lumbar puncture; a cisternal puncture tray contains the necessary equipment. The patient's neck should be flexed forward so that his chin touches his chest. Hold his head firmly in place to bring the brain stem and spinal cord forward and to allow more space for the cisternal needle to enter. If the doctor prefers, the patient may assume a sitting position, with his neck flexed forward.

Posttest care is the same as for lumbar puncture. With an outpatient, instruct a family member to check the puncture site for redness, swelling, and drainage and to watch for signs of complications, such as neck rigidity, irritability, and decreased level of consciousness.

Ventricular puncture

Although rarely performed, a ventricular puncture is the procedure of choice when a spinal puncture may cause brain stem herniation or other complications. A ventricular puncture is usually done in the operating room. The surgeon makes a small incision in the parieto-occipital region of the scalp and then drills a hole in the skull. A short-beveled, hollow needle is inserted through the hole and into a lateral ventricle, and CSF is withdrawn. Complications, such as ventriculitis and hemorrhage from ruptured blood vessels, are rare.

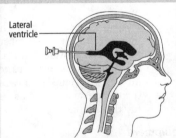

Ventricular puncture into posterior horn of right lateral ventricle

Posttest care is the same as for lumbar puncture, but don't elevate the head of the patient's bed more than 15 degrees. Bed rest for 24 hours is usually prescribed.

TWO TESTS FOR ALZHEIMER'S DISEASE

Two tests are used for patients with symptoms of dementia. One test determines the levels of tau protein and beta-amyloid in the cerebrospinal fluid (CSF) and requires a lumbar puncture. Increased levels of tau protein and decreased levels of beta-amyloid are associated with Alzheimer's disease. The manufacturer claims that this test is 95% accurate in ruling out or confirming Alzheimer's disease in about 60% of symptomatic patients older than 60 years of age.

The second test determines apolipoprotein E (apo E) genotype, which is statistically significant in determining the probability of Alzheimer's. The presence of two copies of the apo E4 allele may increase the probability to over 90%.

Although these tests may prove helpful in diagnosing Alzheimer's disease, experts caution that further studies are necessary to confirm their reliability.

lows to support the spine on a horizontal plane. This position allows full flexion of the spine and easy access to the lumbar subarachnoid space. Help the patient maintain this position by placing one arm around his knees and the other arm around his neck.

- If a sitting position is preferred, have the patient sit up and bend his chest and head toward his knees. Help him maintain this position throughout the procedure. Alternatively, have the patient lean over a bedside stand with a nurse in front of the stand to prevent it from moving.
- After the skin is prepared for injection, the area is draped. Warn the patient that he will probably experience a transient burning sensation when the local anesthetic is injected. Tell him that when the spinal needle is inserted, he may feel some transient local pain as the needle transverses the dura mater. Ask him to report any pain or sensations that differ from this or continue after this expected discomfort because these may indicate irritation or puncture of a nerve root, requiring repositioning of the needle. Instruct the patient to remain still and breathe normally; movement and hyperventilation can alter pressure readings or cause injury.
- The anesthetic is injected, and the spinal needle is inserted in the midline between the spinous processes of the vertebrae (usually between the third and fourth lumbar vertebrae). When the stylet is removed from the needle, CSF will drip from it if the needle is properly positioned. A stopcock and manometer are attached to the needle to measure the initial (opening) CSF pressure.
- After the specimen is collected, label the containers in the order in which they were filled and ask the doctor if there are any specific instructions for the laboratory. A final pressure reading is taken, and the needle is re-

moved. Clean the puncture site with a local antiseptic, such as povidone-iodine solution, and apply a small adhesive bandage.

■ Normally, the doctor records CSF pressure and checks the appearance of the specimen. Three tubes are routinely collected and sent to the laboratory for analysis of protein and glucose as well as RBCs and WBCs for serologic testing, for example, the Venereal Disease Research Laboratory test for neurosyphilis. A separate specimen is also sent to the laboratory for culture and sensitivity testing. Electrolyte analysis and Gram stain may be ordered as supplementary tests. CSF electrolyte levels are of special interest in patients with abnormal serum electrolyte levels or CSF infection and in those receiving hyperosmolar agents.

Precautions

■ Infection at the puncture site contraindicates removal of CSF.

CLINICAL ALERT In a patient with increased intracranial pressure, CSF should be removed with extreme caution because the rapid reduction in pressure that follows withdrawal of fluid can cause cerebellar tonsillar herniation and medullary compression.

■ During the procedure, observe closely for signs of an adverse reaction, such as elevated pulse rate, pallor, or clammy skin. Alert the doctor immediately to any significant changes.

■ Record the collection time on the laboratory request. Send the form and labeled specimens to the laboratory immediately.

Reference values and implications of results

For the implications of abnormal CSF analysis findings, see *Interpreting CSF findings.*

Posttest care

■ Find out if the patient must lie flat or if the head of his bed may be slightly elevated. In most cases, you will be instructed to keep the patient lying flat for 8 hours after lumbar puncture, but some doctors allow a 30-degree elevation. Remind the patient that, although he must not raise his head, he can turn from side to side.

■ Encourage the patient to drink fluids, and provide a flexible straw.

■ Check the puncture site for redness, swelling, and drainage every hour for the first 4 hours, then every 4 hours for the first 24 hours.

■ If CSF pressure is elevated, assess neurologic status every 15 minutes for 4 hours. If the patient is stable, as-

INTERPRETING CSF FINDINGS

The following tests on cerebrospinal (CSF) have widespread diagnostic significance.

Test	Normal	Abnormal	Implications
Pressure	50 to 180 mm H_2O	Increase	Increased intracranial pressure from hemorrhage, tumor, or edema caused by trauma
		Decrease	Spinal subarachnoid obstruction above puncture site
Appearance	Clear, colorless	Cloudy	Infection (elevated white blood cell [WBC] count and protein, or many microorganisms)
		Xanthochromic or bloody	Subarachnoid, intracerebral, or intraventricular hemorrhage; spinal cord obstruction; traumatic lumbar puncture (usually noted only in initial specimen)
		Brown, orange	Elevated protein levels, red blood cell (RBC) breakdown (blood present for at least 3 days)
Protein	15 to 45 mg/dl	Marked increase	Tumors, trauma, hemorrhage, diabetes mellitus, polyneuritis, blood in CSF
		Marked decrease	Rapid CSF production
Gamma globulin	3% to 12% of total protein	Increase	Demyelinating disease (such as multiple sclerosis), neurosyphilis, Guillain-Barré syndrome
Glucose	50 to 80 mg/dl	Increase	Systemic hyperglycemia
		Decrease	Systemic hypoglycemia, bacterial or fungal infection, meningitis, mumps, post-subarachnoid hemorrhage
Cell count	0 to 5 WBCs	Increase	Active disease: meningitis, acute infection, onset of chronic illness, tumor, abscess, infarction, demyelinating disease
	No RBCs	RBCs	Hemorrhage or traumatic lumbar puncture
Venereal Disease Research Laboratories test for syphilis and other serologic tests	Nonreactive	Positive	Neurosyphilis

(continued)

INTERPRETING CSF FINDINGS (continued)			
Test	Normal	Abnormal	Implications
Chloride	118 to 130 mEq/L	Decrease	Infected meninges (as in tuberculosis or meningitis)
Gram stain	No organisms	Gram-positive or gram-negative organisms	Bacterial meningitis

sess every hour for 2 hours, then every 4 hours or according to pretest schedule.

■ Watch for complications of lumbar puncture, such as a reaction to the anesthetic, meningitis, bleeding into the spinal canal, and cerebellar tonsillar herniation and medullary compression. Signs of meningitis include fever, neck rigidity, and irritability; signs of herniation include decreased level of consciousness, changes in pupil size and equality, altered vital signs (including widened pulse pressure, decreased pulse rate, and irregular respirations), and respiratory failure.

Interfering factors

■ The patient's position and activity can alter CSF pressure. Crying, coughing, or straining may increase pressure.

■ Delay between collection time and laboratory testing can invalidate results, especially cell counts.

Ceruloplasmin test, serum

This test measures serum levels of ceruloplasmin, an alpha$_2$-globulin that binds about 95% of serum copper, usually in the liver. Little copper exists in the body in a free state. Because ceruloplasmin catalyzes oxidation of ferrous compounds to ferric ions, it is thought to regulate iron uptake by transferrin, making iron available to reticulocytes for heme synthesis. The usual clinical indications for this assay are Menkes' kinky-hair syndrome, suspected copper deficiency from total parenteral nutrition, and suspected Wilson's disease.

Purpose

To aid diagnosis of Wilson's disease, Menkes' kinky-hair syndrome, and copper deficiency.

Patient preparation

Explain to the patient that this test helps determine the copper content of the blood. Tell the patient the test requires a blood sample, explain who will perform the venipuncture and when, and note that the needle puncture and the tourniquet may cause transient discomfort. Check the patient's medication history for drugs that may influence ceruloplasmin levels.

Procedure

Perform a venipuncture and collect the sample in a 7-ml clot-activator tube.

Precautions

Send the sample to the laboratory immediately.

Reference values

Serum ceruloplasmin levels for adults normally range from 22.9 to 43.1 mg/dl.

Implications of results

Low ceruloplasmin levels usually indicate Wilson's disease; this is confirmed by Kayser-Fleischer rings (copper deposits in the corneas that form green-gold rings) or by liver biopsy results that show 250 μg of copper per gram of dry weight. Low ceruloplasmin levels may also occur in Menkes' kinky-hair syndrome, nephrotic syndrome, and hypocupremia caused by total parenteral nutrition. Elevated levels may indicate certain hepatic diseases and infections.

Posttest care

If a hematoma develops, apply warm soaks.

Interfering factors

■ Estrogen, methadone, and phenytoin may elevate serum ceruloplasmin levels.
■ Pregnancy may elevate serum ceruloplasmin levels.

Cervical punch biopsy

Cervical punch biopsy is the excision by sharp forceps of a tissue specimen from the cervix for histologic examination. Generally, multiple biopsies are done to obtain specimens from all areas with abnormal tissue or from the squamocolumnar junction and other sites around the cervical circumference.

This procedure is indicated for women with suspicious cervical lesions and should be performed when the cervix is least vascular (usually 1 week after menses). Biopsy sites are selected by direct visualization of the cervix with a colposcope, which is the most accurate method, or by Schiller's test, which stains normal squamous epithelium a dark mahogany but fails to color abnormal tissue. (For information on other biopsies done

ENDOMETRIAL AND OVARIAN BIOPSIES

This chart lists purposes and special considerations for two types of biopsy.

Method	Purpose	Special considerations
Endometrial biopsy ■ Dilation and curettage (D&C) ■ Endometrial washing (by jet irrigation, aspiration, or brushing)	■ To evaluate uterine bleeding ■ To diagnose suspected endometrial cancer ■ To diagnose a missed abortion	■ Time of menstrual cycle affects accuracy of biopsy results. ■ Type of specimen obtained depends on patient's age and disorder. ■ Endometrial washing requires no anesthesia and can be done in a doctor's office.
Ovarian biopsy ■ Transrectal or transvaginal fine-needle biopsy ■ Aspiration biopsy during laparoscopy	■ To detect an ovarian tumor ■ To determine the spread of cancer	■ D&C by endometrial washing may follow a negative biopsy. ■ Specimens obtained by D&C may be processed as frozen sections. ■ Fine-needle biopsy may follow palpation, laparoscopy, or computed tomography that detects an abnormal ovary. ■ Aspiration during laparoscopy is particularly useful for young women who are infertile or who have lesions that appear benign.

to detect gynecologic disorders, see *Endometrial and ovarian biopsies*.)

Purpose
■ To evaluate suspicious cervical lesions
■ To diagnose cervical cancer.

Patient preparation
Describe the procedure to the patient and explain that it provides a cervical tissue specimen for microscopic study. Tell her who will perform the biopsy and where and that it takes about 15 minutes. Tell the patient that she may experience mild discomfort during and after the biopsy. Advise the outpatient to have someone accompany her home after the biopsy. Make sure the patient has signed a consent form. Just before the biopsy, ask her to void.

Procedure
■ Place the patient in the lithotomy position. Tell her to relax as the unlubricated speculum is inserted.
■ For direct visualization: The colposcope is inserted through the speculum, the biopsy site is located, and the cervix is cleaned with a swab soaked in 3% acetic acid solution. The biopsy forceps are then inserted through the speculum or the colposcope and tissue is removed from any lesion or from selected sites, starting from the posterior lip to avoid obscuring other sites with blood.

Each specimen is immediately put in 10% formalin solution in a labeled bottle. To control bleeding after biopsy, the cervix is swabbed with 5% silver nitrate solution (cautery or sutures may be used instead). If bleeding persists, the examiner may insert a tampon.

■ For Schiller's test: An applicator stick saturated with iodine solution is inserted through the speculum. This stains the cervix to identify lesions for biopsy.

■ Record the names of the patient and clinician as well as the biopsy sites on the laboratory request.

Precautions

Send the specimens to the laboratory immediately.

Normal findings

Cervical tissue should be composed of columnar and squamous epithelial cells, loose connective tissue, and smooth-muscle fibers, with no dysplasia or abnormal cell growth.

Implications of results

Histologic examination of a cervical tissue specimen identifies abnormal cells and differentiates the tissue as intraepithelial neoplasia or invasive cancer. If the cause of an abnormal Papanicolaou (Pap) test is not demonstrated by cervical biopsy or if the specimen shows advanced dysplasia or carcinoma in situ, a cone biopsy is performed in the operating room under general anesthesia. A cone biopsy garners a larger tissue specimen and allows a more accurate evaluation of dysplasia.

Posttest care

■ Instruct the patient to avoid strenuous exercise for 8 to 24 hours after the biopsy. Encourage the outpatient to rest briefly before leaving the office.

■ If a tampon was inserted after the biopsy, tell the patient to leave it in place for 8 to 24 hours. Inform her that some bleeding may occur, but tell her to report heavy bleeding (heavier than menstrual) to the doctor. Warn the patient to avoid using additional tampons, which can irritate the cervix and provoke bleeding, according to her doctor's directions.

■ Tell the patient to avoid douching and to refrain from intercourse for up to 2 weeks, or as directed, if she has undergone such treatments as cryotherapy or laser treatment during the procedure.

■ Inform the patient that a foul-smelling, gray-green vaginal discharge is normal for several days after the biopsy and may persist for 3 weeks.

Interfering factors

Failure to obtain representative specimens or to place them in the preservative immediately may alter results.

Chlamydia trachomatis *culture*

The most common cause of sexually transmitted disease in the United States is *Chlamydia trachomatis*, an obligate intracellular parasite organism that must be cultivated in the laboratory by infection of susceptible cells.

In this procedure, the elementary bodies of *C. trachomatis* attach to specific receptor sites on McCoy cells and are engulfed by the cytoplasm of the cells where the organisms divide within inclusion bodies. After 48 hours of incubation, chlamydia-infected cells can be detected by fluorescein isothiocyanate-conjugated monoclonal antibodies (FITC-MoAb) or by iodine stain. Optimal conditions for recovery of *C. trachomatis* include infection of McCoy cells in shell vials, centrifugation at 700 × G, incubation for 48 hours, and staining with FITC-MoAb rather than iodine.

Recovery of *C. trachomatis* is considered the laboratory method of choice, although rapid nonculture (antigen detection) procedures are available for processing specimens from most clinical sites. Strains of *C. psittaci* and *C. pneumoniae* aren't detected in these cell cultures without specific technical manipulations and reagents for detecting these species. (See *DNA detection of* Chlamydia trachomatis.)

Purpose

To confirm infection caused by *C. trachomatis*.

Patient preparation

Explain the purpose of the test and the procedure for collecting the specimen. If the specimen will be collected from the genital tract, instruct the patient not to urinate for 3 to 4 hours before the specimen is taken. Instruct a female patient not to douche for 24 hours before the test. Tell a male patient that he may experience some burning and pressure as the culture is taken but that the discomfort will subside after a few minutes.

Equipment

Gloves ■ sterile cotton swabs ■ wire bacteriologic loop or thin urogenital alginate swabs (for male patient) ■ vaginal speculum ■ sucrose phosphate (2SP) transport medium ■ microbiologic transport swab or cytobrush.

Procedure

■ Obtain a specimen of the epithelial cells from the infected site. In adults, these sites may include the eye,

---

DNA DETECTION OF *CHLAMYDIA TRACHOMATIS*

The Food and Drug Administration has approved a test that will detect *Chlamydia trachomatis* deoxyribonucleic acid (DNA) in cervical specimens: Digene Corporation's Hybrid Capture II Chlamydia test. The test is indicated to identify or confirm the presence of *C. trachomatis* in women who may be susceptible to the infection, whether they have symptoms or not.

---

urethra, endocervix, or rectum. Epithelial cells are collected from the urethra rather than from the purulent exudate that may be present.

■ You can obtain a urethral specimen by inserting a cotton-tipped applicator ⅖" to 2" (2 to 5 cm) into the urethra. To collect a specimen from the endocervix, use a microbiologic transport swab or cytobrush. Then extract the specimen into sucrose phosphate (2SP) transport medium. Specimens collected from the throat, eye, and nasopharynx and aspirates from infants should be extracted into 2SP transport medium. Send the specimens to the laboratory at 39.2° F (4° C).

■ If the anticipated time between specimen collection and inoculation into cell culture is more than 24 hours, freeze the 2SP transport medium and send it to the laboratory with dry ice.

CLINICAL ALERT If you suspect that your patient has been sexually abused, test all specimens for *C. trachomatis* by culture rather than antigen detection methods.

■ If the culture confirms infection, provide counseling for the patient regarding treatment of sexual partners.

■ Advise the patient to avoid all sexual contact until test results are available.

Precautions

■ Place the male patient in the supine position to prevent him from falling if he develops vasovagal syncope when the cotton swab or wire loop is introduced into the urethra. Observe him for profound hypotension, bradycardia, pallor, and sweating.

■ Use gloves when performing procedures and handling specimens.

■ Collect a urethral specimen at least 1 hour after the patient has voided to prevent loss of urethral secretions.

■ After collecting the specimens, carefully dispose of gloves, swabs, and speculum to prevent staff exposure to the organism.

Normal findings

No pathogens should appear in the culture.

Implications of results

A positive culture confirms *C. trachomatis*.

Interfering factors

■ Use of an antimicrobial within a few days before collection of the specimen may prevent recovery of *C. trachomatis*.

■ Improper collection technique may provide an unrepresentative or contaminated specimen.

■ Fecal material may contaminate a rectal culture.

■ In males, voiding within 1 hour before specimen collection washes secretions out of the urethra, making fewer organisms available for culture.

■ In females, douching within 24 hours before specimen collection can interfere with results by washing out cervical secretions, making fewer organisms available for culture.

Chloride test, serum

This test, a quantitative analysis, measures serum levels of chloride, the major extracellular fluid anion. Interacting with sodium, chloride helps maintain the osmotic pressure of blood and therefore helps regulate blood volume and arterial pressure. Chloride levels also affect acid-base balance. Serum concentrations of this electrolyte are regulated by aldosterone secondarily to regulation of sodium. Chloride is absorbed from the intestines and is excreted primarily by the kidneys.

Purpose

To detect acid-base imbalance (acidosis and alkalosis) and to aid evaluation of fluid status and extracellular cation-anion balance.

Patient preparation

Explain to the patient that this test evaluates the chloride content of blood. Tell him this test requires a blood sample, discuss who will perform the venipuncture and when, and note that he may feel some transient discomfort from the needle puncture and the pressure of the tourniquet. Check the patient history for use of drugs that influence chloride levels.

Procedure

Perform a venipuncture and collect the sample in a 7-ml clot-activator tube.

Precautions

Handle the sample gently to prevent hemolysis.

Reference values

Normal serum chloride levels range from 100 to 108 mEq/L.

Implications of results

Chloride levels relate inversely to those of bicarbonate and thus reflect acid-base balance. Excessive loss of gastric juices or of other secretions containing chloride may cause hypochloremic metabolic alkalosis; excessive chloride retention or ingestion may lead to hyperchloremic metabolic acidosis.

Elevated serum chloride levels (hyperchloremia) may result from bicarbonate loss caused by diarrhea, severe dehydration, complete renal shutdown, head injury (producing neurogenic hyperventilation), or primary aldosteronism.

Low chloride levels (hypochloremia) are usually associated with low sodium and potassium levels. Possible underlying causes include prolonged vomiting, gastric suctioning, intestinal fistula, chronic renal failure, and Addison's disease. Congestive heart failure or edema resulting in excess extracellular fluid can cause dilutional hypochloremia.

Both hypochloremia and hyperchloremia require treatment of the underlying condition for correction.

Posttest care

If a hematoma develops, apply warm soaks.

CLINICAL ALERT Observe a patient with hypochloremia for hypertonicity of muscles, tetany, and depressed respirations. In a patient with hyperchloremia, be alert for signs of developing stupor, rapid deep breathing, and weakness that may lead to coma.

Interfering factors

■ Elevated serum chloride levels may result from administration of ammonium chloride, cholestyramine, boric acid, oxyphenbutazone, or phenylbutazone or from excessive I.V. infusion of sodium chloride.

■ Serum chloride levels are decreased by thiazide diuretics, ethacrynic acid, furosemide, bicarbonates, or prolonged I.V. infusion of dextrose 5% in water.

■ Hemolysis caused by rough handling of the sample may interfere with accurate determination of test results.

Cholesterol test, total

The quantitative analysis of serum cholesterol measures the circulating levels of free cholesterol and cholesterol esters; it reflects the level of the two forms in which this biochemical compound appears in the body.

Cholesterol, a structural component in cell membranes and plasma lipoproteins, is absorbed from the diet and synthesized in the liver and other body tissues from those saturated fats in the diet. The body uses cholesterol for numerous functions, including steroid and hormone synthesis (sex hormones as well as adrenal steroids), cell membrane biogenesis, and formation of bile acids.

The human body can produce all the cholesterol it requires, although researchers estimate that 20% to 40% is obtained through diet. A diet high in saturated fat raises cholesterol levels by stimulating absorption of lipids, including cholesterol, from the intestine; a diet low in saturated fat lowers cholesterol levels. High serum cholesterol levels may be associated with an increased risk of atherosclerosis-related diseases, especially coronary artery disease (CAD).

A total serum cholesterol level should be screened at least once every 5 years in people age 21 and older.

Purpose

- To assess the risk of atherosclerosis and CAD
- To evaluate fat metabolism
- To aid in monitoring the effects of other disease processes such as nephrotic syndrome, diabetes mellitus, pancreatitis, hepatic disease, and hypothyroidism and hyperthyroidism
- To assess the efficacy of lipid-lowering drug therapy.

Patient preparation

Explain that this test determines the body's fat metabolism by measuring the amount of cholesterol in the blood. Fasting isn't needed for isolated cholesterol checks or screening but is required if the test is part of a lipid profile.

If fasting is required, instruct the patient to abstain from food and drink for 12 hours before the test. Tell him the test requires a blood sample, who will perform the venipuncture and when, and that he may experience transient discomfort from the needle puncture and the pressure of the tourniquet. Withhold drugs that may affect test results.

Procedure

Perform a venipuncture and collect the sample in a 7-ml tube containing EDTA. The patient should be in a sitting position for 5 minutes before the blood is drawn. Fingersticks can also be used for initial screening when using an automated analyzer. Always observe universal precautions. Document any drugs the patient is taking.

Precautions

Send the sample to the laboratory immediately.

Reference values

Total cholesterol levels vary with age and sex. Total cholesterol values for adults and children are as follows:
- adults: desirable: < 209 mg/dl for women and <191 mg/dl for men; borderline-high: up to 239 mg/dl, depending on sex; high: > 240 mg/dl
- children 12 to 18 years of age: desirable: < 170 mg/dl; high: > 200 mg/dl.

Implications of results

The cholesterol level needs to be evaluated in the context of an entire risk factor analysis for each individual patient. If the level is abnormal, a second cholesterol test should be completed in 1 week to verify the results. Marked fluctuations can occur from day to day. A decision to begin treatment will be based on the number of risk factors and a patient's prior cardiovascular history.

An elevated serum cholesterol level (hypercholesterolemia) may indicate an increased risk for CAD as well as incipient hepatitis, lipid disorders, bile duct blockage, nephrotic syndrome, obstructive jaundice, pancreatitis, and hypothyroidism. Hypercholesterolemia associated with increased intake of fats and cholesterol-rich foods requires dietary changes and, possibly, medication to retard absorption of cholesterol.

Diet therapy can decrease cholesterol levels 10% to 15%. A dietitian referral is helpful. The patient will need to replace saturated fats with polyunsaturated fats. In addition, increasing soluble fiber in the diet may help to decrease cholesterol levels. Weight loss and exercise programs should also be instituted.

A low serum cholesterol level (hypocholesterolemia) is commonly associated with malnutrition, cellular necrosis of the liver, or hyperthyroidism.

Abnormal cholesterol levels commonly require further testing to pinpoint the causative disorder, depending on the type of abnormality and the presence of overt signs. Abnormal levels associated with cardiovascular diseases, for example, may require lipoprotein phenotyping.

Posttest care
- If a hematoma develops, apply warm soaks.
- Resume diet and medications discontinued before the test.

Interfering factors
- Failure to follow dietary restrictions may interfere with test results.
- Cholesterol levels are lowered by cholestyramine, clofibrate, colestipol, dextrothyroxine, haloperidol, neomycin, niacin, and chlortetracycline.
- Levels are raised by epinephrine, chlorpromazine, trifluoperazine, oral contraceptives, and trimethadione.
- Androgens may have a variable effect on cholesterol levels. Some antibiotics may cause falsely low readings.
- Some vitamins (such as vitamin E) may cause false elevations.
- Pregnancy may increase levels.
- Seasonal variation in levels has been observed with higher values in winter and fall and lower values in spring and summer.
- Emotional stress and menstrual cycle may also affect the levels.
- If a genetic lipid disorder is discovered, family members should be screened for cholesterol abnormalities.
- Cholesterol levels shouldn't be measured immediately after a myocardial infarction (MI) because of falsely low readings. In these patients, cholesterol levels should be evaluated 3 months after the MI.

Cholinesterase test

The cholinesterase test measures the amounts of two similar enzymes that hydrolyze acetylcholine: acetylcholinesterase (or true cholinesterase) and pseudocholinesterase (also known as serum cholinesterase). Acetylcholinesterase is present in nerve tissue, red cells of the spleen, and the gray matter of the brain. It inactivates acetylcholine at nerve junctions and helps transmit impulses across nerve endings to muscle fibers.

Pseudocholinesterase is produced primarily in the liver and appears in small amounts in the pancreas, intestine, heart, and white matter of the brain. Although pseudocholinesterase has no known function, its measurement is significant because certain chemicals that inactivate acetylcholinesterase also affect pseudocholinesterase.

Two groups of anticholinesterase chemicals — organophosphates and muscle relaxants — are important. Organophosphates, which are used by the military as nerve gases and are common ingredients in many insecticides, inactivate acetylcholinesterase directly. Muscle relaxants (such as succinylcholine chloride), which interfere with acetylcholine-mediated transmission across nerve endings, are normally destroyed by pseudocholinesterase.

When poisoning by an organophosphate (such as parathion) is suspected, either cholinesterase may be measured. For technical reasons, pseudocholinesterase is generally tested (although this analysis is less sensitive than the one for acetylcholinesterase).

In muscle relaxant poisoning, prolonged apnea develops not from the drug itself but because the patient lacks adequate pseudocholinesterase, which normally inactivates the muscle relaxant. In this case, measurement of pseudocholinesterase is required.

Purpose

■ To evaluate, preoperatively or before electroconvulsive therapy, the patient's potential response to succinylcholine, which is hydrolyzed by cholinesterase
■ To detect atypical forms of pseudocholinesterase to identify those patients who may have adverse reactions to muscle relaxants
■ To assess overexposure to insecticides containing organophosphates
■ To assess liver function and aid diagnosis of liver disease (rarely).

Patient preparation

Explain to the patient that this test assesses muscle function or the extent of exposure to poisoning. Inform him that he needn't restrict food or fluids. Tell him the test requires a blood sample, who will perform the venipuncture and when, and that he may experience transient discomfort from the needle puncture and the pressure of the tourniquet.

Withhold substances that affect serum cholinesterase levels. If such substances must be continued, note this on the laboratory request.

Procedure

Perform a venipuncture, and collect the sample in a 7-ml red-top tube.

Precautions

■ Handle the collection tube gently to prevent hemolysis.

■ If the sample can't be sent to the laboratory within 6 hours after being drawn, refrigerate it.

Reference values

Pseudocholinesterase levels range from 5 to 12 U/ml (when determined by kinetic colorimetric technique).

Implications of results

Very low pseudocholinesterase levels suggest a congenital deficiency or organophosphate insecticide poisoning; levels near zero necessitate emergency treatment.

Pseudocholinesterase levels are usually normal in early extrahepatic obstruction and decreased in hepatocellular damage, such as hepatitis or cirrhosis. Levels also decline in acute infections, chronic malnutrition, anemia, myocardial infarction, obstructive jaundice, and metastasis.

Posttest care

■ If a hematoma develops, apply warm soaks.
■ Resume administration of medications that were discontinued before the test.

Interfering factors

■ Serum cholinesterase levels can be falsely depressed by cyclophosphamide, echothiophate iodide, monoamine oxidase inhibitors, succinylcholine, neostigmine, quinine, quinidine, chloroquine, caffeine, theophylline, epinephrine, ether, barbiturates, atropine, morphine, codeine, phenothiazines, vitamin K, and folic acid.
■ Hemolysis caused by rough handling of the sample may alter test results.
■ Pregnancy or recent surgery may affect test results.

Chromosome analysis

Chromosomes are threadlike bodies in the cell nucleus that are made up of deoxyribonucleic acid (DNA), the basic genetic material. Each chromosome contains thousands of genes that determine biochemical programs for cell function. Chromosome analysis, an integral facet of cytogenetics, studies the relationship between the microscopic appearance of chromosomes and the person's phenotype — the expression of the genes in physical, biochemical, and physiologic traits.

Light microscopy can visualize the chromosomes, but no available technology can directly visualize individual genes. Ideally, chromosomes should be studied during metaphase, the middle phase of mitosis, when new cell poles appear. Only rapidly dividing cell lines, such as bone marrow or neoplastic cells, permit direct, immedi-

PERCUTANEOUS UMBILICAL BLOOD SAMPLING

Useful in chromosomal analysis, percutaneous umbilical blood sampling (PUBS) provides a fetal blood sample for karyotype, direct Coombs' test, or complete blood count. PUBS, sometimes called cordocentesis, can also be used to determine fetal blood type, check blood gas levels and acid-base status, and identify and treat isoimmunization.

To obtain a percutaneous umbilical blood sample:
- A needle is inserted transabdominally (using ultrasound guidance) into a fetal umbilical vessel.
- A blood sample is then tested by Kleihauer-Betke method to verify that fetal and not maternal blood has been drawn.

Possible complications include blood leakage at the puncture site, fetal bradycardia, or infection.

ate study. Most other cell types require stimulation of mitosis by addition of phytohemagglutinin to the culture. Subsequently, the addition of colchicine (a cell poison) arrests the cell division in metaphase. Harvested, stained, and viewed under a microscope, the cells are finally photographed to provide a karyotype, the systematic arrangement of chromosomes in groupings according to size and shape.

Indications for the test determine the type of specimen required (blood, bone marrow, amniotic fluid, skin, and placental or tumor tissue) and the procedure. Umbilical cord sampling may also be used to perform chromosome analysis. (See *Percutaneous umbilical blood sampling*.)

Purpose

To identify chromosomal abnormalities, such as hypoploidy (fewer than 46 chromosomes) or hyperploidy (more than 46 chromosomes), as the underlying cause of malformation, maldevelopment, or disease.

Patient preparation

Explain to the patient or to his parents, if appropriate, that this test identifies the underlying cause of maldevelopment or disease due to a chromosomal abnormality. Tell him who will perform the test and what kind of specimen will be required. Inform him when results will be available, according to the specimen required. For example, test results on a blood sample are generally available 72 to 96 hours after stimulation; analysis of skin biopsy specimens or amniotic fluid cells may take several weeks.

Procedure

- As appropriate, collect a blood sample (in a 5- to 10-ml heparinized tube), a tissue specimen, 1 ml of bone marrow, or at least 20 ml of amniotic fluid.
- Explain the test results and their implications to the patient or to the parents of a child with a chromosomal abnormality.
- If necessary, recommend appropriate genetic or other counseling and follow-up care, such as an infant stimulation program for a child with Down syndrome.

Precautions

- Keep all specimens sterile, especially those requiring a tissue culture.
- To facilitate interpretation of test results, send the specimen to the laboratory immediately, with a brief patient history and the indication for the test. If transport must be delayed, refrigerate the specimen but don't freeze it.
- Before a skin biopsy, make sure the povidone-iodine solution is thoroughly removed with alcohol. This solution could prevent cell growth in the tissue culture.

Normal findings

The normal cell contains 46 chromosomes: 22 pairs of nonsex chromosomes (autosomes) and 2 sex chromosomes (XY in males, XX in females). On a karyotype, chromosomes are arranged according to size and the location of their primary constrictions, or centromeres. The centromere may be medial (metacentric), slightly to one end of the chromosome (submetacentric), or entirely to one end (acrocentric). The largest chromosomes are displayed first; the others are arranged in order of decreasing size; the two sex chromosomes are traditionally placed last, but they may be separated and arranged with the other chromosomes in order of size.

By convention, the centromere is always placed at the top in a karyotype. Thus, if the two pairs of chromosomal arms are of unequal length, the arm above the centromere will be shorter. The letter *p* designates the short arm; the letter *q*, the long arm.

Special stains identify individual chromosomes and locate and enumerate particular portions of chromosomes. Trypsin, alkali, heat denaturation, and Giemsa stain are used for visible light microscopy; quinacrine stain, for ultraviolet microscopy. These staining techniques produce nonuniform staining of each chromosome in a repetitive, banded pattern. The mechanism of chromosome banding is unknown but seems related to primary DNA sequence and protein composition of the chromosome.

Implications of results

Chromosomal abnormalities may be numerical or structural. Numerical deviation from the norm of 46 chromosomes is called aneuploidy. Fewer than 46 chromosomes is called hypoploidy; more than 46, hyperploidy. Special designations exist for whole multiples of the haploid number 23: diploidy for the normal somatic number of 46, triploidy for 69, tetraploidy for 92, and so forth. When the deviation occurs within a single pair of chromosomes, the suffix -somy is used, as in trisomy for the presence of three chromosomes instead of the usual pair, or monosomy for the presence of only one chromosome.

Aneuploidy most commonly follows failure of the chromosomal pair to separate (nondisjunction) during anaphase, the mitotic stage that follows metaphase. It may also result from anaphase lag, in which one of the normally separated chromosomes fails to move to a pole and is left out of the daughter cells. If nondisjunction or anaphase lag occurs during meiosis, the cells of the zygote will all be the same. Errors in mitotic division after the formation of the zygote will produce more than one cell line in an individual (mosaicism).

Structural chromosomal abnormalities result from chromosome breakage. Intrachromosomal rearrangement occurs within a single chromosome in the following forms:

■ deletion: loss of an end (terminal) or middle (interstitial) portion of a chromosome

■ inversion: end-to-end reversal of a chromosome segment, which may be pericentric inversion (including the centromere) or paracentric inversion (occurring in only one arm of the chromosome)

■ ring chromosome formation: breakage of both ends of a chromosome and reunion of the ends

■ isochromosome formation: abnormal splitting of the centromere in a transverse rather than longitudinal plane.

Interchromosomal rearrangements (of more than one chromosome, usually two) also occur. The most common rearrangement is translocation (exchange) of genetic material between two chromosomes. Translocations occur in the following ways:

■ balanced, in which the cell neither loses nor gains genetic material

■ unbalanced, in which a piece of genetic material is gained or lost from each cell

CHROMOSOME ANALYSIS FINDINGS

Specimens for chromosome analysis can be obtained from blood, bone marrow, skin, amniotic fluid, placental tissue, and tumor tissue. This chart lists the indications for chromosome analysis, the possible findings, and the implications of such findings.

Specimen and indication	Possible findings	Implications
Blood To evaluate abnormal appearance of development suggesting chromosomal irregularity	Abnormal chromosome number (aneuploidy) or arrangement	Identifies specific chromosomal abnormality
To evaluate couple with history of miscarriages or to identify balanced translocation carriers having unbalanced offspring	Normal chromosomes	Miscarriage unrelated to parental chromosomal abnormality
	Parental balanced translocation carrier	Increased risk of repeated abortion or unbalanced offspring indicates need for amniocentesis in future pregnancies
To detect chromosomal rearrangements in rare genetic diseases predisposing patient to malignant neoplasms	Chromosomal rearrangements, gaps, and breaks	Occurs in Bloom syndrome, Fanconi's syndrome, telangiectasia; patient predisposed to malignant neoplasms
Blood and bone marrow To identify Philadelphia chromosome and confirm chronic myelogenous leukemia	Translocation of chromosome 22q (long arm) to another chromosome (often chromosome 9)	Aids diagnosis of chronic myelogenous leukemia
	Aneuploidy (usually associated with abnormalities in chromosomes 8 and 12)	Occurs in acute myelogenous leukemia
	Trisomy 21	Occasionally occurs in chronic lymphocytic leukemia cells
Skin To evaluate abnormal appearance or development suggesting chromosomal irregularity	All chromosomal abnormalities are possible	Same as chromosomal abnormality in blood; in rare cases, mosaic individual has normal blood but abnormal skin chromosomes
Amniotic fluid To evaluate developing fetus with possible chromosomal abnormality	All chromosomal abnormalities are possible	Same as chromosomal abnormality in blood or fetus

(continued)

CHROMOSOME ANALYSIS FINDINGS (continued)		
Specimen and indication	**Possible findings**	**Implications**
Placental tissue To evaluate products of conception after a miscarriage to determine if abnormality is fetal or placental in origin	All chromosomal abnormalities are possible	Over 50% of aborted tissue is chromosomally abnormal
Tumor tissue For research purposes only	Many chromosomal abnormalities are possible	Although malignant tumors aren't associated with specific chromosomal aberrations, most are aneuploid (usually hyperploid)

■ reciprocal (in children), in which two chromosomes exchange material
■ robertsonian, in which two chromosomes fuse to form one large chromosome with little or no loss of material.
  Implications of chromosome analysis results depend on the type of specimen and the indications for the test. (See *Chromosome analysis findings.*)

Posttest care
■ Depending on the procedure used, provide post-test care, as appropriate. (See "Bone marrow aspiration and biopsy," page 116; "Amniotic fluid analysis," page 51; and *Percutaneous umbilical blood sampling*, page 163.)
■ Resume administration of medications that were discontinued before the test.

Interfering factors
■ Chemotherapy may cause implications of results, such as chromosome breaks.
■ Contamination of tissue with bacteria, fungus, or a virus may inhibit growth of the culture.
■ Inclusion of maternal cells in a specimen obtained by amniocentesis, with subsequent culturing, may cause false results.

Cold agglutinin test
Cold agglutinins are antibodies (usually of the IgM type) that cause red blood cells (RBCs) to aggregate at low temperatures. Transient elevations of these antibodies develop during certain infectious diseases, notably primary atypical pneumonia. Small amounts may also occur in healthy people. This test reliably detects such pneumonia within 1 to 2 weeks after onset.

Although cold agglutinins are inert at inner body temperatures, some become active in exposed areas of skin at 82.4° to 89.6° F (28° to 32° C), producing pallor and acrocyanosis (Raynaud's phenomenon) and numbness of hands and feet. Intense agglutination of a whole blood sample occurs on cooling to temperatures between 32° and 68° F (0° and 20° C), peaking at 39.2° F (4° C), and is reversible by rewarming to 98.6° F (37° C). However, after rewarming, complement remains on the cell and may produce hemolysis. Consequently, patients with high cold agglutinin titers, such as those with primary atypical pneumonia, may develop acute transient hemolytic anemia after repeated exposure to cold; patients with persistently high titers may develop chronic hemolytic anemia.

Purpose

- To help confirm diagnosis of primary atypical pneumonia
- To provide additional diagnostic evidence for cold agglutinin disease associated with many viral infections or lymphoreticular malignancy.

Patient preparation

Explain to the patient that this test detects antibodies in the blood that attack RBCs after exposure to low temperatures. If appropriate, inform him that the test will be repeated to monitor his response to therapy. Advise him that it isn't necessary to restrict food or fluids. Tell him that the test requires a blood sample, who will perform the venipuncture and when, and that he may experience transient discomfort from the needle puncture and the pressure of the tourniquet.

If the patient is receiving antimicrobial drugs, note this on the laboratory request because these drugs may interfere with the development of cold agglutinins.

Procedure

- Perform a venipuncture and collect the sample in a 7-ml tube without additives that has been prewarmed to 98.6° F (37° C).
- If cold agglutinin disease is suspected, keep the patient warm. If the patient is exposed to low temperatures, agglutination may occur within peripheral vessels, possibly leading to frostbite, anemia, Raynaud's phenomenon or, in rare cases, focal gangrene.
- Watch for signs of vascular abnormalities, such as mottled skin, purpura, jaundice, or pallor; pain or swelling of extremities; and cramping of fingers and toes. Hemoglobinuria may result from severe intravascular hemolysis on exposure to severe cold.

Precautions

■ Handle the sample gently to prevent hemolysis and send it to the laboratory immediately.

CLINICAL ALERT Do not refrigerate the sample; cold agglutinins will coat the RBCs, leaving none in the serum.

Reference values

Results are reported as positive or negative. Positive results are titered. Normal titers are less than 1:64, but they may be higher in elderly persons.

Implications of results

High titers may occur as primary phenomena or secondary to infections or lymphoreticular malignancy. Elevations may be present in infectious mononucleosis, cytomegalovirus infection, hemolytic anemia, multiple myeloma, scleroderma, malaria, cirrhosis, congenital syphilis, peripheral vascular disease, pulmonary embolism, trypanosomiasis, tonsillitis, staphylococcemia, scarlatina, influenza and, occasionally, in pregnancy. Chronically elevated titers are most commonly associated with pneumonia and lymphoreticular malignancy; an acute transient elevation commonly accompanies many viral infections.

In primary atypical pneumonia, cold agglutinins appear in serum in one-half to two-thirds of all patients during the first week of acute infection, even before antimycoplasmal antibodies can be detected by complement fixation or metabolic inhibition tests. Thus, titers usually become positive at 7 days, peak above 1:32 in 4 weeks, and disappear rapidly after 6 weeks. When sequential titers verify this pattern and clinical evidence of pneumonia exists, the diagnosis is confirmed.

Extremely high titers (1:2000 or higher) can occur with idiopathic cold agglutinin disease that precedes development of lymphoma. Patients with titers this high are susceptible to intravascular agglutination, which causes significant clinical problems.

Posttest care

If a hematoma develops, apply warm soaks.

Interfering factors

■ Antimicrobials can interfere with the development of cold agglutinins.

■ Hemolysis caused by rough handling of the sample can falsely depress titers, as can refrigeration of the sample before serum is separated from RBCs.

Complement assays

Complement is a collective term for a system of at least 15 serum proteins that work together to destroy foreign cells and to help remove foreign materials. The system may be triggered by contact with antigen-antibody complexes or clotting factor XIIa. A cascade of events follows, resulting in the formation of a complex that ruptures cell membranes.

Complement components are numerically designated as C1 through C9, with C1 having three subcomponents: C1q, C1r, and C1s. These components constitute 3% to 4% of total serum globulins and play a key role in antibody-mediated immune reactions.

Complement can function as a defense by promoting removal of infectious agents or as a threat by triggering destructive reactions in host tissues. Therefore, complement deficiency can increase susceptibility to infection and can predispose a person to other diseases. Complement assays are thus indicated in patients with known or suspected immune-mediated disease or repeatedly abnormal response to infection.

Normally, complement is present in serum in an inactive state until "fixed," or activated, in the classical pathway by binding to an antibody-coated surface. In the classical pathway, a specific antibody identifies and coats an antigen that enters the body. C1 then recognizes and binds with this specific antibody, activating the complement cascade — a series of enzymatic reactions involving all complement components — and producing a coordinated inflammatory response, which usually results in cell lysis or some other damaging outcome.

In the alternative pathway, substances such as polysaccharides, bacterial endotoxins, and aggregated immunoglobulins react with properdin and factors B, D, H, and I, producing an enzyme that activates C3. In turn, C3 activates the remainder of the complement cascade.

In both pathways, specific inhibitors regulate the sequential activation of complement components. The C1 esterase inhibitor, the most commonly studied inhibitor, regulates the classic pathway; the C3b inhibitor can regulate either pathway because C3 is a pivotal component of both.

Although various laboratory methods are used to evaluate and measure total complement and its components, hemolytic assay, laser nephelometry, and radial immunodiffusion are the most common.

■ Hemolytic assay evaluates the lytic capacity of complement and is expressed as hemolytic units per millimeter (the dilution of serum needed to lyse 50% of the erythrocytes in the assay). In this test, sheep red blood cells (RBCs) are mixed with a specific antiserum that lacks complement. Antibody-antigen complexes form, but because complement is absent, lysis can't occur. After the patient's serum sample is serially diluted, equal volumes of these sensitized sheep RBCs are added to each dilution. Complement activity, reported in CH50 units, is the dilution capable of lysing 50% of available RBCs.

■ Laser nephelometry measures C1 esterase inhibitor. The serum sample is mixed with monospecific antiserum for C1 esterase inhibitor. It reacts to form a precipitate that scatters light from a laser beam directed through it. The amount of light scattered reflects the amount of C1 esterase inhibitor in the serum.

■ Radial immunodiffusion measures C3, C4, C5, properdin, factor B, and C1 inhibitor. In this test, an agar slide is impregnated with monospecific antibody for the factor to be studied. Known standards of complement and the patient's serum are placed in appropriate wells punched in the agar. Within 24 hours, a precipitation ring forms around the well where antigen and antibody react; its diameter is proportional to the concentration of complement component.

Although complement assays provide valuable information about the patient's immune system, the results must be considered in light of serum immunoglobulin and autoantibody tests for a definitive diagnosis of immune-mediated disease or abnormal response to infection.

Purpose

■ To help detect immune-mediated disease or genetic complement deficiency
■ To monitor effectiveness of therapy.

Patient preparation

Explain to the patient that this test measures a group of proteins that fight infection. Advise him that he needn't restrict food or fluids. Tell him the test requires a blood sample, who will perform the venipuncture and when, and that he may experience transient discomfort from the needle puncture and the pressure of the tourniquet.

If the patient is scheduled for C1q assay, check his history for recent heparin therapy. Report such therapy to the laboratory because it may affect test results.

Procedure

Perform a venipuncture and collect the sample in a 7-ml tube without additives.

Precautions

- Handle the sample gently to prevent hemolysis.
- Send it to the laboratory immediately because complement is heat labile and deteriorates rapidly.

Reference values

Normal values for complement range as follows:

- total complement: 25 to 110 U
- C1 esterase inhibitor: 8 to 24 mg/dl
- C3: 70 to 150 mg/dl
- C4: 14 to 40 mg/dl.

Implications of results

Complement abnormalities may be genetic or acquired; acquired abnormalities are most common. Depressed total complement levels (which are clinically more significant than elevations) may result from excessive formation of antigen-antibody complexes, insufficient synthesis of complement, inhibitor formation, or increased complement catabolism; decreased levels are characteristic in such conditions as systemic lupus erythematosus (SLE), acute poststreptococcal glomerulonephritis, and acute serum sickness. Low levels may also occur in some patients with advanced cirrhosis of the liver, multiple myeloma, hypogammaglobulinemia, and rapidly rejecting allografts.

Elevated total complement may occur in obstructive jaundice, thyroiditis, acute rheumatic fever, rheumatoid arthritis, acute myocardial infarction, ulcerative colitis, and diabetes.

C1 esterase inhibitor deficiency is characteristic in hereditary angioedema, the most common genetic abnormality associated with complement; C3 deficiency is characteristic in recurrent pyogenic infection; C4 deficiency is characteristic in SLE.

Posttest care

CLINICAL ALERT Because many patients with complement defects have a compromised immune system, keep the venipuncture site clean and dry.

If a hematoma develops, apply warm soaks.

Interfering factors

- Recent heparin therapy can affect test results.
- Hemolysis caused by rough handling of the sample or failure to send the sample to the laboratory immediately may affect the accuracy of test results.

Copper test, urine

This test measures the urine level of copper, an essential trace element and a component of several metalloenzymes and proteins necessary for hemoglobin synthesis and oxidation reduction. Urine normally contains only a small amount of free copper; plasma, only trace amounts. Most copper in plasma is bound to and transported by an alpha$_2$ globulin (plasma protein) called ceruloplasmin. When copper is unbound, the ions can inhibit many enzyme reactions, resulting in copper toxicity.

Urine copper levels are frequently measured to detect Wilson's disease, a rare, inborn error of metabolism that's most common among persons of eastern European Jewish, southern Italian, or Sicilian ancestry. Wilson's disease is marked by decreased ceruloplasmin, increased urinary excretion of copper, and accumulation of copper in the interstitial tissues of the liver and brain. The cause of this disorder is unclear. Early detection and treatment (with a low-copper diet and D-penicillamine) are vital to prevent irreversible changes, such as nerve tissue degeneration and cirrhosis of the liver.

Purpose

■ To help detect Wilson's disease, chronic active hepatitis, or environmental exposure
■ To screen infants with a family history of Wilson's disease.

Patient preparation

Explain to the patient that this test determines the amount of copper in urine. Inform him that no special restrictions are necessary and that the test requires a 24-hour urine specimen. If it's to be collected at home, explain the proper collection technique.

Procedure

Collect a 24-hour urine specimen with no preservative.

Precautions

Tell the patient not to contaminate the urine specimen with toilet tissue or stool.

Reference values

Normal urinary excretion of copper ranges from 15 to 60 µg/24 hours.

Implications of results

Elevated urine copper levels usually indicate Wilson's disease (a liver biopsy helps establish this diagnosis). High copper levels may also occur in nephrotic syn-

drome, chronic active hepatitis, biliary cirrhosis, and
rheumatoid arthritis.

Interfering factors

■ Administration of D-penicillamine causes elevated
urine levels of copper.
■ Failure to collect all urine during the test period may
affect the accuracy of test results.

Corticotropin test

This test measures the plasma levels of corticotropin
(also known as adrenocorticotropic hormone or ACTH)
by radioimmunoassay. Corticotropin stimulates the
adrenal cortex to secrete cortisol and, to a lesser degree,
androgens and aldosterone. It also has some melanocyte-
stimulating activity, increases the uptake of amino acids
by muscle cells, promotes lipolysis by fat cells, stimulates pancreatic beta cells to secrete insulin, and may
contribute to the release of growth hormone. Corticotropin levels vary diurnally, peaking between 6 a.m.
and 8 a.m. and ebbing between 6 p.m. and 11 p.m.

The corticotropin test may be ordered for patients
with signs of adrenal hypofunction (insufficiency) or hyperfunction (Cushing's syndrome). Corticotropin suppression or stimulation testing is usually necessary to
confirm diagnosis. However, the instability and unavailability of corticotropin greatly limit this test's diagnostic
significance and reliability.

Purpose

■ To facilitate differential diagnosis of primary and secondary adrenal hypofunction
■ To aid differential diagnosis of Cushing's syndrome.

Patient preparation

Explain to the patient that this test helps determine if
his hormonal secretion is normal. Advise him that he
must fast and limit his physical activity for 10 to 12
hours before the test. Tell him that the test requires a
blood sample, and explain who will perform the venipuncture and when. Inform him that he may experience
some transient discomfort from the needle puncture and
the tourniquet.

Check the patient's drug history for the use of medications that may affect the accuracy of test results such as
corticosteroids and medications that affect cortisol levels, such as estrogens, amphetamines, spironolactone,
lithium carbonate, calcium gluconate, and alcohol
(ethanol). Withhold these medications for 48 hours or

longer before the test. If they must be continued, note this on the laboratory slip.

Arrange with the dietary department to provide a low-carbohydrate diet for 2 days before the test. This requirement may vary, depending on the laboratory.

Procedure

■ For a patient with suspected adrenal hypofunction, perform the venipuncture for a baseline level between 6 a.m. and 8 a.m. (peak secretion).

■ For a patient with suspected Cushing's syndrome, perform the venipuncture between 6 p.m. and 11 p.m. (low secretion).

■ Collect the sample in a plastic tube (corticotropin may adhere to glass) or in a tube with EDTA (sodium metabisulfite solution) added. The tube must be full because excess anticoagulant will affect results.

■ Pack the sample in ice and send it to the laboratory immediately, where plasma must be rapidly separated from blood cells at 39.2° F (4° C). The collection technique may vary, depending on the laboratory.

■ Resume diet and administration of medications that were discontinued before the test.

Precautions

Because proteolytic enzymes in plasma degrade corticotropin, a temperature of 39.2° F (4° C) is necessary to retard enzyme activity. Immediate transfer of the sample, packed in ice, to the laboratory is essential for reliable test results.

Reference values

Mayo Medical Laboratories sets baseline values at less than 60 pg/ml, but these values may vary in different laboratories.

Implications of results

A higher-than-normal corticotropin level may indicate primary adrenal hypofunction (Addison's disease), in which the pituitary gland attempts to compensate for the unresponsiveness of the target organ by releasing excessive corticotropin. The underlying cause of adrenocortical hypofunction may be idiopathic atrophy of the adrenal cortex or partial destruction of the gland by granuloma, neoplasm, amyloidosis, or inflammatory necrosis.

A low-normal corticotropin level suggests secondary adrenal hypofunction resulting from pituitary or hypothalamic dysfunction. The primary determinant may be panhypopituitarism, absence of corticotropin-releasing hormone in the hypothalamus, or chronic blunting of corticotropin levels by long-term corticosteroid therapy.

In suspected Cushing's syndrome, an elevated corticotropin level suggests Cushing's disease, in which pituitary dysfunction (due to adenoma) causes continuous hypersecretion of corticotropin and, consequently, continuously elevated cortisol levels without diurnal variations. Moderately elevated corticotropin levels suggest pituitary-dependent adrenal hyperplasia and nonadrenal tumors, such as oat cell carcinoma of the lungs.

A low-normal corticotropin level implies adrenal hyperfunction due to adrenocortical tumor or hyperplasia.

Posttest care

If a hematoma develops, apply warm soaks.

Interfering factors

■ Corticosteroids, including cortisone and its analogues, can decrease corticotropin levels.
■ Drugs that increase endogenous cortisol secretion, such as estrogens, calcium gluconate, amphetamines, spironolactone, and ethanol, can decrease corticotropin levels.
■ Lithium carbonate decreases cortisol levels and may interfere with corticotropin secretion.
■ Failure to observe pretest restrictions, menstrual cycle, pregnancy, radioactive scan performed within 1 week before the test, and acute stress (including hospitalization and surgery) or depression can interfere with test results.

Corticotropin test, rapid

The rapid corticotropin test (also known as the rapid ACTH test or cosyntropin test) is gradually replacing the 8-hour corticotropin stimulation test as the most effective diagnostic tool for evaluating adrenal hypofunction. Using cosyntropin, the rapid corticotropin test provides faster results and causes fewer allergic reactions than the 8-hour test, which uses natural corticotropin from animal sources.

This test requires prior determination of baseline cortisol levels to evaluate the effect of cosyntropin administration on cortisol secretion. An unequivocally high morning cortisol level rules out adrenal hypofunction and makes further testing unnecessary.

Purpose

To aid in identification of primary and secondary adrenal hypofunction.

Patient preparation

Explain to the patient that this test helps determine if his condition is caused by a hormonal deficiency. Inform him that he may be required to fast for 10 to 12 hours before the test and must be relaxed and resting quietly for 30 minutes before the test. Tell him that the test takes at least 1 hour to perform. Inform the patient that he may experience transient discomfort from the needle puncture and the tourniquet.

If the patient is in a facility, withhold corticotropin and all steroid medications before the test. If he is an outpatient, tell him to refrain from taking these drugs, unless instructed otherwise by his doctor. If the drugs must be continued, note this on the laboratory slip.

Procedure

- Draw 5 ml of blood for a baseline value. Collect the sample in a 5-ml heparinized tube. Label this sample "preinjection" and send it to the laboratory.
- Inject 250 µg (0.25 mg) of cosyntropin I.V. or I.M. (I.V. administration provides more accurate results because ineffective absorption after I.M. administration may cause wide variations in response.) Direct I.V. injection should take about 2 minutes.
- Draw another 5 ml of blood at 30 and 60 minutes after the cosyntropin injection. Collect the samples in 5-ml heparinized tubes. Label the samples "30 minutes postinjection" and "60 minutes postinjection" and send them to the laboratory. Include the actual collection times on the laboratory slip.

Precautions

Handle the samples gently to prevent hemolysis.

Reference values

Normally, cortisol levels rise 7 µg/dl or more above the baseline value to a peak of 18 µg/dl or more 60 minutes after the cosyntropin injection. Generally, a doubling of the baseline value indicates a normal response.

Implications of results

A normal result excludes adrenal hypofunction (insufficiency). In patients with primary adrenal hypofunction (Addison's disease), cortisol levels remain low. Thus, the rapid corticotropin test provides an effective method of screening for adrenal hypofunction. If test results show subnormal increases in cortisol levels, prolonged stimulation of the adrenal cortex may be required to differentiate between primary and secondary adrenal hypofunction.

Posttest care

■ If a hematoma develops, apply warm soaks.

CLINICAL ALERT Observe the patient for signs of allergic reaction to cosyntropin, such as hives, itching, and tachycardia. Such allergic reaction is rare.

■ Instruct the patient to resume a normal diet.

■ Resume administration of medications discontinued before the test.

Interfering factors

■ Estrogens and amphetamines increase plasma cortisol levels.

■ Lithium carbonate decreases plasma cortisol levels.

■ Smoking and obesity may increase plasma cortisol levels.

■ Failure to observe pretest restrictions, hemolysis caused by rough handling of the sample, and a radioactive scan performed within 1 week before the test may interfere with test results.

Cortisol test, plasma

Cortisol, the principal glucocorticoid secreted by the zona fasciculata of the adrenal cortex, primarily in response to adrenocorticotropic hormone (ACTH) stimulation, helps metabolize nutrients, mediate physiologic stress, and regulate the immune system. Cortisol secretion normally follows a diurnal pattern: Levels rise during the early morning hours and peak around 8 a.m., then decline to very low levels in the evening and during the early phase of sleep. (See *Diurnal variations in cortisol secretion.*) Production of this hormone is influenced by physical or emotional stress, which activates ACTH. Thus, intense heat or cold, infection, trauma, exercise, obesity, and debilitating disease influence cortisol secretion.

This radioimmunoassay, a quantitative analysis of plasma cortisol levels, is usually ordered for patients with signs of adrenal dysfunction, but dynamic tests, suppression tests for hyperfunction, and stimulation tests for hypofunction are generally required to confirm the diagnosis.

Purpose

To aid in the diagnosis of Cushing's disease, Cushing's syndrome, Addison's disease, and secondary adrenal insufficiency.

Patient preparation

Explain to the patient that this test helps determine if his symptoms are due to improper hormonal secretion.

DIURNAL VARIATIONS IN CORTISOL SECRETION

Cortisol secretion rises in the early morning, peaking after the patient awakens. Levels decline sharply in the evening and during the early phase of sleep. They rise again during the night and peak by the next morning.

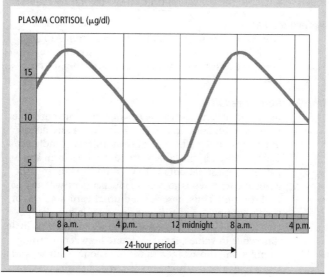

PLASMA CORTISOL (μg/dl)

Instruct him to maintain a normal-sodium diet for 3 days before the test and to fast and limit physical activity for 10 to 12 hours before the test. Tell him a blood sample is required, who will perform the venipuncture and when, and that he may experience some discomfort from the needle puncture. Advise him that the laboratory requires at least 2 days to complete the analysis.

Withhold all medications that may interfere with plasma cortisol levels, such as estrogens, androgens, and phenytoin, for 48 hours before the test. If the patient is receiving replacement therapy and is dependent on exogenous steroids for survival, note this on the laboratory request as well as any other medications that must be continued.

Make sure the patient is relaxed and recumbent for at least 30 minutes before the test.

Procedure

■ Between 6 and 8 a.m., perform a venipuncture. Collect the sample in a 7-ml heparinized tube, label it appropriately, and send it to the laboratory immediately.
■ For diurnal variation testing, draw another sample between 4 and 6 p.m. Collect it in a heparinized tube, label

it appropriately, and send it to the laboratory immediately.

Precautions
- Handle the sample gently to prevent hemolysis.
- Record the collection time on the laboratory request.

Reference values
Normally, plasma cortisol levels range from 7 to 28 µg/dl in the morning and from 2 to 18 µg/dl in the afternoon; the afternoon level is usually half the morning level.

Implications of results
Increased plasma cortisol levels may indicate adrenocortical hyperfunction in Cushing's disease (a rare disease due to basophilic adenoma of the pituitary gland) or in Cushing's syndrome (glucocorticoid excess from any cause). In most patients with Cushing's syndrome, the adrenal cortex tends to secrete independently of any natural rhythm. Thus, absence of diurnal variations in cortisol secretion is a significant finding in almost all patients with Cushing's syndrome; in these patients, little difference in values, if any, is found between morning samples and those taken in the afternoon. Diurnal variations may also be absent in otherwise healthy persons who are under considerable emotional or physical stress.

Decreased cortisol levels may indicate primary adrenal hypofunction (Addison's disease), usually due to idiopathic glandular atrophy (a presumed autoimmune process). Tuberculosis, fungal invasion, and hemorrhage can cause adrenocortical destruction. Low cortisol levels resulting from secondary adrenal insufficiency may occur in conditions of impaired ACTH secretion, such as hypophysectomy, postpartum pituitary necrosis, craniopharyngioma, or chromophobe adenoma.

Posttest care
- If a hematoma develops, apply warm soaks.
- Resume diet and administration of medications that were discontinued before the test.

Interfering factors
- Failure to observe restrictions of diet, medications, or physical activity may interfere with accurate determination of test results.
- Plasma cortisol levels are falsely elevated by estrogens (during pregnancy or in oral contraceptives), which increase plasma proteins that bind with cortisol. Obesity, stress, or severe hepatic or renal disease may also increase these levels.

■ Plasma cortisol levels may be decreased by androgens and phenytoin, which decrease cortisol-binding proteins.
■ A radioactive scan performed within 1 week before the test may influence the results.
■ Hemolysis caused by rough handling of the sample may interfere with accurate determination of test results.

Creatine kinase test

Creatine kinase (CK) is an enzyme that catalyzes the creatine-creatinine metabolic pathway in muscle cells and brain tissue. Because of its important role in energy production, CK levels reflect normal tissue catabolism; above-normal serum levels indicate trauma to cells with high CK content. CK may be separated into three isoenzymes with distinct molecular structures: CK-BB (CK1), found primarily in brain tissue; CK-MB (CK2), found primarily in cardiac muscle (a small amount also appears in skeletal muscle); and CK-MM (CK3), found mainly in skeletal muscle.

Total serum CK levels were once widely used to detect acute myocardial infarction (MI), but elevated levels caused by skeletal muscle damage reduce the test's specificity for this disorder. Fractionation and measurement of CK isoenzymes has replaced total CK assay to accurately localize the site of increased tissue destruction. In addition, subunits of CK-MM and CK-MB, called isoforms, can be assayed to increase the sensitivity of the test.

Purpose

■ To detect and diagnose acute MI and reinfarction (CK-MB primarily used)
■ To evaluate possible causes of chest pain and to monitor the severity of myocardial ischemia after cardiac surgery, cardiac catheterization, or cardioversion (CK-MB primarily used)
■ To detect early dermatomyositis and skeletal muscle disorders that aren't neurogenic in origin, such as Duchenne's muscular dystrophy (total CK primarily used).

Patient preparation

Explain to the patient that this test helps assess heart and skeletal muscle function and that multiple blood samples are required to detect fluctuations in serum levels. Inform him that he need not restrict food or most fluids before the test. If the patient is being evaluated for skeletal muscle disorders, advise him to avoid exercising for 24 hours before the test. Tell him who will perform the venipuncture and when and that he may feel some discomfort from the needle or the tourniquet.

Before the test, withhold alcohol, aminocaproic acid, lithium, clofibrate, codeine, dexamethasone, digoxin, lithium, morphine, succinylcholine, furosemide, glutethimide, halothane, heroin, imipramine, meperidine, and phenobarbital. If these substances must be continued, note this on the laboratory request.

Procedure

Perform a venipuncture and collect the sample in a 7-ml tube without additives.

Precautions

■ Draw the sample before giving an I.M. injection, or wait at least 1 hour after the injection, because muscle trauma raises total CK levels.

■ Obtain the sample as scheduled. Because timing is important to the diagnosis, recording the date and time the sample was drawn and the number of hours that elapsed since the onset of chest pain is critical.

■ Handle the collection tube gently to prevent hemolysis.

■ Send the sample to the laboratory immediately because CK activity diminishes significantly after 2 hours at room temperature.

Reference values

Total CK values determined by ultraviolet or kinetic measurement normally range from 38 to 190 U/L for men and from 10 to 150 U/L for women. CK levels may be significantly higher in very muscular people. Infants up to age 1 have levels two to four times higher than adults, possibly reflecting birth trauma and striated muscle development.

The normal range for troponin is 0.0 to 0.4 μg/ml. The normal ranges for isoenzyme levels are as follows: CK-BB, undetectable; CK-MB, < 4% to 6%; CK-MM, 90% to 100%.

Implications of results

CK-MM constitutes over 99% of total CK normally present in serum. Detectable CK-BB levels may indicate brain tissue injury, certain widespread malignant tumors, severe shock, or renal failure. However, such elevations don't confirm a specific diagnosis.

CK-MB levels greater than 5% of total CK (or more than 10 U/L) indicate MI, especially if the lactate dehydrogenase 1 and 2 (LD1/LD2) isoenzyme ratio is greater than 1 (flipped LD). In acute MI and after cardiac surgery, CK-MB levels begin to rise in 2 to 4 hours, peak in 12 to 24 hours, and usually return to normal in 24 to 48 hours; persistent elevations or increasing levels indicate ongoing myocardial damage. (See *Enzyme and isoenzyme changes after MI*, page 184.) Total CK follows roughly the same pattern but rises slightly later. CK-MB levels don't rise in congestive heart failure or during angina pectoris not accompanied by myocardial cell necrosis, although not all researchers agree about this.

Serious skeletal muscle injury that occurs in certain muscular dystrophies, polymyositis, and severe myoglobinuria may produce mildly elevated CK-MB levels because a small amount of this isoenzyme is present in some skeletal muscles.

Rising CK-MM values follow skeletal muscle damage from trauma, such as surgery and I.M. injections, or from diseases, such as dermatomyositis and muscular dystrophy (values may be 50 to 100 times normal). A moderate rise in CK-MM levels develops in patients with hypothyroidism; sharp elevations occur with muscular activity caused by agitation, such as an acute psychotic episode.

Total CK levels may be elevated in patients with severe hypokalemia, carbon monoxide poisoning, malignant hyperthermia, or alcoholic cardiomyopathy; in those who have recently had a seizure; and occasionally in those who have suffered pulmonary or cerebral infarctions.

Troponin I (cTn I) and cardiac troponin C (cTnC) are present in the contractile cells of cardiac myocardial tissue. When injury occurs to the myocardial tissue, these proteins are released. Troponin levels increase within 1 hour of the infarction and may remain elevated for up to 14 days. As long as myocardial tissue injury occurs, the levels will remain high and may increase to over 50 µg/ml.

Posttest care
- If a hematoma develops, apply warm soaks.
- Resume medications discontinued before the test.

Interfering factors
- Halothane and succinylcholine, alcohol, lithium, and large doses of aminocaproic acid raise total CK values.
- I.M. injections, cardioversion, invasive diagnostic procedures, recent vigorous exercise or muscle massage, and severe coughing and trauma raise total CK values.
- Surgery through skeletal muscle will raise total CK levels.
- Hemolysis may alter test results.

ENZYME AND ISOENZYME CHANGES AFTER MI

Because they're released by damaged tissue, serum enzymes and isoenzymes—catalytic proteins that vary in concentration in specific organs—can help identify the compromised organ and assess the extent of damage. The graph below shows how serum levels of the enzymes and isoenzymes that are most significant in myocardial infarction (MI) fluctuate in the days following an MI.

Enzymes
- Hydroxybutyric dehydrogenase (HBD): an indirect measurement of lactate dehydrogenase 1 and 2 (LD^1, LD^2)
- Aspartate aminotransferase (AST): found primarily in heart muscle and liver; less extensively in skeletal muscles, kidneys, pancreas, and red blood cells (RBCs)
- Troponin I and troponin C : proteins that are present in the contractile cells of myocardial tissue

Isoenzymes
- Creatine kinase-MB (CK-MB): found primarily in heart muscle; a small amount in skeletal muscle
- LD^1 and LD^2: found in the heart, brain, kidneys, liver, skeletal muscles, and RBCs

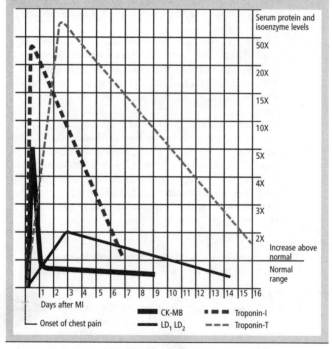

- Failure to send the sample to the laboratory immediately or to refrigerate the serum if testing will be delayed for more than 2 hours may decrease the concentration and affect test results.

■ Failure to draw the samples at the scheduled time may miss peak levels.

Creatine kinase isoform test

An enzyme found in muscle tissue, creatine kinase has three variants (isoenzymes or isoforms): CK-MM (CK3), CK-MB (CK2), and CK-BB (CK1). CK-MM and CK-MB are found primarily in skeletal and heart muscle. CK-BB, most prevalent in brain tissue, is not usually seen in serum. Isoforms, or subforms, of CK-MM and CK-MB are called CK-MM1, CK-MM2, CK-MB1, and CK-MB2. Isoforms are determined by high-voltage electrophoresis or isoelectric focusing.

Cardiac muscle damage releases CK-MM, CK-MB, and lactate dehydrogenase isoenzymes into serum. An increase in CK-MB levels indicates myocardial infarction (MI). Serum levels begin to rise 2 to 4 hours after myocardial damage; isoform levels, 4 to 6 hours after. Evaluating these increases speeds diagnosis and treatment of MI.

Purpose

■ To detect or provide early confirmation of MI
■ To evaluate reperfusion therapy.

Patient preparation

Explain that the test will help to confirm or rule out MI. Tell the patient that it will require a blood test, with specimens drawn at timed intervals. Tell him who will perform the venipunctures and when and that he may feel discomfort from the tourniquet and the needle.

Procedure

■ Perform a venipuncture and collect blood in a 7-ml tube with EDTA (sodium metabisulfite solution) or a clot activator, depending on the laboratory's protocol. Record the time the specimen was drawn.
■ Obtain another specimen every 2 hours, as indicated, and note the time on each. Place each specimen on ice, and deliver it to the laboratory at once.

Precautions

■ Obtain each specimen on schedule, and note the collection time and date on each.
■ Handle the specimens gently; rough handling can cause hemolysis.

Reference values

Normally, CK-MB2 concentrations are less than 1 U/L. The CK-MB2/CK-MB1 ratio is less than 1.5.

Implications of results

Within 2 to 4 hours after MI, more than 50% of patients will have a CK-MB2/CK-MB1 ratio greater than 1.5. By 6 hours after MI, more than 90% of patients will have a ratio of 1.5 or greater.

Giving thrombolytic drugs may restore coronary perfusion. The increased blood flow through the damaged area removes accumulated CK isoenzymes and causes the CK-MB2/CK-MB1 ratio to peak sooner.

Posttest care

- If a hematoma develops, apply warm soaks.
- Resume medications discontinued before the test.

Interfering factors

- Hemolysis may alter test results.
- Failure to draw the samples at the scheduled times may result in missing peak levels.

Creatinine test, serum

A quantitative analysis of serum creatinine levels, this test provides a more sensitive measure of renal damage than blood urea nitrogen levels because renal impairment is virtually the only cause of creatinine elevation. Creatinine is a nonprotein end product of creatine metabolism. Similar to creatine, creatinine appears in serum in amounts proportional to the body's muscle mass; unlike creatine, it is easily excreted by the kidneys, with minimal or no tubular reabsorption. Creatinine levels, therefore, are directly related to the glomerular filtration rate.

Because creatinine levels normally remain constant, elevated levels usually indicate diminished renal function. Determination of serum creatinine is commonly based on the Jaffe reaction or on coupled enzymatic reactions.

Purpose

- To assess renal glomerular filtration
- To screen for renal damage.

Patient preparation

Explain to the patient that this test evaluates kidney function. Tell him that the test requires a blood sample, who will perform the venipuncture and when, and that he may feel some discomfort from the needle puncture and the pressure of the tourniquet. Tell the patient that restriction of food or fluids isn't necessary before the test. Check the patient's medication history for drugs that may interfere with test results.

Procedure

Perform a venipuncture and collect the sample in a 7-ml clot-activator tube.

Precautions

Handle the specimen gently to prevent hemolysis and send it to the laboratory immediately.

Reference values

Serum creatinine levels in males normally range from 0.8 to 1.2 mg/dl; in females, from 0.6 to 0.9 mg/dl.

Implications of results

Elevated serum creatinine levels generally indicate renal disease that has seriously damaged 50% or more of the nephrons. They may also be associated with gigantism and acromegaly.

Posttest care

If a hematoma develops, apply warm soaks.

Interfering factors

■ Ascorbic acid, barbiturates, and diuretics may raise serum creatinine levels.
■ Sulfobromophthalein or phenolsulfonphthalein given within the previous 24 hours can elevate creatinine levels.
■ Patients with exceptionally large muscle mass, such as athletes, may have above-average creatinine levels, even with normal renal function.
■ Hemolysis may elevate results.

Creatinine test, urine

This test measures urine levels of creatinine, the chief metabolite of creatine. Produced in amounts proportional to total body muscle mass, creatinine is removed from the plasma primarily by glomerular filtration and is excreted in the urine.

Because creatinine isn't recycled in the body, it has a relatively high, constant clearance rate, making it an efficient indicator of renal function. However, the creatinine clearance test, which measures both urine and plasma creatinine clearance, is a more precise index than this test. A standard method of determining urine creatinine levels is based on the Jaffe reaction, in which creatinine treated with an alkaline picrate solution yields a bright orange-red complex.

Purpose

■ To help assess glomerular filtration

■ To check the accuracy of 24-hour urine collection based on the relatively constant levels of creatinine excretion.

Patient preparation

Explain to the patient that this test helps evaluate kidney function. Inform him that he needn't restrict fluids but shouldn't eat an excessive amount of meat before the test and should avoid strenuous physical exercise during the collection period. Tell him the test usually requires a 24-hour urine specimen, and teach him the proper collection technique.

Check the patient's medication history for drugs that may affect creatinine levels. Review your findings with the laboratory, and then notify the doctor, who may restrict such drugs before the test.

Procedure

Collect a 24-hour urine specimen in a refrigerated specimen bottle without a preservative.

Precautions

Refrigerate the specimen or keep it on ice during the collection period. When the collection is completed, send the specimen to the laboratory immediately.

Reference values

The normal range for urine creatinine levels in adults is 14 to 26 mg/kg/24 hours. In men, the range is 800 to 2,000 mg/24 hours and, in women, 600 to 1,800 mg/24 hours.

Implications of results

Lower than normal urine creatinine levels may result from impaired renal perfusion (associated with shock, for example) or from renal disease due to urinary tract obstruction. Chronic bilateral pyelonephritis, acute or chronic glomerulonephritis, and polycystic kidney disease may also depress creatinine levels. Increased urine creatinine levels generally have little diagnostic significance.

Posttest care

■ Resume medications withheld before the test.
■ Tell the patient that he may resume his diet and normal activities.

Interfering factors

■ Drugs that may affect urine creatinine levels include corticosteroids, gentamicin, tetracyclines, diuretics, and amphotericin B.

■ Failure to observe pretest restrictions, to collect all urine during the test period, or to store the specimen properly may interfere with test results.

Creatinine clearance test

Creatinine, the main end product of creatine metabolism, is formed and excreted in constant amounts by an irreversible reaction and functions solely as the main end product of creatine. Creatinine production is proportional to total muscle mass and is relatively unaffected by normal physical activity, diet, or urine volume.

An excellent diagnostic indicator of renal function, the creatinine clearance test determines how efficiently the kidneys are clearing creatinine from the blood. The rate of clearance is expressed in terms of the volume of blood (in milliliters) that can be cleared of creatinine in 1 minute.

To arrive at this determination, the equation $C = (U \times V) \div P$ is used; C represents the clearance rate; U, the urine concentration of creatinine; V, the volume of urine collected during the test period (converted to ml/minute); and P, the plasma concentration of creatinine. Naturally, urine and plasma concentrations of creatinine must be expressed in the same units (usually mg/dl), so they cancel each other out in the equation.

A final adjustment must be made to allow for renal parenchymal mass, which differs in each patient. To do this, the clearance rate established in the previous equation is multiplied by $(1.73 \div A)$, where 1.73 equals the body surface area (in square meters) of the average person, and A equals the patient's body surface area. Creatinine levels become abnormal when more than 50% of the total nephron units have been damaged.

Purpose

■ To assess renal function (primarily glomerular filtration)
■ To monitor progression of renal insufficiency.

Patient preparation

Explain to the patient that this test assesses kidney function. Inform him that he needn't restrict fluids but shouldn't eat an excessive amount of meat before the test and should avoid strenuous physical exercise during the collection period. Tell him the test requires a timed urine specimen and at least one blood sample. Tell him how the urine specimen will be collected, who will perform the venipuncture and when, and that he may feel some discomfort from the needle puncture. Explain that more than one venipuncture may be necessary.

Check the patient's medication history for drugs that may affect creatinine clearance. Review your findings with the laboratory, and then notify the doctor, who may want to restrict these medications before the test.

Procedure
■ Collect a timed urine specimen at 2, 6, 12, or 24 hours in a bottle containing a preservative to prevent degradation of the creatinine.
■ Perform a venipuncture anytime during the collection period, and collect the sample in a 7-ml tube without additives.

Precautions
Refrigerate the specimen or keep it on ice during the collection period. When the collection is completed, send the specimen to the laboratory at once.

Reference values
At age 20, creatinine clearance normally ranges from 85 to 146 ml/minute/1.73 m^2 for men and from 81 to 134 ml/minute/1.73 m^2 for women. Creatinine clearance normally decreases by 6 ml/minute for each decade after age 20.

Implications of results
Low creatinine clearance may result from reduced renal blood flow (associated with shock or renal artery obstruction), acute tubular necrosis, acute or chronic glomerulonephritis, advanced bilateral chronic pyelonephritis, advanced bilateral renal lesions (as in polycystic kidney disease, cancer, or renal tuberculosis), or nephrosclerosis. Congestive heart failure and severe dehydration may also cause creatinine clearance to fall below normal.

High creatinine clearance rates generally have little diagnostic significance.

Posttest care
■ Resume administration of medications withheld before the test.
■ Tell the patient that he may resume his diet and normal activity.
■ If a hematoma develops, apply warm soaks.

Interfering factors
■ A high-protein diet before the test and strenuous physical exercise during the collection period may increase creatinine excretion.

■ Drugs that may affect creatinine clearance include am-photericin B, thiazide diuretics, furosemide, and amino-glycosides.
■ Failure to observe pretest restrictions, to collect all urine during the test period, or to store the specimen properly may affect the accuracy of test results.

Crossmatching

Crossmatching establishes the compatibility or incompatibility of a donor's and a recipient's blood. It's the best antibody detection test available for avoiding lethal transfusion reactions.

After the donor's and the recipient's ABO blood type and Rh factor type are determined, major crossmatching establishes compatibility between the donor's red blood cells (RBCs) and the recipient's serum. They're compatible if the recipient's serum has no antibodies that would destroy transfused cells and possibly cause an acute hemolytic reaction. Minor crossmatching establishes compatibility between the donor's serum and the recipient's RBCs. This crossmatch is less important, however, because the donor's antibodies are greatly diluted in the recipient's plasma. Indeed, because the antibody-screening test is routinely performed on all blood donors, minor crossmatching is often omitted.

Blood is always crossmatched before a transfusion, except in emergencies. Because a complete crossmatch may take from 45 minutes to 2 hours, an incomplete (10-minute) crossmatch may be acceptable in some emergencies, such as severe blood loss due to trauma. In such cases, transfusion can begin with limited amounts of group O-packed RBCs while crossmatching is completed.

CLINICAL ALERT An emergency transfusion must proceed with special awareness of the complications that may arise because of incomplete typing and crossmatching. After crossmatching, compatible units of blood are labeled, and a compatibility record is completed.

Purpose

To serve as the final check for compatibility between the donor's blood and the recipient's blood.

Patient preparation

Explain to the patient that this test ensures that the blood he receives correctly matches his own to prevent a transfusion reaction. Inform him that he needn't fast before the test. Tell him the test requires a blood sample, who will perform the venipuncture and when, and that he may experience some transient discomfort from the needle puncture and the pressure of the tourniquet.

Check the patient's history for recent administration of blood, dextran, or I.V. contrast media.

Procedure

■ Perform the venipuncture and collect the sample in a 10-ml tube without additives or with EDTA (sodium metabisulfite solution). ABO typing, Rh typing, and crossmatching are all done together.
■ Label the sample with the patient's name, the hospital or blood bank number, the date, and the initials of the phlebotomist.
■ Indicate on the laboratory request the amount and type of blood component needed.
■ Send the sample to the laboratory immediately.

Precautions

■ Handle the sample gently to prevent hemolysis, which can mask hemolysis of the donor RBCs.
■ Crossmatching must be performed on the sample within 72 hours.
■ Before a transfusion, if more than 72 hours have elapsed since a previous transfusion, previously cross-matched donor blood must be crossmatched again with a new recipient serum sample to detect newly acquired incompatibilities.
■ If the patient is scheduled for surgery and has received a transfusion or been pregnant within the past 3 months, antibodies may develop and linger. The patient's blood will need to be crossmatched again if his surgery is rescheduled to detect recently acquired incompatibilities.

Normal findings

Absence of agglutination indicates compatibility between the donor's and recipient's blood, which means that the transfusion of donor blood can proceed.

Implications of results

A positive crossmatch indicates incompatibility between the donor's blood and the recipient's blood, which means the donor's blood can't be transfused to the recipient. The sign of a positive crossmatch is agglutination, or clumping, when the donor's RBCs and the recipient's serum are correctly mixed and incubated. Agglutination indicates an undesirable antigen-antibody reaction. The donor's blood must be withheld and the crossmatch continued to determine the cause of the incompatibility and to identify the antibody.

A negative crossmatch (the absence of agglutination) indicates probable compatibility between the donor's blood and the recipient's blood, which means the transfusion of donor blood can proceed. It doesn't guarantee a safe transfusion, but it's the best method available to prevent an acute hemolytic reaction.

Posttest care

If a hematoma develops, apply warm soaks.

Interfering factors

- Previous administration of dextran or I.V. contrast media causes aggregation resembling agglutination. A previous blood transfusion may produce antibodies to the donor blood that could interfere with compatibility testing.
- The administration of certain drugs may produce antibodies that could interfere with testing.
- Hemolysis may affect results.

Cryoglobulin test

Cryoglobulins are abnormal serum proteins that precipitate at low laboratory temperatures (39.2° F [4° C]) and redissolve after being warmed. Their presence in the blood (cryoglobulinemia) is usually associated with immune disorders, but cryoglobulins can also occur in the absence of known immunopathology. (See *Diseases associated with cryoglobulinemia*, page 194.)

Cryoglobulinemia occurs in three forms:

- Type I, which involves the reaction of a single monoclonal immunoglobulin
- Type II, in which a monoclonal immunoglobulin shows antibody activity against a polyclonal immunoglobulin
- Type III, in which both components are polyclonal immunoglobulins.

If patients with cryoglobulinemia are subjected to cold, they may experience Raynaud-like symptoms (pain, cyanosis, and coldness of fingers and toes), which generally result from precipitation of cryoglobulins in cooler parts of the body. In some patients, for example, cryoglobulins may precipitate in peripheral blood vessels at temperatures as high as 86° F (30° C).

The cryoglobulin test involves refrigerating a serum sample at 33.8° F (1° C) for at least 72 hours and observing for formation of a heat-reversible precipitate. Such a precipitate requires further study by immunoelectrophoresis or double diffusion to identify cryoglobulin components.

DISEASES ASSOCIATED WITH CRYOGLOBULINEMIA

This chart indicates typical serum levels and diseases associated with the three types of cryoglobulins.

Type of cryoglobulin	Serum level	Associated diseases
Type I Monoclonal cryoglobulin	> 5 mg/ml	■ Myeloma ■ Waldenström's macroglobulinemia ■ Chronic lymphocytic leukemia
Type II Mixed cryoglobulin	> 1 mg/ml	■ Rheumatoid arthritis ■ Sjögren's syndrome ■ Mixed essential cryoglobulinemia
Type III Mixed polyclonal cryo-globulin	< 1 mg/ml (50% below 80 µg/ml)	■ Systemic lupus erythematosus ■ Rheumatoid arthritis ■ Sjögren's syndrome ■ Infectious mononucleosis ■ Cytomegalovirus infections ■ Acute viral hepatitis ■ Chronic active hepatitis ■ Primary biliary cirrhosis ■ Poststreptococcal glomerulonephritis ■ Infective endocarditis ■ Leprosy ■ Kala-azar ■ Tropical splenomegaly syndrome

Purpose

To detect cryoglobulinemia in patients with Raynaud-like vascular symptoms.

Patient preparation

Explain to the patient that this test detects antibodies in blood that may cause sensitivity to low temperatures. Instruct him to fast for 4 to 6 hours before the test. Tell him that the test requires a blood sample, who will perform the venipuncture and when, and that he may experience transient discomfort from the needle puncture and the pressure of the tourniquet.

Procedure

Perform a venipuncture and collect the sample in a warmed 10-ml tube without additives.

Precautions

■ Warm the collection tube to 98.6° F (37° C) before venipuncture and keep it at that temperature to prevent loss of cryoglobulins.
■ Send the sample to the laboratory immediately.

Normal findings

Serum is negative for cryoglobulins. Positive results are reported as a percentage based on the amount of sample cryoprecipitation.

Implications of results

Specific levels of cryoglobulins are characteristic of certain diseases. However, cryoglobulinemia doesn't always mean that clinical disease is present.

Posttest care

- Tell the patient to resume his usual diet.
- If the test is positive for cryoglobulins, tell the patient to avoid cold temperatures and contact with cold objects.
- If a hematoma develops, apply warm soaks.
- Observe for intravascular coagulation (decreased color and temperature in distal extremities and increased pain).

Interfering factors

- Failure to adhere to dietary restrictions may affect the accuracy of test results.
- Failure to keep the sample at 98.6° F (37° C) before centrifugation may cause loss of cryoglobulins.
- Reading the sample before the end of the 72-hour precipitation period may cause test results to be reported incorrectly because some cryoglobulins take several days to precipitate.

Cyclic adenosine monophosphate (cAMP) test

Formed from adenosine triphosphate by the action of the enzyme adenylate cyclase, the nucleotide cyclic adenosine monophosphate (cAMP) influences the protein synthesis rate within cells. Measuring urinary excretion of cAMP after I.V. infusion of a standard dose of parathyroid hormone (PTH) can show renal tubular resistance in a patient with hypoparathyroid symptoms and high levels of PTH. Such findings suggest type I pseudohypoparathyroidism. This rare inherited disorder results from tissue resistance to PTH and produces hypocalcemia, hyperphosphatemia, and skeletal and constitutional abnormalities.

`CLINICAL ALERT` This test is contraindicated in patients with high calcium levels because PTH further raises calcium levels. It should be used cautiously in patients receiving cardiac glycosides and in those with sarcoidosis or renal or cardiac disease.

Purpose

To aid differential diagnosis of pseudohypoparathyroidism.

Patient preparation

Explain to the patient that this test evaluates parathyroid function. Tell him it requires a 15-minute I.V. infusion of PTH and collection of a 3- to 4-hour urine specimen.

Perform a skin test to detect a possible allergy to PTH; keep epinephrine readily available in case of an adverse reaction. Just before the procedure is performed, instruct the patient not to touch the I.V. line or exert pressure on the arm receiving the infusion. Tell him he may experience transient discomfort from the needle puncture. Ask him to notify you if he feels severe burning or if the site becomes inflamed or swollen.

Equipment

PTH (300 units in refrigerated ampules) ■ vial of sterile water (saline solution causes precipitate to form) ■ urine collection container with hydrochloric acid as a preservative.

Procedure

■ Instruct the patient to empty his bladder. If he has an indwelling urinary catheter in place, change the collection bag. If ordered, send this specimen to the laboratory; otherwise, discard it.
■ Prepare the PTH for infusion as directed, using sterile water for dilution. Start the I.V. infusion with dextrose 5% in water, and infuse the PTH over 15 minutes. Record the start of the infusion as time zero.
■ Discontinue the infusion.
■ Collect a urine specimen 3 to 4 hours after the infusion.

Precautions

■ Tell the patient not to contaminate the specimen with toilet tissue or stool.
■ Send the specimen to the laboratory immediately or refrigerate it if transport is delayed. If the patient is catheterized, keep the collection bag on ice.
■ This test is contraindicated in patients with a positive PTH test as well as in patients with hypercalcemia because PTH will further increase calcium levels.
■ Use this test with caution in patients on cardiac glycosides and in patients with renal impairment, cardiac disease, or sarcoidosis.

Reference values

A 10- to 20-fold increase (3.6 to 4 μmol) in cAMP demonstrates a normal response or hypoparathyroidism.

Implications of results

Failure to respond to PTH, indicated by normal urinary excretion of cAMP, suggests type I pseudohypoparathyroidism.

Posttest care

CLINICAL ALERT Observe for symptoms of hypercalcemia: lethargy, anorexia, nausea, vomiting, vertigo, and abdominal cramps.

If a hematoma or irritation develops at the venipuncture site, apply warm soaks.

Interfering factors

Contamination or improper storage of the specimen or failure to acidify the urine with hydrochloric acid may alter test results.

Cytomegalovirus antibody screening test

After primary infection, cytomegalovirus (CMV) remains latent in white blood cells (WBCs). The presence of CMV antibodies indicates past infection with this virus. In an immunocompromised patient, CMV can be reactivated to cause active infection. Administration of blood or tissue from a seropositive donor may cause active CMV infection in CMV-seronegative organ transplant recipients or neonates, especially those born prematurely.

Antibodies to CMV can be detected by several methods, including passive hemagglutination, latex agglutination, enzyme immunoassay, and indirect immunofluorescence. The complement fixation test is only 60% sensitive compared with other assays and shouldn't be used to screen for CMV antibodies. Screening tests for CMV antibodies are qualitative; they detect the presence of antibody at a single low dilution. In quantitative methods, several dilutions of the serum sample are tested to indicate acute infection with CMV.

Purpose

■ To detect past CMV infection in donors and recipients of organs and blood
■ To screen for CMV infection in infants who require blood transfusions or tissue transplants
■ To detect past CMV infection in immunocompromised patients.

Patient preparation

As appropriate, explain the purpose of the test to the patient or the parents of an infant. Tell the patient that the test requires a blood sample and who will perform the venipuncture and when. Provide reassurance that, although the needle puncture and the tourniquet may cause transient discomfort, collecting the sample takes less than 3 minutes.

Procedure

- Perform a venipuncture and collect the sample in a 5-ml tube without additives.
- Allow the blood to clot for at least 1 hour at room temperature.

Precautions

- Handle the sample gently to prevent hemolysis.
- Transfer the serum to a sterile tube or vial and send it to the laboratory.
- If transfer must be delayed, store the serum at 39.2° F (4° C) for 1 to 2 days or at –4° F (–20° C) for longer periods to avoid contamination.

Normal findings

Patients who have never been infected with CMV have no detectable antibodies to the virus. Immunoglobulin G (IgG) and IgM are normally negative.

Implications of results

A serum sample collected early during the acute phase or late in the convalescent stage of CMV infection may not contain detectable IgG or IgM antibodies to CMV. Therefore, a negative result doesn't preclude recent infection. More than a single sample is needed to ensure accurate results.

A serum sample that tests positive for antibodies at this single dilution indicates that the patient has been infected with CMV and that his WBCs contain latent virus capable of being reactivated in an immunocompromised host. Immunosuppressed patients who lack antibodies to CMV should receive blood products or organ transplants from donors who are also seronegative. Patients with CMV antibodies don't require seronegative blood products.

Post-test care

If a hematoma develops, apply warm soaks.

Interfering factors

- Rough handling of the sample can cause hemolysis.
- Failure to store serum at the proper temperature can affect test results.

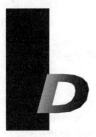

D-Dimer test

A D-dimer is an asymmetrical carbon compound fragment formed after thrombin converts fibrinogen to fibrin, factor XIIIa stabilizes it into a clot, and plasma acts on the cross-linked, or clotted, fibrin. The test is specific for fibrinolysis because it confirms the presence of fibrin split products.

Purpose

■ To diagnose disseminated intravascular coagulation (DIC)
■ To differentiate subarachnoid hemorrhage from a traumatic lumbar puncture in spinal fluid analysis.

Patient preparation

Obtain the patient's history of hematologic diseases, recent surgery, and the results of other tests performed. Explain to the patient that the test is used to determine if the blood is clotting normally. Tell him that the test requires a blood sample. Explain who will perform the venipuncture and when. Reassure him that drawing a blood sample will take less than 3 minutes. Explain that he may feel slight discomfort from the tourniquet pressure and the needle puncture.

Procedure

■ Perform a venipuncture and collect the sample in a 5-ml tube with sodium citrate added.
■ For a spinal fluid analysis, the sample is collected during a lumbar puncture and placed in a plastic vial. (See "Cerebrospinal fluid analysis" for details of the procedure.)

Precautions

Completely fill the collection tube, invert it gently several times, and send it to the laboratory immediately.
CLINICAL ALERT For a patient with coagulation problems, you may need to apply additional pressure at the venipuncture site to control bleeding.

Reference values

Normal D-dimer test results are negative or less than 250 µg/ml.

Implications of results

Increased D-dimer values may indicate DIC, pulmonary embolism, arterial or venous thrombosis, neoplastic disease, pregnancy (late and postpartum), surgery performed during the 2 days before testing, subarachnoid hemorrhage (spinal fluid only), or secondary fibrinolysis.

Posttest care

■ Apply pressure to the venipuncture site for 5 minutes or until bleeding stops.
■ If a hematoma develops at the venipuncture site, apply warm soaks.

Interfering factors

■ Failure to fill the collection tube completely or to send the sample to the laboratory immediately can alter test results.
■ Rough handling of the sample can cause hemolysis.
■ High rheumatoid factor titers or increased CA-125 levels can cause false-positive results.
■ False-negative results can occur with spinal fluid analysis in infants under age 6 months.

Delta-aminolevulinic acid test, urine

Using the colorimetric technique, this quantitative analysis of urine delta-aminolevulinic acid (ALA) levels helps diagnose porphyrias, hepatic disease, and lead poisoning. In an emergency, a simple qualitative screening test can be performed. ALA, the basic precursor of the porphyrins, normally converts to porphobilinogen through the action of the enzyme ALA-dehydrase during heme synthesis. Impaired conversion, as in porphyrias and lead poisoning, causes urine ALA levels to rise before other chemical or hematologic changes occur.

Purpose

■ To screen for lead poisoning
■ To aid diagnosis of porphyrias and certain hepatic disorders, such as hepatitis and hepatic carcinoma.

Patient preparation

Explain to the patient that this test detects abnormal hemoglobin formation. If lead poisoning is suspected, tell the patient (or the parents, as the patient in these cases is usually a child) that the test helps detect the presence of excessive lead in the body. Inform the patient (or parents) that restriction of food or fluids isn't necessary.

Tell him that the test requires a 24-hour urine specimen and provide instruction on the proper collection technique.

Check the patient's medication history for recent use of drugs that may alter ALA levels. Review your findings with the clinician, who may want to restrict these medications before the test.

Procedure

Collect a 24-hour urine specimen in a light-resistant bottle containing a preservative (usually glacial acetic acid) to prevent degradation of ALA.

Precautions

■ Refrigerate the specimen or keep it on ice during the collection period. When the collection is completed, send the specimen to the laboratory at once.
■ Protect the specimen from direct sunlight. If the patient has an indwelling urinary catheter in place, insert the collection bag into a dark plastic bag.

Reference values

Normal urine ALA values range from 1.5 to 7.5 mg/dl/24 hours.

Implications of results

Elevated urine ALA levels occur in lead poisoning, acute porphyria, hepatic carcinoma, and hepatitis.

Posttest care

Resume administration of medications withheld before the test.

Interfering factors

■ Barbiturates and griseofulvin cause porphyrins to accumulate in the liver and thus raise urine ALA levels. Vitamin E in pharmacologic doses may lower urine ALA levels.
■ Failure to observe medication restrictions, to collect all urine during the test period, or to store the specimen properly may alter test results.

Dexamethasone suppression test

A standard screening test for Cushing's syndrome, the dexamethasone suppression test also helps diagnose major depression and monitor its treatment. Certain patients with major depression have high levels of circulating adrenal steroid hormones in their blood. Administration of an oral corticosteroid such as dexamethasone suppresses these levels in normal people but fails to suppress them in patients with Cushing's syndrome or some forms of depression.

Purpose
- To diagnose Cushing's syndrome
- To aid diagnosis of clinical depression.

Patient preparation
Explain the purpose of the test. Inform the patient that the test requires two blood samples drawn after administration of dexamethasone. Tell him who will perform the venipuncture and when and that he may experience transient discomfort from the needle puncture and the pressure of the tourniquet. Restrict food and fluids for 10 to 12 hours before the test.

Procedure
- Give the patient 1 mg of dexamethasone at 11 p.m.
- On the following day, collect blood samples at 4 p.m. and 11 p.m. More frequent sampling may increase the likelihood of measuring a nonsuppressed cortisol peak.

Precautions
Many medications, including corticosteroids, oral contraceptives, lithium, methadone, aspirin, diuretics, morphine, and monoamine oxidase (MAO) inhibitors, may affect the accuracy of test results. If possible, don't administer any of these medications after midnight the night before the test.

Reference values
A cortisol level of 5 g/dl (140 nmol/L) or more indicates failure of dexamethasone suppression.

Implications of results
A normal test result doesn't rule out major depression, but an abnormal result strengthens a clinically based diagnosis. Failure of suppression occurs in patients with Cushing's syndrome, severe stress, and depression that's likely to respond to treatment with antidepressants.

The dexamethasone suppression test has proved disappointing in differentiating dysthymic disorder from major affective illness. It may be useful in patients with other psychiatric disorders (such as schizoaffective disorder) to establish the need to treat coexisting depression.

Posttest care
If a hematoma develops at the venipuncture site, apply warm soaks.

Interfering factors

■ False-positive results can occur if caffeine was ingested after midnight the night before the test.
■ False-positive results can follow the use of certain drugs, particularly barbiturates or phenytoin, within 3 weeks of the test.
■ False-positive results can occur in diabetes mellitus, pregnancy, and severe stress (such as trauma, severe weight loss, dehydration, and acute alcohol withdrawal).
■ Failure to withhold corticosteroids, oral contraceptives, lithium, methadone, aspirin, diuretics, morphine, or MAO inhibitors for 24 to 48 hours before the test may interfere with test results.

Direct antiglobulin test

Also known as the direct Coombs' test, the direct antiglobulin test detects immunoglobulins (antibodies) on the surfaces of red blood cells (RBCs). These immunoglobulins coat RBCs when they become sensitized to an antigen, such as Rh factor.

In this test, addition of antiglobulin (Coombs') serum to saline-washed RBCs results in agglutination if immunoglobulins or complement is present. This test is "direct" because it requires only one step — the addition of Coombs' serum to washed cells.

Purpose

■ To diagnose hemolytic disease of the newborn (HDN)
■ To investigate hemolytic transfusion reactions
■ To aid differential diagnosis of hemolytic anemias, which may be congenital or may result from an autoimmune reaction or use of certain drugs.

Patient preparation

If the patient is a neonate, explain to the parents that this test helps diagnose HDN. If the patient is suspected of having hemolytic anemia, explain that this test determines whether the condition results from an abnormality in the body's immune system, from the use of certain drugs, or from some unknown cause.

Inform the adult patient that fasting isn't necessary. Tell the patient (or the infant's parents) that the test requires a blood sample, who will perform the venipuncture and when, and that the needle puncture may cause transient discomfort.

Withhold medications that may induce autoimmune hemolytic anemia.

Procedure

- For an adult, perform a venipuncture and collect the sample in two 5-ml tubes with EDTA added.
- For a neonate, draw 5 ml of cord blood into a tube with EDTA or no additives after the cord is clamped and cut.

Precautions

- Handle the sample gently to prevent hemolysis.
- Send the sample to the laboratory immediately. The test must be performed within 24 hours.

Normal findings

A negative test, in which neither antibodies nor complement is present on the RBCs, is normal.

Implications of results

- A positive test on umbilical cord blood indicates that maternal antibodies have crossed the placenta and have coated fetal RBCs, causing HDN.
- Transfusion of compatible blood lacking the antigens to these maternal antibodies may be necessary to prevent anemia. Notify the doctor or clinician immediately so that prompt action can be taken.
- In other patients, a positive test result may suggest hemolytic anemia and may help differentiate between autoimmune and secondary hemolytic anemia, which can be drug-induced or associated with an underlying disease such as lymphoma. A positive test result can also indicate sepsis.
- A borderline or slightly positive test result may suggest a transfusion reaction in which the patient's antibodies react with transfused RBCs containing the corresponding antigen.

Posttest care

- If a hematoma develops at the venipuncture site, apply warm soaks.
- Resume administration of medications withheld before the test.
- Tell the patient or the parents of an infant with HDN that further testing will be necessary to monitor anemia.

Interfering factors

- Positive results may follow use of quinidine, methyldopa, cephalosporins, sulfonamides, chlorpromazine, diphen-ylhydantoin, dipyrone, ethosuximide, hydralazine, levodopa, mefenamic acid, melphalan, penicillin, procainamide, rifampin, streptomycin, tetracyclines, or isoniazid. A positive test caused by these drugs may or may not be associated with immune hemolysis.

■ Hemolysis caused by rough handling of the sample may alter test results.

Duodenal contents culture

This test requires duodenal intubation, aspiration of duodenal contents, and cultivation of any microbes present to isolate and identify a duodenal or biliary pathogen. Occasionally, a specimen may be obtained during surgery (such as a cholecystectomy) or duodenoscopy. Duodenal contents (pancreatic and duodenal enzymes and bile) are normally almost sterile, but they're subject to infection by many bacterial pathogens, such as *Escherichia coli, Staphylococcus aureus*, and Salmonella species, as well as parasites, such *as Giardia lamblia* and *Strongyloides stercoralis*. Infection of the biliary tract and duodenum can cause duodenitis, cholecystitis, or cholangitis.

Purpose

■ To detect bacterial infection of the biliary tract and duodenum; to differentiate between such infection and gallstones

■ To rule out bacterial infection as the cause of persistent GI symptoms (epigastric pain, nausea, vomiting, and diarrhea).

Patient preparation

Explain to the patient that this test helps to determine the cause of his symptoms. Instruct him to restrict food and fluids for 12 hours before the test. Tell him who will perform the procedure and where it will be done.

Describe the intubation procedure to the patient. Assure him that although this procedure is uncomfortable, it isn't dangerous. Explain that passage of the tube may make him gag, but following the examiner's instructions about proper positioning, breathing, swallowing, and relaxing will minimize discomfort. Suggest to the patient that he empty his bladder before the procedure to increase his comfort.

Equipment

Gloves ■ double-lumen tube with olive tip ■ water-soluble lubricating jelly ■ 30-ml sterile syringe ■ emesis basin ■ sterile specimen container ■ adhesive tape.

Procedure

■ After the nasoenteric tube is inserted, place the patient in the left lateral decubitus position with his feet elevated to allow peristalsis to move the tube into the duodenum. The pH of a small amount of aspirated fluid determines tube position: If the tube is in the stomach,

pH is lower than 7.0; if the tube is in the duodenum, pH is higher than 7.0. Correct tube position can also be confirmed by fluoroscopy. After confirmation, duodenal contents are aspirated.
■ Transfer the specimen to a sterile container and label it with the patient's name, doctor's name, date and time of collection, and collector's initials.

Precautions
■ Use gloves when performing procedures and handling specimens.
■ Duodenal intubation is contraindicated in pregnancy, acute pancreatitis or cholecystitis, esophageal disorders (varices, stenosis, diverticula, or malignant neoplasms), recent severe gastric hemorrhage, aortic aneurysm, congestive heart failure, or myocardial infarction.
■ Collect the specimen for culture before antimicrobial therapy begins.
■ Withdraw the tube slowly (6″ to 8″ [15 to 20 cm] every 10 minutes) until it reaches the esophagus; then clamp the tube and remove it quickly. Notify the doctor if the tube can't be withdrawn easily; never force the tube.
■ Send the specimen to the laboratory immediately.

Reference values
A duodenal contents culture normally contains small amounts of polymorphonuclear leukocytes and epithelial cells with no pathogens. The bacterial count is usually less than 100,000/ml.

Implications of results
■ Generally, bacterial counts of 100,000/ml or more or the presence of any number of pathogens, such as Salmonella, indicates infection. Susceptibility testing may be required.
■ Numerous polymorphonuclear leukocytes, copious mucous debris, and bile-stained epithelial cells in the bile fluid suggest inflammation of the biliary tract.
■ Many segmented neutrophils and exfoliated epithelial cells suggest inflammation of the pancreas, the duodenum, or bile ducts.
■ The presence of bile sand indicates cholelithiasis or calculi in the biliary tract.

Differential diagnosis requires further testing, including oral or I.V. cholecystography; white blood cell count; cholangiography; measurement of serum bilirubin, alkaline phosphatase, serum amylase, and urine urobilinogen; and culture of surgical material.

Posttest care

CLINICAL ALERT After duodenal intubation or duodenoscopy, observe the patient carefully for signs of perforation from tube passage, such as dysphagia, epigastric
or shoulder pain, dyspnea, or fever.

■ After duodenoscopy, monitor vital signs until the patient is stable; keep the bed rails up, and enforce bed rest
until the patient is fully alert.

■ Resume diet discontinued before the test.

Interfering factors

■ Failure to observe a 12-hour fast can dilute the specimen, which decreases the bacterial count.

■ Improper collection technique can contaminate the
specimen.

Duodenal contents examination

This test evaluates duodenal contents for the presence
of parasites in a specimen obtained by duodenal intubation and aspiration or by the string (Entero) test. Such
parasites include trophozoites of *Giardia lamblia;* the
ova and larvae of *Strongyloides stercoralis;* and the ova
of *Necator americanus* or *Ancylostoma duodenale* in
various stages of cleavage. This test can also detect ova
of the liver flukes *Clonorchis sinensis* and *Fasciola hepatica* in the biliary tract. Liver fluke infestations are
rare in the United States, but they may occur in people
who have spent time in tropical third world countries.

Examination of duodenal contents for ova and parasites is performed only in a symptomatic patient with
negative stool examinations.

Purpose

To detect parasitic infection when stool examinations
are negative

Patient preparation

Explain to the patient that this test detects parasitic infection of the GI tract. Instruct him to restrict food and
fluids for 12 hours before the test. Tell him who will
perform the test and when. If the test will be done with
a nasoenteric tube, warn him that he may gag during the
tube's passage but reassure him that following the examiner's instructions about positioning, breathing, and
swallowing will minimize discomfort. Just before the
procedure, instruct the patient to empty his bladder.

Equipment

Gloves ■ double-lumen tube with olive tip (or weighted
gelatin capsule with string attached, for string test) ■

water-soluble jelly ■ 30-ml sterile syringe ■ emesis basin
■ sterile specimen container ■ ½" (1.2 cm) adhesive tape.

Procedure

If using a nasoenteric tube:
■ After inserting the tube, place the patient in a left lateral decubitus position, with his feet elevated, to allow peristalsis to move the tube into the duodenum.
■ The pH of a small amount of aspirated fluid determines tube position: If the tube is in the stomach, pH is lower than 7.0; if it's in the duodenum, pH is higher than 7.0. Fluoroscopy can also determine correct positioning.
■ When tube position is confirmed, residual duodenal contents are aspirated. Transfer the entire specimen to a sterile container; label it appropriately.
If using an Entero test capsule with string:
■ Tape the free end of the string to the patient's cheek. Then tell him to swallow the capsule (on the other end of the string) with water.
■ Leave the string in place for 4 hours; then pull it out gently and place it in a sterile container. Label the container appropriately.
■ Dispose of equipment properly.

Precautions

■ Use gloves when performing the procedure and handling specimens.
■ Duodenal intubation is contraindicated during pregnancy and in patients with acute cholecystitis, acute pancreatitis, esophageal disorders (varices, stenosis, diverticula, or malignant neoplasms), recent severe gastric hemorrhage, aortic aneurysm, or congestive heart failure.
■ When possible, obtain the specimen before the start of drug therapy.
■ Send the specimen to the laboratory immediately.
■ Withdraw the tube slowly (6" to 8" [15 to 20 cm] every 10 minutes) to the esophagus; then clamp the tube and remove it quickly. Never force the tube.

Normal findings

No ova or parasites should be present.

Implications of results

Finding *G. lamblia* suggests giardiasis, which may cause malabsorption syndrome
■ *S. stercoralis* suggests strongyloidiasis
■ *A. duodenale* and *N. americanus* imply hookworm disease

■ *C. sinensis* and *F. hepatica* signify histopathologic changes in the bile ducts.

Posttest care

■ Provide mouth care and offer water.
■ After duodenal intubation or duodenoscopy, observe the patient carefully for signs of perforation from tube passage, such as dysphagia, epigastric or shoulder pain, dyspnea, or fever.
■ After duodenoscopy, monitor vital signs until the patient is stable; keep the bed rails up, and enforce bed rest until the patient is fully alert.
■ Resume diet discontinued before the test.

Interfering factors

■ Failure of the patient to observe the 12-hour fast can dilute the specimen.
■ Previous drug therapy or delay in sending the specimen may alter results.

D-xylose absorption test

One of the most important tests for malabsorption, D-xylose absorption gives important information about patients with such symptoms as weight loss and generalized malnutrition, weakness, and diarrhea. In this test, the patient ingests a standard dose of D-xylose—a pentose sugar that's absorbed in the small intestine without the aid of pancreatic enzymes, passed through the liver without being metabolized, and excreted in the urine. The amounts of D-xylose in the urine and blood reflect the absorptive capacity of the small intestine. Normally, blood levels of D-xylose peak 2 hours after ingestion; 80% to 95% of the dose is excreted in 5 hours and the remainder within 24 hours.

To make sure results will be accurate, the patient must fast overnight and remain in bed during the specimen collection period. His renal function must be adequate for the absorption and excretion of D-xylose.

Purpose

■ To aid differential diagnosis of malabsorption
■ To determine the cause of malabsorption syndrome.

Patient preparation

Explain to the patient that this test helps evaluate digestive function by analyzing blood and urine specimens after ingestion of a sugar solution. Advise him to fast overnight before the test. Instruct him to abstain from all food and fluids and to remain in bed during the entire test period because activity affects test results.

Tell him that the test requires several blood samples, who will perform the venipunctures and when, and that he may experience some discomfort from the needle punctures and the pressure of the tourniquet. Reassure him that collecting each blood sample takes less than 3 minutes. Inform him that all his urine will be collected for 5 or 24 hours.

Withhold aspirin and indomethacin, which alter test results, and record any medications the patient is taking on the laboratory request.

Equipment

Tourniquet ■ venipuncture equipment ■ 10-ml tube without additives ■ sterile urine specimen container ■ specimen labels ■ gloves ■ biohazard transport bags.

Procedure

■ Perform a venipuncture to obtain a fasting blood sample, and collect the sample in a 10-ml tube without additives. Then collect a first-voided morning urine specimen. Label these specimens and send them to the laboratory immediately to serve as a baseline.

■ Give the patient 25 g of D-xylose dissolved in 8 oz (240 ml) of water followed by an additional 8 oz of water. If the patient is a child, administer 0.5 g of D-xylose per pound of body weight, up to 25 g. Record the time of D-xylose ingestion.

■ In an adult, draw a blood sample 2 hours after D-xylose ingestion; in a child, 1 hour. Collect the sample in a 10-ml tube without additives.

■ Occasionally, a 5-hour blood sample may be drawn to support the findings of the 1- or 2-hour sample.

■ Collect and pool all urine during the 5 or 24 hours following D-xylose ingestion.

Precautions

■ Check with the doctor or clinician to determine how long the collection period should be because patients age 65 and older and those with borderline or elevated creatinine levels tend to have low 5-hour urine levels but normal 24-hour levels.

■ Handle the blood collection tubes gently to prevent hemolysis.

■ Tell the patient not to contaminate the urine specimens with toilet tissue or stool.

■ Be sure to collect all urine and refrigerate the specimen during the collection period.

■ At the end of the collection period, send the specimens to the laboratory immediately.

■ Keep the patient on bed rest and withhold food and fluids (other than D-xylose and water) throughout the test period.

Reference values

The following are normal values for the D-xylose absorption test:

■ adults: blood concentration, 25 to 40 mg/dl in 2 hours; urine, more than 3.5 g excreted in 5 hours (age 65 or older, more than 5 g in 24 hours)

■ children: blood concentration, more than 30 mg/dl in 1 hour; urine, 16% to 33% of ingested D-xylose excreted in 5 hours.

Implications of results

Depressed blood and urine D-xylose levels most commonly result from malabsorptive disorders that affect the proximal small intestine, such as sprue and celiac disease. However, depressed D-xylose levels may also result from regional enteritis involving the jejunum, Whipple's disease, multiple jejunal diverticula, myxedema, diabetic neuropathic diarrhea, rheumatoid arthritis, alcoholism, severe congestive heart failure, and ascites.

Posttest care

■ If a hematoma develops at the venipuncture site, ease discomfort by applying warm soaks.

■ Observe the patient for abdominal discomfort or mild diarrhea caused by D-xylose ingestion.

■ Resume administration of medications discontinued before the test.

■ Tell the patient to resume a normal diet.

Interfering factors

■ Aspirin decreases D-xylose excretion by the kidneys; indomethacin depresses its intestinal absorption.

■ Failure to adhere to dietary and activity restrictions affects absorption of D-xylose.

■ Failure to obtain a complete urine specimen or to collect blood samples at designated times interferes with accurate testing.

■ Intestinal overgrowth of bacteria, renal insufficiency, or renal retention of urine may decrease urine levels.

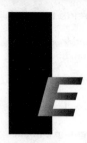

Epstein-Barr virus antibody test

Epstein-Barr virus (EBV), a member of the herpesvirus group, is the causative agent in heterophile-positive infectious mononucleosis, Burkitt's lymphoma, and nasopharyngeal carcinoma. Although the virus doesn't replicate in standard cell cultures, most EBV infections can be recognized by testing the patient's serum for heterophile antibodies (monospot test), which usually appear within the first 3 weeks of illness and then decline rapidly within a few weeks. In about 10% of adults and a larger percentage of children, the monospot test is negative despite primary infection with EBV. (See *Monospot test for infectious mononucleosis.*)

EBV has also been associated with lymphoproliferative processes in immunosuppressed people. These disorders occur with reactivated, rather than primary, EBV infections and, thus, are also monospot-negative.

Alternatively, EBV-specific antibodies, which develop to several antigens of the virus during active infection, can be measured with high sensitivity and specificity by indirect immunofluorescence tests. The test profile results of immunoglobulin (Ig) G, IgM, and IgA class antibodies directed to the EBV antigens, viral capsid antigen (VCA) and Epstein-Barr nuclear antigen (EBNA), can help determine whether the patient was infected recently or in the remote past.

Purpose

- To provide a laboratory diagnosis of heterophile- (or monospot-) negative cases of infectious mononucleosis
- To determine the antibody status to EBV of immunosuppressed patients with lymphoproliferative processes.

Patient preparation

Explain the purpose of the test. Inform the patient that this test requires a blood sample, who will perform the venipuncture and when, and that he may experience transient discomfort from the needle puncture and the pressure of the tourniquet.

MONOSPOT TEST FOR INFECTIOUS MONONUCLEOSIS

Several screening tests can detect the heterophil infectious mononucleosis (IM) antibody. One of these—the monospot test—converts the Paul-Bunnell and the Davidsohn's differential absorption tests into one rapid slide test without titration. Monospot rivals the classic heterophil agglutination test for sensitivity.

The monospot test relies on agglutination of horse red blood cells (RBCs) by heterophil antibodies. Because horse RBCs contain both Forssman and IM antigens, differential absorption of the patient's serum is necessary to distinguish between them. This is done by mixing the serum sample with guinea pig kidney antigen (containing only Forssman antigen) on one end of a slide and with beef RBC stroma (containing only IM antigen) on the other. Each absorbs only the heterophil antibody specific to it. After addition of horse RBCs to each spot, agglutination on the beef cell end of the slide indicates the presence of the IM heterophil antibody and confirms IM.

False-positive results may occur in lymphoma, hepatitis A and hepatitis B, leukemia, and pancreatic cancer.

Procedure

Perform a venipuncture and collect 5 ml of sterile blood in a clot-activator tube. Allow the blood to clot for at least 1 hour at room temperature.

Precautions

- Handle the sample gently because excessive agitation will cause hemolysis of the sample.
- Transfer the serum to a sterile tube or vial and send it to the laboratory promptly. If transfer must be delayed, store the serum at 39.2° F (4° C) for 1 or 2 days or at –4° F (–20° C) for longer periods to prevent bacterial contamination.

Normal findings

Serum from patients who have never been infected with EBV will have no detectable antibodies to the virus measured by either the monospot or indirect immunofluorescence test. The monospot test is positive only during the acute phase of EBV infection; the indirect immunofluorescence test will detect and discriminate between acute and past infection.

Implications of results

- EBV infection can be ruled out if no antibodies to EBV antigens are detected in the indirect immunofluorescence test.

■ A positive monospot test or an indirect immunofluorescence test that is either IgM-positive or EBNA-negative indicates acute EBV infection.

■ A negative monospot result doesn't necessarily rule out acute or past infection with EBV. IgG class antibody to VCA and EBNA antigens (IgM-negative) indicates remote (more than 2 months) infection with EBV. (Most cases of monospot-negative infectious mononucleosis are caused by cytomegalovirus infections.)

■ Notify the clinician if the test indicates an active infection because the patient will need immediate medical attention.

Posttest care

If a hematoma develops at the venipuncture site, apply warm soaks.

Interfering factors

Hemolysis will alter test results.

Erythrocyte sedimentation rate test

The erythrocyte sedimentation rate (ESR) measures the degree of erythrocyte (red blood cell [RBC]) settling during a specified time period. As the RBCs descend in the tube, they displace an equal volume of plasma upward, which retards the downward progress of other settling blood elements. Factors affecting ESR include red cell volume, surface area, density, aggregation, and surface charge. Plasma proteins (notably fibrinogen and globulin) encourage aggregation, increasing the sedimentation rate.

The ESR is a sensitive but nonspecific test that is frequently the earliest indicator of disease when other chemical or physical signs are normal. It often rises significantly in widespread inflammatory disorders due to infection or autoimmune mechanisms; such elevations may be prolonged in localized inflammation and malignancy.

Purpose

■ To monitor inflammatory or malignant disease
■ To aid detection and diagnosis of occult disease, such as tuberculosis, tissue necrosis, or connective tissue disease.

Patient preparation

Explain to the patient that this test evaluates the condition of RBCs. Inform him that he need not restrict food or fluids. Tell him the test requires a blood sample, who will perform the venipuncture and when, and that he may experience transient discomfort from the needle puncture and the pressure of the tourniquet.

Procedure

Perform a venipuncture and collect the sample in a 7-ml tube with EDTA added or a 4.5-ml tube with sodium citrate added. (Check with the laboratory to determine preference.)

Precautions

- Completely fill the collection tube and invert it gently several times to adequately mix the sample and the anticoagulant.
- Because prolonged standing decreases the ESR, send the sample to the laboratory immediately after examining it for clots or clumps. The sample must be tested within 2 to 4 hours.
- Handle the sample gently to prevent hemolysis.

Reference values

Normal ESR ranges from 0 to 10 mm/hour in males and from 0 to 20 mm/hour in females; rates gradually increase with age.

Implications of results

- The ESR rises in pregnancy, acute or chronic inflammation, tuberculosis, paraproteinemias (especially multiple myeloma and Waldenström's macroglobulinemia), rheumatic fever, rheumatoid arthritis, and some cancers.
- Anemia also tends to raise ESR, because less upward displacement of plasma occurs to retard the relatively few sedimenting RBCs.
- Polycythemia, sickle cell anemia, hyperviscosity, or low plasma fibrinogen or globulin levels tend to depress ESR.

Posttest care

If a hematoma develops at the venipuncture site, apply warm soaks.

Interfering factors

- Failure to use the proper anticoagulant in the collection tube, to adequately mix the sample and anticoagulant, or to send the sample to the laboratory immediately may affect test results.
- Hemolysis caused by rough handling or excessive mixing of the sample may affect the sedimentation.
- Prolonged tourniquet constriction may cause hemoconcentration.

Erythropoietin test

This test of renal hormone production measures erythropoietin by immunoassay. It's used to evaluate anemia, polycythemia, and kidney tumors. It's also used to evaluate abuse of commercially prepared erythropoietin by athletes who believe the drug enhances performance.

A glycoprotein hormone, erythropoietin is secreted by the kidneys in adults. The hormone acts on stem cells in the bone marrow to stimulate production of red blood cells. It's regulated by a feedback loop involving red cell volume and oxygen saturation of the blood, especially in the brain.

Purpose

- To aid diagnosis of anemia and polycythemia
- To aid diagnosis of kidney tumors
- To detect abuse of erythropoietin by athletes.

Patient preparation

Explain to the patient that this test determines whether hormonal secretion is causing changes in his red blood cells. Instruct him to fast for 8 to 10 hours before the test. Tell him that this test requires a blood sample, who will perform the venipuncture and when, and that he may feel transient discomfort from the puncture. Advise him that the laboratory requires up to 4 days to complete the analysis. Keep the patient relaxed and recumbent for 30 minutes before the test.

Procedure

- Perform a venipuncture, and collect the sample in a 5-ml clot-activator tube.
- If a hematocrit is requested at the same time, collect an additional sample in a 2-ml tube with EDTA added.

Precautions

Handle the specimen gently to prevent hemolysis.

Reference values

The normal range is up to 24 mU/ml.

Implications of results

- Low levels of erythropoietin appear in anemic patients with inadequate or absent hormone production and may occur in severe renal disease.
- Congenital absence of erythropoietin also can occur.
- Elevated levels occur in anemias as a compensatory mechanism in the reestablishment of homeostasis.
- Inappropriate elevations (when the hematocrit level is normal to high) occur in polycythemia and erythropoietin-secreting tumors.

■ Erythropoietin can be produced for sale by recombinant gene technology and is used by some athletes as a performance enhancer. The increased red cell volume conveys additional oxygen-carrying capacity to the blood. Adverse reactions from such use may include clotting abnormalities, headache, seizures, hypertension, nausea, vomiting, diarrhea, and rash.

Posttest care

If a hematoma develops at the venipuncture site, apply warm soaks.

Interfering factors

■ Failure to collect a fasting sample will affect test results.
■ Hemolysis may affect results.

Estrogen tests

Estrogens are secreted by the ovaries. They are responsible for the development of secondary female sexual characteristics and for normal menstruation. Levels are usually undetectable in children. These hormones are secreted by ovarian follicular cells during the first half of the menstrual cycle and by the corpus luteum during the luteal phase and during pregnancy. In menopause, estrogen secretion drops to a constant, low level.

This radioimmunoassay measures serum levels of estradiol, estrone, and estriol (the only estrogens that appear in serum in measurable amounts) and has diagnostic significance in evaluating female gonadal dysfunction. (See *Predicting premature labor*, page 218.) Tests of hypothalamic-pituitary function may be required to confirm the diagnosis.

Purpose

■ To determine sexual maturation and fertility
■ To aid diagnosis of gonadal dysfunction, such as precocious or delayed puberty, menstrual disorders (especially amenorrhea), and infertility
■ To determine fetal well-being
■ To aid diagnosis of tumors known to secrete estrogen.

Patient preparation

Explain to the patient that this test helps determine if secretion of female hormones is normal and that the test may be repeated during the various phases of the menstrual cycle. Tell her that she need not restrict food or fluids. Inform her that the test requires a blood sample and tell her who will perform the venipuncture and when. Explain that she may experience transient discomfort from the needle puncture and tourniquet but

PREDICTING PREMATURE LABOR

A simple salivary test can help determine whether a pregnant woman is at risk for premature labor, a complication that is detrimental to the health of the premature infant. The test, known as the SalEst test, measures salivary levels of estriol, an estrogen that increases 1,000-fold during pregnancy. For women determined to be at risk, the SalEst test is 98% accurate in ruling out or predicting premature labor and delivery.

The test is performed on women between weeks 22 and 36 of gestation using their saliva and the SalEst test kit. Estriol levels rise 2 to 3 weeks before the spontaneous onset of labor and delivery. A positive test indicates that the patient is at risk for premature labor. With this knowledge and evaluation by a doctor, precautions can be instituted to decrease the risk of preterm labor and maintain fetal viability.

that collecting the sample takes only a few minutes. Withhold all steroid and pituitary-based hormones. If they must be continued, note this on the laboratory slip.

Procedure

- Procedure and posttest care may vary slightly, depending on whether plasma or serum is being measured.
- Perform a venipuncture and collect the sample in a 10-ml clot-activator tube.
- If the patient is premenopausal, indicate the phase of her menstrual cycle on the laboratory slip.

Reference values

- Normal serum estrogen levels for premenopausal women vary widely during the menstrual cycle, from 30 to 400 pg/ml.
- The range for postmenopausal women is 0 to 30 pg/ml.
- The normal range in men is 10 to 50 pg/ml.
- In children under age 6, the normal level is less than 10 pg/ml.

Implications of results

- Low estrogen levels may indicate primary hypogonadism, or ovarian failure, as in Turner's syndrome (XO karyotype) or ovarian agenesis; secondary hypogonadism, such as in hypopituitarism; or menopause.
- Abnormally high estrogen levels suggest estrogen-producing tumors, precocious puberty, or severe hepatic disease, such as cirrhosis, that prevents clearance of plasma estrogens.

■ High levels may also result from congenital adrenal hyperplasia (increased conversion of androgens to estrogen).

Posttest care

■ If a hematoma develops at the venipuncture site, apply warm soaks.
■ Resume administration of medications discontinued before the test.

Precautions

■ Handle the sample gently to prevent hemolysis.
■ Send the sample to the laboratory immediately.

Interfering factors

■ Pregnancy and pre-test use of estrogens, such as oral contraceptives (possible increase)
■ Clomiphene, an estrogen antagonist (possible decrease)
■ Steroids and pituitary-based hormones, such as dexamethasone
■ Hemolysis caused by rough handling of the sample

Estrogens test, total urine

The total urine estrogens test is a quantitative analysis of total urine levels of estradiol, estrone, and estriol—the major estrogens present in significant amounts in urine. A common assay for total urine estrogen levels uses purification by gel filtration followed by spectrophotofluorometry. Supplementary tests that may provide further information about ovarian function include cytologic examination of vaginal smears, measurement of urinary pregnanediol and follicle-stimulating hormone, and evaluation of response to an injection of progesterone.

Purpose

■ To evaluate ovarian activity and to help determine the cause of amenorrhea and female hyperestrogenism
■ To aid diagnosis of tumors of ovarian, adrenocortical, or testicular origin
■ To assess fetoplacental status.

Patient preparation

Explain to the nonpregnant female patient that this test helps evaluate ovarian function; to the pregnant patient that this test helps evaluate fetal development and placental function; and to the male patient that this test helps evaluate testicular function. Inform the patient that the test requires collection of urine over a 24-hour period. Advise the patient that no pretest restrictions of food or fluids are necessary. If the 24-hour specimen is to be collected at home, teach the patient the proper collection technique.

Procedure

- Collect the patient's urine over a 24-hour period. Use a bottle containing a preservative to keep the specimen at a pH of 3.0 to 5.0.
- If the patient is pregnant, note the approximate week of gestation on the laboratory slip.
- If the patient is not pregnant, note the stage of her menstrual cycle.

Precautions

Refrigerate the specimen or keep it on ice during the collection period.

Reference values

- Total urine estrogen levels rise and fall during the menstrual cycle, peaking shortly before midcycle, decreasing immediately after ovulation, increasing through the life of the corpus luteum, and decreasing greatly as the corpus luteum degenerates and menstruation begins. Total estrogen levels range from 4 to 60 µg/24 hours.
- During pregnancy, urine levels rise steadily as follows: First trimester: 0 to 800 µg/24 hours; second trimester: 800 to 5000 µg/24 hours; third trimester: 5000 to 50,000 µg/24 hours.
- After menopause, values are less than 10 µg/24 hours.
- In males, total estrogen levels range from 4 to 25 µg/24 hours.

Implications of results

- Decreased total urine estrogen levels may reflect ovarian agenesis, primary ovarian insufficiency (due to Stein-Leventhal syndrome, for example), or secondary ovarian insufficiency (due to pituitary or adrenal hypofunction or metabolic disturbances).
- Elevated total estrogen levels in nonpregnant females may indicate tumors of ovarian or adrenocortical origin, adrenocortical hyperplasia, or a metabolic or hepatic disorder. In males, elevated total estrogen levels are associated with testicular tumors.
- High total urine estrogen levels are normal during pregnancy; serial determinations should show a rising titer.

Interfering factors

Drugs that may influence total urine estrogen levels include steroid hormones, methenamine mandelate, phenazopyridine hydrochloride, phenothiazines, tetracyclines, phenolphthalein, ampicillin, meprobamate, senna, cascara sagrada, and hydrochlorothiazide.

Extractable nuclear antigen antibody tests

Extractable nuclear antigen (ENA) is a complex of at least two and possibly three antigens: ribonucleoprotein (RNP)—which is susceptible to degradation by ribonuclease; Smith (Sm) antigen—an acidic nuclear protein that resists ribonuclease degradation; and Sjögren's (SS-B) antigen—which forms a precipitate when antibody is present. Antibodies to these antigens are associated with certain autoimmune disorders.

Assays for ENA antibodies (ribonucleoprotein, anti-Smith, and Sjögren's antibodies) help differentiate autoimmune disorders with similar signs and symptoms.

■ RNP autoantibodies are associated with systemic lupus erythematosus (SLE), progressive systemic sclerosis, and other rheumatic disorders. This test aids in the differential diagnosis of systemic rheumatic disease and is a useful follow-up test for collagen vascular autoimmune disease.

■ Sm autoantibodies are a specific marker for SLE. This test, too, helps monitor collagen vascular autoimmune disease.

■ SS-B autoantibodies are produced in Sjögren's syndrome, an immunologic abnormality sometimes associated with rheumatic arthritis and SLE. However, this test doesn't confirm a diagnosis of Sjögren's syndrome.

Sheep red blood cells are sensitized with ENA extracted from rabbit thymus and then incubated with serum samples; ENA antibodies present in the serum will agglutinate the cells. If agglutination occurs, differential double immunoassays are performed to determine which antibody is present. Anti-ENA tests are most useful in tandem with anti-DNA, serum complement, and antinuclear antibody tests.

Purpose

■ To aid differential diagnosis of autoimmune disease
■ To distinguish between anti-RNP and anti-Sm antibodies
■ To screen for anti-RNP antibodies (common in mixed connective tissue disease)
■ To screen for anti-Sm antibodies (common in SLE)
■ To support diagnosis of collagen vascular autoimmune diseases
■ To monitor response to therapy.

Patient preparation

Explain to the patient that this test detects certain antibodies and that test results help determine diagnosis and treatment. Or, when indicated, explain that the test assesses the effectiveness of treatment. Advise him that he need not restrict food or fluids. Tell him the test requires a blood sample, who will perform the venipuncture and when, and that he may experience transient discomfort from the needle puncture and the pressure of the tourniquet.

Procedure

- Perform a venipuncture and collect the sample in a 7-ml tube without additives.
- Because a patient with an autoimmune disease has a compromised immune system, check the venipuncture site for infection and report any change promptly.

Precautions

Send the sample to the laboratory immediately.

Normal findings

Serum should be negative for anti-RNP, anti-Sm, and SS-B antibodies.

Implications of results

- The presence of anti-Sm strongly suggests a diagnosis of SLE.
- A high titer of anti-RNP with a low titer of anti-Sm suggests mixed connective tissue disease.
- SS-B antibodies are associated with primary Sjögren's disease. Their presence doesn't confirm the diagnosis of this disorder; however, a positive test mandates further testing.

Posttest care

- Keep a clean, dry bandage over the site for at least 24 hours.
- If a hematoma develops at the venipuncture site, apply warm soaks.

Interfering factors

Failure to send the sample to the laboratory immediately may affect the accuracy of test results.

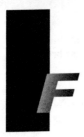

Febrile agglutination tests

Bacterial infections such as tularemia, brucellosis, and the disorders caused by Salmonella and rickettsial infections (including Rocky Mountain spotted fever and typhus) sometimes cause a fever of undetermined origin (FUO). In these infections and others in which microorganisms are difficult to isolate from blood or excreta, febrile agglutination tests can provide important diagnostic information.

The Weil-Felix reaction for rickettsial disease, Widal's test for Salmonella, and tests for brucellosis and tularemia are essentially the same. In these tests, a serum sample is mixed with a few drops of prepared antigens in normal saline solution on a slide; the reaction is observed with the unaided eye. If agglutination occurs, antigen is added to serial dilutions of the patient's serum. Antibody titer is expressed as the reciprocal of the last dilution showing visible agglutination.

The Weil-Felix reaction establishes rickettsial antibody titers. Unlike other febrile agglutination tests, the Weil-Felix reaction doesn't use the causal agent as the antigen; instead it uses three forms of Proteus antigens (OX-19, OX-2, and OX-K) that cross-react with the various strains of rickettsiae.

In Salmonella infection — gastroenteritis and extraintestinal focal infections, both caused by Salmonella enteritidis, and enteric (typhoid) fever, caused by Salmonella typhosa — the Salmonella organism presents flagellar (H) and somatic (O) antigens; Widal's test establishes their titers. Antibodies that agglutinate with H antigens form coarse, unstable aggregates that return to solution easily; those that agglutinate with O antigens form finer, more stable aggregates. The O antigens are considered more specific for Salmonella than H antigens. A third antigen — Vi, or envelope, antigen — may indicate typhoid carrier status, which often tests negative for H and O antigens. Widal's test isn't recommended for diagnosing Salmonella gastroenteritis because symptoms subside before the titer rises.

Slide-agglutination and tube dilution tests, using killed suspensions of the disease organism as antigens, establish titers for the gram-negative coccobacilli Brucella and *Francisella tularensis*, which cause brucellosis and tularemia, respectively.

Purpose

■ To support clinical findings in diagnosing disorders caused by *Salmonella, Rickettsieae, F. tularensis*, or *Brucella* species
■ To identify the cause of FUO.

Patient preparation

Explain to the patient that the test detects and measures microorganisms that may cause fever and other symptoms. Inform him that he need not restrict food or fluids. Tell him that this test requires a blood sample, who will perform the venipuncture and when, and that he may experience transient discomfort from the needle puncture and the pressure of the tourniquet.

Explain to the patient that this test requires a series of blood samples to detect a pattern of titers that is characteristic of the suspected disorder.

Note on the laboratory request when antimicrobial therapy (if any) began.

Procedure

Perform a venipuncture and collect the sample in a 7-ml clot-activator tube.

Precautions

Send samples to the laboratory immediately.

Reference values

Normal dilutions are as follows:
■ Salmonella antibody: <1:80
■ Brucella antibody: <1:80
■ Francisella antibody: <1:40
■ Rickettsia antibody: <1:40.

Implications of results

Observation of rising and falling titers is crucial for detecting active infection. If this isn't possible, certain titer levels can suggest the disorder. For all febrile agglutinins, a fourfold increase in titers is strong evidence of infection.

RICKETTSIA

■ The Weil-Felix reaction is positive for rickettsiae with antibodies to Proteus 6 to 12 days after infection; titers peak in 1 month and usually drop to negative in 5 or 6 months.

■ This test can't be used for diagnosing rickettsial pox or Q fever, because the antibodies of these diseases don't cross-react with Proteus antigens.

SALMONELLA

■ H and O agglutinins usually appear in serum after 1 week, and titers rise for 3 to 6 weeks.

■ O agglutinins usually fall to insignificant levels in 6 to 12 months; H agglutinins may remain elevated for years.

BRUCELLOSIS

■ Titers usually rise after 2 or 3 weeks and reach their highest levels between 4 and 8 weeks.

■ Absence of Brucella agglutinins doesn't rule out brucellosis.

TULAREMIA

■ Titers usually become positive in the second week of infection, exceed 1:320 by the third week, peak in 4 to 7 weeks, and decline gradually during 1 year after recovery.

Posttest care

■ If a hematoma develops at the venipuncture site, apply warm soaks.

■ In FUO and suspected infection, contact the hospital infection control department. Isolation may be necessary.

Interfering factors

■ Patients taking antibiotics show depressed titers early in the course of the disorder.

■ Patients with elevated immunoglobulin levels due to hepatic disease, or those who use drugs excessively, often have high Salmonella titers.

■ Patients who have had skin tests with Brucella antigen may show elevated Brucella titers.

■ Failure to send the sample to the laboratory immediately may alter results.

■ Vaccination or continuous exposure to bacterial or rickettsial infection (resulting in immunity) causes high titers.

■ Many antibodies cross-react with bacteria that cause other infectious diseases. For example, tularemia antibodies cross-react with Brucella antigens.

■ Immunodeficient patients may show infectious symptoms but be unable to produce antibodies. In such cases, titers remain negative, even during infection.

■ Patients with Proteus infections may show positive Weil-Felix titers for rickettsial disease.

Ferritin test

Ferritin, a major iron-storage protein found in reticulo-endothelial cells, normally appears in small quantities in serum. In healthy adults, serum ferritin levels are directly related to the amount of available iron stored in the body and can be measured accurately by radioimmunoassay. Unlike many other blood studies, the serum ferritin test isn't affected by moderate hemolysis of the sample or by the patient's use of any known drugs.

Purpose

- To screen for iron deficiency and iron overload
- To measure iron storage
- To distinguish between iron deficiency (a condition of low iron storage) and chronic inflammation (a condition of normal storage).

Patient preparation

Explain to the patient that this test assesses the amount of available iron stored in the body. Inform him that he need not restrict food, fluids, or medications before the test. Tell him that the test requires a blood sample, who will perform the venipuncture and when, and that he may experience transient discomfort from the needle puncture and the pressure of the tourniquet. Review the patient's history for a recent transfusion.

Procedure

Perform a venipuncture and collect the sample in a 10-ml tube without additives.

Reference values

Normal serum ferritin values vary with age, as follows:
- adults: 20 to 300 ng/ml in men and 20 to 120 ng/ml in women
- 6 months to 15 years: 7 to 140 ng/ml
- 2 to 5 months: 50 to 200 ng/ml
- 1 month: 200 to 600 ng/ml
- neonates: 25 to 200 ng/ml.

Implications of results

- High serum ferritin levels suggest acute or chronic hepatic disease, iron overload, leukemia, acute or chronic infection or inflammation, Hodgkin's disease, or chronic hemolytic anemias; in these disorders, iron stores in the bone marrow may be normal or significantly increased.
- Serum ferritin levels are characteristically normal or slightly elevated in patients who have chronic renal disease.
- Low serum ferritin levels indicate chronic iron deficiency.

Posttest care

If a hematoma develops at the venipuncture site, apply warm soaks.

Interfering factors

A recent transfusion may cause elevated serum ferritin levels.

Fetal-maternal erythrocyte distribution test

Some transfer of red blood cells (RBCs) from fetal to maternal circulation occurs during most spontaneous or elective abortions and most normal deliveries. Usually, the amount of blood transferred is minimal and has no clinical significance. But transfer of significant amounts of blood from an Rh-positive fetus to an Rh-negative mother can cause maternal immunization to the $Rh_o(D)$ antigen and the development of anti-Rh-positive antibodies in maternal circulation. During a subsequent pregnancy, the maternal immunization subjects an Rh-positive fetus to potentially fatal hemolysis and erythroblastosis.

To prevent maternal $Rh_o(D)$ immunization, $Rh_o(D)$ immune globulin is given to an unsensitized Rh-negative mother shortly after the birth of an Rh-positive infant or after an abortion. The amount needed depends on the volume of fetal blood transferred. This test measures the number of fetal RBCs in maternal circulation to allow calculation of the $Rh_o(D)$ immune globulin dose.

This test, usually a modification of the Kleihauer-Betke technique, uses a maternal blood smear fixed with ethanol. The adult hemoglobin is eluted from the RBCs with a citric acid phosphate buffer. Removing hemoglobin doesn't destroy the RBCs; thus they can be counted and differentiated from the normally stained fetal RBCs. (A counterstain, such as aniline blue, may help visualize the eluted adult RBCs by giving them a light gray-blue color.) The percentage of fetal RBCs counted is used to calculate the approximate fetal-maternal erythrocyte volume, based on average total RBC volume.

Purpose

■ To detect and measure fetal-maternal blood transfer
■ To determine the amount of $Rh_o(D)$ immune globulin needed to prevent maternal immunization to the $Rh_o(D)$ antigen.

Patient preparation

Explain that this test determines or verifies the number of fetal RBCs in maternal circulation and that it allows the clinicians to calculate how many doses of $Rh_o(D)$ immune globulin she'll require to prevent immunization as a result of this pregnancy. Inform the patient that she need not fast before the test. Tell her that the test requires a blood sample, who will perform the venipuncture and when, and that she may feel transient discomfort from the needle puncture and the pressure of the tourniquet.

Check the patient's history for recent administration of dextran, I.V. contrast media, or drugs that may alter results.

Procedure
■ Perform the venipuncture and collect the sample in a 10-ml tube with EDTA added.
■ Label the sample with the patient's name, the hospital or blood bank number, the date, and the initials of the phlebotomist.

Precautions
Send the sample to the laboratory immediately with a properly completed laboratory request.

Normal findings
Maternal whole blood should contain no fetal RBCs.

Implications of results
■ The number of vials needed is determined by dividing the calculated fetomaternal hemorrhage by 30 (a single vial of $Rh_o[D]$ immune globulin will provide protection against a 30-ml fetomaternal hemorrhage). (See *Recommended RhIg dose after fetomaternal hemorrhage.*)
■ An elevated fetal RBC volume in maternal circulation necessitates administration of more than one dose of $Rh_o(D)$ immune globulin.

Posttest care
If a hematoma develops at the venipuncture site, apply warm soaks.

Interfering factors
■ Hemolysis caused by improper temperature or rough handling may alter test results.
■ Delays of more than 72 hours after collection may yield inaccurate results and will prevent timely administration of $Rh_o(D)$ immune globulin.

Fibrin split products test
After a fibrin clot forms in response to vascular injury, the fibrinolytic system acts to degrade the clot by converting plasminogen into the enzyme plasmin. Plasmin

RECOMMENDED RhIg DOSE AFTER FETOMATERNAL HEMORRHAGE

Dose of Rh immune globulin (RhIg) is determined by estimated volume of feto-maternal hemorrhage.

| Fetal cells (%) | Hemorrhage volume (ml whole blood) | | Vials of RhIg |
	Average	Range*	
0.3-0.5	20	<50	2
0.6-0.8	35	15-80	3
0.9-1.1	50	22-110	4
1.2-1.4	65	30-140	5
1.5-2.0	88	37-200	6
2.1-2.5	115	52-250	6

*The range provides for the poor precision of acid separation elution test.

Source: Fischbach, F., *A Manual of Laboratory & Diagnostic Tests*, 6th edition, Lippincott Williams & Wilkins Co., 2000.

breaks down fibrin and fibrinogen into fragments known as fibrin split products (FSP) or fibrin degradation products. The fragments are labeled X, Y, D, and E, in order of decreasing molecular weight. An excess of FSP in the circulation may combine with fibrin monomers to prevent polymerization; that is, the fragments cause anticoagulant activity. This excess may lead to coagulation disorders, which may be due to fibrinogenolysis or clotting excesses such as disseminated intravascular coagulation (DIC).

FSP are detected by an immunoprecipitation reaction, in which diluted serum is mixed on a slide with latex particles that carry antibodies to D and E split products. The latex particles clump if FSP are present in the serum dilution.

Purpose

■ To detect FSP in the circulation
■ To help determine the presence and approximate severity of a hyperfibrinolytic state that may be associated with primary fibrinogenolysis or hypercoagulability such as DIC. (See *Causes of disseminated intravascular coagulation*, page 230.)

Patient preparation

Explain to the patient that this test helps determine if his blood clots normally. Tell him that he need not restrict food or fluids before the test. Inform him that the

CAUSES OF DISSEMINATED INTRAVASCULAR COAGULATION

Obstetric:	Amniotic fluid embolism, eclampsia, retained dead fetus, retained placenta, abruptio placentae, and toxemia
Neoplastic:	<ul><li>sarcoma</li><li>metastatic carcinoma</li><li>acute leukemia</li><li>prostate cancer</li><li>giant hemangioma</li></ul>
Infectious:	<ul><li>acute bacteremia</li><li>septicemia</li><li>rickettsemia</li><li>viral, fungal, or protozoal infection</li></ul>
Necrotic:	<ul><li>trauma</li><li>destruction of brain tissue</li><li>extensive burns</li><li>heat stroke</li><li>rejection of transplant</li><li>hepatic necrosis</li></ul>
Cardiovascular:	<ul><li>fat embolism</li><li>acute venous thrombosis</li><li>cardiopulmonary bypass surgery</li><li>hypovolemic shock</li><li>cardiac arrest and hypotension</li></ul>
Other:	<ul><li>snakebite</li><li>cirrhosis</li><li>transfusion of incompatible blood</li><li>purpura</li><li>glomerulonephritis</li></ul>

test requires a blood sample, who will perform the venipuncture and when, and that he may experience transient discomfort from the needle puncture and the pressure of the tourniquet.

Check the patient history for use of any medications (especially heparin) that may affect the accuracy of test results.

Procedure

■ Perform a venipuncture, and draw 2 ml of blood into a plastic syringe. Transfer the sample to the tube provided by the laboratory, which contains a soybean trypsin inhibitor and bovine thrombin. Evacuated tubes are available in kits designed to provide a rapid semiquantitative analysis of FSP. Follow the manufacturer's directions for specimen collection and handling.

Precautions

CLINICAL ALERT Drawing the sample before administering heparin will help avoid false-positive test results.
■ Gently invert the collection tube several times to mix the contents adequately. The blood clots within 2 seconds and must then be sent to the laboratory immediately to be incubated at 98.6° F (37° C) for 30 minutes before testing proceeds.

Reference values

Normal serum contains less than 10 μg/ml of FSP.

Implications of results

■ FSP levels rise in primary fibrinolytic states because of increased levels of circulating profibrinolysin; in secondary states, because of DIC and subsequent fibrinolysis.
■ Levels also increase in alcoholic cirrhosis, preeclampsia, premature separation of the placenta, congenital heart disease, sunstroke, burns, intrauterine death, pulmonary embolus, deep vein thrombosis (transient increase), and myocardial infarction (after 1 or 2 days). FSP levels usually exceed 100 μg/ml in patients with active renal disease or during kidney transplant rejection.

Posttest care

If a hematoma develops at the venipuncture site, apply warm soaks.

Interfering factors

■ Pre-test administration of heparin causes false-positive results.
■ Leaving the tourniquet on the arm longer than 1 minute may affect test result.
■ Fibrinolytic drugs, such as urokinase, streptokinase, and tissue plasminogen activator and large doses of barbiturates increase FSP levels.
■ Failure to fill the collection tube completely, to mix the sample and additive adequately, or to send the sample to the laboratory immediately may affect the accuracy of test results.
■ Hemolysis caused by rough handling of the sample may alter test results.

Fibrinogen test, plasma

The plasma fibrinogen test measures the plasma concentration of fibrinogen available for coagulation. Fibrinogen (factor I), a plasma protein originating in the liver, isn't normally present in serum; it's converted to fibrin by thrombin during clotting. Because fibrin is a necessary part of a blood clot, fibrinogen deficiency can produce mild to severe bleeding disorders. When fibrinogen levels drop below 100 mg/dl, accurate interpretation of all coagulation tests that have a fibrin clot as an end point becomes difficult.

Purpose

To aid the diagnosis of suspected clotting or bleeding disorders caused by fibrinogen abnormalities.

Patient preparation

Explain to the patient that this test helps determine if his blood clots normally. Inform him that he need not restrict food or fluids before the test. Tell him that a blood sample is required, who will perform the venipuncture and when, and that he may experience discomfort from the needle puncture and the pressure of the tourniquet. Check the patient history for use of heparin and oral contraceptives. Note such drugs on the laboratory request.

Procedure

Perform a venipuncture and collect the sample in a 7-ml tube with sodium citrate added.

Precautions

■ This test is contraindicated in patients with active bleeding or acute infection or illness, and in those who have received a blood transfusion within the past 4 weeks.

CLINICAL ALERT If the patient is receiving heparin therapy, notify the laboratory; such therapy requires use of a different reagent.

■ Completely fill the collection tube, invert it gently several times and send it to the laboratory immediately.

■ Avoid excessive probing during the venipuncture, and handle the sample gently.

Reference values

Fibrinogen levels normally are 150 to 350 mg/dl.

Implications of results

■ Depressed fibrinogen levels may suggest congenital afibrinogenemia, hypofibrinogenemia or dysfibrinogenemia, disseminated intravascular coagulation, fibrinolysis, severe hepatic disease, bone marrow lesions, or cancer of the prostate, pancreas, or lung. Obstetric complications or trauma may also cause low levels.

■ Elevated levels suggest cancer of the stomach, breast, or kidney, or inflammatory disorders, such as pneumonia or membranoproliferative glomerulonephritis.

■ Prolonged activated partial thromboplastin time, prothrombin time, and thrombin time may also reflect a fibrinogen deficiency.

Posttest care

If a hematoma develops at the venipuncture site, apply warm soaks. Ensure that subdermal bleeding has stopped before removing pressure. If the hematoma is large, monitor pulses distal to the phlebotomy site.

Interfering factors

■ Fibrinogen levels may be elevated during the third trimester of pregnancy and in postoperative patients.
■ Hemolysis caused by traumatic venipuncture or rough handling of the sample may affect test results.
■ Failure to fill the collection tube completely, to mix the sample and anticoagulant adequately, or to send the sample to the laboratory promptly may affect the accuracy of test results.

Fibrinolysis/euglobulin lysis time test

This test measures the interval between clot formation and dissolution in the euglobulin fraction of plasma. In the laboratory, a precipitated plasma extract is clotted with thrombin. The time required for this clot to lyse is then recorded.

Purpose

■ To assess the fibrinolytic system
■ To help detect abnormal fibrinolytic states.

Patient preparation

Explain to the patient that this test evaluates the clotting mechanism. Tell him that the test requires a blood sample, who will perform the venipuncture and when, and that he may have some discomfort from the needle puncture and the tourniquet pressure.

Procedure

Perform a venipuncture. Collect a 4.5-ml sample in a tube with sodium citrate or in a chilled tube with 0.5 ml sodium oxalate.

Precautions

■ When drawing the sample, be careful not to rub the area over the vein too vigorously, not to pump the fist excessively, and not to leave the tourniquet in place too long. Avoid excessive probing during venipuncture, and handle the sample gently.
■ If a tube containing sodium citrate and citric acid is used, mix the sample and anticoagulant thoroughly. If a

chilled tube containing 0.5 ml sodium oxalate is used, mix the sample and preservative adequately, pack the sample in ice, and send it to the laboratory immediately.

Normal findings

Lysis normally occurs in 2 to 4 hours.

Implications of results

■ Clot lysis within 1 hour indicates increased plasminogen activator activity (abnormal fibrolytic activity).
■ In pathologic fibrinolysis, lysis time may be as brief as 5 to 10 minutes.

Posttest care

If a hematoma develops at the venipuncture site, apply warm soaks.

Interfering factors

■ Decreased lysis time with administration of thrombolytic therapy, dextran, and clofibrate.
■ Prolonged tourniquet constriction, vigorous vein preparation, or excessive pumping of the fist shortens lysis time.
■ Hemolysis resulting from excessive probing during venipuncture or from rough handling of the sample may alter test results.
■ Failure to follow appropriate precautions for the type of collection tube used may affect the accuracy of test results.
■ Depressed fibrinogen levels (less than 100 mg/dl) can shorten lysis time.

Fluorescent treponemal antibody absorption test

The fluorescent treponemal antibody absorption (FTA-ABS or FTA) test uses indirect immunofluorescence to detect antibodies to the spirochete *Treponema pallidum* — the cause of syphilis — in serum. In this test, prepared *T. pallidum* is fixed on a slide; a preparation of Reiter treponema, which adsorbs to most nonsyphilitic antibodies, is added; and then the patient's serum is added. This addition to the test serum prevents interference by antibodies from almost all nonsyphilitic treponemas and thereby makes the FTA-ABS test specific for *T. pallidum*.

If syphilitic antibodies are present in the test serum, they will coat the treponemal organisms on the slide. The slide is then stained with fluorescein-labeled antiglobulin. This antiglobulin attaches to the coated

OTHER TESTS FOR *TREPONEMA PALLIDUM*

The microhemagglutination assay for *Treponema pallidum* antibody increases the specificity of syphilis testing by eliminating methodologic interference. In this assay, tanned sheep red blood cells are coated with *T. pallidum* antigen and are combined with adsorbed test serum. Hemagglutination occurs in the presence of specific anti-*T. pallidum* antibodies in the serum.

In the enzyme-linked immunosorbent assay, tubes coated with *T. pallidum* are washed and then treated with enzyme-labeled anti-human globulin. After the substrate for the enzymes is added to the tubes, the enzymatic activity is measured by quantitating the reaction product formed.

spirochetes and makes them fluoresce when viewed under a microscope with ultraviolet light.

The FTA-ABS test is generally performed on a serum sample to detect primary or secondary syphilis. Diagnosis of tertiary syphilis requires a cerebrospinal fluid (CSF) specimen. Because antibody levels remain constant for long periods, the FTA-ABS test isn't recommended for monitoring response to therapy.

Two other tests can also detect *T. pallidum.* (See *Other tests for* Treponema pallidum.)

Purpose
- To confirm primary or secondary syphilis
- To screen for suspected false-positive results of the Venereal Disease Research Laboratory (VDRL) test.

Patient preparation
Explain to the patient that this test can confirm or rule out syphilis and doesn't require food or fluid restrictions. Tell him that the test requires a blood sample, who will perform the venipuncture and when, and that he may experience transient discomfort from the needle puncture and the pressure of the tourniquet.

Procedure
Perform a venipuncture and collect the sample in a 7-ml clot-activator tube.

Precautions
Handle the sample gently to prevent hemolysis.

Normal findings
Reaction to the FTA-ABS test should be negative (no fluorescence).

Implications of results

■ The presence of treponemal antibodies in the serum—a reactive test result—doesn't indicate the stage or the severity of infection. (However, the presence of these antibodies in CSF is strong evidence of tertiary neurosyphilis.)

■ Elevated antibody levels are present in 80% to 90% of patients with secondary syphilis and persist for years, with or without treatment.

■ The absence of treponemal antibodies—a nonreactive test—doesn't necessarily rule out syphilis. T. pallidum causes no detectable immunologic changes in the blood for 14 to 21 days after initial infection. (A dark-field microscope may detect organisms earlier.)

■ Low antibody levels or other nonspecific factors produce borderline findings. In such cases, repeated testing and a thorough review of the patient history may be productive.

■ Although the FTA-ABS test is specific, some patients with nonsyphilitic conditions, such as systemic lupus erythematosus, genital herpes, or increased or abnormal globulins, and pregnant women, may show minimally reactive levels.

■ In addition, the FTA-ABS test doesn't always distinguish between T. pallidum and certain other treponemas, such as those that cause pinta, yaws, and bejel.

Posttest care

■ If a hematoma develops at the venipuncture site, apply warm soaks.

■ If the test is reactive, explain the nature of syphilis, and stress the importance of proper treatment and the need to find and treat the patient's sexual partners. Also, prepare him for inquiries from public health authorities.

■ If the test is nonreactive, or findings are borderline but syphilis hasn't been ruled out, instruct the patient to return for follow-up testing; explain that inconclusive results don't necessarily indicate he is free of the disease.

Interfering factors

Hemolysis caused by rough handling of the sample may affect test results.

Folic acid test

A quantitative analysis of serum folic acid levels by radioisotopic assay of competitive binding, this test is often performed concomitantly with serum vitamin B_{12} determinations. Like vitamin B_{12}, folic acid (also known as pteroylglutamic acid, folacin, or folate) is a water-soluble vitamin that influences hematopoiesis, deoxyribonucleic acid (DNA) synthesis, and overall body growth. Women of child-bearing age whose diets are deficient in folic acid have an increased risk of having a child with spina bifida or other neural tube defects. The parent compound of folate vitamins, folic acid is biologically inactive and requires enzymatic breakdown in the small intestine for absorption into the bloodstream and subsequent rapid absorption into the tissues.

Normally, diet supplies folic acid in liver, kidney, yeast, fruits, leafy vegetables, eggs, and milk. Because the body stores only small amounts of folic acid (mostly in the liver), inadequate dietary intake causes a deficiency, especially during pregnancy, when the metabolic demand for folic acid rises. Because of folic acid's vital role in hematopoiesis, the usual indication for this test is a suspected hematologic abnormality.

Purpose

- To aid differential diagnosis of megaloblastic anemia, which may result from deficiency of folic acid or vitamin B_{12}
- To assess folate stores in pregnancy.

Patient preparation

Explain to the patient that this test determines the folic acid level in the blood. Instruct him to observe an overnight fast before the test. Tell him the test requires a blood sample, who will perform the venipuncture and when, and that he may experience some discomfort from the needle puncture and the pressure of the tourniquet.

Check the patient's medication history for drugs that may affect test results.

Procedure

Perform a venipuncture, and collect the sample in a 7-ml tube without additives.

Precautions

- Handle the sample gently to prevent hemolysis.
- Protect the sample from light and send it to the laboratory immediately.

Reference values

Normal serum folic acid values are 3 to 16 ng/ml.

Implications of results

- Low serum levels (less than 2 ng/ml) may indicate hematologic abnormalities, such as anemia (especially megaloblastic anemia), leukopenia, or thrombocytope-

nia. The Schilling test is often performed to rule out vitamin B_{12} deficiency, which also causes megaloblastic
anemia (pernicious anemia).

■ Decreased folic acid levels can also result from hypermetabolic states (such as hyperthyroidism), inadequate
dietary intake, chronic alcoholism, small-bowel malabsorption syndrome, or pregnancy.

■ High serum levels (more than 20 ng/ml) may indicate
excessive dietary intake of folic acid or folic acid supplements. This vitamin is nontoxic in humans, even when
taken in large doses.

Posttest care

■ If a hematoma develops at the venipuncture site, apply
warm soaks.

■ Tell the patient that he may resume his normal diet.

Interfering factors

■ Alcohol and phenytoin interfere with folic acid absorption and lower serum folic acid.

■ Pyrimethamine (an antimalarial) can cause folate deficiency.

■ Other drugs that may decrease levels include anticonvulsants such as primidone, antineoplastics, antimalarials, and oral contraceptives.

■ Hemolysis may alter test results.

■ Folate deterioration may occur if the specimen isn't
protected from light.

Follicle-stimulating hormone test, serum

This test of gonadal function, performed more often in
females than in males, measures follicle-stimulating
hormone (FSH) levels by radioimmunoassay and is vital
to infertility studies. Its overall diagnostic significance
often depends on the results of related hormone tests
(for luteinizing hormone, estrogen, or progesterone, for
example).

A glycoprotein secreted by the anterior pituitary, FSH
stimulates gonadal activity in both sexes. In females, it
spurs development of primary ovarian follicles into
Graafian follicles for ovulation. Secretion varies diurnally and fluctuates during the menstrual cycle, peaking at
ovulation. In males, continuous secretion of FSH (and
testosterone) stimulates and maintains spermatogenesis.
Plasma levels fluctuate widely in females; to obtain a
true baseline level, daily testing may be necessary (for 3
to 5 days), or multiple samples may be drawn on the
same day.

Purpose

- To aid in the diagnosis of infertility and disorders of menstruation, such as amenorrhea
- To aid in the diagnosis of precocious puberty in girls (before age 9) and in boys (before age 10)
- To aid in the differential diagnosis of hypogonadism.

Patient preparation

Explain to the patient that this test helps determine if her hormonal secretion is normal. Inform her that she need not fast or limit physical activity before the test. Tell her a blood sample will be drawn and that she may feel some discomfort from the needle puncture. Advise her that the laboratory requires at least 3 days to complete the analysis.

Withhold medications that may interfere with accurate determination of test results, such as estrogens and progestogen, for 48 hours before the test. If these medications must be continued, note this on the laboratory request.

Make sure the patient is relaxed and recumbent for 30 minutes before the test.

Procedure

Perform a venipuncture, preferably between 6 a.m. and 8 a.m., using a 7-ml clot-activator tube. Send the sample to the laboratory immediately.

Precautions

- Handle the sample gently to prevent hemolysis.
- If the patient is a female, note her menstrual cycle phase or if she is menopausal on the laboratory request.

Reference values

Values vary greatly, depending on the patient's age, stage of sexual development and, for a female, the phase of her menstrual cycle. Approximate values are as follows:

- follicular phase: 5 to 20 mIU/ml
- ovulatory phase: 15 to 30 mIU/ml
- luteal phase: 5 to 15 mIU/ml
- postmenopause: 50 to 100 mIU/ml
- adult males: 5 to 20 mIU/ml.

Implications of results

- Low FSH secretion may cause male or female infertility: aspermatogenesis in males and anovulation in females.
- Low FSH levels may reflect hypogonadotropic states secondary to anorexia nervosa, panhypopituitarism, or hypothalamic lesions.

- High FSH levels in females suggest ovarian failure associated with Turner's syndrome (primary hypogonadism, XO karyotype) or Stein-Leventhal syndrome (polycystic ovary syndrome).
- Levels also may be high in patients with precocious puberty (idiopathic or with central nervous system lesions) and in postmenopausal women.
- In males, abnormally high FSH levels reflect destruction of the testes (from mumps orchitis or X-ray exposure), testicular failure, seminoma, or male climacteric.
- Congenital absence of the gonads and early-stage acromegaly may cause high FSH levels in both sexes.

Posttest care

- If a hematoma develops at the venipuncture site, apply warm soaks.
- Resume medications that were discontinued before the test.

Interfering factors

- Failure to observe restriction of medications may hinder accurate determination of test results. Ovarian steroid hormones, such as estrogen or progesterone, and related compounds may, through negative feedback, inhibit the flow of releasing hormones from the hypothalamus and pituitary; phenothiazines (such as chlorpromazine) may exert a similar effect.
- Radioactive scan performed within 1 week before the test may affect results.
- Hemolysis due to rough handling of the sample may interfere with accurate determination of test results.

Fractionated erythrocyte porphyrins test

This test measures erythrocyte porphyrins (also known as erythropoietic porphyrins); specifically, protoporphyrin, coproporphyrin, and uroporphyrin. Porphyrins, pigments that are present in all protoplasm, have a significant role in energy storage and use. Protoporphyrin, coproporphyrin, and uroporphyrin are produced during heme biosynthesis. Small amounts of these porphyrins or their precursors normally appear in blood, urine, and feces. Production and excretion of porphyrins or their precursors increase in porphyrias, which are separated into erythropoietic and hepatic types. This test detects erythropoietic porphyrias.

Total porphyrins can be quantitated and separated by high-performance liquid chromatography into uroporphyrin, coproporphyrin, and protoporphyrin. Elevated levels suggest the need for further enzyme testing, which can identify the specific porphyria present.

Purpose
- To aid diagnosis of congenital or acquired erythropoietic porphyrias
- To help confirm diagnosis of disorders affecting red blood cell (RBC) activity.

Patient preparation
Explain to the patient that this test helps detect RBC disorders. Tell him that the test requires a blood sample, who will perform the venipuncture and when, and that he may feel some transient discomfort from the needle puncture and from the pressure of the tourniquet.

Procedure
Perform a venipuncture and collect the sample in a 5-ml or larger heparinized tube. Label the sample, place it on ice, and send it to the laboratory immediately.

Precautions
- Handle the sample gently to prevent hemolysis.
- Send the sample to the laboratory promptly.

Reference values
- Total porphyrins: 16 to 60 μg/dl of packed RBCs
- Protoporphyrin: 16 to 60 μg/dl
- Coproporphyrin and uroporphyrin: less than 2 μg/dl.

Implications of results
- Elevated protoporphyrin levels suggest erythropoietic protoporphyria, infection, increased erythropoiesis, thalassemia, sideroblastic anemia, iron deficiency anemia, or lead poisoning.
- Increased coproporphyrin levels suggest congenital erythropoietic porphyria, erythropoietic protoporphyria or coproporphyria, or sideroblastic anemia.

Posttest care
If a hematoma develops at the venipuncture site, apply warm soaks.

Interfering factors
Hemolysis due to rough handling of the sample may interfere with test results.

Free cortisol test, urine
Used as a screen for adrenocortical hyperfunction, this test measures urine levels of the portion of cortisol not bound to the corticosteroid-binding globulin transcortin. It's one of the best diagnostic tools for detecting Cushing's syndrome.

The major glucocorticoid secreted by the adrenal cortex in response to adrenocorticotropic hormone (ACTH) stimulation, cortisol helps regulate fat, carbohydrate, and protein metabolism; it also helps promote glyconeo-genesis, anti-inflammatory response, and cellular permeability. Only about 10% of this hormone is unbound and physiologically active; this small portion is known as free cortisol. Urine cortisol concentrations increase significantly when the amount secreted exceeds the binding capacity of transcortin, which is normally almost saturated.

Radioimmunoassay determinations of free cortisol levels in a 24-hour urine specimen—unlike a single measurement of plasma cortisol—reflect overall secretion levels instead of diurnal variations. Concurrent measurements of plasma cortisol and ACTH, urine 17-hydroxycorticosteroids, and the dexamethasone suppression test, may confirm the diagnosis.

Purpose

To aid diagnosis of Cushing's syndrome.

Patient preparation

Explain to the patient that this test helps evaluate adrenal gland function. Advise him that he need not restrict food or fluids before the test but should avoid stressful situations and excessive physical exercise during the collection period. Tell him the test requires collection of a 24-hour urine specimen, and teach him the proper collection technique.

Check the patient's recent drug history for medications that may interfere with test results, such as reserpine, phenothiazines, morphine, amphetamines, and prolonged steroid use. Review your findings with the clinician.

Procedure

Collect a 24-hour specimen in a bottle containing a preservative to keep the specimen at a pH of 4.0 to 4.5.

Precautions

Refrigerate the specimen or place it on ice during the collection period.

Reference values

Normal free cortisol values are 24 to 108 µg/24 hours.

Implications of results

■ Elevated free cortisol levels suggest Cushing's syndrome resulting from adrenal hyperplasia, adrenal or pituitary tumor, or ectopic ACTH production.

- Hepatic disease and obesity, which can raise plasma cortisol levels, generally don't appreciably raise urine levels of free cortisol.
- Monitor for thromboembolic problems, glucose intolerance, nutritional status, early signs and symptoms of infection, hypertension, and bleeding tendencies.
- This test is designed to screen for excessive secretion of free cortisol. Low levels have little diagnostic significance and don't necessarily indicate adrenocortical hypofunction.

Posttest care

- Tell the patient that he may resume normal activity restricted during the test.
- Resume administration of medications discontinued before the test.

Interfering factors

- Reserpine, phenothiazines, morphine, amphetamines, oral contraceptives, danazol, aldactone, and prolonged corticosteroid therapy may elevate free cortisol levels.
- Dexamethasone, ethacrynic acid, thiazides, and ketoconazole may decrease free cortisol levels.
- Failure to collect all urine during the test period or to store the specimen properly may affect the accuracy of test results.
- Pregnancy causes increased free cortisol levels.

Free thyroxine and free triiodothyronine tests

These tests measure serum levels of free thyroxine (FT_4) and free triiodothyronine (FT_3), the minute portions of T_4 and T_3 not bound to thyroxine-binding globulin (TBG) and other serum proteins. As the active components of T_4 and T_3, these unbound hormones enter target cells and are responsible for the thyroid's effects on cellular metabolism. Because levels of circulating FT_4 and FT_3 are regulated by a feedback mechanism that compensates for changes in binding protein concentrations by adjusting total hormone levels, measurement of free hormone levels is the best indicator of thyroid function. Of the two tests, FT_3 is the better indicator. This test may be useful in the 5% of patients in whom the standard T_3 or T_4 tests fail to produce diagnostic results.

Purpose

- To measure the metabolically active form of the thyroid hormones
- To aid diagnosis of hypothyroidism or hyperthyroidism when TBG levels are abnormal.

Patient preparation

Explain to the patient that this special test helps evaluate thyroid function. Tell him the test requires a blood sample, who will perform the venipuncture and when, and that he may feel transient discomfort from the needle puncture.

Procedure

Draw venous blood into a 7-ml clot-activator tube.

Precautions

Handle the sample gently to prevent hemolysis.

Reference values

■ Normal range for FT_4 is 0.8 to 3.3 ng/dl; for FT_3, 0.2 to 0.6 ng/dl.
■ Values vary, depending on the laboratory. (See *Measuring FT_3.*)

Implications of results

■ Elevated FT_4 and FT_3 levels indicate hyperthyroidism, unless peripheral resistance to thyroid hormone is present.
■ T_3 toxicosis, a distinct form of hyperthyroidism, yields high FT_3 and normal or low FT_4 values.
■ Low FT_4 levels usually indicate hypothyroidism, except in patients receiving replacement therapy with T_3.
■ Patients receiving thyroid hormone replacement therapy may have varying levels of FT_4 and FT_3, depending on the preparation used and the time of sample collection.

Posttest care

If a hematoma develops at the venipuncture site, apply warm soaks.

Interfering factors

■ Rough handling of the sample can cause hemolysis.
■ Recent administration of radioisotopes can affect test results.
■ Test results may be inaccurate at high altitudes.
■ Depending on the dosage, thyroid therapy may increase FT_4 or FT_3 levels. However, these medications shouldn't be withheld.

Fungal serology test

Most fungal organisms enter the body as spores inhaled into the lungs or infiltrated through wounds in the skin or mucosa. If the body's defenses can't destroy the organisms initially, the fungi multiply to form lesions; blood and lymph vessels may then spread the fungal infection,

---

MEASURING FT₃

Free triiodothyronine (FT_3) levels can be determined by procedures using monoclonal antibodies. These engineered antibodies are highly specific and permit rapid testing.

Free T_3 reacts with the antibody, which is coupled to a chromogenic (color-producing) enzyme or a fluorescent marker. Under test conditions, a color is produced or fluorescence is detected in proportion to the FT_3 concentration.

---

called mycosis, through the body. Mycosis may be deep-seated or superficial. Deep-seated mycosis occurs primarily in the lungs; superficial mycosis, in the skin or the mucosal linings.

Most healthy people easily overcome initial mycotic infection, but the elderly and others with deficient immune systems are more susceptible to acute or chronic mycotic infection and to disorders secondary to such infection.

Although cultures are usually performed to diagnose mycosis by identifying the causative organism, serologic tests occasionally provide the sole evidence of mycosis. These tests are used to detect blastomycosis, coccidioidomycosis, histoplasmosis, aspergillosis, sporotrichosis, and cryptococcosis. Fungal serologic tests use immunodiffusion, complement fixation, precipitin, latex agglutination, or agglutination methods to demonstrate the presence of mycotic antibodies.

Purpose
- To rapidly detect the presence of antifungal antibodies, aiding in the diagnosis of mycoses
- To monitor the effectiveness of therapy for mycoses

Patient preparation
Explain to the patient that this test aids diagnosis of certain fungal infections. If appropriate, explain that the test monitors his response to therapy and that it may be repeated during his illness. Instruct him to fast and go without fluids for 12 to 24 hours before the test. Tell him that this test requires a blood sample, who will perform the venipuncture and when, and that he may experience transient discomfort from the needle puncture and the pressure of the tourniquet.

Procedure
Perform a venipuncture and collect the sample in a 10-ml sterile clot-activator tube.

IMPLICATIONS OF ABNORMAL FUNGAL SEROLOGIC TESTS

Disease and normal values	Clinical significance of abnormal results
Blastomycosis: Complement fixation: titers <1:8	Titers ranging from 1:8 to 1:16 suggest infection; titers >1:32 denote active disease. A rising titer in serial samples taken every 3 to 4 weeks indicates disease progression; a falling titer indicates regression. This test has limited diagnostic value because of the high percentage of false-negatives.
Immunodiffusion: negative	A more sensitive test for blastomycosis; detects 80% of infections.
Coccidioidomycosis: Complement fixation: titers <1:2	Most sensitive test for this fungus. Titers ranging from 1:2 to 1:4 suggest active infection; titers >1:16 usually denote active disease. Test may remain negative in mild infections.
Immunodiffusion: negative	Most useful for screening, followed by complement fixation test for confirmation.
Precipitin: titers <1:16	Good screening test; titers >1:16 usually indicate infection. About 80% of infected people show positive titers by 2 weeks; most revert to negative by 6 months. Early primary disease is shown by positive precipitin and negative complement fixation test. A positive complement fixation and negative precipitin test indicate chronic disease.
Histoplasmosis Complement fixation (histoplasmin): titers <1:8	Titers ranging from 1:8 to 1:16 suggest infection; titers >1:32 indicate active disease. Antibodies generally appear 10 to 21 days after initial infection. Test is positive in 10% to 15% of cases.
Complement fixation (yeast): titers <1:18	Titers ranging from 1:8 to 1:16 suggest infection; titers >1:32 indicate active disease. More sensitive than histoplasmin complement fixation test; gives positive results in 75% to 80% of cases. Both histoplasmin and yeast antigens are positive in 10% of cases. A rising titer in serial samples taken every 2 to 3 weeks indicates progressive infection; a decreasing titer indicates regression.
Immunodiffusion (histoplasmin): negative	Appearance of both H and M bands indicates active infection. If the M band appears first and lasts longer than the H band, the infection may be regressing. The M band alone may indicate early infection, chronic disease, or a recent skin test.
Aspergillosis Complement fixation: titers <1:8	Titers of >1:8 suggest infection; 70% to 90% of patients with known pulmonary aspergillosis or aspergillus allergy present antibodies, as does about 5% of the general population. This test can't detect invasive aspergillosis because patients with this disease don't present antibodies; a biopsy is required.
Immunodiffusion: negative	One or more precipitin bands suggests infection; precipitins appear in 95% of patients with pulmonary fungus balls and in 50% of those with allergic bronchopulmonary disorders. The number of bands is related to complement fixation titers; the more precipitin bands, the higher the titer.

(continued)

IMPLICATIONS OF ABNORMAL FUNGAL SEROLOGIC TESTS
(continued)

Disease and normal values	Clinical significance of abnormal results
Sporotrichosis Agglutination: titers <1:40	Titers >1:80 usually indicate active disease. The test usually is negative in cutaneous infections and positive in extracutaneous infections.
Cryptococcosis Latex agglutination for cryptococcal antigen: negative	About 90% of patients with cryptococcal meningoencephalitis present capsular antigen in cerebrospinal fluid (CSF) or serum. Serum is positive less frequently than CSF. Culturing is definitive because false-positive results do occur. Presence of rheumatoid factor may cause a positive reaction. Serum antigen tests are positive in 33% of patients with pulmonary cryptococcosis; a biopsy is usually required.

Precautions

Send the sample to the laboratory immediately. If transport must be delayed, store the sample at 39.2° F (4° C).

Normal findings

Depending on the test method, a negative finding or normal titer usually indicates the absence of mycosis. (See *Implications of abnormal fungal serologic tests.*)

Implications of results

The clinical significance of abnormal serologic test values varies, depending on which technique is used.

Posttest care

If a hematoma develops at the venipuncture site, apply warm soaks.

Interfering factors

- A nonfasting specimen may alter test results.
- Some antigens, such as the blastomycosis and histoplasmosis antigens, may cross-react with each other to produce false-positive results or high titers.
- Recent skin testing with fungal antigens may cause high titers.
- Many mycoses depress the immune system, causing low titers or false-negative test results.
- Failure to send a sterile sample to the laboratory immediately or to store the sample properly if transport is delayed may affect test results.

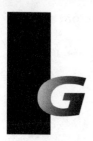

Galactose-1-phosphate uridyltransferase test

This enzyme (commonly known as GPUT), galactokinase, and uridine diphosphate glucose 4-epimerase, convert galactose to glucose during lactose metabolism. Deficiency of one of these enzymes causes galactosemia, an autosomal recessive disorder marked by elevated serum galactose and decreased serum glucose. Unless detected and treated soon after birth, galactosemia can impair eye, brain, and liver development, causing irreversible cataracts, mental retardation, and cirrhosis.

A deficiency of GPUT causes the most common and severe form of galactosemia, detected by both qualitative and quantitative tests. Some hospitals require the simple, qualitative screening test for all neonates. Blood collected on specially treated filter paper is checked for fluorescence after 1- and 2-hour exposures under an ultraviolet light. Normal blood fluoresces; GPUT-deficient blood doesn't.

The quantitative test requires a blood sample and measures the amount of a fluorescent substance generated during a coupled enzyme reaction. This is generally ordered as soon as possible after a positive screening test and may occasionally be ordered for an adult to detect a carrier state.

Prenatal testing of amniotic fluid can also detect GPUT deficiency, but it's rarely performed because neonatal screening can detect the deficiency in time to prevent irreversible damage.

Purpose
- To screen infants for galactosemia
- To detect heterozygous carriers of galactosemia.

Patient preparation
When testing a neonate, explain to the parents that the test screens for galactosemia, a potentially dangerous enzyme deficiency. If a blood sample wasn't taken from the umbilical cord at birth, tell the parents that a small amount of blood will be drawn from the infant's heel.

Explain that the procedure is safe and quickly performed.

When testing an adult, explain that the test identifies carriers of galactosemia, a genetic disorder that may be transmitted to his offspring. Tell the patient that the test requires a blood sample, who will perform the venipuncture and when, and that he may feel discomfort from the needle puncture and the tourniquet.

Procedure

■ For a qualitative (screening) test, collect cord blood or blood from a heelstick on special filter paper, saturating all three circles.
■ For a quantitative test, perform a venipuncture and collect a 4-ml sample in a heparinized or EDTA tube, depending on the laboratory method used.
■ Indicate the patient's age on the laboratory request. Check his history for a recent exchange transfusion. Note this on the laboratory request or postpone the test.

Precautions

■ Handle the collection tube gently to prevent hemolysis.
■ Send the collection tube to the laboratory on wet ice.

Reference values

■ Normally, the qualitative test is negative (fluorescence is strong 1 and 2 hours after the test begins).
■ The normal range for the quantitative test is 18.5 to 28.5 U/g of hemoglobin. Check the normal range for your laboratory if it uses a different method.

Implications of results

■ A positive qualitative test, in which no fluorescence is observed, may indicate GPUT deficiency. A follow-up quantitative test should be performed as soon as possible.
■ Quantitative test results less than 5 U/g of hemoglobin indicate galactosemia; levels between 5 U/g and 18.5 U/g may indicate a carrier state.

Posttest care

■ If a hematoma develops at the venipuncture site, apply warm soaks.
■ If test results indicate galactosemia, provide nutritional counseling for the parents and a galactose- and lactose-free diet for their infant. A soybean- or meat-based formula may replace milk.
■ If one or both parents are carriers, stress the importance of having a screening test performed on their infant at birth.

Interfering factors

■ Failure to use the proper tube or to send the sample on wet ice may cause a false-positive result because heat inactivates the transferase.

■ A total exchange transfusion causes a transient false-negative result because normal transfused blood contains the transferase.

■ Hemolysis caused by rough handling of the sample may affect test results.

Gamma glutamyl transferase test

Gamma glutamyl transferase (GGT), also known as gamma glutamyl transpeptidase, participates in the transfer of amino acids across cellular membranes and, possibly, in glutathione metabolism. Highest concentrations of GGT exist in the renal tubules, where amino acids are reabsorbed from glomerular filtrate, but this enzyme also appears in the liver, biliary tract epithelium, pancreas, lymphocytes, brain, and testes. At least four isoenzymes exist, but fractionation isn't clinically useful or practical.

Because GGT isn't elevated during bone growth or pregnancy, this test is a somewhat more sensitive indicator of hepatic necrosis than the aspartate aminotransferase assay and is as sensitive as or more sensitive than the alkaline phosphatase (ALP) assay. However, the test is nonspecific, providing little data about the type of hepatic disease, because increased levels also occur in renal, cardiac, and prostatic disease and with use of certain medications. GGT is particularly sensitive to the effects of alcohol in the liver; levels may be elevated after moderate alcohol intake and in chronic alcoholism, even without clinical evidence of hepatic injury. (See *Bilirubin and enzyme changes in hepatobiliary disease.*)

Purpose

■ To provide information about hepatobiliary disease, to assess liver function, and to detect alcohol ingestion

■ To distinguish between skeletal disease and hepatic disease when serum ALP levels are elevated. (Normal GGT levels suggest that ALP elevation stems from skeletal disease.)

Patient preparation

Explain to the patient that this test evaluates liver function. Tell him who will perform the venipuncture and when, and that he may experience discomfort from the needle puncture and the pressure of the tourniquet.

BILIRUBIN AND ENZYME CHANGES IN HEPATOBILIARY DISEASE

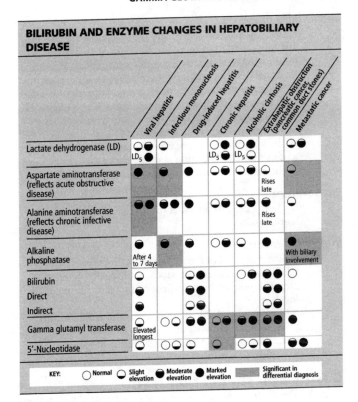

	Viral hepatitis	Infectious mononucleosis	Drug-induced hepatitis	Chronic hepatitis	Alcoholic cirrhosis	Extrahepatic obstruction (pancreatic cancer, common duct stones)	Metastatic cancer
Lactate dehydrogenase (LD)	◐◕ ○ LD₅ ●	○		◐● LD₅ ◐	○● LD₅ ○		◐●
Aspartate aminotransferase (reflects acute obstructive disease)	●		●	◐	◐●	○ Rises late	◐
Alanine aminotransferase (reflects chronic infective disease)	◐●	◐●	●	◐●	◐●	○ Rises late	○
Alkaline phosphatase	◐ After 4 to 7 days	◐	●	○◐	○	●	◐● With biliary involvement
Bilirubin	○		◐●		○◐	◐●	○
Direct	◐		◐●			◐●	
Indirect	◐		◐●			◐●	
Gamma glutamyl transferase	○ Elevated longest	○◐	◐●	◑◐	◐●	◐●	●
5'-Nucleotidase	○	○◐	◐		◐	○◐	◐●

KEY: ○ Normal ◐ Slight elevation ◑ Moderate elevation ● Marked elevation ▓ Significant in differential diagnosis

Procedure

Perform a venipuncture and collect the sample in a 7-ml tube without additives.

Precautions

■ Handle the collection tube gently to prevent hemolysis.

■ GGT activity is stable in serum at room temperature for 2 days.

Reference values

Serum GGT values vary with the assay method used (kinetic or end-point method). Normal levels range as follows:

■ Males: 16 years of age and older, 6 to 38 U/L; younger than 16 years of age, 10 to 50 U/L

■ Females: between 16 and 45 years of age, 4 to 27 U/L; younger than 16 years of age, 10 to 40 U/L; 45 years of age and older, 6 to 37 U/L.

Implications of results

Serum GGT levels rise in any acute hepatic disease as enzyme production increases in response to hepatocellular injury. Moderate increases occur in acute pancreatitis, renal disease, prostatic metastases, in some patients with epilepsy or brain tumors, and postoperatively. Levels also increase after alcohol ingestion. The sharpest elevations occur in patients with obstructive jaundice or hepatic metastatic infiltrations. GGT may increase 5 to 10 days after acute myocardial infarction, either as a result of tissue granulation and healing or as an indication of the effects of cardiac insufficiency on the liver.

Posttest care

If a hematoma develops at the venipuncture site, apply warm soaks.

Interfering factors

- Clofibrate and oral contraceptives decrease serum GGT levels. Aminoglycosides, barbiturates, phenytoin, glutethimide, and methaqualone increase serum GGT levels.
- Moderate intake of alcohol causes increased serum GGT levels that may persist for at least 60 hours.
- Hemolysis caused by rough handling of the sample may alter test results.

Gastric acid stimulation test

The gastric acid stimulation test measures the secretion of gastric acid for 1 hour after subcutaneous injection of pentagastrin or a similar drug that stimulates gastric acid output. It's indicated when the basal secretion test suggests abnormal gastric secretion and is usually performed immediately after that test.

Pentagastrin stimulates the parietal cells to secrete hydrochloric acid. If these cells are damaged or destroyed, acid secretion decreases or is absent; if the cells are hyperactive, acid secretion increases. Although this test detects abnormal gastric secretion, radiographic studies and endoscopy are necessary to determine the cause.

Purpose

To aid diagnosis of duodenal ulcer, Zollinger-Ellison syndrome, pernicious anemia, and gastric carcinoma.

Patient preparation

Explain to the patient that this test determines if the stomach is secreting acid properly. Instruct him to refrain from eating, drinking, and smoking from midnight before the test. Tell him who will perform the test and that it takes 1 hour.

Tell the patient that the test requires passing a tube through the nose and into the stomach and injecting pentagastrin subcutaneously. Describe the possible adverse effects—abdominal pain, nausea, vomiting, flushing, transitory dizziness, faintness, and numbness of the extremities—and instruct him to report such symptoms immediately.

Check the patient's history for hypersensitivity to pentagastrin. Withhold antacids, anticholinergics, adrenergic blockers, histamine-2 (H_2) blockers, corticosteroids, proton pump inhibitors, and reserpine before the test. If these drugs must be continued, note this on the laboratory request. Record baseline vital signs before beginning the procedure.

Procedure

- After basal gastric secretions have been collected, keep the nasogastric (NG) tube in place. Pentagastrin is then injected subcutaneously. Wait 15 minutes, and then collect a specimen every 15 minutes for 1 hour.
- Record the color and odor of each specimen, and note the presence of food, mucus, bile, or blood. Label all specimens "Stimulated Contents," and number them 1 through 4. If the NG tube is to be left in place, clamp it or attach it to low intermittent suction.

Precautions

- The gastric acid stimulation test is contraindicated in patients with hypersensitivity to pentagastrin or with conditions that prohibit NG intubation.
- Observe for adverse effects of pentagastrin.
- To prevent contamination of the specimens with saliva, instruct the patient to expectorate excess saliva.
- Send the specimens to the laboratory as soon as the collection is completed.

Reference values

- Males: 18 to 28 mEq/hour
- Females: 11 to 21 mEq/hour

Implications of results

- Elevated gastric secretion suggests duodenal ulcer.
- Markedly elevated secretion suggests Zollinger-Ellison syndrome.
- Depressed secretion suggests gastric carcinoma.
- Achlorhydria suggests pernicious anemia.

Posttest care

- Watch for nausea, vomiting, and abdominal distention and pain after removal of the NG tube.
- If the patient complains of a sore throat, provide soothing lozenges.
- The patient may resume his usual diet and medications withheld before the test.

Interfering factors

- Gastric acid levels are elevated by cholinergics, adrenergic blockers, and reserpine.
- Gastric acid levels are depressed by antacids, anticholinergics, H2 blockers, and proton pump inhibitors.
- Failure to adhere to pretest restrictions may affect the accuracy of test results.

Gastric culture

Gastric culture requires aspiration of gastric contents and cultivation of any microbes present to identify mycobacterial infection. Performed in conjunction with a chest radiograph and a purified protein derivative skin test, gastric culture is especially useful when a sputum sample can't be obtained by expectoration or nebulization. Gastric aspiration also provides a specimen for rapid presumptive identification of bacteria (by Gram stain) in neonatal septicemia.

Purpose

- To aid diagnosis of mycobacterial infections
- To identify the infecting bacteria in neonatal septicemia.

Patient preparation

Explain to the patient (or to the parents if the patient is a child) that gastric culture helps diagnose tuberculosis. Instruct him to fast for 8 hours before the test. Tell him who will perform the procedure and that it may have to be performed on three consecutive mornings. Instruct the patient to remain in bed each morning until the specimen has been collected to prevent premature emptying of stomach contents.

Describe the procedure to the patient. Tell him the nasogastric (NG) tube may make him gag but passes more easily if he relaxes and follows instructions about breathing and swallowing. Just before the procedure, obtain baseline heart rate and rhythm, and place the patient in high-Fowler's position.

Inform the patient (or his parents) that test results may take 2 months because acid-fast bacteria generally grow slowly. Check his history for recent antimicrobial therapy.

Equipment

Water-soluble lubricating gel ■ sterile water ■ size 16 or 18 French disposable, plastic NG tube ■ 50-ml sterile syringe ■ sterile specimen container ■ sterile gloves ■ emesis basin ■ stethoscope ■ clamp (if necessary).

Procedure

■ As soon as the patient awakens in the morning, put on gloves, perform NG intubation, and obtain gastric washings. Clamp the tube before quickly removing it.

■ Note recent antimicrobial therapy on the laboratory request, along with the site and time of collection.

■ Label the specimens with the patient's name, the doctor's name, and the hospital number.

Precautions

■ Gastric intubation is contraindicated in pregnancy, esophageal disorders (varices, stenosis, diverticula, or malignant neoplasms), recent severe gastric hemorrhage, aortic aneurysm, heart failure, and myocardial infarction.

■ If possible, obtain the specimen before the start of antimicrobial therapy.

■ Use gloves when performing the procedure and handling specimens.

■ Make sure the specimen container is tightly capped. Wipe the outside of the container with disinfectant and send it to the laboratory (upright in a plastic bag) immediately.

■ Handle the NG tube with gloved hands, and dispose of all equipment carefully to prevent staff contamination.

CLINICAL ALERT Watch for signs that the tube has entered the trachea—coughing, cyanosis, or gasping.

CLINICAL ALERT Never inject fluid into an NG tube unless you're sure the tube is correctly placed in the patient's stomach. During lavage, use sterile, distilled water to decrease risk of contamination with saprophytic mycobacteria.

CLINICAL ALERT Because some patients develop arrhythmias during this procedure, check the pulse rate for irregularities.

Normal findings

The culture specimen should be free of pathogenic mycobacteria.

Implications of results

■ Isolation and identification of the organism *Mycobacterium tuberculosis* indicates the presence of active tuberculosis.

■ Other species of Mycobacterium, such as *M. bovis*, *M. kansasii*, and *M. aviumintracellulare* complex, may cause pulmonary disease that is clinically indistinguishable from tuberculosis. Treatment of these mycobacterial diseases may be difficult and commonly requires susceptibility studies to determine effective antimicrobial therapy.

■ Pathogenic bacteria that cause neonatal septicemia may also be identified through culture.

Posttest care

■ Resume administration of medications discontinued before the test.

■ Instruct the patient not to blow his nose for at least 4 hours to prevent bleeding.

■ Tell the patient that he may resume his normal diet.

Interfering factors

■ Failure to observe an 8-hour fast before the test may decrease the amount of bacteria by diluting stomach contents or removing contents through digestion.

■ Certain drugs, such as tetracycline and aminoglycosides, can weaken bacilli, causing false-negative culture results.

■ The presence of saprophytic mycobacteria in gastric contents may cause false-positive acid-fast smears because these bacteria can't be microscopically distinguished from pathogenic mycobacteria.

Gastrin test

Gastrin is a polypeptide hormone produced and stored primarily by specialized G cells in the antrum of the stomach and, to a lesser degree, by the islets of Langerhans in the pancreas. The main function of gastrin is to facilitate digestion of food by triggering gastric acid secretion in the parietal area of the stomach in response to food (especially proteins), vagal stimulation, or decreased stomach acidity. Secondarily, gastrin stimulates the release of pancreatic enzymes and the gastric enzyme pepsin, increases gastric and intestinal motility, and stimulates bile flow from the liver.

Through a strong negative feedback control mechanism, acid in the gastric antrum inhibits gastrin release in response to all stimuli. However, abnormal secretion of gastrin can result from tumors (gastrinomas) and from

GASTRIN STIMULATION TESTS

Because some patients with duodenal or gastric ulcers have normal fasting gastrin levels, provocative testing is necessary to identify them; a protein-rich test meal serves this purpose. In a patient with duodenal or gastric ulcers, gastrin levels increase markedly after such a meal; in a healthy person, they rise only moderately.

Provocative testing is also necessary to distinguish a patient with duodenal or gastric ulcers from one suspected of having Zollinger-Ellison syndrome, as both may show similar baseline gastrin levels. One effective test involves I.V. infusion of calcium gluconate in a dosage of 5 mg/kg of body weight over 3 hours. After the infusion, 10 ml of venous blood is drawn and sent to the laboratory. In a patient with Zollinger-Ellison syndrome, gastrin levels double, rising to about 500 pg/ml; in a patient with duodenal or gastric ulcers, levels rise only moderately or don't change at all.

A third indication for provocative testing is an abnormally — but not strikingly — high fasting serum gastrin level. This is possible in both Zollinger-Ellison syndrome and in pernicious anemia. To distinguish between the two, hydrochloric acid may be infused into the stomach through a nasogastric tube. Such infusion causes a sharp drop in gastrin levels in patients with pernicious anemia but not in patients with Zollinger-Ellison syndrome.

pathologic disorders affecting the stomach, pancreas and, less commonly, the esophagus and small bowel.

This radioimmunoassay, a quantitative analysis of gastrin levels, is diagnostically significant in patients suspected of having gastrinomas (Zollinger-Ellison syndrome). In doubtful situations, provocative testing may be necessary. However, gastrin estimation has limited value in persons with duodenal ulcer because the role of gastrin in peptic ulcers is unclear.

Purpose

■ To confirm diagnosis of gastrinoma, the gastrin-secreting tumor in Zollinger-Ellison syndrome
■ To aid differential diagnosis of gastric and duodenal ulcers and pernicious anemia. (See *Gastrin stimulation tests.*)

Patient preparation

Explain to the patient that this test helps determine the cause of his GI symptoms. Instruct him to abstain from alcohol for at least 24 hours before the test and to fast for 12 hours before it (water is permitted). Tell him the test requires a blood sample, who will perform the venipuncture and when, and that he may feel some transient discomfort from the needle puncture.

Withhold all medications that may interfere with test results, especially anticholinergics (such as atropine and belladonna) and insulin. If these medications must be continued, note this on the laboratory request.

Because stress can increase gastrin levels, make sure the patient is relaxed and recumbent for at least 30 minutes before the test.

Procedure

Perform a venipuncture and collect the sample in a 10- to 15-ml clot-activator tube.

Precautions

- Handle the sample gently to avoid hemolysis.
- To prevent destruction of serum gastrin by proteolytic enzymes, send the sample to the laboratory immediately to have the serum separated and frozen.

Reference values

Normal serum gastrin levels are less than 300 pg/ml.

Implications of results

- Strikingly high serum gastrin levels (over 1,000 pg/ml) confirm Zollinger-Ellison syndrome. (Levels as high as 450,000 pg/ml have been reported.)
- Gastrin levels may be high in various conditions, but the concomitant findings of very low gastric juice pH and a very high serum gastrin level indicate autonomous hormone secretion not governed by a negative feedback mechanism.
- Increased serum levels of gastrin may occur in a few patients with duodenal ulceration (less than 1%) and in patients with achlorhydria (with or without pernicious anemia) or with extensive stomach carcinoma (because of hyposecretion of gastric juices and hydrochloric acid).

Posttest care

- If a hematoma develops at the venipuncture site, apply warm soaks.
- Resume diet and medications that were discontinued before the test.

Interfering factors

- Gastrin secretion is increased by amino acids (especially glycine), calcium carbonate, acetylcholine, calcium chloride, and ethanol, and by insulin-induced hypoglycemia.
- Gastrin secretion is decreased by anticholinergics (atropine), hydrochloric acid, and secretin (a strongly basic polypeptide).
- Failure to observe restrictions of diet, medications, or physical activity may interfere with accurate determination of test results.

■ Hemolysis caused by rough handling of the sample may interfere with accurate determination of test results.

Glucagon test, plasma

Glucagon, a polypeptide hormone, is secreted by alpha cells of the islets of Langerhans in the pancreas. It acts primarily on the liver to promote glucose production and control glucose. This test is a quantitative analysis of plasma glucagon by radioimmunoassay.

Purpose

To aid diagnosis of glucagonoma and hypoglycemia due to chronic pancreatitis or idiopathic glucagon deficiency.

Patient preparation

Explain to the patient that this test helps to evaluate pancreatic function. Instruct the patient to fast for 10 to 12 hours before the test. Tell the patient that the test requires a blood sample. Inform him who will perform the venipuncture and when. Explain that he may experience transient discomfort from the needle puncture and tourniquet but that collecting the sample takes only a few minutes. Withhold insulin, catecholamines, and other drugs that could influence the test results. If they must be continued, note this on the laboratory slip. Have the patient lie down and relax for 30 minutes before the test.

Procedure

Perform a venipuncture and collect the sample in a chilled, 10-ml lavender-top tube.

Precautions

■ Place the sample on ice and send it to the laboratory immediately.
■ Handle the sample gently to prevent hemolysis.

Reference values

Normal fasting glucagon level is less than 60 pg/ml.

Implications of results

■ Elevated fasting glucagon levels (900 to 7800 pg/ml) can occur in glucagonoma, diabetes mellitus, acute pancreatitis, and pheochromocytoma.
■ Abnormally low glucagon levels are associated with idiopathic glucagon deficiency and hypoglycemia due to chronic pancreatitis.

Posttest care

- If a hematoma develops at the venipuncture site, apply warm soaks.
- Instruct the patient to resume his normal diet and medications withheld before the test.

Interfering factors

- Failure to observe Posttest care restrictions
- Hemolysis caused by rough handling of the sample
- Failure to pack the sample in ice and send it to the laboratory immediately
- Exercise, stress, prolonged fasting, insulin, or catecholamines (increase)
- Radioactive scans and tests performed within 48 hours of the test.

Glucose fasting test, plasma

Commonly used to screen for diabetes mellitus, the fasting plasma glucose test (also known as the fasting blood sugar test) measures plasma glucose levels following a 12- to 14-hour fast.

In the fasting state, plasma glucose levels decrease, stimulating release of the hormone glucagon. Glucagon then acts to raise plasma glucose by accelerating glycogenolysis, stimulating glyconeogenesis, and inhibiting glycogen synthesis. Normally, secretion of insulin checks this rise in glucose levels. In diabetes, however, absence or deficiency of insulin allows persistently high glucose levels. (See *Recognizing symptoms of diabetes*.)

Purpose

- To screen for diabetes mellitus
- To monitor drug or dietary therapy in patients with diabetes mellitus.

Patient preparation

Explain to the patient that this test detects disorders of glucose metabolism and aids diagnosis of diabetes. Advise him to fast for 12 to 14 hours before the test. Tell him that this test requires a blood sample, who will perform the venipuncture and when, and that he may experience transient discomfort from the needle puncture and the pressure of the tourniquet.

Withhold drugs that affect test results. If these medications must be continued, note this on the laboratory request. Advise the patient with diabetes that he'll receive his medication after the test.

Alert the patient to the symptoms of hypoglycemia — weakness, restlessness, nervousness, hunger, and sweat-

---

RECOGNIZING SYMPTOMS OF DIABETES

When you suspect diabetes, observe the patient carefully for the following classic symptoms:
■ *Polyuria:* Excessive plasma glucose overflows into the urine and exerts an osmotic pressure because of its concentration. This inhibits normal reabsorption of water by the renal tubules and leads to osmotic diuresis and dehydration.
■ *Polydipsia:* Frequent urination leads to dehydration and severe thirst.
■ *Weight loss:* Depletion of fat and protein stores to satisfy energy requirements causes severe, unexplained weight loss.
■ *Polyphagia:* In some patients, tissue destruction raises metabolic requirements and produces severe hunger.

---

ing—and tell him to report such symptoms immediately.

Procedure

Perform a venipuncture and collect the sample in a 5-ml clot-activator tube.

Precautions

■ Send the sample to the laboratory immediately because blood glucose levels decrease when the sample is left at room temperature. If transport is delayed, refrigerate the sample.
■ Specify on the laboratory request the time that the patient last ate, the sample collection time, and the time that he received the last pretest dose of insulin or oral antidiabetic drug (if applicable).

Reference values

■ The normal range for fasting plasma glucose varies according to the laboratory procedure.
■ Generally, normal values after at least an 8-hour fast are 70 to 110 mg of true glucose/dl of blood when measured by the glucose oxidase and hexokinase methods.

Implications of results

■ A fasting plasma glucose level of 126 mg/dl or higher obtained on two or more occasions confirms provisional diabetes mellitus. An impaired blood glucose level is 125 mg/dl. A borderline or transiently elevated level requires the 2-hour postprandial plasma glucose test or the oral glucose tolerance test to confirm the diagnosis.
■ Although increased fasting plasma glucose levels most commonly occur in diabetes, they can also result from pancreatitis, recent acute illness (such as myocardial infarction), Cushing's syndrome, acromegaly, and pheochromocytoma.

■ Hyperglycemia may also be associated with hyperlipoproteinemia (especially type III, IV, or V), chronic hepatic disease, nephrotic syndrome, brain tumor, sepsis, or gastrectomy with dumping syndrome, and is typical in eclampsia, anoxia, and seizure disorders.

■ Depressed plasma glucose levels can result from hyperinsulinism, insulinoma, von Gierke's disease, functional or reactive hypoglycemia, myxedema, adrenal insufficiency, congenital adrenal hyperplasia, hypopituitarism, malabsorption syndrome, and some cases of hepatic insufficiency.

CLINICAL ALERT When using fasting plasma glucose tests to monitor drug or diet therapy in patients with diabetes mellitus, results may require immediate action. Most patients develop symptoms when blood glucose is between 50 to 60 mg/dl. Symptoms include fatigue, malaise, nervousness, mood changes, irritability, trembling, tension, headache, hunger, cold sweats, rapid heart rate, and palpitations. Without immediate reversal of the hypoglycemia with parenteral or I.V. glucose, the blood glucose level will continue to fall. Evidence of progressive central nervous system disturbance includes blurry or double vision, inability to concentrate, confusion, motor weakness, hemiplegia, seizures, loss of consciousness, irreversible brain damage, and death.

■ Plasma glucose levels higher than 300 mg/dl can require immediate treatment with appropriate doses of insulin.

Posttest care

■ If a hematoma develops at the venipuncture site, apply warm soaks.

■ Provide a balanced meal or a snack.

■ Resume administration of medications withheld before the test.

Interfering factors

■ Failure to observe dietary restrictions may elevate plasma glucose levels.

■ False-positive findings may be caused by acetaminophen when the glucose oxidase or hexokinase method is used. Other drugs known to elevate plasma glucose levels are chlorthalidone, thiazide diuretics, furosemide, triamterene, oral contraceptives (estrogen-progestogen combination), benzodiazepines, phenytoin, phenothiazines, lithium, epinephrine, arginine, phenolphthalein, dextrothyroxine, diazoxide, large doses of nicotinic acid, corticosteroids, and recent I.V. glucose infusions. Ethacrynic acid may also cause hyperglycemia, but large doses can produce hypoglycemia in patients with uremia.

■ Decreased plasma glucose levels may be caused by beta-adrenergic blockers, ethanol, clofibrate, insulin, oral antidiabetic agents, and monoamine oxidase inhibitors.

■ Recent illness, infection, or pregnancy can elevate plasma glucose levels; strenuous exercise can depress them.

■ Glycolysis due to failure to refrigerate the sample or to send it to the laboratory immediately can result in false-negative results.

Glucose oxidase test

The glucose oxidase test, which involves the use of commercial, plastic-coated reagent strips (Clinistix, Diastix or Tes-Tape) is a specific, qualitative test for glycosuria. Although part of routine urinalysis, this test is used primarily to monitor urine glucose levels in patients with diabetes. Patients can perform this simple, convenient test at home.

Purpose
■ To detect glycosuria
■ To monitor urine glucose level during insulin therapy.

Patient preparation
Explain to the patient that this test determines urine glucose levels. If the patient is newly diagnosed with diabetes, teach him how to perform the test himself. (See *Interpreting glucose oxidase test results*, page 264.) Have the patient void, then give him a drink of water. After 30 to 45 minutes, collect a second-voided urine specimen.

Equipment
Specimen container ■ glucose test strips ■ reference color blocks.

Procedure
Collect a second-voided specimen, and use one of the following procedures:

■ Clinistix test: Dip the test area of the reagent strip in the specimen for 2 seconds. Remove excess urine by tapping the strip against a clean surface or the side of the container, and begin timing. Hold the strip in the air, and "read" the color exactly 10 seconds after taking the strip out of the urine by comparing it with the reference color blocks on the container label. Record the results. Ignore color changes that develop after 10 seconds.

■ Diastix test: Dip the reagent strip in the specimen for 2 seconds. Remove excess urine by tapping the strip

INTERPRETING GLUCOSE OXIDASE TEST RESULTS

Until recently, all glucose oxidase tests used the plus (+) symbol to indicate glycosuria. However, because the plus symbol didn't reflect a standard glucose value, regulating insulin dosages was difficult. Therefore, some manufacturers stopped using the plus symbol. As the chart below shows, Diastix doesn't use the plus symbol, but Tes-Tape does. These tests are semiquantitative. Clinistix (not shown) has no quantitative value; it is strictly qualitative. Results for this test are reported as negative, light, medium, or dark.

Test	0%	0.1%	0.25%	0.5%	1%	≥2%
Diastix	Negative	100 mg/dl	250 mg/dl	500 mg/dl	1,000 mg/dl	≥2,000 mg/dl
Tes-Tape	Negative	+	++	+++		++++

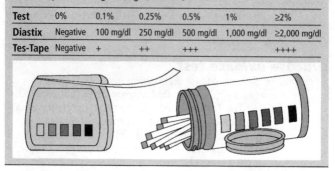

against the container, and begin timing. Hold the strip in the air, and compare the color to the color chart exactly 30 seconds after taking the strip out of the urine. Record the results. Ignore color changes that develop after 30 seconds.

■ Tes-Tape: Withdraw about 1½" (4 cm) of the reagent tape from the dispenser; dip ¼" (0.6 cm) in the specimen for 2 seconds. Remove excess urine by tapping the strip against the side of the container, and begin timing. Hold the tape in the air, and compare the color of the darkest part of the tape to the color chart exactly 60 seconds after taking the strip out of the urine. If the tape indicates 0.5% or higher, wait an additional 60 seconds to make the final color comparison. Record the results.

■ Provide written guidelines and a flow sheet so the patient can record the test results and insulin dosage taken at home.

■ Tell the patient when the next specimen is needed.

Precautions

■ Instruct the patient not to contaminate the urine specimen with toilet tissue or stool.

■ Keep the test strip container tightly closed to prevent deterioration of strips by exposure to light or moisture. Store it in a cool place (under 86° F [30° C]) to avoid heat degradation.

■ Don't use discolored or darkened Clinistix or Diastix strips, or dark yellow or yellow-brown Tes-Tape strips.

Normal findings

Glucose shouldn't be present in urine.

Implications of results

■ Glycosuria occurs in diabetes mellitus, adrenal and thyroid disorders, hepatic and central nervous system diseases, Fanconi's syndrome and other conditions involving low renal threshold, toxic renal tubular disease, heavy metal poisoning, glomerulonephritis, nephrosis, pregnancy, and total parenteral nutrition.

■ Other causes include administration of large amounts of glucose or niacin, prolonged use of phenothiazines, and use of certain other drugs, such as asparaginase, corticosteroids, carbamazepine, ammonium chloride, thiazide diuretics, dextrothyroxine, and lithium carbonate.

Interfering factors

■ Reducing substances, such as levodopa, ascorbic acid, phenazopyridine, methyldopa, and salicylates, may cause false-negative results.

■ Tetracyclines also produce false-negative results.

■ Diluted, stale urine or bacterial contamination of the specimen may affect test results.

■ Use of reagent strips after the expiration date, failure to keep the reagent strip container tightly closed, or failure to record the reagent strip method used may alter test results.

Glucose tolerance test, oral

The oral glucose tolerance test (OGTT), the most sensitive method of evaluating borderline cases of diabetes mellitus in selected patients, measures carbohydrate metabolism after ingestion of a challenge dose of glucose. (See *Administering oral glucose solutions*, page 266.) The body absorbs this dose rapidly, causing plasma glucose levels to rise and peak within 30 minutes to 1 hour. The pancreas responds by secreting more insulin, causing glucose levels to return to normal after 2 to 3 hours.

During this period, plasma and urine glucose levels are monitored to assess insulin secretion and the body's ability to metabolize glucose. Occasionally, glucose levels are monitored an additional 2 to 3 hours to aid diagnosis of hypoglycemia and malabsorption syndrome. However, such extended testing is contraindicated when insulinoma is strongly suspected because prolonged fasting in such a patient can lead to fainting and coma.

In a patient with mild or diet-controlled diabetes, fasting plasma glucose levels may be in the normal range; however, insufficient secretion of insulin after ingestion

ADMINISTERING ORAL GLUCOSE SOLUTIONS

The oral glucose load in a glucose tolerance test usually varies from 50 to 100 g. The American Diabetes Association recommends a glucose dose of 40 g/m² of body surface area, as calculated by a nomogram based on height and weight. Others advocate a glucose load of 1.75 g/kg of body weight, which is especially useful in testing pediatric patients.

Many patients become nauseated after drinking the overly sweet glucose solution. One way to make the solution more palatable is to dissolve it in water, flavor it with lemon juice, and chill it. Another is to substitute Glucola, a carbonated drink, or Gel-a-dex, a cherry-flavored gelatin, for the appropriate amount of glucose.

of carbohydrates causes plasma glucose levels to rise sharply and return to normal slowly. This decreased tolerance for glucose helps to confirm mild diabetes.

The OGTT isn't usually used in patients with fasting plasma glucose values above 140 mg/dl or postprandial plasma glucose above 200 mg/dl. Two other tests are also used to confirm or sensitize OGTT findings. (See *Supplementary glucose tolerance tests.*)

Purpose
- To confirm diabetes mellitus in selected patients
- To aid diagnosis of hypoglycemia and malabsorption syndrome.

Patient preparation
Explain to the patient that this test evaluates glucose metabolism. Instruct him to maintain a high-carbohydrate diet for 3 days and then to fast for 10 to 16 hours before the test. Advise him not to smoke, drink coffee or alcohol, or exercise strenuously for 8 hours before or during the test. Tell him this test usually requires five blood samples and five urine specimens, who will perform the venipunctures and when, and that he may experience transient discomfort from the needle punctures and the pressure of the tourniquet. Suggest that he bring a book or other quiet diversions with him to the test because the procedure usually takes 3 hours but can last as long as 6 hours.

Withhold drugs that may affect test results. If these drugs must be continued, note this on the laboratory request. Alert the patient to the symptoms of hypoglycemia—weakness, restlessness, nervousness, hunger, and sweating—and tell him to report such symptoms immediately.

SUPPLEMENTARY GLUCOSE TOLERANCE TESTS

Although the oral glucose tolerance test (OGTT) is the most effective test for detecting diabetes, two other tests are sometimes used as research tools to sensitize or confirm OGTT findings.

I.V. glucose tolerance test

This test measures blood glucose after the patient receives an I.V. infusion of 50% glucose over 3 or 4 minutes. Blood samples are then drawn at $1/2$-, 1-, 2-, and 3-hour intervals. After an immediate glucose peak of 300 to 400 mg/dl (accompanied by glycosuria), the normal glucose curve falls steadily, reaching fasting levels within 1 to $1 1/2$ hours.

Failure to reach fasting glucose levels within 2 to 3 hours generally confirms diabetes. A similarly delayed return to fasting glucose levels may result from fever, stress, old age, inactivity, carbohydrate deprivation, neoplasms, cirrhosis, or steroid-producing endocrine diseases.

Nevertheless, the I.V. glucose tolerance test (IVGTT) has the following advantages over the OGTT:

- GI hormones that cause insulin secretion won't affect IVGTT glucose tolerance curves.
- Patients with intestinal absorption syndromes won't present abnormal curves.
- The IVGTT provides an alternative to flat OGTT curves resulting from hypopituitarism, hypoparathyroidism, or Addison's disease.
- This test doesn't require the patient to ingest an unpalatable oral glucose load.

Cortisone glucose tolerance test

This test is occasionally used for patients with borderline carbohydrate-tolerance deficiencies or a strong familial predisposition to diabetes who produce a normal OGTT curve. After a 3-day high-carbohydrate diet, oral cortisone acetate is administered 8 and 2 hours before the standard OGTT. Cortisone promotes glyconeogenesis and may accentuate carbohydrate intolerance in latent or mild diabetes.

Although this test is used primarily for research, values that rise approximately 20 mg/dl above those of the standard OGTT after 2 hours indicate probable diabetes in some people with only minimally decreased carbohydrate intolerance.

Procedure

- Between 7 a.m. and 9 a.m., draw a fasting blood sample in a 7-ml clot-activator tube. Collect a urine specimen at the same time, if your institution includes this as part of the test. After collecting these samples, administer the test load of oral glucose, and record the time of ingestion. Encourage the patient to drink the entire glucose solution within 5 minutes.
- Draw blood samples 30 minutes, 1 hour, 2 hours, and 3 hours after giving the loading dose, using 7-ml clot-activator tubes. Collect urine specimens at the same intervals. Tell the patient to lie down if he feels faint from

the numerous venipunctures. Encourage him to drink water throughout the test to promote adequate urine excretion.

Precautions

Send blood and urine samples to the laboratory immediately or refrigerate them. Specify when the patient last ate and the blood and urine collection times. As appropriate, record the time that the patient received his last pretest dose of insulin or oral antidiabetic drug.

CLINICAL ALERT If the patient develops severe hypoglycemia, notify the clinician. Draw a blood sample, record the time on the laboratory request, and discontinue the test. Have the patient drink a glass of orange juice or administer glucose I.V. to reverse the reaction.

Reference values

Normal plasma glucose levels peak at 160 to 180 mg/dl 30 minutes to 1 hour after administration of an oral glucose test dose and return to fasting levels or lower in 2 to 3 hours. (See *Interpreting results of the OGTT*.) Urine glucose tests remain negative throughout.

Implications of results

■ Depressed glucose tolerance, in which levels peak sharply before falling slowly to fasting levels, may confirm diabetes or may result from Cushing's disease, hemochromatosis, pheochromocytomas, or central nervous system lesions.

■ Increased glucose tolerance, in which levels may peak at less than normal, may indicate insulinoma, malabsorption syndrome, adrenocortical insufficiency (Addison's disease), hypothyroidism, or hypopituitarism.

Posttest care

■ If a hematoma develops at the venipuncture site, apply warm soaks.
■ Provide a balanced meal or a snack, but observe for a hypoglycemic reaction.
■ Resume administration of medications withheld before the test.

Interfering factors

■ Carbohydrate deprivation before the test can produce a diabetic response (abnormal increase in plasma glucose with a delayed decrease) because the pancreas is unaccustomed to responding to high-carbohydrate load.
■ Elevated plasma glucose levels may result from chlorthalidone, thiazide diuretics, furosemide, triamterene, oral contraceptives (estrogen-progestogen combination), benzodiazepines, phenytoin, phenothiazines, lithium,

INTERPRETING RESULTS OF THE OGTT

Because plasma glucose levels in the oral glucose tolerance test (OGTT) can be measured in various ways, inconsistent results and misinterpretation are common. Age, race, inactivity, and obesity may also affect established OGTT criteria. The American Diabetes Association recommends using the reference values obtained by the Wilkerson point system, the Fajans-Conn system, or the National Institutes of Health (NIH) system, depending on whether the patient is a child or is pregnant.

Method	Hour	Whole blood	Plasma	Points
Wilkerson point system Two or more total points confirm the diagnosis of diabetes.	Fasting	≥ 110 mg/dl	≥ 130 mg/dl	1
	1	≥ 170 mg/dl	≥ 195 mg/dl	½
	2	≥ 120 mg/dl	≥ 140 mg/dl	½
	3	≥ 110 mg/dl	≥ 130 mg/dl	1
Fajans-Conn system If all levels equal or exceed established values, the diagnosis of diabetes is confirmed.	1	≥ 160 mg/dl	≥ 185 mg/dl	
	1½	≥ 140 mg/dl	≥ 165 mg/dl	
	2	≥ 120 mg/dl	≥ 140 mg/dl	
NIH system If all levels exceed established values, the diagnosis of diabetes is confirmed.	Fasting		> 140 mg/dl	
	2		> 200 mg/dl	

epinephrine, phenolphthalein, caffeine, arginine, dextrothyroxine, diazoxide, large doses of nicotinic acid, corticosteroids, and recent I.V. glucose infusions.

■ Depressed glucose levels may be caused by ingestion of beta-adrenergic blockers, amphetamines, ethanol, clofibrate, insulin, oral antidiabetic drugs, and monoamine oxidase inhibitors.

■ Failure to adhere to dietary and exercise restrictions may alter test results.

■ A recent infection, fever, pregnancy, or acute illness such as myocardial infarction may elevate glucose levels.

■ People over age 50 tend to exhibit decreasing carbohydrate tolerance; their upper limits of glucose tolerance rise by about 1 mg/dl for every year over age 50.

Glucose test, 2-hour postprandial, plasma

The 2-hour postprandial glucose test is a valuable screening tool for detecting diabetes mellitus. This procedure is performed on patients who have symptoms of diabetes (polydipsia and polyuria) or on patients whose fasting plasma glucose test results suggest diabetes.

The 2-hour postprandial test reliably reflects the body's insulin response to carbohydrate ingestion. It re-

PREFERRED SCREENING TEST FOR DIABETES MELLITUS

Because the 2-hour postprandial test is a simpler procedure than the oral glucose tolerance test or the fasting plasma glucose test, it's often the preferred test for diabetes screening in patients with any of the following conditions:
■ obesity
■ family history of diabetes
■ transient glycosuria or hyperglycemia (especially during pregnancy, surgery, or use of adrenal steroids) or after trauma, emotional stress, myocardial infarction, or cerebrovascular accident
■ unexplained hypoglycemia, neuropathy, retinopathy, nephropathy, or peripheral vascular disease
■ pregnancy resulting in abortion, premature labor, stillbirth, neonatal death, or a very large infant
■ recurrent infection, especially boils and abscesses.

lies solely on the 2-hour glucose level, avoiding the multiple venipunctures required for the oral glucose tolerance test (OGTT). If postprandial test results are borderline, the OGTT may confirm the diagnosis. (See *Preferred screening test for diabetes mellitus*.)

Purpose
■ To aid diagnosis of diabetes mellitus
■ To monitor drug or diet therapy in patients with diabetes mellitus.

Patient preparation
Explain to the patient that this test evaluates glucose metabolism and helps detect diabetes. Tell him to eat a balanced meal or one containing 100 g of carbohydrate (recommended by the American Diabetes Association) before the test and then to fast for 2 hours. Instruct him to avoid smoking and strenuous exercise after the meal. Tell him this test requires a blood sample, who will perform the venipuncture and when, and that he may experience transient discomfort from the needle puncture and the pressure of the tourniquet.

Procedure
Perform a venipuncture and collect the sample in a 5-ml clot-activator tube.

Precautions
■ Send the sample to the laboratory immediately or refrigerate it.
■ Specify on the laboratory request the time that the patient last ate, the sample collection time, and the time

TWO-HOUR POSTPRANDIAL GLUCOSE LEVELS BY AGE

The greatest difference in normal and diabetic insulin responses and, thus, in plasma glucose level, occurs about 2 hours after a glucose challenge. Normal glucose values can fluctuate according to the patient's age (as shown below). After age 50, for example, normal levels rise markedly and steadily, sometimes reaching 160 mg/dl or higher. In younger patients, glucose levels over 145 mg/dl suggest incipient diabetes and require further evaluation.

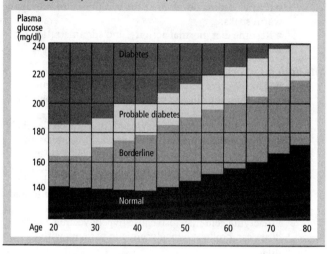

that he received the last pretest dose of insulin or oral antidiabetic drug (if applicable).

■ If the sample is to be drawn by a technician, tell him the exact time the venipuncture must be performed.

Reference values

In a person without diabetes, normal postprandial glucose values are less than 145 mg/dl by the glucose oxidase or hexokinase method; normal levels are slightly elevated in people over age 50. (See *Two-hour postprandial glucose levels by age.*)

Implications of results

■ Two-hour postprandial plasma glucose values of 150 mg/dl or more suggest diabetes mellitus. Values greater than 200 mg/dl confirm the diagnosis.

■ High levels may also result from pancreatitis, Cushing's syndrome, acromegaly, or pheochromocytoma.

■ Hyperglycemia may also be associated with hyperlipoproteinemia (especially type III, IV, or V), chronic hepatic disease, nephrotic syndrome, brain tumor, sepsis, gastrectomy with dumping syndrome, eclampsia, anoxia, or convulsive disorders.

■ Depressed glucose levels can result from hyperinsulinism, insulinoma, von Gierke's disease, functional or reactive hypoglycemia, myxedema, adrenal insufficiency, congenital adrenal hyperplasia, hypopituitarism, malabsorption syndrome, and some cases of hepatic insufficiency.

Posttest care

■ If a hematoma develops at the venipuncture site, apply warm soaks.
■ Resume diet, normal activity, and administration of medications that were discontinued before the test.

Interfering factors

■ False-positive results may be caused by acetaminophen when the glucose oxidase or hexokinase method is used.
■ Other drugs known to elevate plasma glucose levels are chlorthalidone, thiazide diuretics, furosemide, triamterene, oral contraceptives (estrogen-progestogen combination), benzodiazepines, phenytoin, phenothiazines, lithium, epinephrine, arginine, phenolphthalein, dextrothyroxine, diazoxide, large doses of nicotinic acid, corticosteroids, and recent I.V. glucose infusions. Ethacrynic acid may also cause hyperglycemia, but large doses can produce hypoglycemia in patients with uremia.
■ Depressed glucose levels may result from the use of beta blockers, amphetamines, ethanol, clofibrate, insulin, oral antidiabetic drugs, and monoamine oxidase inhibitors.
■ Recent illness, infection, or pregnancy may raise glucose levels; strenuous exercise or stress may depress them.
■ Glycolysis caused by failure to refrigerate the sample or to send it to the laboratory immediately can depress glucose levels.

Glucose-6-phosphate dehydrogenase test

Glucose-6-phosphate dehydrogenase (G6PD), an enzyme found in most body cells, is part of the pentose phosphate pathway (hexose monophosphate shunt) that metabolizes glucose. Measuring serum G6PD levels detects deficiency of this enzyme. Such deficiency is a hereditary, sex-linked condition carried on the female X chromosome (clinical disease occurs mostly in males). The deficiency impairs the stability of the red cell membrane and makes red cells susceptible to hemolysis by strong oxidizing agents. Drugs that can precipitate this reaction include antimalarials, sulfonamides, aspirin, nonsteroidal anti-inflammatory drugs (NSAIDs), nitrofurantoin, and quinidine.

Red cell enzyme levels normally decrease as cells age, but G6PD deficiency accelerates this process, so that older red cells are more prone to destruction than younger ones. In mild deficiency, young red cells retain enough G6PD to survive; in severe deficiency, all red cells are destroyed.

About 10% of all black males in the United States inherit a mild G6PD deficiency; some people of Mediterranean origin inherit a severe deficiency in which fava beans may produce hemolytic episodes. Although deficiency of G6PD provides partial immunity to falciparum malaria, it precipitates an adverse reaction to antimalarials.

Purpose

■ To detect hemolytic anemia caused by G6PD deficiency
■ To aid differential diagnosis of hemolytic anemia.

Patient preparation

Explain to the patient that this test detects an inherited enzyme deficiency that may affect the life span of red blood cells. Inform him that he need not restrict food or fluids. Tell him that the test requires a blood sample, who will perform the venipuncture and when, and that he may experience some transient discomfort from the needle puncture and the pressure of the tourniquet.

Check the patient history, and report a recent blood transfusion or ingestion of aspirin, sulfonamides, phenacetin, nitrofurantoin, vitamin K derivatives, antimalarials, or fava beans, which cause hemolysis in G6PD-deficient persons.

Procedure

Perform a venipuncture and collect the sample in a 7-ml tube with EDTA.

Precautions

■ Completely fill the collection tube, and invert it gently several times to mix the sample and the anticoagulant.
■ Handle the sample gently to prevent hemolysis.
■ If you can't send the sample to the laboratory immediately, refrigerate it.

Reference values

Serum G6PD values vary with the measurement method used but usually range from 8.6 to 18.6 U/g of hemoglobin. They may also be reported simply as normal or abnormal.

Implications of results

■ Fluorescent spot testing or staining for Heinz bodies or erythrocytes can screen for G6PD deficiency. If results are positive, the kinetic quantitative assay for G6PD may be performed.

■ Electrophoretic techniques assess genetic variants of G6PD deficiency, which may cause lifelong mild, or asymptomatic anemia. Some variants are symptomatic only when the patient experiences stress or illness or is exposed to drugs or agents that elicit hemolytic episodes.

Posttest care

If a hematoma develops at the venipuncture site, apply warm soaks.

Interfering factors

■ The following substances decrease G6PD enzyme activity and precipitate hemolytic episodes: aspirin, sulfonamides, nitrofurantoin, vitamin K derivatives, primaquine, and fava beans.

■ Performing the test after a hemolytic episode or a blood transfusion can cause false-negative results.

■ Failure to use a collection tube containing the proper anticoagulant or to adequately mix the sample and anticoagulant may alter test results.

■ Hemolysis caused by rough handling of the sample may affect test results.

Glycosylated hemoglobin test

The glycosylated hemoglobin test (also known as the total fasting hemoglobin or glycohemoglobin test) helps to monitor the effectiveness of diabetes therapy. The three minor hemoglobins (Hb) measured in this test — Hb A1a, A1b, and A1c — are variants of Hb A formed by glycosylation, a nearly irreversible molecular process in which glucose becomes chemically incorporated in Hb A. Because glycosylation occurs at a constant rate during the 120-day life span of an erythrocyte, glycosylated hemoglobin levels reflect the average blood glucose level during the preceding 2 to 3 months and thus are useful in evaluating the long-term effectiveness of diabetes therapy.

The glycosylated hemoglobin test has distinct advantages over traditional blood and urine glucose tests. Blood glucose testing requires repeated venipunctures;

each measurement reflects glucose control only at the moment the sample was taken. Measuring urinary glucose excretion also reflects glucose control only at the time of collection. In contrast, the glycosylated hemoglobin test requires only one venipuncture every 6 to 8 weeks. In addition, because this test measures glucose within an erythrocyte, levels are more stable than those of plasma glucose, which reflect metabolic processes.

Glycosylated hemoglobin is measured by processing red cell hemolysates through a cation exchange chromatography column to separate glycosylated hemoglobins from Hb A.

Purpose

To assess control of diabetes mellitus.

Patient preparation

Explain to the patient that this test evaluates the effectiveness of diabetes therapy. Advise him that he need not restrict food or fluids, and instruct him to maintain his prescribed medication or diet regimen. Tell him the test requires a blood sample, who will perform the venipuncture and when, and that he may experience transient discomfort from the needle puncture and the pressure of the tourniquet.

Procedure

Perform a venipuncture and collect the sample in a 5-ml tube with EDTA added.

Precautions

Fill the collection tube completely, and invert it gently several times to mix the sample and anticoagulant adequately.

Reference values

Glycosylated hemoglobin values are reported as a percentage of the total hemoglobin within an erythrocyte. Because Hb A1c is present in a larger quantity than the other minor hemoglobins, it's commonly measured and reported separately.

■ Hb A1a and Hb A1b account for about 1.6% and 0.8%, respectively; Hb A1c accounts for approximately 5%; and total glycosylated hemoglobin accounts for 4% to 7%.

Implications of results

■ Good diabetic control is indicated when the glycosylated hemoglobin value is less than 8%.

■ A value greater than 10% indicates poor control.

■ Glycosylated hemoglobin levels approach normal range as therapy begins to control diabetes.

Posttest care
■ If a hematoma develops at the venipuncture site, apply warm soaks.
■ Schedule the patient for an appointment in 6 to 8 weeks for appropriate follow-up testing.

Interfering factors
■ Failure to mix the sample and the anticoagulant adequately may affect the accuracy of test results.
■ Results can be lower if the patient has hemolytic anemia, chronic blood loss, or abnormal hemoglobins (S, C, or D).
■ Results can be elevated if the patient has hyperglycemia, thalassemia, or chronic renal failure; is on dialysis; had a splenectomy; or has elevated triglyceride or hemoglobin F levels.

Gonorrhea culture

Although a stained smear of genital exudate can confirm gonorrhea in 90% of males with characteristic symptoms, a culture is often necessary, especially in asymptomatic females. Possible culture sites include the urethra (usual site in males), endocervix (usual site in females), anal canal, and oropharynx.

Gonorrhea, the most prevalent venereal disease, almost always results from sexual transmission of *Neisseria gonorrhoeae*. Its most common effect in females is a greenish yellow cervical discharge. Other symptoms include dysuria and possibly bleeding, but in many females, it causes no signs or symptoms at all—a factor that contributes to the epidemic prevalence of this infection. In males, gonorrhea generally causes painful urination and a mucopurulent urethral discharge, symptoms of acute anterior urethritis. In both sexes, it may also cause pharyngitis.

Purpose
To confirm gonorrhea.

Patient preparation
Describe the procedure to the patient, and explain that this test confirms gonorrhea. Inform the patient who will perform the test and when and that results are usually available within 24 to 72 hours.

Instruct the female patient not to douche for 24 hours before the test. Tell the male patient not to void for an hour before the test. Warn him that males sometimes experience nausea, sweating, weakness, and fainting from fear or discomfort when the cotton swab or wire loop is introduced into the urethra.

Equipment

Sterile gloves ■ sterile cotton swabs or sterile gauze ■ wire bacteriologic loop or thin urogenital alginate swabs (for male patient) ■ vaginal speculum ■ modified Thayer-Martin medium in plates (or Transgrow medium in specimen bottles if laboratory isn't readily available) ■ ring forceps ■ cotton balls.

Procedure

ENDOCERVICAL CULTURE

■ Place the patient in the lithotomy position, drape her, and instruct her to take deep breaths.

■ Using gloved hands, insert a vaginal speculum that has been lubricated only with warm water. Clean mucus from the cervix, using cotton balls in ring forceps.

■ Insert a dry, sterile cotton swab into the endocervical canal, and rotate it from side to side. Leave the swab in place for several seconds for optimum absorption of organisms.

ENDOMETRIAL CULTURE

In cases of deep pelvic inflammatory disease, cultures of the endometrium or aspirations by laparoscopy or culdoscopy may be necessary. Endometrial specimens are obtained by inserting stents through a narrow-bore catheter introduced into the cervical canal.

URETHRAL CULTURE

■ Place the patient in the supine position, and drape him appropriately. Clean the urinary meatus with sterile gauze or a cotton swab; then insert a thin urogenital alginate swab or a wire bacteriologic loop ⅜" to ¾" (1 to 2 cm) into the urethra, and rotate it from side to side. Leave it in place for several seconds for optimum absorption of organisms.

■ If permitted by the clinician, the patient may "milk" his urethra, bringing urethral secretions to the meatus for collection on a cotton swab.

RECTAL CULTURE

■ After obtaining an endocervical or urethral specimen (while the patient is still on the examining table), insert a sterile cotton swab about 1" (2.5 cm) into the anal canal, move it from side to side, and leave it in place for several seconds for optimum absorption.

■ If the swab is contaminated with feces, discard it and repeat the procedure with a clean swab.

THROAT CULTURE

Position the patient with his head tilted back and his eyes closed. Check his throat for inflamed areas, using a tongue blade. Rub a sterile swab from side to side over the tonsillar areas, including any inflamed or purulent sites. Be careful not to touch the teeth, cheeks, or tongue with the swab.

AFTER COLLECTING SPECIMEN

■ Roll the swab in a Z pattern in a plate containing modified Thayer-Martin medium. Then cross-streak the medium with a sterile wire loop or the tip of the swab, and cover the plate. Label the specimen with the patient's name and room number (if applicable), the doctor's name, and the date and time of collection.

■ Direct smears of obtained material should be made immediately to prepare the Gram stain. Remaining material must be quickly inoculated into selective culture media or into a transport system. A culturette transport tube or a swab transport medium containing charcoal can be used. Charcoal helps to neutralize toxic materials in the specimen.

■ If laboratory facilities aren't readily available, uncap the Transgrow medium specimen bottle just before inserting the swab of test material into the bottle. Keep the bottle upright to minimize loss of carbon dioxide. With the swab, absorb the excess moisture in the bottle; then roll the swab across the Transgrow medium. Discard the swab, and place the lid on the bottle. Label the bottle appropriately.

Precautions

■ Use gloves when performing procedures and handling specimens.

■ Place the male patient in the supine position to prevent falling if vasovagal syncope occurs during introduction of the cotton swab or wire loop into the urethra. Observe him for profound hypotension, bradycardia, pallor, and sweating.

■ Collect a urethral specimen at least 1 hour after the patient has voided to prevent loss of urethral secretions.

■ After collecting the specimens, carefully dispose of gloves, swabs, and speculum to prevent staff exposure to any organisms.

■ Immediately send the specimen to the laboratory or arrange for transport of the Transgrow bottle because the specimen must be subcultured within 24 to 48 hours.

Normal findings

No *Nisseria gonorrhoeae* organisms should appear in the culture.

Implications of results

■ A positive culture confirms a diagnosis of gonorrhea. Stress the importance of completing the entire course of antibiotic therapy even after symptoms subside. Emphasize abstinence from sexual activity until the patient is disease-free. Trace all potentially exposed sex partners to institute treatment for them as well. Advise patients to use condoms during future intercourse, to wash genitalia before and after intercourse, and to avoid sharing washcloths and douche equipment.

■ Administration of silver nitrate or erythromycin in the eyes of all neonates immediately after birth is a routine precaution. Newborns of infected mothers should be checked for signs and symptoms of gonorrhea.

Posttest care

■ Advise the patient to avoid intercourse and all sexual contact until test results are available. Explain that treatment usually begins after confirmation of a positive culture, except in a patient with symptoms of gonorrhea or in a person who has had intercourse with someone known to have gonorrhea.

■ Advise the patient that a repeat culture is required 1 week after treatment is completed to evaluate the effectiveness of therapy.

■ Inform the patient that positive culture findings must be reported to the local health department.

Interfering factors

■ Improper collection technique may provide a nonrepresentative or contaminated specimen.

■ Fecal material may contaminate a rectal culture.

■ In males, voiding within 1 hour of specimen collection washes secretions out of the urethra, making fewer organisms available for culture.

■ In females, douching within 24 hours of specimen collection washes out cervical secretions, making fewer organisms available for culture.

Growth hormone suppression test

This test, also known as the glucose loading test, evaluates excessive baseline levels of growth hormone (hGH) from the anterior pituitary by measuring the secretory response to a loading dose of glucose. Normally, hGH raises plasma glucose and fatty acid concentrations; in response, insulin secretion increases to counteract these effects. Consequently, a glucose load should suppress hGH secretion. In a patient with excessive hGH levels, failure of suppression reflects anterior pituitary dysfunction and confirms a diagnosis of acromegaly or gigantism.

Purpose

■ To assess elevated baseline hGH levels
■ To confirm a diagnosis of gigantism in children and acromegaly in adults.

Patient preparation

Explain to the patient and to his family (if the patient is a child) that this test helps determine the cause of his abnormal growth. Instruct him to fast and limit physical activity for 10 to 12 hours before the test. Tell him two blood samples will be drawn, and warn that he may experience nausea after drinking the glucose solution and feel some discomfort from the needle punctures. Inform him that the test takes about 1 hour but that the laboratory requires at least 2 days to complete the analysis.

Before the test, withhold all steroids — including estrogens and progestogens — and other pituitary-based hormones. If these or other medications must be continued, note this on the laboratory request.

Because hGH levels rise after exercise or excitement, make sure the patient is relaxed and recumbent for 30 minutes before the test.

Procedure

■ Between 6 a.m. and 8 a.m., draw 6 ml of venous blood (basal sample) into a 7-ml clot-activator tube. Label the tube and send it to the laboratory immediately after drawing the sample. Administer 100 g of glucose solution orally. To prevent nausea, advise the patient to drink the glucose slowly.
■ About an hour later, draw venous blood into a second 7-ml clot-activator tube. Label the tube and send it to the laboratory immediately after drawing the sample.

Precautions

■ Handle the samples gently to prevent hemolysis.
■ Send each sample to the laboratory immediately because hGH has a half-life of only 20 to 25 minutes.

Reference values

■ Normally, glucose suppresses hGH to levels ranging from undetectable to 3 ng/ml in 30 minutes to 2 hours.
■ In children, rebound stimulation may occur after 2 to 5 hours.

Implications of results

■ In a patient with active acromegaly, basal hGH levels are elevated (75 ng/ml) and aren't suppressed to less than 5 ng/ml during the test.

■ Unchanged or increased hGH levels in response to glucose loading suggest hGH hypersecretion and may confirm suspected acromegaly or gigantism. This response may be verified by repeating the test after a 1-day rest.

Posttest care

■ If a hematoma develops at the puncture sites, apply warm soaks.

■ Resume diet and medications that were discontinued before the test.

Interfering factors

■ Failure to observe restrictions of diet, medications, and physical activity may interfere with accurate determination of test results. Release of hGH may be impaired by corticosteroids and phenothiazines (chlorpromazine), and may be increased by arginine, levodopa, amphetamines, glucagon, niacin, or estrogens.

■ A radioactive scan performed within 1 week before the test may affect results, because hGH levels are determined by radioimmunoassay.

■ Hemolysis due to rough handling of the sample may interfere with accurate determination of test results.

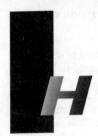

Ham test

The Ham test (also known as the acidified serum lysis test) is performed to determine the cause of undiagnosed hemolytic anemia, hemoglobinuria, or bone marrow aplasia. The Ham test relies on the susceptibility of red blood cells (RBCs) to lysis. It helps establish a diagnosis of paroxysmal nocturnal hemoglobinuria (PNH), a rare hematologic disease. RBCs from patients with PNH are unusually susceptible to lysis by complement.

In the laboratory, washed RBCs are mixed with ABO-compatible normal serum and acid. After incubation at 98.6°F (37°C), the cells are examined for hemolysis. In the presence of acidified human serum, a substantial portion of PNH cells are lysed, whereas normal RBCs show no hemolysis.

Purpose

To help establish a diagnosis of PNH.

Patient preparation

Explain to the patient that this test helps determine the cause of his anemia or other signs. Advise him that he needn't restrict food or fluids. Tell him that this test requires a blood sample, who will perform the venipuncture and when, and that he may experience transient discomfort from the needle puncture and the pressure of the tourniquet.

Procedure

Because the blood sample must be defibrinated immediately, laboratory personnel will perform the venipuncture and collect the sample.

Precautions

None.

Normal findings

RBCs do not normally undergo hemolysis.

Implications of results

Hemolysis of RBCs indicates PNH.

Posttest care

If a hematoma develops at the venipuncture site, apply warm soaks.

Interfering factors

- Blood containing large numbers of spherocytes may produce false-positive results.
- Blood from patients with congenital dyserythropoietic anemia will produce false-positive results.

Haptoglobin test

By means of radial immunodiffusion or nephelometry, this test measures serum levels of haptoglobin, a glycoprotein produced in the liver. Free hemoglobin binds haptoglobin, preventing its accumulation in plasma, permitting its clearance by reticuloendothelial cells, and conserving body iron. Hemoglobin circulates inside erythrocytes (or red blood cells); when aged erythrocytes die, they release free hemoglobin into plasma. Certain anemias, bacterial toxins, mechanical disruptions (from a prosthetic heart valve, for example), or antibodies can increase intravascular hemolysis. In acute intravascular hemolysis, haptoglobin levels fall rapidly; low levels may last for 5 to 7 days, until the liver synthesizes more glycoprotein.

Purpose

- To serve as an index of hemolysis
- To distinguish between hemoglobin and myoglobin in plasma because haptoglobin doesn't bind with myoglobin
- To investigate hemolytic transfusion reactions
- To establish proof of paternity, using genetic (phenotypic) variations in haptoglobin structure.

Patient preparation

Explain to the patient that this test helps determine the condition of red blood cells. Inform him that he needn't restrict food or fluids. Tell him the test requires a blood sample, who will perform the venipuncture and when, and that he may experience transient discomfort from the needle puncture and the pressure of the tourniquet. Check the patient's medication history for drugs that may influence haptoglobin levels, such as corticosteroids or androgens.

Procedure

Draw a venous blood sample into a 7-ml clot-activator tube.

Precautions

Handle the sample gently.

Normal findings

Serum haptoglobin concentrations, measured in terms of the protein's hemoglobin-binding capacity, normally range from 38 to 270 mg/dl. Nephelometric procedures yield lower results.

Implications of results

Markedly depressed serum haptoglobin levels are characteristic of acute and chronic hemolysis, severe hepatocellular disease, infectious mononucleosis, and transfusion reactions. Hepatocellular disease inhibits the synthesis of haptoglobin. In hemolytic transfusion reactions, haptoglobin levels begin falling after 6 to 8 hours and drop to 40% of pretransfusion levels after 24 hours.

If serum haptoglobin values are very low, watch for symptoms of hemolysis: chills, fever, back pain, flushing, distended neck veins, tachycardia, tachypnea, and hypotension.

Although haptoglobin is absent in 90% of neonates, levels usually rise to normal by age 4 months. However, in about 1% of the general population—including 4% of blacks—haptoglobin is permanently absent; this disorder is known as congenital ahaptoglobinemia.

Markedly elevated serum haptoglobin levels occur in diseases marked by chronic inflammatory reactions or tissue destruction, such as rheumatoid arthritis and malignant neoplasms.

Posttest care

If a hematoma develops at the venipuncture site, apply warm soaks.

Interfering factors

■ Corticosteroids and androgens can elevate haptoglobin levels and mask hemolysis in patients with inflammatory disease.
■ Hemolysis caused by rough handling of the sample can alter test results.

Heinz body test

Heinz bodies are particles of denatured hemoglobin that have precipitated out of the cytoplasm of red blood cells (RBCs) and have collected in small masses attached to the cell membranes. They form as a result of drug injury to RBCs, the presence of unstable hemoglobins, unbalanced globin chain synthesis associated with thalassemia, or a red cell enzyme deficiency (such as glucose-6-

IDENTIFYING HEINZ BODIES

After special supravital staining, Heinz bodies (particles of denatured hemoglobin that are usually attached to the cell membrane) appear as small, purple inclusions at cell margins. Heinz bodies are present in certain hemolytic anemias.

phosphate dehydrogenase deficiency). Although Heinz bodies are rapidly removed from RBCs in the spleen, they are a major factor in causing hemolytic anemias. (See *Identifying Heinz bodies.*)

Heinz bodies can be detected in whole blood by phase microscopy or with supravital stains, such as crystal violet, brilliant cresyl blue, or new methylene blue. However, when Heinz bodies do not form spontaneously, addition of various oxidant drugs to the whole blood sample may induce their formation.

Purpose

To help detect the cause of hemolytic anemia.

Patient preparation

Explain to the patient that this test helps determine the cause of anemia. Inform him that he needn't restrict food or fluids before the test. Tell him the test requires a blood sample, who will perform the venipuncture and when, and that he may experience transient discomfort from the needle puncture and the pressure of the tourniquet.

Review the patient's drug history for medications that may alter test results. Withhold antimalarials, furazolidone, nitrofurantoin, phenacetin, procarbazine, and sulfonamides. If these medications must be continued, note this on the laboratory request.

Procedure

Perform a venipuncture and collect the sample in a 7-ml tube containing EDTA.

Precautions

Completely fill the sample collection tube and invert it gently several times to adequately mix the sample and the anticoagulant.

Normal findings

Absence of Heinz bodies is the normal (negative) test result.

Implications of results

The presence of Heinz bodies (positive test result) suggests the presence of an inherited red cell enzyme deficiency, unstable hemoglobins, thalassemia, or drug-induced red cell injury. Heinz bodies may also be present after splenectomy.

Posttest care

- If a hematoma develops at the venipuncture site, apply warm soaks.
- Resume administration of medications withheld before the test.

Interfering factors

- Antimalarials, furazolidone (in infants), nitrofurantoin, phenacetin, procarbazine, and sulfonamides can cause false-positive results.
- Failure to use the appropriate anticoagulant in the collection tube, to fill the collection tube completely, to adequately mix the sample and the anticoagulant, or to send the sample to the laboratory immediately may affect the accuracy of test results.
- A recent transfusion may affect test results.

Helicobacter pylori *antibody test*

Helicobacter pylori is a spiral, gram-negative bacterium associated with chronic gastritis and chronic duodenal ulceration. Although a gastric specimen can be obtained by endoscopy and cultured for *H. pylori*, the *H. pylori* antibody blood test is a more useful noninvasive screening procedure that may be performed with the enzyme-linked immunosorbent assay (ELISA) test. (See *Other tests to diagnose* H. pylori.)

Purpose

To help diagnose *H. pylori* infection in patients with GI symptoms.

Patient preparation

Inform the patient that this test is used to diagnose the infection that may cause ulcers. Tell him that he need not restrict food or fluids. Explain that a blood sample will be taken and who will perform the venipuncture and when. Explain to him that he may experience transient discomfort from the needle puncture and the tourniquet, but the test takes less than 3 minutes.

Procedure

- Perform a venipuncture and collect the sample in a 7-ml clot-activator tube.
- Send the sample to the laboratory immediately.

> ### OTHER TESTS TO DIAGNOSE *H. PYLORI*
>
> #### Fecal antigen
> An enzyme immunoassay (HpSA) for detecting *H. pylori* antigens in stool, the fecal antigen test has recently been approved by the FDA for diagnosis of *H. pylori* infection.
>
> #### Urea breath tests
> In the carbon-14–urea breath test (C-14) and the carbon-13–urea breath test (C-13), the patient swallows a small amount of carbon isotope-labeled urea, which is converted into carbon dioxide and ammonia in the presence of *H. pylori*. After the lungs excrete the carbon dioxide, it can be detected as C-13 urea by mass spectrometry and as C-14 by scintillation counting. The FDA has approved these tests for screening for *H. pylori*, although they are most effectively used to confirm bacterial eradication.

Precautions

This test should be performed only on patients with GI symptoms because a large number of healthy people have *H. pylori* antibodies.

Normal findings

Normally, no antibodies to *H. pylori* are present. Test results are reported as negative or positive.

Implications of results

A positive *H. pylori* test result indicates that the patient has antibodies to the bacterium. The serologic results should be interpreted in light of the clinical findings.

Posttest care

If a hematoma develops at the venipuncture site, apply warm soaks.

Interfering factors

None significant.

Hematocrit

Hematocrit (HCT), a common, reliable test, may be done by itself or as part of a complete blood count. It measures the percentage by volume of packed red blood cells (RBCs) in a whole blood sample; for example, an HCT of 40% means that a 100-ml sample contains 40 ml of packed RBCs. This packing is achieved by centrifugation of anticoagulated whole blood in a capillary tube, so that RBCs are tightly packed without hemolysis.

Most commonly, HCT is measured electronically, producing results 3% lower than when HCT is measured manually. Manual measurement traps plasma in the column of packed RBCs. Test results may be used to calculate two erythrocyte indices: mean corpuscular volume (MCV) and mean corpuscular hemoglobin concentration (MCHC).

Purpose
- To aid diagnosis of abnormal states of hydration, polycythemia, and anemia
- To aid in calculating erythrocyte indices.

Patient preparation
Explain to the patient that this test detects anemia and other abnormal conditions of the blood. Inform him that he needn't restrict food or fluids before the test. Tell him the test requires a blood sample, who will perform the venipuncture and when, and that he may experience transient discomfort from the needle puncture and the pressure of the tourniquet. If the patient is an infant or child, explain to the parents (and to the child if he's old enough to understand) that a small amount of blood will be drawn from his finger or earlobe.

Procedure
Perform a fingerstick using a heparinized capillary tube with a red band on the anticoagulant end.

Precautions
Fill the capillary tube from the red-banded end to about two-thirds capacity, and seal this end with clay. Send the sample to the laboratory immediately. Or, if you perform the test, place the tube in the centrifuge, with the red-banded end pointing outward.

Normal findings
Hematocrit values vary, depending on the patient's sex and age, type of sample, and the laboratory performing the test. (See *Normal hematocrit values by age.*)

Implications of results
Low HCT suggests anemia, hemodilution, or massive blood loss; high HCT indicates polycythemia or hemoconcentration resulting from blood loss and dehydration.

Posttest care
If a hematoma develops at the venipuncture site, apply warm soaks.

Interfering factors
- Failure to use the proper anticoagulant in the collection tube, to fill the tube appropriately, or to adequately

NORMAL HEMATOCRIT VALUES BY AGE	
Newborns	55% to 68%
1 week	47% to 65%
1 month	37% to 49%
3 months	30% to 36%
1 year	29% to 41%
10 years	36% to 40%
Adult males	42% to 54%
Adult females	38% to 46%

mix the sample and the anticoagulant may alter test results.

■ Hemolysis caused by rough handling of the sample may affect test results.

■ Tourniquet constriction for longer than 1 minute causes hemoconcentration and typically raises HCT by 2.5% to 5%.

■ Taking the blood sample from the same arm that is being used for I.V. infusion causes hemodilution.

■ Failure to adequately mix the sample with the anticoagulant may hinder accurate determination of test results.

Hemoglobin electrophoresis test

Contained in red blood cells (RBCs), hemoglobin consists of heme, an iron-protoporphyrin complex, and globin, a polypeptide. Hemoglobin combines with oxygen and carbon dioxide to allow RBCs to transport these gases between the lungs and the tissues. Aging RBCs are constantly being destroyed by normal mechanisms in the reticuloendothelial system. However, when RBC destruction occurs in circulating blood, as in intravascular hemolysis, free hemoglobin enters the plasma and binds with haptoglobin, a plasma alpha$_2$ globulin.

Hemoglobin (Hb) electrophoresis is probably the most useful laboratory method for separating and measuring normal and certain abnormal hemoglobins. Electrophoresis apparatus consists of an anode (+) and a cathode (−), separated by buffered cellulose acetate on which hemoglobin molecules migrate when an electrical current is passed through the medium. Different types of hemoglobin migrate toward the anode at different speeds, creating a series of distinctive pigmented bands in the medium.

The laboratory may change the medium (from cellulose acetate to starch gel) or its pH (from 8.6 to 6.2), depending on the types of hemoglobins being detected. This variation expands the range of this test beyond those hemoglobins routinely checked: Hb A, Hb A$_2$, Hb S, and Hb C.

Purpose

■ To measure the amount of Hb A and to detect abnormal hemoglobins

■ To aid diagnosis of thalassemias.

Patient preparation

Explain to the patient that this test evaluates hemoglobin. Tell the patient he needn't restrict food or fluids. Inform him that the test requires a blood sample, who will perform the venipuncture and when, and that he may experience transient discomfort from the needle puncture and the pressure of the tourniquet. If the patient is an infant or child, explain to the parents (and to the child if he's old enough to understand) that a small amount of blood will be drawn from the patient's finger or earlobe. Check for a recent blood transfusion (within the past 4 months).

Procedure

Perform a venipuncture and collect the sample in a 7-ml tube containing EDTA. For younger children, collect capillary blood in a microcollection device.

Precautions

Completely fill the collection tube and invert it gently several times to mix the sample and anticoagulant adequately. Do not shake the tube vigorously.

Normal findings

In adults, Hb A accounts for more than 95% of all hemoglobins; Hb A$_2$, 2% to 3%; and Hb F, less than 1%. In neonates, Hb F normally accounts for half the total; Hb S and Hb C are normally absent.

Implications of results

Hemoglobin electrophoresis allows identification of various types of hemoglobins, many of which may suggest the presence of a hemolytic disease. (See *Hemoglobin types and distribution.*)

Posttest care

If a hematoma develops at the venipuncture site, apply warm soaks.

Interfering factors

■ A blood transfusion within the past 4 months may invalidate test results.

■ Failure to use the proper anticoagulant in the collection tube, to fill the tube completely, or to mix the sam-

HEMOGLOBIN TYPES AND DISTRIBUTION

This chart shows the distribution pattern and clinical effects associated with some types of hemoglobin.

Hemoglobin	Total hemoglobin (%)	Clinical implications
Hb A	95% to 100%	Normal
Hb A$_2$	4% to 5.8%	β-thalassemia minor
	2% to 3%	Normal
	Less than 2%	Hb H disease
Hb F	Less than 1%	Normal
	2% to 5%	β-thalassemia minor
	10% to 90%	β-thalassemia major
	5% to 15%	β-δ-thalassemia minor
	5% to 35%	Heterozygous hereditary persistence of fetal hemoglobin (HPFH)
	100%	Homozygous HPFH
	15%	Homozygous Hb S
Homozygous Hb S	70% to 98%	Sickle cell disease
Homozygous Hb C	90% to 98%	Hb C disease
Heterozygous Hb C	24% to 44%	Hb C trait

ple and the anticoagulant adequately may alter test results.

■ Hemolysis caused by rough handling of the sample may affect the accuracy of test results.

Hemoglobin test, total

Contained in red blood cells (RBCs), hemoglobin consists of heme, an iron-protoporphyrin complex, and globin, a polypeptide. Hemoglobin combines with oxygen and carbon dioxide to allow RBCs to transport these gases between the lungs and the tissues. Aging RBCs are constantly being destroyed by normal mechanisms in the reticuloendothelial system. However, when RBC destruction occurs in circulating blood, as in intravascular hemolysis, free hemoglobin enters the plasma and binds with haptoglobin, a plasma alpha$_2$ globulin.

This test measures the grams of hemoglobin (Hb) found in a deciliter (100 ml) of whole blood. Hemoglobin concentration correlates closely with the red blood cell (RBC) count and affects the Hb:RBC ratio (mean corpuscular hemoglobin [MCH] and mean corpuscular hemoglobin concentration [MCHC]). In the laboratory, hemoglobin is chemically converted to pigmented compounds and is measured by either spectrophotometric or colorimetric technique.

The test is usually performed as part of a complete blood count.

Purpose
■ To measure the severity of anemia or polycythemia and to monitor response to therapy
■ To supply figures for calculating MCH and MCHC.

Patient preparation
Explain to the patient that this test helps determine if he has anemia or polycythemia (or, if appropriate, that it assesses his response to treatment). Inform him that he needn't restrict food or fluids. Tell him the test requires a blood sample, who will perform the venipuncture and when, and that he may experience transient discomfort from the needle puncture and the pressure of the tourniquet. If the patient is an infant or child, explain to the parents (and to the child if he's old enough to understand) that a small amount of blood will be drawn from the patient's finger or earlobe.

Procedure
■ For adults and older children, perform a venipuncture and collect the sample in a 7-ml tube containing EDTA.
■ For younger children and infants, collect the sample by fingerstick or heelstick in a microcollection device containing EDTA.

Precautions
■ Completely fill the collection tube, and invert it gently several times to adequately mix the sample and the anticoagulant.
■ Handle the sample gently to prevent hemolysis.

Normal findings
Hemoglobin concentration varies, depending on the patient's age and sex and on the type of blood sample drawn. (See *Normal hemoglobin values by age.*)

Implications of results
Low hemoglobin concentration may indicate the presence of anemia, recent hemorrhage, or hemodilution caused by fluid retention; elevated hemoglobin suggests hemoconcentration caused by polycythemia or dehydration.

Posttest care
If a hematoma develops at the venipuncture site, apply warm soaks.

NORMAL HEMOGLOBIN VALUES BY AGE

The hemoglobin values below reflect the number of grams per deciliter.

Newborns	17 to 22
1 week	15 to 20
1 month	11 to 15
Children	11 to 13
Males	14 to 18
Males after middle age	12.4 to 14.9
Females	12 to 16
Females after middle age	11.7 to 13.8

Interfering factors

■ Failure to use the proper anticoagulant in the collection tube or to adequately mix the sample and anticoagulant may affect test results.

■ Hemolysis due to rough handling may adversely affect the test results.

■ Prolonged tourniquet constriction may cause hemoconcentration.

■ Very high white cell counts, lipemia, or red cells that are resistant to lysis will falsely elevate hemoglobin values.

Hemoglobin test, urine

Free hemoglobin in the urine, an abnormal finding, may occur in hemolytic anemias, infection, or severe intravascular hemolysis from a transfusion reaction. It may also follow strenuous exercise. Contained in red blood cells (RBCs), hemoglobin consists of heme, an iron-protoporphyrin complex, and globin, a polypeptide. Hemoglobin combines with oxygen and carbon dioxide to allow RBCs to transport these gases between the lungs and the tissues.

Aging RBCs are constantly being destroyed by normal mechanisms in the reticuloendothelial system. However, when RBC destruction occurs in circulating blood, as in intravascular hemolysis, free hemoglobin enters the plasma and binds with haptoglobin, a plasma alpha$_2$ globulin. If the plasma level of hemoglobin exceeds that of haptoglobin, the excess of unbound hemoglobin is excreted in the urine (hemoglobinuria).

This test is based on the fact that heme proteins act like enzymes that catalyze oxidation of organic substances, such as guaiac or orthotolidine. The reaction produces a blue color that varies in intensity with the amount of hemoglobin present. Microscopic examination is required to identify intact RBCs in urine (hematuria), which can occur in the presence of unbound hemoglobin.

BEDSIDE TESTING FOR URINE BLOOD PIGMENTS

To test a patient's urine for blood pigments at bedside, use one of the following methods. Because these methods detect only blood pigments, immunochemical studies are necessary to differentiate hemoglobin from other blood pigments, such as myoglobin.

Dipstick, Multistix, or Chemstrips
- Collect a urine specimen.
- Dip the stick into the specimen and withdraw it.
- After 30 seconds, compare the stick to the color chart. Blue indicates a positive reaction; the intensity of color indicates pigment concentration.

Occult tablet
- Collect a urine specimen.
- Put one drop of urine on the filter paper. Place the tablet on the urine, and then put two drops of water on the tablet.
- After 2 minutes, inspect the filter paper around the tablet. Blue indicates a positive reaction; the intensity of color indicates pigment concentration.

Occult solution
- Collect a urine specimen.
- After placing one drop of urine on the filter paper, close the package and turn it over. Open the opposite side, and place two drops of solution on the filter paper.
- After 30 seconds, inspect the filter paper. Blue indicates a positive reaction; the intensity of color indicates pigment concentration.

Testing for urine blood pigments can also be performed at the patient's bedside. (See *Bedside testing for urine blood pigments*.)

Purpose

To aid diagnosis of hemolytic anemias, infection, or severe intravascular hemolysis from transfusion reaction.

Patient preparation

Explain to the patient that this test detects excessive RBC destruction. Inform him that he needn't restrict food or fluids. Tell him the test requires a random urine specimen, and teach him the proper collection technique. If the female patient is menstruating, reschedule the test because contamination of the specimen with menstrual blood will alter test results.

Check the patient's medication history for drugs that may affect free hemoglobin levels, such as large doses of vitamin C, drugs that contain vitamin C as a preservative (certain antibiotics), nephrotoxic drugs (such as amphotericin B), or anticoagulants (such as warfarin). Review your findings with the laboratory, then notify the doctor; he may want to restrict these medications before the test.

Procedure

Collect a random urine specimen.

Precautions

Send the specimen to the laboratory immediately.

Normal findings

Hemoglobin should not be present in the urine.

Implications of results

Hemoglobinuria may result from severe intravascular hemolysis during a blood transfusion reaction, burns, or crushing injuries; from acquired hemolytic anemias caused by chemical or drug intoxication or malaria; or from the hemolytic anemia known as paroxysmal nocturnal hemoglobinuria. Hemoglobinuria may also result from congenital hemolytic anemias (such as hemoglobinopathies) or enzyme defects and, less commonly, from cystitis, ureteral calculi, or urethritis.

Hemoglobinuria and hematuria occur in patients with renal epithelial damage (as in acute glomerulonephritis or pyelonephritis), renal tumor, or tuberculosis.

Posttest care

Resume administration of medications discontinued before the test.

Interfering factors

■ Large doses of vitamin C or of drugs that contain vitamin C as a preservative (such as certain antibiotics) can inhibit reagent activity, producing false-negative results.
■ Nephrotoxic drugs (such as amphotericin B) or anticoagulants (such as warfarin) may cause a false positive result for hemoglobinuria or hematuria.
■ Lysis of RBCs in stale or alkaline urine and contamination of the specimen with menstrual blood will cause false-positive test results.
■ Bacterial peroxidases in highly infected specimens can produce false-positive test results.

Hemoglobin test, unstable

Unstable hemoglobins are rare, congenital red cell defects caused by amino acid substitutions in the normally stable structure of hemoglobin. These abnormal replacements produce a molecule that spontaneously denatures into clumps and aggregations called Heinz bodies (see page 284), which separate from the red cell cytoplasm and accumulate at the cell membrane. Although Heinz bodies are usually efficiently removed by the spleen or

SIGNS AND SYMPTOMS OF UNSTABLE HEMOGLOBINS

More than 60 varieties of unstable hemoglobins exist, each named after the city in which it was discovered. Their effects vary according to the amount present, degree of instability, condition of the spleen, and oxygen-binding capacity.

A patient with an unstable hemoglobin typically exhibits:
- pallor
- jaundice
- fatigue
- shortness of breath
- splenomegaly
- in those with a severely unstable hemoglobin: cyanosis, pigmenturia, and hemoglobinuria.

Thalassemia often causes similar signs and symptoms, but the molecular bases of the two diseases differ greatly.

liver, they may cause mild to severe hemolysis. (See *Signs and symptoms of unstable hemoglobins*.)

Unstable hemoglobins are best detected by precipitation tests (heat stability or isopropanol solubility) performed in the laboratory. Although a hemoglobin electrophoresis and the Heinz body test can detect certain unstable hemoglobins, the tests don't always confirm the presence of such hemoglobins. Globin-chain analysis identifies them more reliably, but this procedure is time-consuming and technically complex and, therefore, is not performed routinely.

Purpose

To detect unstable hemoglobins.

Patient preparation

Explain to the patient that this test detects abnormal hemoglobins in the blood. Inform him that he needn't restrict food or fluids. Tell him the test requires a blood sample, who will perform the venipuncture and when, and that he may experience transient discomfort from the needle puncture and the pressure of the tourniquet.

Withhold antimalarials, furazolidone (from infants), nitrofurantoin, phenacetin, procarbazine, and sulfonamides before the test because these drugs may induce hemolysis. If these medications must be continued, note this on the laboratory request.

Procedure

Perform a venipuncture and collect the sample in a 7-ml tube containing EDTA.

Precautions

Completely fill the collection tube, and invert it gently several times to mix the sample and the anticoagulant adequately. Don't shake the tube vigorously because hemolysis may result.

Normal findings

When no unstable hemoglobins are present in the sample, the heat stability test is reported as negative; the isopropanol solubility test, as stable.

Implications of results

A positive heat stability or unstable solubility test, especially with hemolysis, strongly suggests the presence of unstable hemoglobins.

Posttest care

■ If a hematoma develops at the venipuncture site, apply warm soaks.
■ Resume administration of medications withheld before the test.

Interfering factors

■ Antimalarials, furazolidone (in infants), nitrofurantoin, phenacetin, procarbazine, and sulfonamides can induce Heinz body formation and result in a positive or unstable test.
■ High levels of hemoglobin F may cause a false-positive isopropanol test.
■ Failure to use the proper anticoagulant in the collection tube, to fill the tube completely, or to mix the sample and the anticoagulant adequately may interfere with test results.
■ Hemolysis caused by rough handling of the sample or hemoconcentration caused by prolonged tourniquet constriction may influence test results.
■ A recent blood transfusion may affect results.

Hemosiderin test, urine

This test measures the urine level of hemosiderin, a colloidal iron oxide and one of the two forms of storage iron deposited in body tissue. When iron overload exceeds the capacity of iron storage mechanisms, excess iron may accumulate in cells not equipped with the mechanisms to handle high iron concentrations and thereby cause toxic effects. Particularly vulnerable to such toxicity are the liver, myocardium, bone marrow, pancreas, kidneys, and skin, which are likely to develop tissue damage known as hemochromatosis. This disorder may occur in a rare hereditary form known as primary hemochromatosis and in exogenous forms. Elevated tissue storage of iron without associated tissue damage is called hemosiderosis and is often confused with hemochromatosis.

Purpose

To aid diagnosis of hemochromatosis.

Patient preparation

Explain to the patient that this test helps determine if the body is accumulating excessive amounts of iron. Inform him that no special restrictions are necessary and that the test requires a urine specimen.

Procedure

Collect a urine specimen of approximately 30 ml, preferably from the first void of the morning.

Precautions

Seal the container securely and send the specimen to the laboratory at once.

Normal findings

The presence of hemosiderin in urine is a positive test.

Implications of results

The presence of hemosiderin, appearing as yellow-brown granules in urinary sediment, suggests hemochromatosis; liver or bone marrow biopsy is necessary to confirm primary disease. A positive hemosiderin assay may also suggest pernicious anemia, chronic hemolytic anemia, multiple blood transfusions, or paroxysmal nocturnal hemoglobinuria associated with excessive iron injections or dietary intake of iron.

Interfering factors

Failure to send the specimen to the laboratory immediately may alter test results.

Hepatitis B surface antigen test

Hepatitis B surface antigen (HBsAg) appears in the serum of patients infected with hepatitis B virus, formerly called serum hepatitis or long-incubation hepatitis. This antigen can be detected by radioimmunoassay or, less commonly, by reverse passive hemagglutination during the extended incubation period and usually during the first 3 weeks of acute infection or if the patient is a carrier.

Because transmission of hepatitis is one of the gravest complications associated with blood transfusions, all donors must be screened for hepatitis B before their blood is stored. This test, required by the Food and Drug Administration, has helped reduce the incidence of hepatitis, but it doesn't screen for hepatitis A (infectious hepatitis).

(For information on related tests, see *Viral hepatitis test panel*, page 300, and *Serodiagnosis of acute viral hepatitis*, page 301.)

Purpose

- To screen blood donors for hepatitis B
- To screen persons at high risk for contracting hepatitis B, such as hemodialysis nurses
- To aid differential diagnosis of viral hepatitis.

Patient preparation

Explain that the test helps identify a type of viral hepatitis. Inform the patient that he needn't restrict food or fluids before the test. Tell him that this test requires a blood sample, who will perform the venipuncture and when, and that he may experience transient discomfort from the needle puncture and the pressure of the tourniquet. Check the patient's history for hepatitis B vaccine. If the patient is giving blood, explain the donation procedure to him.

Procedure

Perform a venipuncture and collect the sample in a 10-ml clot-activator tube.

Precautions

Be sure to observe CDC Standard Precautions.

Normal findings

Serum should be negative for HBsAg.

Implications of results

The presence of HBsAg in a patient with hepatitis confirms hepatitis B. In chronic carriers and persons with chronic active hepatitis, HBsAg may be present in serum several months after the onset of acute infection. It may also occur in more than 5% of patients with other diseases, such as hemophilia, Hodgkin's disease, and leukemia. If the antigen is found in donor blood, the blood must be discarded because of the high risk of transmitting hepatitis. Blood samples that test positive should be retested because inaccurate results do occur.

Notify the blood donor if test results are positive. Report confirmed viral hepatitis to public health authorities; this is a reportable disease in most states.

Interfering factors

Patients who have received the hepatitis B vaccine may test positive.

VIRAL HEPATITIS TEST PANEL

The several types of viral hepatitis produce similar symptoms but differ in transmission mode, course of treatment, prognosis, and carrier status. When clinical history is insufficient for differentiation, serologic tests can aid diagnosis. Hepatitis A, B, and C antigens induce type-specific antibodies detectable by a variety of methods. The timing of the appearance and disappearance of these antibodies, in conjunction with clinical symptoms, helps diagnose and stage acute and chronic forms of these distinct diseases.

Typical sequence of hepatitis A markers after exposure

Testing for hepatitis A: Present in blood and feces only briefly before symptoms appear, hepatitis A virus (HAV) may elude detection. However, anti-HAV, the antibody to hepatitis A virus, appears early in the acute phase of the disease, persists for many years after recovery, and ultimately gives the patient immunity. A single positive anti-HAV test may indicate previous exposure to the virus, but because this antibody persists so long in the bloodstream, only evidence of *rising* anti-HAV titers confirms hepatitis A as the cause of current or very recent infection. Determining recent infection relies on identifying the antibody as IgM (associated with recent infection). A negative anti-HAV test rules out hepatitis A.

Typical sequence of hepatitis B and C markers after exposure

Testing for hepatitis B: Hepatitis B viruses are composed of a core protein and a surface protein. The surface antigen (HBsAg) appears in serum during the long incubation period (up to 26 weeks) or during the early acute phase of infection (2 to 3 weeks) and normally peaks after symptoms begin. High levels of HBsAg continuing 3 or more months after onset of acute infection suggest chronic hepatitis or carrier status. Potential blood donors are screened for this antigen to prevent transmission of hepatitis B to recipients.

Another antibody that develops after exposure to hepatitis B is anti-HBc, induced by the core component of the B antigen. An early indicator of acute infection, antibody (IgM) to core antigen (anti-HBc IgM) is rarely detected in chronic infection. Thus, it is also useful in distinguishing acute from chronic infection.

Anti-HBs, antibody to the surface component of the B virus, appears long after symptoms have subsided and after the HBsAg has disappeared from blood. Detection of this antibody signals late convalescence or recovery from infection. Anti-HBs remains in the blood to provide immunity.

Testing for hepatitis C: A single-stranded RNA virus causes hepatitis C. To detect the virus by amplifying the number of RNA particles, most major laboratories use polymerase chain reaction (PCR). The test can be conducted as soon as 2 weeks after exposure. Another test, using a serologic assay, can detect an antibody to a nonstructural protein of the virus. This antibody has been designated anti-HCV. Anti-HCV can appear relatively late in the infection, usually 16 to 24 weeks after the initial elevation of liver enzyme levels. The progress of the infection can be monitored by periodic analysis of alanine aminotransferase and anti-HCV levels. The clinical symptoms and epidemiology are similar to those of hepatitis B, but the rate of chronic infection is much higher. The plasma of chronically infected HCV patients remains infectious.

SERODIAGNOSIS OF ACUTE VIRAL HEPATITIS

The chart below helps evaluate positive test results in acute viral hepatitis

Test results			Interpretation
HBsAg	Anti-HBc IgM	Anti-HAV IgM	
–	–	+	Recent acute hepatitis A infection
+	+	–	Acute hepatitis B infection
+	–	–	Early acute hepatitis B infection or chronic hepatitis B
–	+	–	Confirms acute or recent infection with hepatitis B virus
–	–	–	Possible hepatitis C (formerly non-A, non-B) infection, other viral infection, or liver toxin
+	+	+	Recent probable hepatitis A infection and superimposed acute hepatitis B infection; uncommon profile

KEY: + = positive   – = negative

Reprinted with permission of Abbott Laboratories, Abbott Park, Ill.

Herpes simplex antibody test

Herpes simplex virus (HSV), a herpesvirus, produces a wide spectrum of disorders, including keratitis, gingivostomatitis, encephalitis, and commonly, disseminated disease in immunocompromised persons. It can also cause lesions on the glans penis, vulva, perineum, buttocks, and cervix.

Of the two closely related antigenic types, type 1 usually causes infections above the waistline; type 2 primarily involves the external genitalia. Primary contact with this virus occurs in early childhood as acute stomatitis or, more commonly, as an inapparent infection. More than 50% of adults have antibodies to HSV.

Sensitive assays, such as indirect immunofluorescence or enzyme immunoassay (but not complement fixation), are used to demonstrate IgM class antibodies to HSV or to detect a fourfold or greater increase in IgG class antibodies between acute- and convalescent-phase serum.

Purpose

To confirm infections caused by HSV.

Patient preparation

Explain the purpose of the test, and inform the patient that it will require a blood sample, who will perform the venipuncture and when, and that he may experience transient discomfort from the needle puncture and the pressure of the tourniquet.

Procedure

Perform a venipuncture and collect 5 ml of sterile blood in a tube of the type designated by the local laboratory. Allow the blood to clot for at least 1 hour at room temperature.

Precautions

- Handle the sample gently to prevent hemolysis.
- Transfer the serum to a sterile tube or vial, and send it to the laboratory promptly. If transfer must be delayed for 1 or 2 days, store the serum at 39.2°F (4°C); if it must be delayed longer, store at –4°F (–20°C) to avoid bacterial contamination.

Normal findings

Serum from patients who have never been infected with HSV will have no detectable antibodies (less than 1:5). Patients with primary HSV infection will show both IgM and IgG class antibodies. Reportedly, over 50% of adults have IgG class antibodies to HSV because of prior infection. Reactivated infections caused by HSV can be recognized serologically only by an increase in IgG class antibodies between acute- and convalescent-phase serum.

Implications of results

HSV infection can be ruled out in patients whose serum shows no detectable antibodies to the virus. The presence of IgM antibodies or a fourfold or greater increase in IgG antibodies indicates active HSV infection.

Posttest care

If a hematoma develops at the venipuncture site, apply warm soaks.

Interfering factors

Hemolysis will alter results.

Herpes simplex virus culture

Herpes simplex virus (HSV), a herpesvirus, produces a wide spectrum of disorders, including keratitis, gingivo-stomatitis, encephalitis, and commonly, disseminated disease in immunocompromised persons. It can also cause lesions on the glans penis, vulva, perineum, buttocks, and cervix.

Of the eight viruses of the herpesvirus group (Epstein-Barr virus, cytomegalovirus [CMV], varicella-zoster virus [VZV], human herpesvirus-6, herpesvirus-7, herpesvirus-8, and the two closely related serotypes of HSV — type 1 and type 2), only CMV, VZV, and HSV replicate in the standard cell cultures used in diagnostic laboratories. Of these herpesviruses, HSV replicates most rapidly in cell cultures. Approximately 50% of HSV strains can be detected by characteristic cytopathic effects (CPE) within 24 hours after the laboratory receives the specimen; the rest require 5 to 7 days to be detected because they're present in low titers in specimens.

Alternatively, early antigens of HSV can be detected by monoclonal antibodies in shell vial cell cultures within 16 hours after receipt of the specimen with the same sensitivity and specificity as standard tube cell cultures.

Purpose

To confirm diagnosis of HSV infection by culturing the virus from specimens.

Patient preparation

Explain that this test will be performed to detect infection by HSV. Specimens should be collected from suspected lesions during the prodromal and acute stages of clinical infection to ensure the best chance of recovering a virus in cell cultures.

Procedure

■ Collect a specimen for culture in the appropriate collection device. Vesicle fluid can be obtained with a 27-gauge needle on a tuberculin syringe. If the fluid is scant, the base of the ulcer can be scraped with a swab to remove cells.
■ Throat, skin, eye, or genital area: Use a microbiologic transport swab. Body fluids or other respiratory specimens (washings, lavage): Use a sterile screw-capped jar.
■ Specimens should be transported to the laboratory as soon as possible after collection. If the anticipated time between collection and inoculation of cell cultures is more than 3 hours, the specimen should be stored and transported at 39.2°F (4°C).

Precautions

■ Be sure to observe CDC standard precautions. (See *Precautions*, pages 3 and 4.)
■ Do not allow the specimen to become dry.

Normal findings

HSV is rarely recovered from immunocompetent patients who show no overt signs of disease. However, like other herpesviruses, HSV can be shed intermittently from immunocompromised patients without apparent disease. For epidemiologic purposes, HSV detected by CPE in standard tube cell cultures must be confirmed and identified by transfer of infected cells to slides and subsequent immunologic serotyping as type 1 or type 2. In the shell vial assay, this step occurs as part of the initial detection of the virus.

Implications of results

■ HSV detected in specimens taken from dermal lesions, the eye, cerebrospinal fluid, or tissue are highly significant.

■ Specimens from the upper respiratory tract may be associated with intermittent shedding of the virus, particularly in an immunocompromised patient.

Interfering factors

Administration of antiviral drugs before specimen collection may interfere with detection of the virus.

Heterophil antibody tests

Heterophil antibody tests detect and identify two immunoglobulin M (IgM) antibodies in human serum that react against foreign red blood cells (RBCs): Epstein-Barr virus (EBV) antibodies and Forssman antibodies.

In the Paul-Bunnell test—also called the presumptive test—EBV antibodies in the sera of patients with infectious mononucleosis agglutinate with sheep RBCs in a test tube. Forssman antibodies, present in the sera of some normal persons as well as in the sera of patients with conditions such as serum sickness, also agglutinate with sheep RBCs, thus rendering test results inconclusive for infectious mononucleosis.

If the Paul-Bunnell test establishes a presumptive titer, Davidsohn's differential absorption test can then distinguish between EBV antibodies and Forssman antibodies. (See *Monospot test for infectious mononucleosis*.)

Purpose

To aid differential diagnosis of infectious mononucleosis.

Patient preparation

Explain to the patient that this test helps detect infectious mononucleosis. Tell him that the test requires a blood sample, who will perform the venipuncture and when, and that he may experience transient discomfort from the needle puncture and the pressure of the tourniquet.

MONOSPOT TEST FOR INFECTIOUS MONONUCLEOSIS

Several screening tests can detect the heterophil infectious mono-nucleosis (IM) antibody. One of these tests, the monospot test, con-verts the Paul-Bunnell and Davidsohn's differential absorption tests into one rapid slide test without titration. Monospot relies on ag-glutination of horse red blood cells (RBCs) by heterophil antibodies.

Distinguishing antibodies

Because horse RBCs contain both Forssman and IM antigens, differ-ential absorption of the patient's serum is necessary to distinguish between them. This is done by mixing the serum sample with guinea pig kidney antigen (containing only Forssman antigen) on one end of a slide and with beef RBC stroma (containing only IM antigen) on the other end of the slide. Each absorbs only the het-erophil antibody specific to it. After addition of horse RBCs to each spot, agglutination on the beef cell end of the slide demonstrates the presence of the IM heterophil antibody and confirms the diag-nosis of IM.

The monospot test rivals the classic heterophil agglutination test for sensitivity. False-positives may occur in the presence of lym-phoma, hepatitis A and hepatitis B, leukemia, and pancreatic cancer.

Procedure

Perform a venipuncture and collect the sample in a 7-ml clot-activator tube.

Precautions

Handle the sample gently to prevent hemolysis.

Normal findings

Normally, the titer is less than 1:56 but may be higher in elderly people. Some laboratories refer to a normal titer as "negative" or as having "no reaction."

Implications of results

Although heterophil antibodies are present in the sera of about 80% of patients with infectious mononucleosis 1 month after onset, a positive finding—a titer higher than 1:56—doesn't confirm this diagnosis. A high titer can also result from systemic lupus erythematosus, syphilis, cryoglobulinemia, or the presence of antibodies to nonsyphilitic treponemata (such as yaws, pinta, and bejel). A gradual increase in titer during week 3 or 4 fol-lowed by a gradual decrease during weeks 4 to 8 proves most conclusive for infectious mononucleosis. A nega-tive titer doesn't always rule out this disorder; occasion-ally, the titer becomes reactive 2 weeks later. Therefore, if symptoms persist, the test should be repeated in 2 weeks.

Confirmation of infectious mononucleosis depends on heterophil agglutination tests and hematologic tests that show absolute lymphocytosis, with 10% or more atypical lymphocytes.

Posttest care

If a hematoma develops at the venipuncture site, apply warm soaks.

Interfering factors

- Use of narcotics or phenytoin therapy can produce false-positive results.
- Hemolysis caused by rough handling of the sample will alter results.
- Patients with lymphoma, hepatitis, or leukemia may have false-positive results.

Hexosaminidase A and B tests

This fluorometric test measures the hexosaminidase A and B content of serum samples drawn by venipuncture, collected from a neonate's umbilical cord, or from samples of amniotic fluid obtained by amniocentesis. Hexosaminidase deficiency can also be identified by testing cultured skin fibroblasts; however, this procedure is costly and technically complex. A reference center for congenital disease should be consulted for the preferred screening method and specimen.

Hexosaminidase is a group of enzymes necessary for the metabolism of gangliosides, water-soluble glycolipids found primarily in brain tissue. A deficiency of hexosaminidase A (one of the two hexosaminidase isoenzymes) causes Tay-Sachs disease. In this autosomal recessive disorder, GM_2 ganglioside builds up in brain tissue, resulting in progressive destruction and demyelination of central nervous system cells and, usually, death before age 5.

In the United States each year, fewer than 100 infants are born with Tay-Sachs disease. This disorder strikes people of Eastern European Jewish ancestry about 100 times more often than the general population; about 1 in 30 persons of this ancestry in New York City carries this defective gene. If two carriers have a child, this child and subsequent offspring have a 25% chance of inheriting Tay-Sachs disease. Sandhoff's disease, which results from total hexosaminidase deficiency (both A and B), is uncommon and not prevalent in any ethnic group.

Purpose

- To confirm or rule out Tay-Sachs disease in neonates
- To screen for Tay-Sachs carriers

■ To establish a prenatal diagnosis of hexosaminidase A deficiency.

Patient preparation

When testing an adult, explain that this test identifies carriers of Tay-Sachs disease. Emphasize the test's importance to a Jewish couple of Eastern European ancestry who plan to have children and explain that both must carry the defective gene to transmit Tay-Sachs disease to their offspring. Tell the patient the test requires a blood sample, who will perform the venipuncture and when, and that he may experience transient discomfort from the needle puncture and the tourniquet.

When testing a neonate, explain to the parents that this test detects Tay-Sachs disease. Tell them blood will be drawn from the neonate's arm, neck, or umbilical cord, and explain that the procedure is safe and quickly performed. Tell them the neonate will have a small bandage on the site of the venipuncture.

Inform the patient or parents that no pretest restrictions of food or fluid are necessary. If the test is being performed prenatally, teach the patient how to prepare for amniocentesis.

Procedure

■ Perform a venipuncture, collect cord blood, or assist with amniocentesis, as appropriate. Collect the sample in a 7-ml clot-activator tube.
■ When testing a neonate, find out the laboratory's preferred method for collecting serum samples. Take the sample from the neonate's arm, neck, or umbilical cord, as appropriate.

Precautions

■ Handle the collection tube gently.
■ This test cannot be done on a pregnant woman's serum, but the father's blood may be tested. If it is negative, the child won't have Tay-Sachs disease. The mother's leukocytes or amniotic fluid may be tested, if necessary.
■ If the test cannot be performed immediately, freeze the sample.

Normal findings

Total serum hexosaminidase levels range from 5 to 12.9 U/L; hexosaminidase A makes up 55% to 76% of the total.

Implications of results

Absence of hexosaminidase A indicates Tay-Sachs disease (total hexosaminidase levels can be normal). Absence of both hexosaminidase A and hexosaminidase B indicates Sandhoff's disease, an uncommon, virulent variant of Tay-Sachs disease that causes faster deterioration.

If both partners are Tay-Sachs carriers, refer them for genetic counseling. Stress the importance of having amniocentesis as early as possible during pregnancy. If only one partner is a carrier, reassure the couple that their offspring cannot inherit the disease (but may be a carrier) because both parents must be carriers to transmit Tay-Sachs disease.

Posttest care

If a hematoma develops at the venipuncture site, apply warm soaks.

Interfering factors

■ Oral contraceptives may falsely increase hexosaminidase levels.
■ Rifampin and isoniazid may increase hexosaminidase levels.
■ Hemolysis may alter test results.

Homocysteine test, total, plasma

Homocysteine, a sulfur-containing amino acid, is a transmethylation product of methionine. It is an intermediate in the synthesis of cysteine, which is produced by the enzymatic or acid hydrolysis of proteins. The test is useful for the biochemical diagnosis of inborn errors of methionine, folate, and vitamins B_6 and B_{12} metabolism. Studies have shown that blood levels of homocysteine correlate with a patient's odds of having a stroke or heart attack.

Purpose

■ Biochemical diagnosis of inborn errors of methionine, folate, and vitamins B_6 and B_{12} metabolism; also is an indicator of acquired folate or cobalamin deficiency
■ Evaluation of risk factors for atherosclerotic vascular disease
■ Evaluation as a contributing factor in the pathogenesis of neural tube defects.

Patient preparation

Inform the patient that this test detects homocysteine levels in plasma. Advise him to fast for 12 to 14 hours before the test. Tell him that this test requires a blood sample, who will perform the venipuncture and when, and that he may experience transient discomfort from the needle puncture and the pressure of the tourniquet.

Procedure

- Perform a venipuncture and collect the sample in a 5-ml tube containing EDTA.
- Immediately send the specimen to the laboratory, where it will be transferred to a plastic vial and frozen on dry ice.

Precautions

Handle the sample gently to prevent hemolysis.

Normal findings

Normal total homocysteine levels are less than or equal to 13 μmol/L.

Implications of results

- Low homocysteine levels are associated with inborn or acquired folate or cobalamine deficiency and inborn B_6 or B_{12} deficiency.
- Elevated homocysteine levels are associated with atherosclerotic vascular disease. In patients with type 2 diabetes mellitus, studies have shown that homocysteine levels increase with even a modest deterioration in renal function.
- Research has shown that when supplemental folate, cobalamin, vitamins B_6 and B_{12} are given to high-risk patients (such as smokers, those with hyperlipidemia, or those with type 2 diabetes mellitus), they have a substantially lower risk for developing vascular disease. This supplementation may prevent the degradation of homocysteine.

Posttest care

If a hematoma develops at the venipuncture site, apply warm soaks.

Interfering factors

- Failure to adhere to dietary restrictions will alter test results.
- Failure to immediately freeze the specimen will alter test results.

Homovanillic acid test, urine

This test measures urine levels of homovanillic acid (HVA), a metabolite of dopamine, one of the three major catecholamines. Synthesized primarily in the brain, dopamine is a precursor of epinephrine and norepinephrine, the other principal catecholamines. The liver breaks down most dopamine into HVA for eventual excretion; a minimal amount of dopamine appears in the urine.

On two-dimensional chromatography, urine HVA levels are usually measured simultaneously with the major catecholamines and other catecholamine metabolites—metanephrine, normetanephrine, and vanillylmandelic acid. The principal indication for this test is suspected neuroblastoma or ganglioneuroma, which usually affects children and adolescents.

Purpose
■ To aid diagnosis of neuroblastoma and ganglioneuroma
■ To rule out pheochromocytoma.

Patient preparation
Explain to the patient that this test assesses hormone secretion. Inform him that he needn't restrict food or fluids before the test but should avoid stressful situations and excessive physical exercise during the collection period. Tell him the test requires collection of a 24-hour urine specimen and teach him the proper collection technique.

Check the patient's history for drugs that may affect test results. Review your findings with the laboratory, and notify the doctor; he may want to withhold these medications before the test.

Procedure
Collect a 24-hour urine specimen in a bottle containing a preservative to keep the specimen at pH 2.0 to 4.0.

Precautions
Refrigerate the specimen or keep it on ice during the collection period. Send the specimen to the laboratory as soon as the collection is completed.

Normal findings
The normal urine HVA value for adults is less than 8 mg/24 hours. Normal values in children vary with age, as follows (values are expressed in micrograms per milligram of creatinine):
■ age 15 to 17: 0.5 to 2
■ age 10 to 15: 0.25 to 12
■ age 5 to 10: 0.5 to 9
■ age 2 to 5: 0.5 to 13.5
■ age 1 to 2: 4 to 23
■ age 0 to 1: 1.2 to 35.

Implications of results
Elevated urine HVA levels suggest neuroblastoma, a malignant soft-tissue tumor that develops in infants and young children, or ganglioneuroma, a tumor of the sym-

pathetic nervous system that develops in older children and adolescents and rarely metastasizes. HVA levels don't usually rise in patients with pheochromocytoma because this tumor mainly secretes epinephrine, which metabolizes primarily into vanillylmandelic acid. Thus, an abnormally high urine HVA level generally rules out pheochromocytoma.

Posttest care

- Resume administration of medications withheld before the test.
- Tell the patient that he may resume activities restricted during the test.

Interfering factors

- Monoamine oxidase inhibitors decrease urine HVA levels by inhibiting dopamine metabolism.
- Aspirin, methocarbamol, and levodopa may increase or decrease HVA levels.
- Failure to observe drug restrictions, to collect all urine during the test period, or to store the specimen properly may affect test results.
- Excessive physical exercise or emotional stress during the collection period may raise HVA levels.

Human chorionic gonadotropin test, serum

Human chorionic gonadotropin (hCG) is a glycoprotein hormone produced by the trophoblastic cells, probably the syncytiotrophoblasts, of the placenta. After conception, placental trophoblastic cells start to produce hCG, a glycoprotein that prevents degeneration of the corpus luteum at the end of the normal menstrual cycle. The corpus luteum then secretes large quantities of progesterone and estrogen, promoting early development of the endometrium, placenta, and fetus. Levels of hCG rise steadily and rapidly during the first trimester, peak around the 10th week of gestation, and subsequently taper off to less than 10% of peak levels. At approximately 2 weeks after delivery, the hormone may no longer be detectable. (See *Production of hCG during pregnancy*, page 312, and *Site of hCG secretion*, page 313.)

A specific assay for hCG, commonly known as the beta-subunit assay, may detect this hormone in the blood as early as 9 days after ovulation. This test is more sensitive (and costly) than the routine pregnancy test using a urine specimen. It can detect pregnancy within 3 days after implantation.

PRODUCTION OF hCG DURING PREGNANCY

Production of human chorionic gonadotropin (hCG) increases steadily during the first trimester, peaking around the 10th week of gestation, as shown below. Levels then fall to less than 10% of the first-trimester levels during the remainder of the pregnancy.

Purpose
- To detect early pregnancy
- To determine the adequacy of hormone production in high-risk pregnancies (for example, habitual abortion)
- To aid diagnosis of trophoblastic tumors, such as hydatidiform mole or choriocarcinoma, and of tumors that ectopically secrete hCG
- To monitor treatment for induction of ovulation and conception.

Patient preparation
Explain to the patient that this test determines if she is pregnant. If detection of pregnancy is not the diagnostic objective, offer the appropriate explanation. Inform her she needn't restrict food or fluids. Tell her the test requires a blood sample, who will perform the venipuncture and when, and that she may feel transient discomfort from the needle puncture and the tourniquet.

Procedure
Perform a venipuncture and collect the sample in a 7-ml clot-activator tube.

Precautions
Handle the sample gently to prevent hemolysis, and send it to the laboratory immediately.

Normal findings
Normal values for hCG in nonpregnant women are less than 4 IU/L. During pregnancy, hCG levels are quite variable and depend partially on the number of days since the last normal menstrual period.

Implications of results
Elevated hCG beta-subunit levels are diagnostic of pregnancy; significantly higher concentrations suggest a multiple pregnancy. Increased levels may also suggest hydatidiform mole, trophoblastic neoplasm of the placenta, or nontrophoblastic carcinomas that secrete hCG (including gastric, pancreatic, and ovarian adenocarcinomas). Beta-subunit levels cannot differentiate between pregnancy and tumor recurrence because levels are high in both conditions.

SITE OF hCG SECRETION

Nine days after ovulation, the trophoblastic cells of the blastocyst begin secreting human chorionic gonadotropin (hCG). Under the influence of hCG, the corpus luteum secretes increasing amounts of estrogen and progesterone — vital for a successful pregnancy. The trophoblastic cells develop into the chorionic villi of the placenta and continue secreting hCG. Levels of hCG peak during the 10th week of gestation.

Low hCG beta-subunit levels can occur in ectopic pregnancy, impending abortion, or pregnancy of less than 9 days.

Posttest care

If a hematoma develops at the venipuncture site, apply warm soaks.

Interfering factors

■ Heparin anticoagulants and EDTA depress plasma hCG levels and may alter test results. Check with the laboratory to find out if the test is to be performed on plasma or serum.
■ Hemolysis caused by rough handling of the sample may affect test results.

Human chorionic gonadotropin test, urine

As a qualitative analysis of urine levels of human chorionic gonadotropin (hCG), this test can detect pregnancy as early as 14 days after ovulation. Quantitative measurements can evaluate suspected hydatidiform mole or hCG-secreting tumors.

After conception, placental trophoblastic cells start to produce hCG, a glycoprotein that prevents degeneration of the corpus luteum at the end of the normal menstrual cycle. The corpus luteum then secretes large quantities of progesterone and estrogen, promoting early development of the endometrium, placenta, and fetus. Levels of hCG rise steadily and rapidly during the first trimester, peak around the 10th week of gestation, and subsequently taper off to less than 10% of peak levels. Urine hCG is detectable 26 to 36 days after onset of the last menstrual period, or 8 to 10 days after conception.

The most common method of evaluating hCG in urine is hemagglutination inhibition. This laboratory procedure, based on an antigen-antibody reaction, can provide both qualitative and quantitative information. The qualitative urine test is easier and less expensive than the serum hCG test (beta-subunit assay), so it is used more frequently to detect pregnancy even though the serum hCG test allows the earliest possible determination of pregnancy (as early as 7 days after conception).

Many women today use home pregnancy tests to initially determine whether they are pregnant. (See *Performing a home pregnancy test*, appendix 671.)

Purpose
■ To detect and confirm pregnancy
■ To aid diagnosis of hydatidiform mole or hCG-secreting tumors.

Patient preparation
Explain to the patient that this test determines whether she is pregnant. If detection of pregnancy is not the purpose of the test, offer an appropriate explanation. Tell her she needn't restrict food but she should restrict fluids for 8 hours before the test. Inform her that the test requires a first-voided morning specimen or a 24-hour urine collection, depending on whether a qualitative or quantitative test will be performed. Check the patient's recent medication history for use of drugs that may affect hCG levels.

Procedure
■ To verify pregnancy (qualitative analysis), collect a first-voided morning specimen. If this is not possible, collect a random specimen.
■ For quantitative analysis of hCG, collect a 24-hour urine specimen.
■ Specify the date of the patient's last menstrual period on the laboratory request. The test should be performed at least 5 days after a missed period to avoid a false-negative result.

Precautions
Refrigerate the 24-hour specimen or keep it on ice during the collection period.

Normal findings
In qualitative analysis, if agglutination fails to occur, test results are positive, indicating pregnancy.

In quantitative analysis, urine hCG levels in the first trimester of a normal pregnancy may be as high as 500,000 IU/24 hours; in the second trimester, they range from 10,000 to 25,000 IU/24 hours; and in the third trimester, from 5,000 to 15,000 IU/24 hours. Levels decline rapidly after delivery and are undetectable within a few days.

Measurable hCG in the urine of males or nonpregnant females is an abnormal result that requires further investigation.

Implications of results

During pregnancy, elevated urine hCG levels may indicate multiple pregnancy or erythroblastosis fetalis; low levels may indicate threatened abortion or ectopic pregnancy.

Measurable hCG levels in males and nonpregnant females may indicate choriocarcinoma, ovarian or testicular tumors, melanoma, multiple myeloma, or gastric, hepatic, pancreatic, or breast cancer.

Posttest care

Resume administration of medications discontinued before the test.

Interfering factors

■ Phenothiazine use may result in false-negative or false-positive results.

■ Gross proteinuria (more than 1 g/24 hours), hematuria, or an elevated erythrocyte sedimentation rate may produce false-positive results, depending on the laboratory method used.

■ Early pregnancy, ectopic pregnancy, or threatened abortion may produce false-negative results.

Human growth hormone test

Human growth hormone (hGH), also known as growth hormone and somatotropin, is a protein secreted by acidophils of the anterior pituitary and is the primary regulator of human growth. Unlike other pituitary hormones, hGH has no easily defined feedback mechanism or single target gland; it affects many body tissues. Like insulin, hGH promotes protein synthesis and stimulates amino acid uptake by cells. It also raises plasma glucose levels by inhibiting glucose uptake and utilization by cells, and increases free fatty acid concentrations by enhancing lipolysis.

Secretion of hGH appears to be regulated by the hypothalamus by means of a growth hormone-releasing factor and a growth hormone release-inhibiting factor (somatostatin). Secretion of hGH is diurnal and varies with such factors as exercise, sleep, stress, and nutritional status. Hyposecretion or hypersecretion of this hormone may induce pathologic states (such as dwarfism or gigantism). Altered hGH levels are common in patients with pituitary dysfunction.

This test, a quantitative analysis of plasma hGH levels, is usually performed as part of an anterior pituitary stimulation or suppression test. Such testing is crucial before clinical manifestations of an hGH deficiency develop because they can rarely be reversed by therapy.

Purpose

- To aid differential diagnosis of dwarfism; retarded growth in children can result from pituitary or thyroid hypofunction
- To confirm a diagnosis of acromegaly and gigantism
- To aid diagnosis of pituitary or hypothalamic tumors
- To help evaluate hGH therapy.

Patient preparation

Explain to the patient or his parents (if the patient is an infant or child) that this test measures hormone levels and helps determine the cause of abnormal growth. Instruct him to fast and limit physical activity for 10 to 12 hours before the test. Tell him the test requires a blood sample, who will perform the venipuncture and when, and that he may experience transient discomfort from the needle puncture and the pressure of the tourniquet. Advise him that another sample may have to be drawn the following day for comparison and that the laboratory requires at least 2 days for analysis.

Withhold all medications that affect hGH levels, such as pituitary-based steroids. If these medications must be continued, note this on the laboratory request. Make sure the patient is relaxed and recumbent for 30 minutes before the test because stress and physical activity elevate hGH levels.

Procedure

Between 6 a.m. and 8 a.m. on 2 consecutive days, or as ordered, draw venous blood into a 7-ml clot-activator tube.

Precautions

- Handle the sample gently to prevent hemolysis.
- Send it to the laboratory immediately because hGH has a half-life of only 20 to 25 minutes.

Normal findings

Normal hGH levels in men range from undetectable to 5 ng/ml; in women, from undetectable to 10 ng/ml. Higher values in women are due to estrogen effects. Children generally have hGH levels that are higher than adult levels; nevertheless, they may range from undetectable to 16 ng/ml.

Implications of results

Increased hGH levels may indicate a pituitary or hypothalamic tumor (frequently an adenoma), which causes gigantism in children and acromegaly in adults and adolescents. Patients with diabetes mellitus sometimes have elevated hGH levels without acromegaly. Suppression testing is necessary to confirm the diagnosis.

Pituitary infarction, metastatic disease, and tumors may reduce hGH levels. Dwarfism may be due to low hGH levels, although only 15% of all cases of growth failure relate to endocrine dysfunction. Confirmation of the diagnosis requires stimulation testing with arginine or insulin.

Posttest care

■ If a hematoma develops at the venipuncture site, apply warm soaks.
■ Resume diet and any medications that were discontinued before the test.

Interfering factors

■ Arginine, beta blockers (propranolol), and estrogens increase hGH secretion and may affect test results.
■ Amphetamines, bromocriptine, levodopa, dopamine, methyldopa, and histamine also increase hGH secretion.
■ Insulin (induced hypoglycemia), glucagon, and nicotinic acid also raise hGH levels.
■ Phenothiazines (chlorpromazine) and corticosteroids reduce hGH secretion.
■ Failure to follow restrictions of diet, medications, or physical activity may alter test results.
■ A radioactive scan performed within 1 week before the test may affect results.
■ Hemolysis caused by rough handling of the sample may interfere with accurate of test results.

Human immunodeficiency virus antibody test

A number of test methods are used to detect antibodies to human immunodeficiency virus (HIV) in serum. Among the most common are enzyme immunoassay, fluorescence immunoassay, and enzyme-linked immuno sorbent assay (ELISA). Each of these methods requires a blood sample. Patient preparation, normal findings, and posttest care are the same for all. (See *Rapid HIV test*, page 318.)

Inform the patient that despite advertisements to the contrary, no home HIV testing kits have been approved by the Food and Drug Administration. Only one home collection system has been approved, but the sample

---

RAPID HIV TEST

For the estimated 700,000 people a year who do not check back for test results, a rapid HIV test may be useful. The *SUDS HIV-1* test is currently the only rapid HIV test with FDA approval. The results are obtained in less than 10 minutes, using a color indicator similar to a home pregnancy test. If it is positive, a confirmatory test must be done to validate the results.

---

must be sent away for analysis. (See *Performing a home HIV test*, appendix 672.)

HIV transmission occurs by direct exposure of a person's blood to body fluids containing the virus. The virus may be transmitted when contaminated blood and blood products are exchanged from one person to another, during sexual intercourse with an infected partner, when I.V. drugs are shared, and during pregnancy or breast-feeding, from an infected mother to her child.

HIV causes acquired immunodeficiency syndrome (AIDS), which may be manifested in many forms. Female patients may present different symptoms than those of males.

Purpose
■ To screen for HIV in high-risk groups
■ To screen donated blood for HIV.

Patient preparation
Inform the patient that this test detects HIV infection. Provide adequate counseling about the reasons for performing the test (usually requested by the patient's doctor). If the patient has questions about his condition, provide full and accurate answers.

Tell the patient that this test requires a blood sample, who will perform the venipuncture and when, and that he may experience transient discomfort from the needle puncture and the pressure of the tourniquet.

Procedure
Perform a venipuncture and collect the sample in a 10-ml barrier tube, which helps prevent contamination when pouring the serum.

Precautions
When drawing a blood sample, use standard precautions. (See *Precautions*, pages 3 and 4.) Use gloves, dispose of needles properly, and use blood-fluid precaution labels on tubes, as necessary.

Normal findings
The normal test result is nonreactive.

Implications of results

This test detects previous exposure to HIV. However, none of the test methods is 100% sensitive or specific; all may produce false results. A negative result doesn't necessarily indicate absence of HIV antibodies. For example, the tests don't identify a person who has been exposed to the virus but hasn't yet developed antibodies. A positive test for the HIV antibody cannot determine whether the person harbors actively replicating virus or when he will present signs and symptoms of AIDS.

A false-positive result may reflect a lack of specificity of the test method used. As a result, the Western blot test for HIV is recommended for all persons with positive antibody tests. The Western blot test for HIV is a confirmatory test because it detects the presence of specific viral proteins present in HIV.

Many apparently healthy people have been exposed to HIV and have circulating antibodies; these are not false-positive results. Also, patients in later stages of AIDS may exhibit no detectable antibodies in their serum because they can no longer mount an antibody response.

Keep test results confidential. When the results are received, give the patient an opportunity to ask questions.

Posttest care

- If a hematoma develops at the venipuncture site, apply warm soaks.
- Encourage the patient with a positive result to seek follow-up care, even if asymptomatic, and to report early signs of AIDS.
- Counsel the patient to assume that he can transmit HIV to others and to use safe-sex precautions; not to share razors, toothbrushes, or utensils that may be contaminated with blood; to clean such items with household bleach diluted 1:10 in water; not to donate blood,. tissues, or organs; and to inform his doctor and dentist so they can take proper precautions

Interfering factors

None reported.

Human leukocyte antigen test

The human leukocyte antigen (HLA) test identifies a group of antigens that are present on the surfaces of all nucleated cells but are most easily detected on lymphocytes. They're essential to immunity and determine the degree of histocompatibility between transplant recipients and donors. Numerous antigenic determinants (for instance, over 60 at the HLA-B locus) exist for each site; one set of each antigen is inherited from each parent.

Three types of HLA (HLA-A, HLA-B, and HLA-C) are measured with a lymphocyte microcytotoxicity assay. A lymphocyte sample is mixed with known antisera to these antigens and complement. Lymphocytes that react with a specific antiserum lyse and allow a dye to enter; they may then be detected by phase microscopy.

A fourth type of HLA, HLA-D, is measured by a mixed leukocyte reaction. Leukocytes from the recipient and the donor are combined in culture to determine HLA-D compatibility. If the leukocytes are incompatible, the culture will demonstrate blast formation, DNA synthesis, and proliferation.

A high incidence of specific HLA types has been linked to specific diseases, such as rheumatoid arthritis and multiple sclerosis, but these findings have little diagnostic significance. Thus, HLA testing is best used as an adjunct to diagnosis. It is also useful in genetic counseling and paternity testing.

HLA typing is generally performed by specialized tissue typing laboratories with highly trained personnel.

Purpose

- To provide histocompatibility typing of tissue recipients and donors
- To aid genetic counseling
- To aid paternity testing.

Patient preparation

Explain to the patient that this test detects antigens on white blood cells. Advise him that he needn't restrict food or fluids before the test. Tell the patient that this test requires a blood sample, who will perform the venipuncture and when, and that he may experience transient discomfort from the needle puncture and the pressure of the tourniquet.

Check the patient's history for recent blood transfusions, and report such transfusions to the doctor. He may want to postpone HLA testing.

Procedure

Perform a venipuncture and collect a 10-24 ml sample in a heparinized collection tube.

Precautions

Handle the sample gently to avoid hemolysis.

Normal findings

In HLA-A, HLA-B, and HLA-C testing, lymphocytes that react with the test antiserum undergo lysis; they're detected by phase microscopy. In HLA-D testing, leukocyte incompatibility manifests as blast formation, DNA synthesis, and proliferation.

Implications of results

Incompatible HLA-A, HLA-B, HLA-C, or HLA-D groups may cause unsuccessful tissue transplantation.

Many diseases have a strong association with certain types of HLA. For example, HLA-DR5 is associated with Hashimoto's thyroiditis; HLA-B8 and HLA-Dw3 with Graves' disease; HLA-B8 alone with chronic autoimmune hepatitis, celiac disease, and myasthenia gravis; HLA-Dw3 alone with Addison's disease, Sjögren's syndrome, dermatitis herpetiformis, and systemic lupus erythematosus.

In paternity testing, a putative father's phenotype (two haplotypes, or antigen pairs: one from the father and one from the mother) with neither haplotype identical to one of the child's excludes paternity. A putative father with one haplotype identical to one of the child's may be the father; the probability varies with the incidence of the haplotype in the population.

Posttest care

If a hematoma develops at the venipuncture site, apply warm soaks.

Interfering factors

■ Hemolysis caused by rough handling of the sample may affect the accuracy of test results.
■ HLA from blood transfused within 72 hours before collection of a blood sample may affect the accuracy of test results.

Human placental lactogen test

During pregnancy, a polypeptide hormone secreted by placental syncytial trophoblasts, human placental lactogen (hPL) has lactogenic and somatotropic (growth hormone) properties. In combination with prolactin, hPL (also known as human chorionic somatomammotropin) prepares the breasts for lactation. It also promotes lipolysis, liberating free fatty acids to provide energy for maternal metabolism and fetal nutrition.

By exerting an anti-insulin effect, hPL causes the pancreas to increase insulin secretion in response to rising blood sugar levels, thus facilitating protein synthesis and mobilization essential to fetal growth. Secretion begins about the fifth week of gestation and declines rapidly after delivery. According to some evidence, this hormone may not be essential for a successful pregnancy.

This radioimmunoassay measures serum hPL levels, which are roughly proportional to placental mass, as evidenced by higher levels in a multiple pregnancy. These assays may be required in high-risk pregnancies (patients with diabetes mellitus, hypertension, or toxemia) or in suspected placental tissue dysfunction. Because values vary widely during the last half of pregnancy, serial determinations over several days provide the most reliable test results. This test, when combined with measurement of estriol levels, is a reliable indicator of placental function and fetal well-being. It may also be useful as a tumor marker in certain malignant states, such as ectopic tumors that secrete hPL.

Purpose

- To assess placental function
- To aid diagnosis and monitor treatment of nontrophoblastic tumors that ectopically secrete hPL
- To aid diagnosis of hydatidiform mole and choriocarcinoma. (Note: human chorionic gonadotropin levels are more diagnostic in these conditions.)

Patient preparation

Explain to the patient that this test helps assess placental function and fetal well-being. If assessing fetal well-being isn't the diagnostic objective, offer an appropriate explanation. Tell her the test requires a blood sample, who will perform the venipuncture and when, and that she may feel transient discomfort from the needle puncture and the tourniquet. Inform the pregnant patient that this test may be repeated during her pregnancy.

Procedure

Perform a venipuncture and collect the sample in a 7-ml clot-activator tube.

Precautions

Handle the sample gently to prevent hemolysis and send it to the laboratory immediately.

Normal findings

During pregnancy, normal hPL values vary with gestational age:

- 5 to 27 weeks: < 4.6 µg/ml
- 28 to 31 weeks: 2.4 to 6.1 µg/ml
- 32 to 35 weeks: 3.7 to 7.7 µg/ml
- 36 weeks to term: 5.0 to 8.6 µg/ml.

At term, diabetic patients may have mean levels of 9 to 11 µg/ml.

Normal levels in males and nonpregnant females are < 0.5 µg/ml.

Implications of results

For reliable interpretation, hPL levels must be correlated with gestational age; for example, after 30 weeks of gestation, levels below 4 µg/ml may indicate placental dysfunction. Subnormal hPL levels are also associated with trophoblastic neoplastic disease, such as hydatidiform mole or choriocarcinoma, and with postmaturity syndrome, intrauterine growth retardation, and toxemia of pregnancy. Although low hPL concentrations don't confirm fetal distress, they may help differentiate incomplete abortion from threatened abortion.

Conversely, hPL levels over 4 µg/ml after 30 weeks of gestation don't guarantee fetal well-being; elevated levels have been reported after fetal death. An hPL value above 6 µg/ml after 30 weeks of gestation may suggest an unusually large placenta, which commonly occurs in patients with diabetes mellitus, multiple pregnancy, or Rh isoimmunization, but it's usefulness as a predictor of fetal death or Rh isoimmunization in such patients is limited.

Abnormal concentrations of hPL have been found in the sera of patients with various types of cancer, including bronchogenic carcinoma, hepatoma, lymphoma, and pheochromocytoma. In these patients, hPL levels are used as tumor markers to evaluate chemotherapy, to monitor tumor growth and recurrence, and to detect residual tissue after excision.

Posttest care

If a hematoma develops at the venipuncture site, apply warm soaks.

Interfering factors

Hemolysis caused by rough handling of the sample may alter test results.

Hydroxyproline test, urine

This test measures total urine levels of hydroxyproline, an amino acid found mainly in collagen (a component of skin and bone). Urine hydroxyproline levels are a good index of bone matrix turnover because levels increase when collagen breaks down during bone resorption.

Bone matrix turnover and hydroxyproline levels normally rise in children during periods of rapid skeletal growth. However, they also rise in patients with disorders that increase bone resorption, such as Paget's disease, metastatic bone tumors, and certain endocrine disorders. This test helps diagnose these disorders, but it's more commonly used to monitor their response to drug therapy.

Hydroxyproline levels are most often determined colorimetrically on a timed urine sample; they may also be determined by ion-exchange or gas-liquid chromatography. A collagen-restricted diet is essential for this test because hydroxyproline levels reflect collagen intake. Free hydroxyproline, a small component of total hydroxyproline and a sensitive indicator of dietary collagen intake, may be measured to validate results.

Purpose

■ To monitor the effectiveness of treatment for disorders characterized by bone resorption, primarily Paget's disease

■ To aid diagnosis of disorders characterized by bone resorption.

Patient preparation

Explain to the patient that this test helps monitor treatment or detect an amino acid disorder related to bone formation. Advise him to avoid eating meat, fish, poultry, and any foods containing gelatin for 24 hours before the test and during the test period itself. Tell him the test requires a 2-hour or 24-hour urine specimen, as appropriate, and teach him the correct collection technique.

Note the patient's age and sex on the laboratory request. Check his medication history for drugs (See Interfering factors, below) that may alter test results, and restrict such drugs.

Procedure

Collect a 2-hour or 24-hour urine specimen in a container that has a preservative to prevent degradation of hydroxyproline.

Precautions

Refrigerate the specimen or keep it on ice during the collection period and send it to the laboratory immediately.

Normal findings

■ In 2-hour specimen: 0.4 to 5 mg/2-hour specimen (males); 0.4 to 2.9 mg/2-hour specimen (females).
■ In 24-hour specimen: 14 to 45 mg/24 hours (adults).
Normal values in children are much higher and peak between ages 11 and 18. Values also rise during the third trimester of pregnancy, reflecting fetal skeletal growth.

Implications of results

Hydroxyproline levels should fall slowly during therapy for bone resorption disorders. Elevated levels suggest bone disease, metastatic bone tumors, or endocrine disorders that stimulate hormonal secretion.

Posttest care

Resume food and drugs withheld before the test.

Interfering factors

■ Ascorbic acid, vitamin D, aspirin, glucocorticoids, antineoplastic agents, calcium gluconate, corticosteroids, estradiol, and propranolol, as well as calcitonin and mithramycin (used to treat Paget's disease), can decrease levels.

■ Growth hormone, parathyroid hormone, phenobarbital, and sulfonylureas can increase levels.

■ Failure to observe restrictions, to collect all urine during the test period, or to store the specimen correctly may alter test results.

■ Psoriasis and burns can promote collagen turnover, elevating urine hydroxyproline levels.

Hypersensitivity skin tests, delayed

Skin testing is one of the most important methods for evaluating the cell-mediated immune response in a patient with severe recurrent infection, infection caused by unusual organisms, or suspected disorders associated with delayed hypersensitivity. Diminished delayed hypersensitivity may reflect a poor prognosis in patients with certain types of cancer. A positive result shows that the afferent, central, and efferent limbs of the immune response are intact and that the patient can maintain a nonspecific inflammatory response to infection.

These skin tests use new and recall antigens. New antigens, those not previously encountered by the patient, such as dinitrochlorobenzene (DNCB), evaluate the patient's primary immune response when a sensitizing dose is given, followed by a challenge dose. Recall antigens, those to which a patient has had or may have had previous exposure or sensitization, evaluate the secondary immune response; these antigens include candidin, trichophytin, streptokinase-streptodornase, purified protein derivative, mumps, and mixed respiratory vaccine, among others.

In these tests, a small amount of antigen (or group of antigens) is injected intradermally or applied topically, and the test site is later examined for a visible reaction. Skin tests have only limited value in infants because their immune systems are immature and inadequately sensitized.

Purpose

- To evaluate primary and secondary immune responses
- To assess effectiveness of immunotherapy when the patient's immune response is augmented by adjuvants (such as bacille Calmette-Guerin [BCG] vaccine) or other means (transfer factor, levamisole)
- To diagnose fungal diseases (coccidioidomycosis, histoplasmosis), bacterial diseases (tuberculosis, brucellosis, leprosy), and viral diseases (infectious mononucleosis)
- To monitor the course of certain diseases, such as Hodgkin's disease and coccidioidomycosis.

Patient preparation

Explain to the patient that this test evaluates how his immune system reacts after application or injection of small doses of antigens. Inform him that he needn't restrict food or fluids before the test. Tell him who will perform the test and where, that it takes about 10 minutes for each antigen to be administered, and that reactions should appear in 48 to 72 hours. Explain that some antigens (such as DNCB) are administered again after 2 weeks and, if the test is negative, that a stronger dose of antigen may be given.

Check the patient's history for hypersensitivity to any of the test antigens; if not listed in his history, ask the patient if he's had a skin test previously and, if so, what his reactions were. Check for a history of tuberculosis or previous BCG vaccination. If the patient's history reveals no sensitivity or hypersensitivity, intermediate-strength antigens are typically used.

Because many antigens are approved by the Food and Drug Administration (FDA) for use as vaccines but not for skin testing, check with the pharmacy about FDA approval for this purpose. If the tests require the patient's informed consent, such as for use of DNCB in research studies, check with the appropriate hospital committee for guidelines.

Equipment

DNCB TEST

DNCB ■ sterile gauze pad and tape ■ gloves ■ surgical mask ■ alcohol swabs ■ acetone ■ cotton swabs.

RECALL ANTIGEN TEST

1-ml tuberculin syringes ■ 25G 5/8″ needles ■ alcohol swabs ■ antigens ■ syringe filled with diluted epinephrine (1:1,000) ■ needle and syringe containing allergy test diluent ■ pen.

Procedure

DNCB TEST

- Wear gloves and a mask to avoid sensitizing yourself to DNCB.
- Dissolve DNCB in acetone.
- Position the patient's forearm comfortably, ventral side up, with his elbow slightly flexed. Clean a small, hairless area midway between the wrist and elbow with an alcohol swab, and allow it to dry.
- Apply the prescribed amount of DNCB (sensitizing dose) with a cotton swab. Allow this to dry, then cover the area with a sterile gauze pad for 24 to 48 hours.
- Instruct the patient to watch for a spontaneous flare reaction 10 to 14 days after application of DNCB. If a reaction occurs, a lower dose of the test solution can be used for the challenge dose.
- After 14 days, apply a challenge dose of DNCB to the same spot and in the same manner. Inspect the site 48 to 96 hours after application of DNCB for reactivity.
- If test results are negative, the challenge dose can be repeated 2 weeks later (1 month after the sensitizing dose).

RECALL ANTIGEN TEST

- Inject each antigen being tested intradermally, using a separate tuberculin syringe, on the patient's forearm. Circle each injection site with a pen, and label each according to the antigen given. Instruct the patient to avoid washing off the circles until the test is completed.
- Then inject the control allergy diluent on the other forearm.
- Inspect injection sites for reactivity after 48 and 72 hours.
- Record induration and erythema in millimeters. A negative test at the first concentration of antigen should be confirmed using a higher concentration.

Precautions

- Store antigens in lyophilized (freeze-dried) form at 39.2°F (4°C), protected from light. Reconstitute them shortly before use, and check their expiration dates. If the patient is suspected of being hypersensitive to the antigens, apply them first in low concentrations.
- Because excess DNCB can burn the patient's skin, apply only the prescribed amount.
- If the forearms aren't free from disease (for example, if the patient has atopic dermatitis), use other sites such as the back.

CLINICAL ALERT Observe the patient carefully for signs of anaphylactic shock: urticaria, respiratory distress, and hypotension. If these signs develop, administer epinephrine and notify the doctor immediately.

EITHER TEST

■ Watch the patient closely for severe local reactions that may occur at the test site, such as pain, blistering, swelling, induration, itching, and ulceration. Scarring and hyperpigmentation also may result. Observe for swelling and tenderness in the lymph nodes at the elbow or axillary region. Check for tachycardia and fever, although these rarely occur. Symptoms typically appear in 15 to 30 minutes.

■ Tell the patient experiencing hypersensitivity that corticosteroids will control the reaction but that skin lesions may persist for 10 to 14 days. Instruct him to avoid scratching or otherwise disturbing the affected area.

Normal findings

■ DNCB test: a positive reaction (erythema, edema, induration) appears 48 to 96 hours after the second (challenge) dose; 95% of the population reacts positively to DNCB.

■ Recall antigen test: a positive response (5 mm or more of induration at the test site) appears 48 hours after injection.

Implications of results

In the DNCB test, failure to react to the challenge dose indicates diminished delayed hypersensitivity. In the recall antigen test, a positive response to less than two of the six test antigens, persistent unresponsiveness to intradermal injection of higher-strength antigens, or a generalized diminished reaction (causing less than 10 mm combined induration) indicates diminished delayed hypersensitivity.

Diminished delayed hypersensitivity may occur in Hodgkin's disease (common); sarcoidosis; liver disease; congenital immunodeficiency disease, such as ataxia-telangiectasia, DiGeorge syndrome, and Wiskott-Aldrich syndrome; uremia; acute leukemia; viral diseases, such as influenza, infectious mononucleosis, measles, mumps, and rubella; fungal diseases, such as coccidioidomycosis and cryptococcosis; bacterial diseases, such as leprosy and tuberculosis; and terminal cancer. Diminished delayed hypersensitivity can also result from immunosuppressive or steroid therapy or viral vaccination.

Interfering factors

■ Use of antigens that have expired or that have been exposed to heat and light or to bacterial contamination interferes with accurate testing.

■ Oral contraceptives may cause false-negative results by inhibiting lymphocyte mitosis.

■ A strong immediate reaction to the antigen at the injection site may cause a false-negative delayed reaction.

■ Poor injection technique (subcutaneous instead of intradermal injection) may produce false-negative results.

■ Inaccurate dilution of antigens or an error in reading or timing test results causes inaccurate test results.

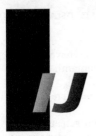

Immune complex test

When immune complexes are produced faster than they can be cleared by the lymphoreticular system, they may cause immune complex—for example, postinfectious syndromes, serum sickness, drug sensitivity, rheumatoid arthritis, and systemic lupus erythematosus (SLE). Immune complexes can form in tissues when a certain ratio of antigen reacts with antibody isotopes IgG 1, 2, 3, or IgM. These complexes fix the first component of complement (C1) and activate the complement cascade. Subsequent complement-mediated activity leads to inflammation and local tissue necrosis. Soluble circulating immune complexes may also activate complement in the blood and eventually cause damage, usually in the renal glomeruli, the aorta, and other large blood vessels.

Histologic examination of tissue obtained by biopsy and the use of fluorescence or peroxidase staining with antibodies specific for immunologic types generally detect immune complexes. However, because tissue biopsies cannot provide information about titers of circulating complexes, serum assays that detect circulating immune complexes indirectly may be required. Due to the inherent variability of these complexes, various serum test methods—using C1, rheumatoid factor, or cellular substrates, such as Raji cells, as reagents—may be appropriate under different circumstances.

Purpose

- To detect circulating immune complexes in serum
- To monitor response to therapy
- To estimate severity of disease.

Patient preparation

Explain to the patient that these tests help evaluate his immune system. If appropriate, inform him that the test will be repeated to monitor his response to therapy. Advise him that he needn't restrict food or fluids before the test. Tell him that this test requires a blood sample, who will perform the venipuncture and when, and that he may experience transient discomfort from the needle puncture and the pressure of the tourniquet.

If the patient is scheduled for a C1q (a component of C1) assay, check his history for recent heparin therapy. Report such therapy to the laboratory because it may affect test results.

Procedure

Perform a venipuncture and collect the sample in a 7-ml clot-activator tube.

Precautions

Send the sample to the laboratory immediately to prevent deterioration of immune complexes.

Normal findings

Normally, immune complexes aren't detectable in serum.

Implications of results

The presence of detectable immune complexes in serum has etiologic importance in many autoimmune diseases, such as SLE and rheumatoid arthritis. However, for a definitive diagnosis, the presence of these complexes must be considered in light of other test results. For example, in SLE, immune complexes are associated with high titers of antinuclear antibodies and circulating antibodies against native deoxyribonucleic acid.

Because of their filtering function, renal glomeruli seem most vulnerable to immune complex deposition, although blood vessel walls and choroid plexuses (vascular folds in the ventricles of the brain) can be affected. A renal biopsy to detect immune complexes can provide conclusive evidence for immune complex (Type III) glomerulonephritis, differentiating it from other types of glomerulonephritis.

Posttest care

■ Because many patients with immune complexes have compromised immune systems, take special care to keep the venipuncture site clean and dry.
■ If a hematoma develops at the venipuncture site, apply warm soaks.

Interfering factors

■ Failure to send the serum sample to the laboratory immediately can result in the deterioration of immune complexes and thus alter test results.
■ The presence of cryoglobulins in the patient's serum can affect test results.
■ Inability to standardize rheumatoid factor inhibition tests and platelet aggregation assays can affect the accuracy of test results.

Immunoglobulin G, A, and M tests

Immunoglobulins, proteins that can function as specific antibodies in response to antigen stimulation, are responsible for the humoral aspects of immunity. They are classified into five groups—IgG, IgA, IgM, IgD, and IgE —that are normally present in serum in predictable percentages.

IgG constitutes about 75% of serum immunoglobulins and includes the warm-temperature type; IgA, about 15% of the total; IgM, 5% to 7% and includes cold agglutinins, rheumatoid factor, and ABO blood group isoagglutinins; and IgD and allergen-specific IgE, less than 2%. Deviations from these normal percentages are characteristic in many immune disorders, such as cancer, hepatic disorders, rheumatoid arthritis, and systemic lupus erythematosus.

Immunoelectrophoresis identifies IgG, IgA, and IgM in a serum sample; the level of each is usually measured by radial immunodiffusion or nephelometry. Some laboratories detect immunoglobulin by indirect immunofluorescence and radioimmunoassay.

In immunoelectrophoresis, serum is placed in a well on a slide containing agar gel, and an electric current is passed through the gel. Immunoglobulins (and other serum proteins) separate according to their different electric charges. Then antiserum is deposited in a shallow trough alongside the separated proteins, from which it diffuses into the agar. Distinct precipitin arcs form wherever the antiserum reacts with specific serum proteins, allowing identification of the immunoglobulins and other proteins.

In radial immunodiffusion, addition of a class-specific antiserum diffuses the serum to form a precipitation ring that is proportional to the immunoglobulin concentration. In nephelometry, photometric measurement of the degree of light scattering caused by the immunoprecipitation reaction provides the relative immunoglobulin concentration.

Purpose

■ To diagnose paraproteinemias, such as multiple myeloma and Waldenström's macroglobulinemia
■ To detect hypogammaglobulinemia and hypergammaglobulinemia, as well as nonimmunologic diseases that are associated with abnormally high immunoglobulin levels, such as cirrhosis and hepatitis
■ To assess the effectiveness of chemotherapy or radiation therapy.

Patient preparation

Explain to the patient that this test measures antibody levels. If appropriate, tell him that the test evaluates the effectiveness of treatment. Instruct him to restrict food and fluids, except for water, for 12 to 14 hours before the test. Tell him the test requires a blood sample, who will perform the venipuncture and when, and that he may experience transient discomfort from the needle puncture and the pressure of the tourniquet.

Check the patient's medication history for drugs that may affect test results. If these medications must be continued, note this on the laboratory request.

Procedure

■ Perform a venipuncture and collect the sample in a 7-ml clot-activator tube.

■ Advise the patient with abnormally low immunoglobulin levels (especially of IgG or IgM) to protect himself against bacterial infection. When caring for such a patient, watch for signs of infection, such as fever, chills, rash, or skin ulcers.

■ Instruct the patient with abnormally high immunoglobulin levels and symptoms of monoclonal gammopathies to report bone pain and tenderness. Such a patient has numerous antibody-producing malignant plasma cells in bone marrow, which hamper production of other blood components. When caring for such a patient, watch for signs of hypercalcemia, renal failure, and spontaneous pathologic fractures.

Precautions

Send the sample to the laboratory immediately to prevent deterioration of immunoglobulins.

Reference values

In assay be nephelometry, serum immunoglobulin levels for adults range as follows:
■ IgG: 700 to 1,500 mg/dl
■ IgA: 60 to 400 mg/dl
■ IgM: 60 to 300 mg/dl.

Implications of results

IgG, IgA, and IgM levels change in various disorders. (See *Immunoglobulin patterns in various disorders,* page 334.) In congenital and acquired hypogammaglobulinemias, myelomas, and macroglobulinemia, the findings confirm the diagnosis. In hepatic and autoimmune diseases, leukemias, and lymphomas, such findings are less important but can support the diagnosis based on other tests, such as biopsies and white blood cell differential, and on physical examination findings.

IMMUNOGLOBULIN PATTERNS IN VARIOUS DISORDERS

The chart below shows the distribution of serum immunoglobulins (IgG, IgA, and IgM) that are associated with certain diseases.

Disorder	IgG	IgA	IgM
Immunoglobulin disorders			
Lymphoid aplasia	D	D	D
Agammaglobulinemia	D	D	D
Type I dysgammaglobulinemia (selective IgG and IgA deficiency)	D	D	N or I
Type II dysgammaglobulinemia (absent IgA and IgM)	N	D	D
IgA globulinemia	N	D	N
Ataxia-telangiectasia	N	D	N
Multiple myeloma, macroglobulinemia, lymphomas			
Heavy chain disease (Franklin's disease)	D	D	D
IgG myeloma	I	D	D
IgA myeloma	D	I	D
Macroglobulinemia	D	D	I
Acute lymphocytic leukemia	N	D	N
Chronic lymphocytic leukemia	D	D	D
Acute myelocytic leukemia	N	N	N
Chronic myelocytic leukemia	N	D	N
Hodgkin's disease	N	N	N
Hepatic disorders			
Hepatitis	I	I	I
Laënnec's cirrhosis	I	I	N
Biliary cirrhosis	N	N	I
Hepatoma	N	N	D
Other disorders			
Rheumatoid arthritis	I	I	I
Systemic lupus erythematosus	I	I	I
Nephrotic syndrome	D	D	N
Trypanosomiasis	N	N	I
Pulmonary tuberculosis	I	N	N

KEY: N = normal   I = increased   D = decreased

Posttest care

■ If a hematoma develops at the venipuncture site, apply warm soaks.

■ Allow the patient to resume his normal diet and any medications withheld before the test.

Interfering factors

■ Radiation therapy or chemotherapy, such as methotrexate, that suppress bone marrow activity may reduce immunoglobulin levels.

■ Aminophenazone, anticonvulsants, asparaginase, hydralazine, hydantoin derivatives, oral contraceptives, and phenylbutazone may raise levels of all immunoglobulins.

■ Methadone raises IgA levels; addiction to narcotics may raise IgM levels.

■ Methotrexate and severe hypersensitivity to bacille Calmette-Guérin vaccine may lower levels of all immunoglobulins.

■ Dextrans and high doses of methylprednisolone lower IgG and IgA levels; dextrans and methylprednisolone lower IgM levels.

Insulin test, serum

This radioimmunoassay is a quantitative analysis of serum insulin levels, which are usually measured concomitantly with glucose levels, because glucose is the primary stimulus for insulin release from pancreatic islet cells. The test helps evaluate patients suspected of having hyperinsulinemia resulting from pancreatic tumor or hyperplasia.

Insulin, a hormone secreted by beta cells of the islets of Langerhans, regulates the metabolism and transport or mobilization of carbohydrates, amino acids, proteins, and lipids. Stimulated by increased plasma levels of glucose, insulin secretion reaches peak levels after meals, when metabolism and food storage are greatest. Insulin insufficiency or resistance is the primary abnormality in diabetes mellitus.

Purpose

■ To aid diagnosis of hypoglycemia resulting from tumor or hyperplasia of pancreatic islet cells, glucocorticoid deficiency, or severe hepatic disease

■ To aid diagnosis of diabetes mellitus and insulin-resistant states. (For information on a related test, see *C-peptide assay*, page 336.)

Patient preparation

Explain that this test helps determine if the pancreas is functioning normally. Instruct the patient to fast for 10 to 12 hours before the test. Questionable results may require a repeat test or, frequently, a simultaneous glucose tolerance test, which requires the patient to drink glucose solution. Tell him that the test requires blood samples, who will perform the venipunctures and when, and that he may experience transient discomfort from the needle puncture and the pressure of the tourniquet.

Withhold corticotropin, corticosteroids (including oral contraceptives), thyroid supplements, epinephrine, and other medications that may interfere with test results. If they must be continued, note this on the laboratory request.

Make sure the patient is relaxed and recumbent for 30 minutes before the test.

C-PEPTIDE ASSAY

Connecting peptide (C-peptide) is a biologically inactive peptide chain formed during the proteolytic conversion of proinsulin to insulin in the pancreatic beta cells. It has no insulin effect, either biologically or immunologically. This is important because circulating insulin is measured by immunologic assay. As insulin is released into the bloodstream, the C-peptide chain splits off from the hormone. Except in patients with islet cell tumors and, possibly, in obese patients, serum C-peptide levels generally parallel those of insulin (normal values range between 0.9 and 4.2 ng/ml).

A C-peptide assay may help to:
■ determine the cause of hypoglycemia by distinguishing between endogenous hyperinsulinism or insulinoma (elevated C-peptide levels) and surreptitious insulin injection (decreased C-peptide levels)
■ indirectly measure insulin secretion in the presence of circulating insulin antibodies, which interfere with insulin assays but not with C-peptide assays
■ detect residual tissue (some C-peptide present) after total pancreatectomy for carcinoma
■ indicate the remission phase (some C-peptide present) of diabetes mellitus
■ determine beta-cell function in patients with diabetes mellitus; absence of C-peptide indicates no beta-cell function, and presence indicates residual beta-cell function.

Procedure

Perform a venipuncture. Collect one sample for insulin testing in a 7-ml tube with EDTA, then collect a sample for glucose testing in a tube with sodium fluoride and potassium oxalate, if requested.

Precautions

■ Make sure that the patient is relaxed before sample collection; agitation or stress may affect insulin levels.
■ Pack the sample for insulin testing in ice, and immediately send it, along with the glucose sample, to the laboratory.
■ In the patient with an insulinoma, fasting for this test may precipitate dangerously severe hypoglycemia. Keep glucose I.V. (50%) available to combat this reaction.
■ Handle the sample gently.

Reference values

Serum insulin levels normally range from 0 to 25 μU/ml.

Implications of results

Insulin levels are interpreted in light of the glucose concentration. A normal insulin level may be inappropriate for the glucose results. High insulin and low glucose levels after a significant fast suggest an insulinoma. Prolonged fasting or stimulation testing may be required to confirm the diagnosis. In insulin-resistant diabetic states, insulin levels are elevated; in non-insulin-resistant diabetes, they are low.

Posttest care

■ If a hematoma develops at the venipuncture site, apply warm soaks.
■ Resume diet and drugs discontinued before the test.

Interfering factors

■ Use of corticotropin, corticosteroids (including oral contraceptives), thyroid hormones, or epinephrine may raise serum insulin levels.
■ Use of insulin by patients who are not insulin-dependent may lower insulin levels.
■ Failure to observe restrictions of diet and activity may affect test results.
■ In patients with type 1 diabetes mellitus, high levels of insulin antibodies may interfere with the test.
■ Failure to pack the insulin sample in ice and send it to the laboratory promptly may affect test results.
■ Hemolysis caused by rough handling of the sample may alter test results.

Insulin tolerance test

This test measures serum levels of human growth hormone (hGH) and corticotropin after administration of a loading dose of insulin. It is more reliable than direct measurement of hGH and corticotropin because many healthy people have undetectable fasting levels of these hormones. Insulin-induced hypoglycemia stimulates hGH and corticotropin secretion in persons with an intact hypothalamic-pituitary-adrenal axis. Failure of stimulation indicates anterior pituitary or adrenal hypofunction, and helps confirm an hGH or corticotropin insufficiency.

Because the insulin tolerance test stimulates an adrenergic response, it's not recommended for patients with cardiovascular or cerebrovascular disorders, epilepsy, and low basal plasma cortisol levels.

Purpose

■ To aid diagnosis of hGH or corticotropin deficiency
■ To identify pituitary dysfunction
■ To aid differential diagnosis of primary and secondary adrenal hypofunction.

Patient preparation

Explain to the patient or to his family that this test evaluates hormonal secretion. Instruct him to fast and to restrict physical activity for 10 to 12 hours before the test. Explain that the test involves I.V. infusion of insulin and the collection of multiple blood samples. Warn him that he may experience an increased heart rate, diaphoresis, hunger, and anxiety after administration of insulin. Reassure him that these symptoms are transient but that if they become severe, the test will be discontinued. Inform him that the test takes about 2 hours and that results are usually available in 2 days.

Because physical activity and excitement increase hGH and corticotropin levels, make sure the patient is relaxed and recumbent for 90 minutes before the test.

Procedure

■ Between 6 a.m. and 8 a.m., collect three 5-ml samples of venous blood for basal levels—one in a tube with sodium fluoride and potassium oxalate for blood glucose (laboratory requirements may vary) and two in heparinized tubes for hGH and corticotropin. Then administer an I.V. bolus of U-100 regular insulin (0.15 U/kg or as ordered) over 1 to 2 minutes.

■ Draw additional blood samples 15, 30, 45, 60, 90, and 120 minutes after administration of insulin. Use an indwelling venous catheter to avoid repeated venipunctures. At each interval, collect three samples: one in a tube with sodium fluoride and potassium oxalate and two in heparinized tubes.

■ Label the tubes appropriately and send them to the laboratory immediately.

Precautions

■ Be sure to have concentrated glucose solution readily avail-able in case the patient has a severe hypoglycemic reaction to insulin. Hypoglycemia can be rapidly and accurately assessed with bedside glucose testing.

■ Note the time of collection on the laboratory request and send all samples to the laboratory immediately.

■ Handle the samples gently to prevent hemolysis.

Reference values

Normally, blood glucose falls to 50% of the fasting level 20 to 30 minutes after insulin administration. This stimulates an increase of 10 to 20 ng/dl over baseline values in both hGH and corticotropin, with peak levels occurring 60 to 90 minutes after insulin administration.

Implications of results

Failure of stimulation or a blunted response suggests dysfunction of the hypothalamic-pituitary-adrenal axis. An increase in hGH levels of less than 10 ng/dl above baseline suggests hGH deficiency. However, a definitive diagnosis requires a supplementary stimulation test, such as the arginine test. Additional testing is necessary to determine the site of the abnormality.

An increase in corticotropin levels of less than 10 ng/dl above baseline suggests adrenal insufficiency. The metyrapone or corticotropin stimulation test then confirms the diagnosis and determines whether insufficiency is primary or secondary.

Posttest care

- If a hematoma develops at the I.V. or venipuncture site, apply warm soaks.
- The patient can resume diet, activity, and drugs.

Interfering factors

- Corticosteroids, such as progestogen and estrogen, and pituitary-based drugs elevate hGH levels; glucocorticoids and beta blockers depress hGH levels.
- Glucocorticoids, estrogens, calcium gluconate, amphetamines, methamphetamines, spironolactone, and ethanol depress corticotropin levels.
- Failure to follow restrictions of diet, physical activity, and medications can prevent reliable test results.
- Hemolysis caused by rough handling of the sample may affect test results.

International normalized ratio test

The international normalized ratio (INR) system is viewed as the best means of standardizing measurement of prothrombin time to monitor oral anticoagulant therapy. It is not used as a screening test for coagulopathies.

Purpose

To evaluate effectiveness of oral anticoagulant therapy.

Patient preparation

Explain to the patient that this test is used to determine the effectiveness of his oral anticoagulant therapy. Tell the patient that a blood sample will be taken, who will perform the venipuncture and when, and that he may experience transient discomfort from the needle puncture and the pressure of the tourniquet. Reassure him that drawing a blood sample will take less than 3 minutes.

Procedure

Perform a venipuncture and collect the sample in a 7-ml tube with sodium citrate added.

Precautions

- Completely fill the collection tube; otherwise, an excess of citrate will appear in the sample.

■ Gently invert the tube several times to thoroughly mix the sample and the anticoagulant.
■ To prevent hemolysis, avoid excessive probing during venipuncture and handle the sample gently.
■ Put the sample on ice and send it to the laboratory promptly.

Reference values

Normal INR for those receiving warfarin therapy is 2.0 to 3.0. For those with mechanical prosthetic heart valves, an INR of 2.5 to 3.5 is suggested.

Implications of results

Elevated INR values may indicate disseminated intravascular coagulation, cirrhosis, hepatitis, vitamin K deficiency, salicylate intoxication, excessive dosage of oral anticoagulant, or massive blood transfusion.

Posttest care

If a hematoma develops at the venipuncture site, apply warm soaks.

Interfering factors

■ Failure to fill the collection tube completely, to adequately mix the sample and the anticoagulant, or to send the sample to the laboratory immediately may affect test results.
■ Hemolysis caused by excessive probing at the venipuncture site or rough handling of the sample may affect test results.

Iron and total iron-binding capacity tests

Iron is essential to the formation and function of hemoglobin as well as many other heme and nonheme compounds. After iron is absorbed by the intestine, it's distributed to various body compartments for synthesis, storage, and transport. (See *Normal iron metabolism*.) Because iron in the plasma is bound to a glycoprotein (transferrin), it's easily sampled and measured. The sample is treated with buffer and color reagents.

Serum iron assay measures the amount of iron bound to transferrin; total iron-binding capacity (TIBC) measures the amount of iron that would appear in plasma if all the transferrin were saturated with iron. The percentage of saturation is obtained by dividing the serum iron result by the TIBC, which reveals the actual amount of saturated transferrin—normally, about 30% saturated.

Serum iron and TIBC are more diagnostically useful when performed with the serum ferritin assay, but these

NORMAL IRON METABOLISM

Ingested iron, absorbed and oxidized in the bowel, binds with the protein transferrin for circulation to bone marrow, where hemoglobin synthesis occurs, and to all iron-hungry body cells. In the spleen, hemoglobin breakdown recycles iron back to the bone marrow or into storage. The body conserves iron, but it loses small amounts through skin, feces, urine, and menses. Storage areas in the liver, spleen, bone marrow, and reticuloendothelial system hold iron as ferritin until the body needs it; the liver alone stores about 60% of the body's iron.

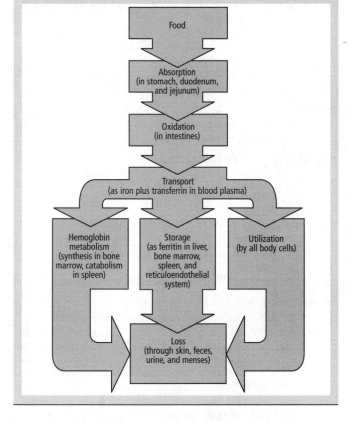

tests may not accurately reflect the state of other iron compartments, such as myoglobin iron and the labile iron pool. Bone marrow or liver biopsy and iron absorption or excretion studies may yield more information.

Purpose

- To estimate total iron storage
- To aid diagnosis of hemochromatosis (See *Siderocyte stain,* page 343.)

■ To help distinguish between iron deficiency anemia and anemia of chronic disease
■ To provide data for evaluating nutritional status.

Patient preparation

Explain to the patient that this test evaluates his body's capacity to store iron. Inform him that he needn't restrict food or fluids before the test. Tell him that the test requires a blood sample, who will perform the venipuncture and when, and that he may experience transient discomfort from the needle puncture and the pressure of the tourniquet.

Review the patient's drug history for medications that may affect test results. Withhold chloramphenicol, corticotropin, iron supplements, and oral contraceptives. If such medications must be continued, note this on the laboratory request.

Procedure

Perform a venipuncture and collect the sample in a 7-ml clot-activator tube.

Precautions

Handle the sample gently to avoid hemolysis, and send it to the laboratory immediately.

Reference values

■ Serum iron: 70 to 150 µg/dl for men; 80 to 150 µg/dl for women
■ TIBC: 300 to 400 µg/dl for men; 300 to 450 µg/dl for women
■ Saturation: 20% to 50% for men and women

Implications of results

In iron deficiency, serum iron levels drop and TIBC increases to decrease the saturation. In cases of chronic inflammation (such as in rheumatoid arthritis), serum iron may be low in the presence of adequate body stores, but TIBC may be unchanged or may drop to preserve normal saturation. Iron overload may not alter serum levels until relatively late, but in general, serum iron increases and TIBC remains the same to increase the saturation.

Posttest care

■ If a hematoma develops at the venipuncture site, apply warm soaks.
■ Ensure subdermal bleeding has stopped before removing pressure. If the hematoma is large, monitor pulses distal to the venipuncture site.
■ Resume administration of any medications that were withheld before the test.

SIDEROCYTE STAIN

Siderocytes are red blood cells (RBCs) that contain particles of non-hemoglobin iron known as siderocytic granules. In neonates, siderocytic granules are normally present in normoblasts and reticulocytes during hemoglobin synthesis. However, the spleen removes most of these granules from normal RBCs, and they disappear rapidly with age.

Clinical associations

In adults, elevated siderocyte levels usually indicate abnormal erythropoiesis, as occurs in congenital spherocytic anemia, chronic hemolytic anemias (such as the thalassemias), pernicious anemia, hemochromatosis, toxicities (such as lead poisoning), infection, and severe burns. Elevated levels may also follow splenectomy because the spleen normally removes siderocytic granules.

Procedure

The siderocyte stain test measures the number of circulating siderocytes.

■ Venous blood is drawn into a 7-ml lavender-top tube or, for infants and children, is collected in a microcollection tube and smeared directly on a 3″ glass slide.

■ When the blood smear is stained, siderocytic granules appear as purple-blue specks clustered around the periphery of mature erythrocytes.

■ Cells containing these granules are counted as a percentage of total RBCs. The results aid differential diagnosis of anemias and hemochromatosis and help detect toxicities.

Values

Normally, siderocyte levels are slightly elevated at birth but reach the normal adult values of 0.5% of total RBCs in 7 to 10 days.

■ Pernicious anemia siderocyte level: 8% to 14%
■ Chronic hemolytic anemia: 20% to 100%
■ Lead poisoning: 10% to 30%
■ Hemochromatosis: 3% to 7%.

An elevated siderocyte level mandates additional testing, including bone marrow examination, to determine the cause of abnormal erythropoiesis.

Interfering factors

■ Chloramphenicol and oral contraceptives can cause false-positive test results; corticotropin can produce false-negative results. Iron supplements can cause false-positive serum iron values but false-negative TIBC.

■ Hemolysis caused by rough handling of the sample or failure to send the sample to the laboratory immediately may alter test results.

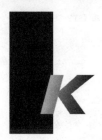

Ketone test, urine

In this routine, semiquantitative screening test, the action of urine on a commercial product (Acetest tablet, Ketostix, or Keto-Diastix) measures the urine level of ketones (also known as ketone bodies). Each product measures a specific ketone. For example, Acetest measures acetone and Ketostix measures acetoacetic acid. Urine determinations reflect serum concentration.

Excessive accumulation of ketones (acetoacetic acid, acetone, and beta-hydroxybutyric acid) — the by-products of fat metabolism — follows carbohydrate deprivation, as occurs in starvation or diabetic ketoacidosis.

Purpose

■ To screen for ketonuria
■ To identify diabetic ketoacidosis and carbohydrate deprivation
■ To distinguish between a diabetic and a nondiabetic coma
■ To monitor control of diabetes mellitus, ketogenic weight reduction, and diabetic ketoacidosis treatment.

Patient preparation

Explain to the patient that this test evaluates fat metabolism. If he's newly diagnosed with diabetes, tell him how to perform the test. Instruct the patient to void; then give him a drink of water. About 30 minutes later, ask him for a second-voided urine specimen.

If the patient is taking levodopa or phenazopyridine or has recently received sulfobromophthalein, Acetest tablets must be used because reagent strips will give inaccurate results.

Procedure

■ Collect a second-voided midstream urine specimen and follow one of these procedures:
– Acetest: Lay the tablet on a piece of white paper, and place one drop of urine on the tablet. After 30 seconds, compare the tablet color (white, lavender, or purple) with the color chart.
– Ketostix: Dip the reagent stick into the specimen and remove it immediately. After 15 seconds, compare the

stick color (buff or purple) with the color chart. Record
the results as negative, small, moderate, or large
amounts of ketones.
– Keto-Diastix: Dip the reagent strip into the specimen,
and remove it immediately. Tap the edge of the strip
against the container or a clean, dry surface to remove
excess urine. Hold the strip horizontally to prevent mixing the chemicals from the two areas. Interpret each
area of the strip separately. After exactly 15 seconds,
compare the color of the ketone section (buff or purple)
with the appropriate color chart; after 30 seconds, compare the color of the glucose section. Ignore color
changes that occur after the specified waiting periods.
Record the results as negative or as positive for small,
moderate, or large amounts of ketones.
■ If the test is to be performed at home, provide written
guidelines and a flow sheet to help the patient record results.
■ Tell the patient when the next specimen is needed.

Precautions

■ Test the specimen within 60 minutes after it is obtained; if this isn't possible, refrigerate specimen and allow it to return to room temperature before testing.
■ Don't use tablets or strips that have become discolored
or darkened.

Normal findings

No ketones present.

Implications of results

Ketonuria occurs in uncontrolled diabetes mellitus and
starvation and as a metabolic complication of total parenteral nutrition.

Interfering factors

■ Levodopa, phenazopyridine, and sulfobromophthalein
produce false-positive test results with Ketostix or Keto-
Diastix.
■ Failure to keep the reagent container tightly closed to
prevent absorption of light or moisture by the test
sticks/strips or bacterial contamination of the specimen
causes false-negative results.

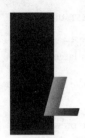

Lactate dehydrogenase test

Lactate dehydrogenase (LD) catalyzes the reversible conversion of muscle lactic acid to pyruvic acid. This essential final step in the Embden-Meyerhof glycolytic pathway provides the metabolic bridge to the Krebs cycle (citric acid or tricarboxylic acid cycle), ultimately producing cellular energy.

Because LD is present in almost all body tissues, cell damage causes total serum LD to rise and thereby limits its diagnostic usefulness. However, immunochemical separation and quantitation or electrophoresis can identify and measure five tissue-specific isoenzymes: LD_1 and LD_2 are present primarily in the heart, red blood cells (RBCs), and kidneys; LD_3, primarily in the lungs; and LD_4 and LD_5, in the liver and the skeletal muscles. Also, the midzone fractions (LD_2, LD_3, LD_4) can be elevated in granulocytic leukemia, lymphomas, and platelet disorders.

The specificity of LD isoenzymes and their distribution pattern are useful in diagnosing hepatic, pulmonary, and erythrocytic damage. However, their widest clinical application is in aiding diagnosis of acute myocardial infarction (MI). An LD isoenzyme assay is useful when creatine kinase (CK) hasn't been measured within 24 hours after an acute MI. The myocardial LD level rises later than CK (12 to 48 hours after infarction begins), peaks in 2 to 5 days, and drops to normal in 7 to 10 days if tissue necrosis doesn't persist. (See *LD isoenzyme variations in disease*.)

Purpose

■ To aid differential diagnosis of MI, pulmonary infarction, anemias, and hepatic disease
■ To support CK isoenzyme test results in diagnosing MI or to provide diagnosis when CK-MB samples are drawn too late to display elevation
■ To monitor patient response to some forms of chemotherapy.

LD ISOENZYME VARIATIONS IN DISEASE

The specificity of LD isoenzymes and their distribution patterns are useful in diagnosing hepatic, pulmonary, and erythrocytic damage. But their widest clinical application is in the diagnosis of acute myocardial infarction (MI).

Disease	LD$_1$	LD$_2$	LD$_3$	LD$_4$	LD$_5$
Cardiovascular					
Myocardial infarction	●	●	○	○	○
Myocardial infarction with hepatic congestion	●	●	○	○	●
Rheumatic carditis	●	●	○	○	○
Myocarditis	●	●	○	○	○
Heart failure (decompensated)	○	○	○	○	●
Shock	●	●	●	●	●
Angina pectoris	●	○	○	○	○
Pulmonary					
Pulmonary embolism	●	○	○	○	○
Pulmonary infarction	○	○	●	○	○
Hematologic					
Pernicious anemia	●	●	○	○	○
Hemolytic anemia	●	●	○	○	○
Sickle cell anemia	●	●	○	○	○
Hepatobiliary					
Hepatitis	○	○	○	○	●
Active cirrhosis	○	○	○	○	●
Hepatic congestion	○	○	○	○	●

KEY: ● Normal ● Diagnostic ○ Not Diagnostic

Adapted with permission from information from Helena Laboratories, 1513 Lindberg Dr., Beaumont, Tex.

Patient preparation

Explain that this test is used primarily to detect tissue alterations. Inform the patient he needn't restrict food or fluids before the test. Tell him that the test requires a blood sample, who will perform the venipuncture and when, and that he may experience transient discomfort from the needle puncture and the pressure of the tourniquet. If an MI is suspected, tell him that the test is likely to be repeated for the next few mornings to monitor progressive changes.

Procedure

Perform a venipuncture and collect the sample in a 7-ml clot-activator tube.

Precautions

■ Draw the samples on schedule to avoid missing peak levels, and mark the collection time on the laboratory request.

■ Handle the sample gently to prevent artifact hemolysis because RBCs contain LD_1.

■ Send the sample to the laboratory immediately or, if transport is delayed, keep the sample at room temperature. Changes in temperature reportedly inactivate LD_5, thus altering isoenzyme patterns.

Reference values

Total LD levels normally range from 35 to 378 U/L, depending on the method used. Normal isoenzyme distribution is as follows:

■ LD_1: 14% to 26% of total
■ LD_2: 29% to 39% of total
■ LD_3: 20% to 26% of total
■ LD_4: 8% to 16% of total
■ LD_5: 6% to 16% of total.

Implications of results

Because many common diseases cause elevations in total LD levels, isoenzyme electrophoresis is usually necessary for diagnosis. In some disorders, total LD may be within normal limits, but abnormal proportions of each isoenzyme indicate specific organ tissue damage. For instance, in acute MI, the concentration of LD_1 is greater than LD_2 within 12 to 48 hours after onset of symptoms. (That is, the LD_1:LD_2 ratio is greater than 1.) This reversal of normal isoenzyme patterns is typical of myocardial damage and is referred to as "flipped LD."

Interfering factors

■ Hemolysis caused by rough handling of the sample may affect results.

■ For diagnosis of acute MI, failure to draw the sample on schedule may interfere with test results.

■ Failure to centrifuge the sample and separate the cells from the serum may affect the results.

■ Failure to send the sample to the laboratory immediately may interfere with accurate determination of LD isoenzyme patterns.
■ Recent surgery or pregnancy can cause elevated LD levels. Prosthetic heart valves may also increase LD levels because of chronic hemolysis.

Lactic acid and pyruvic acid test

Lactic acid, present in blood as lactate ion, is derived primarily from muscle cells and RBCs. It is an intermediate product of carbohydrate metabolism and is normally metabolized by the liver. Blood lactate concentration depends on the rate of production and the rate of metabolism; lactate levels may rise significantly during exercise.

Lactate is the reduction product of pyruvate, a byproduct of carbohydrate metabolism. Together these compounds form a reversible reaction that's regulated by oxygen supply. When oxygen levels are deficient, pyruvate converts to lactate; when they're adequate, lactate converts to pyruvate.

When the hepatic system fails to metabolize lactate sufficiently, or when excess pyruvate converts to lactate because of tissue hypoxia and circulatory collapse, lactic acidosis (lactate levels greater than 2 mEq/L and pH less than 7.35) may result. Measurement of blood lactate levels by enzymatic methods, using lactate dehydrogenase, is recommended for all patients with symptoms of lactic acidosis such as Kussmaul's respirations.

Although arterial or venous blood can be used for lactate analysis, a venous sample is easier to obtain. However, unless the patient rests for 1 hour before the test, venous blood may yield higher values than arterial blood. Comparison of pyruvate and lactate levels reliably mirrors tissue oxidation, but measurement of pyruvate is technically difficult and it's performed infrequently.

Purpose

■ To assess tissue oxidation
■ To help determine the cause of lactic acidosis.

Patient preparation

The patient with acidosis is likely to be comatose or extremely lethargic. Nevertheless, explain to him that this blood test evaluates the oxygen level in tissues. Tell him the test requires a blood sample, who will perform the venipuncture and when, and that he may experience transient discomfort from the needle puncture and the tourniquet pressure. Withhold food overnight, and make sure the patient rests for at least 1 hour before the test.

Procedure

Perform a venipuncture and collect the sample in a 5-ml tube with sodium fluoride and potassium oxalate added.

Precautions

■ Because venostasis may raise blood lactate levels, it's best to avoid using a tourniquet; if you do use one, release it at least 2 minutes before collecting the sample so the blood can circulate. Tell the patient he must not clench his fist during the venipuncture.

■ Because lactate and pyruvate are extremely unstable, place the sample container in an ice-filled cup and send it to the laboratory immediately.

Reference values

Blood lactate values range from 0.93 to 1.65 mEq/L; pyruvate levels, from 0.08 to 0.16 mEq/L. Normally, the lactate:pyruvate ratio is less than 10:1.

Implications of results

Elevated blood lactate levels associated with hypoxia may result from strenuous muscle exercise, shock, hemorrhage, septicemia, myocardial infarction, pulmonary embolism, or cardiac arrest. When no reason for diminished tissue perfusion is apparent, increased lactate levels may result from a systemic disorder (such as diabetes mellitus, leukemias, lymphomas, hepatic disease, and renal failure) or from enzymatic defects (as in von Gierke's disease and fructose 1,6-diphosphatase deficiency).

Lactic acidosis can follow ingestion of large doses of acetaminophen or ethanol as well as I.V. infusion of epinephrine, glucagon, fructose, or sorbitol. Because phenformin causes severe lactic acidosis, the Food and Drug Administration removed it from clinical use as an antidiabetic agent.

Posttest care

■ If a hematoma develops at the venipuncture site, apply warm soaks.

■ Instruct the patient to resume his normal diet.

Interfering factors

■ Failure to adhere to diet and activity restrictions may affect test results.

■ Failure to pack the sample in ice and transport it to the laboratory immediately may elevate blood lactate levels.

Lactose tolerance test, oral

This test measures plasma glucose levels after ingestion of a challenge dose of lactose. It's used to screen for lactose intolerance caused by lactase deficiency.

Lactose, a disaccharide, is found in milk and other dairy products. The intestinal enzyme lactase splits lactose into the monosaccharides glucose and galactose for absorption by the intestinal epithelium. Absence or deficiency of lactase causes undigested lactose to remain in the intestinal lumen, producing abdominal cramps and watery diarrhea.

Congenital lactase deficiency is rare; lactose intolerance is usually acquired as lactase levels decline with age. Secondary lactase deficiency accompanies disorders that damage the intestinal mucosa, such as inflammatory bowel disease, gastroenteritis, and gluten-induced enteropathy.

Purpose

To detect lactose intolerance.

Patient preparation

Explain to the patient that this test determines if his symptoms are associated with an inability to digest lactose. Instruct him to fast and to avoid strenuous activity for 8 hours before the test. Tell him this test requires four blood samples, who will perform the venipunctures and when, and that he may feel transient discomfort from the needle punctures and the pressure of the tourniquet. Explain that the entire procedure may take as long as 2 hours.

Withhold drugs that may affect plasma glucose levels. If these drugs must be continued, note this on the laboratory request.

Procedure

■ After the patient has fasted for 8 hours, perform a venipuncture and collect a blood sample in a 7-ml tube with sodium fluoride and potassium oxalate added.
■ Administer the test load of lactose—for an adult, 50 g of lactose dissolved in 400 ml of water; for a child, 50 g/m^2 of body surface area. Record the time of ingestion.
■ Draw blood samples at 30, 60, and 120 minutes after giving the loading dose, using 7-ml tubes with sodium fluoride and potassium oxalate added. Collect a stool sample 5 hours after the loading dose, if ordered.

Precautions

■ Send blood and stool samples to the laboratory immediately, or refrigerate them if transport is delayed. Note the collection time on the laboratory request.

■ Watch for symptoms of lactose intolerance—abdominal cramps, nausea, bloating, flatulence, and watery diarrhea— caused by the loading dose.

Reference values

Normally, plasma glucose levels rise more than 20 mg/dl over fasting levels within 15 to 60 minutes after ingestion of the lactose loading dose. Stool sample analysis shows normal pH (7 to 8) and low glucose content (less than 1+ on a glucose-indicating dipstick).

Implications of results

A rise in plasma glucose of less than 20 mg/dl indicates lactose intolerance, as do stool acidity (pH of 5.5 or less) and high glucose content (greater than 1+ on the dipstick). Accompanying signs and symptoms provoked by the test also suggest but don't confirm the diagnosis because patients with normal lactase activity may experience such symptoms after a loading dose of lactose. Small-bowel biopsy with lactase assay may be done to confirm the diagnosis.

Posttest care

■ If a hematoma develops at the venipuncture site, apply warm soaks.

■ Instruct the patient to resume diet, activity, and medications withheld before the test.

Interfering factors

■ Delayed emptying of stomach contents can cause depressed glucose levels.

■ Failure to follow diet and exercise restrictions may alter test results.

■ Drugs that affect plasma glucose levels—such as thiazide diuretics, oral contraceptives, benzodiazepines, propranolol, and insulin—may alter test results.

■ Glycolysis may cause false-negative results.

Leucine aminopeptidase test

This test is used to measure serum levels of leucine aminopeptidase (LAP), an isoenzyme of alkaline phosphatase (ALP) that is widely distributed in body tissues. The greatest concentrations appear in the hepatobiliary tissues, pancreas, and small intestine. Serum LAP levels parallel serum ALP levels in hepatic disease.

Purpose

■ To provide information about suspected liver, pancreatic, and biliary diseases
■ To differentiate skeletal disease from hepatobiliary or pancreatic disease
■ To evaluate neonatal jaundice.

Patient preparation

Explain to the patient that this test is used to evaluate liver and pancreatic function. Tell him to fast for at least 8 hours before the test and to stop taking drugs containing estrogen or progesterone for 8 hours before the test. Tell the patient that this test requires a blood sample, who will perform the venipuncture and when, and that he may experience transient discomfort from the needle puncture and the pressure of the tourniquet.

Procedure

Perform a venipuncture and collect the sample in a 7-ml clot-activator tube.

Precautions

■ Handle the sample gently to avoid hemolysis.
■ Transport the sample to the laboratory immediately.

Reference values

Normal values are 80 to 200 U/ml in men and 75 to 185 U/ml in women.

Implications of results

Elevated levels can occur in patients with biliary obstruction, tumors, strictures, and atresia; those in the third trimester of pregnancy; and those undergoing therapy with drugs containing estrogen or progesterone.

Posttest care

■ If a hematoma develops at the venipuncture site, apply warm soaks.
■ Tell the patient that he may resume his usual diet and medications.

Interfering factors

■ Estrogen or progesterone can produce falsely elevated levels.
■ Advanced pregnancy can cause falsely elevated levels.

Leukoagglutinins test

This test detects leukoagglutinins (also known as white cell antibodies or HLA antibodies)—antibodies that react with white blood cells (WBCs) and may cause a transfusion reaction. These antibodies usually develop after exposure to foreign WBCs through transfusions, pregnancies, or allografts.

If a blood recipient has these antibodies, a febrile non-hemolytic reaction may occur 1 to 4 hours after the start of whole blood, red blood cell, platelet, or granulocyte transfusion. (All these blood products contain some granulocytes, which react with the antibodies.) This nonhemolytic reaction (marked by fever and severe chills, sometimes with nausea, headache, and transient hypertension) must be distinguished from a hemolytic reaction before the transfusion can proceed. The presence of these antibodies in a recipient can also cause immune-mediated platelet refractoriness, a condition that is characterized by the failure of platelet count to rise after the transfusion of suitably preserved platelets.

The standard technique used to detect leukoagglutinins is the microlymphocytotoxicity test, in which recipient serum is tested against donor lymphocytes or against a panel of lymphocytes of known HLA phenotype. The antibodies in the recipient serum bind to the corresponding antigen present on the lymphocytes and cause cell membrane injury when complement is added to the test system. Cell injury is detected by examination of the lymphocytes by phase-contrast microscopy to observe dye exclusion (negative test) or dye uptake (positive test).

Purpose

■ To detect leukoagglutinins in blood recipients who develop a transfusion reaction, thus differentiating between hemolytic and febrile nonhemolytic transfusion reactions
■ To detect leukoagglutinins in recipients who develop platelet refractoriness after multiple transfusions of blood products.

Patient preparation

Explain to the patient that this test helps determine the cause of his transfusion reaction. Tell him that the test requires a blood sample, who will perform the venipuncture and when, and that he may feel transient discomfort from the needle puncture and the pressure of the tourniquet.

Note recent administration of blood or dextran or testing with I.V. contrast media on the laboratory request.

Procedure

Perform a venipuncture and collect the sample in a 10-ml clot-activator tube. The laboratory will require 3 to 4 ml of serum for testing.

Precautions

■ If a transfusion recipient has a positive leukoagglutinin test, continued transfusions require premedication with acetaminophen 1 to 2 hours before the transfusion, specially prepared leukocyte-poor blood, or use of leukocyte removal blood filters to prevent further reactions.

■ Tests for these antibodies aren't useful in deciding which patients should receive leukocyte-poor blood components; the decision must be based on clinical experience.

■ The use of leukocyte-poor blood components is becoming routine for patients who require long-term platelet and red blood cell transfusions and is especially important for patients who are likely to become transplant candidates.

■ Label the sample with the patient's name, the hospital or blood bank number, the date, and the initials of the phlebotomist. Be sure to include on the laboratory request the patient's suspected diagnosis and any history of blood transfusions, pregnancies, and drug therapy.

Normal findings

A negative test result is normal. That is, agglutination doesn't occur if the patient's serum contains no antibodies.

Implications of results

A positive result in a blood recipient indicates the presence of agglutinins, identifying his transfusion reaction as a febrile nonhemolytic reaction to these antibodies. Recipients who test positive for HLA antibodies may need HLA-matched platelets to control bleeding episodes caused by thrombocytopenia.

Posttest care

■ If a hematoma develops at the venipuncture site, apply warm soaks.

Interfering factors

None reported.

Lipase test

Lipase is produced in the pancreas and secreted into the duodenum, where it converts triglycerides and other fats into fatty acids and glycerol. Destruction of pancreatic cells, which occurs in acute pancreatitis, releases large amounts of lipase into the blood.

This test measures serum lipase levels by the kinetic turbidimetric technique; it's most useful when performed with a serum or urine amylase test.

Purpose

To aid diagnosis of acute pancreatitis.

Patient preparation

Explain that this test evaluates pancreatic function. Instruct the patient to fast overnight before the test. Tell him that the test requires a blood sample, who will perform the venipuncture and when, and that he may feel transient discomfort from the needle puncture and the pressure of the tourniquet.

Withhold cholinergics, codeine, meperidine, and morphine before the test. If any of these drugs must be continued, note this on the laboratory request.

Procedure

Perform a venipuncture and collect the sample in a 7-ml clot-activator tube.

Precautions

Handle the collection tube gently.

Reference values

Serum levels are method-dependent and are generally less than 300 U/L. When triolein is used for analysis, normal levels are less than 200 U/L; when olive oil is used, normal levels are less than 160 U/L.

Implications of results

High lipase levels lasting up to 14 days suggest acute pancreatitis or pancreatic duct obstruction. Lipase levels may also increase in other pancreatic injuries, such as perforated peptic ulcer with chemical pancreatitis caused by gastric juices, and in patients with a high intestinal obstruction, pancreatic cancer, or renal disease with impaired excretion.

Posttest care

■ If a hematoma develops at the venipuncture site, apply warm soaks.
■ Resume administration of drugs discontinued before the test.

Interfering factors

■ Cholinergics, codeine, meperidine, and morphine cause spasm of the sphincter of Oddi, producing false-positive results.

■ Hemolysis may alter test results.

Lipids test, fecal

Lipids excreted in feces include monoglycerides, diglycerides, triglycerides, phospholipids, glycolipids, soaps (fatty acids and fatty acid salts), sterols, and cholesterol esters. These lipids are derived from sloughed intestinal bacterial cells and epithelial cells, unabsorbed dietary lipids, and GI secretions. Normally, dietary lipids emulsified by bile are almost completely absorbed in the small intestine, provided that biliary and pancreatic secretions are adequate. However, excessive excretion of fecal lipids (steatorrhea) occurs in various malabsorption syndromes.

Both qualitative and quantitative tests can detect excessive excretion of lipids in patients with signs of malabsorption: weight loss, abdominal distention, and scaly skin. In the qualitative test, a specimen from a random stool is stained with Sudan III dye and examined microscopically for evidence of malabsorption — undigested muscle fibers and various fats. In the quantitative test, the entire 72-hour specimen is dried and weighed; the lipids therein are extracted with a solvent, evaporated, and weighed. Only the quantitative test can confirm steatorrhea.

Purpose

To confirm or rule out steatorrhea.

Patient preparation

Explain to the patient that this test evaluates digestion of fats. Instruct him to abstain from alcohol and to maintain a high-fat diet (100 g/day) for 3 days before the test and during the collection period. Tell him the test requires a 72-hour stool collection. Withhold drugs that may affect test results. If these medications must be continued, note this on the laboratory request.

Teach the patient how to collect a timed stool specimen, and provide him with the necessary equipment. Inform him that the laboratory requires 1 or 2 days to complete the analysis.

Procedure

Collect a 72-hour stool specimen.

Precautions

■ Don't use a waxed collection container because the wax may become incorporated in the stool and interfere with accurate testing.

■ Tell the patient to avoid contaminating the stool specimen with toilet tissue or urine.

■ Tell the patient to refrigerate the collection container between defecations, and keep it tightly covered.

Reference values

Fecal lipids normally make up less than 20% of excreted solids, with excretion of less than 7 g/24 hours.

Implications of results

Both digestive and absorptive disorders cause steatorrhea. Digestive disorders may affect the production and release of pancreatic lipase or bile; absorptive disorders may affect the integrity of the intestine. In pancreatic insufficiency, impaired lipid digestion may result from insufficient production of lipase. Pancreatic resection, cystic fibrosis, chronic pancreatitis, or ductal obstruction by stone or tumor may prevent the normal release or action of lipase.

In impaired hepatic function, faulty lipid digestion may result from inadequate production of bile salts. Biliary obstruction, which may accompany gallbladder disease, may prevent the normal release of bile salts into the duodenum. Extensive small-bowel resection or bypass may also interrupt normal enterohepatic circulation of bile salts.

Diseases of the intestinal mucosa affect normal absorption of lipids; regional ileitis and atrophy resulting from malnutrition cause gross structural changes in the intestinal wall, and celiac disease and tropical sprue produce mucosal abnormalities. Scleroderma, radiation enteritis, fistulas, intestinal tuberculosis, small intestine diverticula, and altered intestinal flora may also cause steatorrhea. Whipple's disease and lymphomas cause lymphatic obstruction that may inhibit fat absorption.

Posttest care

Tell the patient he may resume his usual diet and medications withheld before the test.

Interfering factors

■ The following drugs and substances may produce inaccurate test results by inhibiting absorption or affecting chemical digestion: azathioprine, bisacodyl, cholestyramine, kanamycin, neomycin, colchicine, aluminum hydroxide, calcium carbonate, alcohol, potassium chloride, and mineral oil.

■ Failure to observe pretest restrictions, use of a waxed collection container, contamination of the sample, or incomplete stool specimen collection (total weight less than 300 g) will affect the accuracy of test results.

Lipoprotein-cholesterol measurement

Most serum cholesterol is present in the form of low-density lipoprotein (LDL) cholesterol. LDL cholesterol has a strong and direct association with coronary artery disease (CAD). If the total cholesterol is elevated, the LDL is usually also elevated. The LDLs are the cholesterol-rich remnants of the very-low-density lipoprotein (VLDL) lipid-transport vehicle.

Measurement of LDL cholesterol is done because of the extreme difficulty in measuring VLDL. The LDL level isn't measured directly. Most laboratories use the Friedewald equation to calculate the LDL cholesterol level: LDL cholesterol equals total cholesterol minus HDL cholesterol minus triglycerides, divided by 5 (where all concentrations are expressed in mg/dl). However, this formula isn't valid for specimens when triglyceride levels are greater than 400 mg/dl.

Another method, the cholesterol fractionation test, isolates and measures the cholesterol in serum — LDL and HDL — by ultracentrifugation. The ultracentrifugal method isn't readily available and is mostly used by specialized lipoprotein laboratories.

Usually, about 20% of total cholesterol is HDL cholesterol. Some experts have suggested that for every decrease of 5 mg/dl in HDL below mean, the risk for CAD increases 25%. HDL appears to help the enzyme lecithin cholesterol acyltransferase remove cholesterol from arterial walls.

Patients with angina pectoris or myocardial infarction generally have lower HDL levels than do healthy persons. Low HDL levels, which can be hereditary, are not only associated with CAD, but they precede it. Low HDL levels are also connected with diabetes mellitus, hypertension, cigarette smoking, obesity, and lack of exercise.

The higher incidence of heart disease in men and postmenopausal women than in premenopausal women may result from low levels of estrogen, a hormone that helps regulate synthesis of HDL cholesterol. Paradoxically, oral contraceptives and pregnancy elevate HDL levels. Because HDL levels are only 5% to 8% lower in premenopausal women than in men of the same age, the potentially protective action of estrogens against atherosclerosis remains controversial.

APOLIPOPROTEINS AND CAD

Although measurement of apolipoproteins — the protein fractions of lipoprotein molecules — is primarily a research procedure, mounting evidence suggests that it may have important clinical applications as well. Because apolipoproteins can be measured directly in serum, they may reflect risk for coronary artery disease (CAD) more accurately than high-density lipoprotein (HDL) or low-density lipoprotein (LDL) levels, which must be measured indirectly.

Of the eight apolipoproteins so far identified, apolipoprotein A (ApoA, the major protein component of HDL), and apolipoprotein B (ApoB, the major protein component of LDL), are the most clinically significant. Reduced ApoA levels (below 140 mg/dl) occur in ischemic heart disease, whereas elevated ApoB levels (above 135 mg/dl) occur in hyperlipidemia, angina pectoris, and myocardial infarction.

Measurement of apolipoproteins may also be clinically important in determining an individual's risk of CAD. (See *Apolipoproteins and CAD.*)

Purpose

- To assess the risk of CAD
- To assess efficacy of lipid-lowering drug therapy.

Patient preparation

Tell the patient that this test helps determine the risk of CAD. Instruct him to maintain his normal diet for 2 weeks before the test, to abstain from alcohol for 24 hours before the test, and to fast and avoid exercise for 12 to 14 hours before the test. Tell the patient the test requires a blood sample, who will perform the venipuncture and when, and that he may feel transient discomfort from the needle puncture and the pressure of the tourniquet. Withhold thyroid hormone, oral contraceptives, and antilipemic agents, which alter test results.

Procedure

Perform a venipuncture and collect the sample in a 7-ml tube with EDTA.

Precautions

Send the sample to the laboratory immediately to avoid spontaneous redistribution among the lipoproteins. If the sample can't be transported immediately, refrigerate it but don't allow it to freeze.

Reference values

LDL cholesterol: For people who don't have CAD, desirable levels are less than 130 mg/dl; borderline high levels are in the range of 130 to 159 mg/dl; and high levels

DIET AND DRUG TREATMENT RECOMMENDATIONS

Treatment recommendations based on low-density lipoprotein cholesterol levels are as follows:

	Initiation level	Minimal goal
Diet		
■ No coronary artery disease (CAD) and less than two other risk factors	>160 mg/dl	<160 mg/dl
■ No CAD but two or more risk factors	>130 mg/dl	<130 mg/dl
■ With CAD	>100 mg/dl	<100 mg/dl
Drug treatment		
■ No CAD and less than two other risk factors	>190 mg/dl	<160 mg/dl
■ No CAD but two or more risk factors	>160 mg/dl	<130 mg/dl
■ With CAD	>130 mg/dl	<100 mg/dl

are more than 160 mg/dl. For those with CAD, optimal levels are less than 100 mg/dl and higher-than-optimal levels are more than 100 mg/dl.

HDL cholesterol: In males, desirable values range from 37 to 70 mg/dl; in females, from 40 to 85 mg/dl.

Implications of results

Care for patients with elevated LDL levels consists of teaching diet and lifestyle changes to reduce the risk of heart disease. (See *Diet and drug treatment recommendations*, above, and *Risk level for CAD*, page 362.)

Long-term aerobic and vigorous exercise can raise HDL levels. Counsel patients that exercising vigorously, maintaining a low-fat diet, and reducing high blood pressure may raise levels of beneficial HDL cholesterol.

Studies show that 3% of males in the United States have low HDL levels for unknown reasons even though their total cholesterol and triglyceride levels are normal. These males are at increased risk for CAD. Risk levels for CAD associated with HDL values are as follows:

< 25 mg/dl	dangerously high
26 to 35 mg/dl	high
36 to 44 mg/dl	moderate
45 to 59 mg/dl	average
60 to 74 mg/dl	below average
> 75 mg/dl	probable protection.

Decreased LDL levels can occur during acute stress (illness, burns, myocardial infarction), inflammatory joint disease, chronic pulmonary disease, and myeloma. Decreased HDL levels are often seen in patients with hypertriglyceridemia. The HDL level may increase if the elevated triglyceride level is treated.

RISK LEVEL FOR CAD

Clinical laboratories may report a cholesterol:high-density lipoprotein (HDL) ratio. This ratio gives more information than either value alone. The higher the cholesterol:HDL ratio, the greater the risk for developing atherosclerosis. Look for this ratio reported with the total cholesterol values.

Risk level	Cholesterol/HDL ratio	
	Men	Women
Low	3.43	3.27
Average	4.97	4.44
Moderate	9.55	7.05
High	23.99	11.04

High LDL levels increase the risk of CAD. Elevated HDL levels generally reflect a healthy state, but they can also indicate chronic hepatitis, early stage primary biliary cirrhosis, or alcohol consumption. Rarely, a sharp rise (to as high as 100 mg/dl) indicates a second type of HDL (alpha-HDL) that may signal CAD.

Although cholesterol fractionation provides valuable information about the risk for heart disease, other risk factors (such as diabetes mellitus, hypertension, and cigarette smoking) are at least as important.

Posttest care

- If a hematoma develops at the venipuncture site, apply warm soaks.
- Resume diet and medication withheld before the test.

Interfering factors

- Values are lowered by antilipemic medications such as clofibrate, cholestyramine, colestipol, niacin, and gemfibrozil.
- Oral contraceptives, disulfiram, alcohol, miconazole, and high doses of phenothiazines may increase values.
- Estrogens usually increase but may decrease values.
- The presence of bilirubin, hemoglobin, salicylates, iodine, and vitamins A and D may affect test results.
- Failure to send the sample to the laboratory immediately may allow spontaneous redistribution of the lipoproteins and alter test results.
- Collecting the sample in a heparinized tube may produce false elevations of values through activation of the enzyme lipase, which, in turn, causes the release of fatty acids from triglycerides.

■ Concurrent illness, especially if accompanied by fever, recent surgery, or myocardial infarction, may interfere with test results.

Lipoprotein electrophoresis test

Electrophoresis of a blood sample helps determine lipoprotein levels. The density of the four major lipoproteins varies, depending on their relative percentages of triglyceride and protein:

■ chylomicrons, which are very light lipid aggregates, consist of 85% to 95% triglycerides, 5% to 10% phospholipids, 3% to 5% cholesterol, and 1% to 2% protein

■ very-low-density (prebeta) lipoproteins (VLDL) consist of 45% to 65% triglycerides, 7% to 14% phospholipids, 7% to 14% cholesterol, and 2% to 13% protein

■ low-density (beta) lipoproteins (LDL) consist of 7% to 10% triglycerides, 20% to 30% phospholipids, 35% to 45% cholesterol, and 15% to 38% protein

■ high-density (alpha) lipoproteins (HDL) consist of about 1% to 7% triglycerides, 28% to 30% phospholipids, 17% to 20% cholesterol, and 49% to 50% protein.

For transport through the blood, most lipids must combine with water-soluble proteins (apoproteins) to form lipoproteins. Several types of lipoproteins normally exist in the body, but in certain familial disorders, the blood levels of these types change. Classification of patients by the pattern of their lipoprotein levels identifies hyperlipoproteinemias and hypolipoproteinemias.

Purpose

To classify hyperlipoproteinemia.

Patient preparation

Explain to the patient that this test helps determine how his body metabolizes fats. Instruct him to abstain from alcohol for 24 hours before the test, to eat a low-fat meal the night before the test, and to fast after midnight before the test. Tell him that this test requires a blood sample, who will perform the venipuncture and when, and that he may experience transient discomfort from the needle puncture and the pressure of the tourniquet.

Check the patient's drug history for use of heparin. Withhold antilipemics, such as cholestyramine, for about 2 weeks before the test.

Notify the laboratory if the patient is hospitalized for any other condition that might significantly alter lipoprotein metabolism, such as diabetes mellitus, nephrosis, or hypothyroidism.

Procedure

Perform a venipuncture and collect the sample in a 7-ml tube with EDTA.

Precautions

- When drawing multiple samples, collect the sample for lipoprotein phenotyping first, if possible, because venous obstruction by the tourniquet for 2 minutes (while other blood samples are being drawn) can affect test results.
- Fill the collection tube completely, and invert it gently several times to mix the sample and the anticoagulant.
- Handle the sample gently to prevent hemolysis, which can alter test results.

Reference values

- Chylomicrons: 0–2%
- LDL: 33–52% mass fraction of total lipoprotein
- VLDL: 7–28% mass fraction of total lipoprotein
- HDL: 10–30% mass fraction of total lipoprotein

The types of hyperlipoproteinemias or hypolipoproteinemias are identified by their characteristic electrophoretic patterns. The laboratory reports the type of lipoproteinemia present.

Implications of results

Familial lipoprotein disorders are classified as either hyperlipoproteinemias or hypolipoproteinemias. (See *Familial hyperlipoproteinemias*, pages 366 and 367.)

The hyperlipoproteinemias break down into six types—I, IIa, IIb, III, IV, and V. Types IIa, IIb, and IV are relatively common. In contrast, all hypolipoproteinemias are rare; they include hypobetalipoproteinemia, abetalipoproteinemia (Bassen-Kornzweig syndrome), and alpha-lipoprotein deficiency (Tangier disease).

Posttest care

- If a hematoma develops at the venipuncture site, apply warm soaks.
- Instruct the patient to resume his normal diet.
- Resume administration of medications withheld before the test.

Interfering factors

- Hemolysis caused by rough handling of the sample may affect test results.
- Failure to observe dietary and alcohol restrictions or recent use of drugs that lower lipid levels may affect the accuracy of test results.

■ Administration of heparin (which activates the enzyme lipase, producing fatty acids from triglycerides) or collection of the sample in a heparinized tube may falsely elevate values.

Liver biopsy, percutaneous

Percutaneous biopsy of the liver is the needle aspiration of a core of tissue for histologic analysis. This procedure is performed under local or general anesthesia using a special needle. Such analysis can identify hepatic disorders after ultrasonography, computed tomography scans, and radionuclide studies have failed to detect them. Because many patients with hepatic disorders have coagulation defects, testing for hemostasis should precede liver biopsy.

Purpose

To diagnose hepatic parenchymal disease, malignant tumors, and granulomatous infections.

Patient preparation

Describe the procedure to the patient, and ask if he has any questions. Explain that this test helps diagnose liver disorders. Instruct the patient to restrict food and fluids for 4 to 8 hours before the test. Tell him who will perform the biopsy and where, that the biopsy needle remains in the liver about 1 second, and that the entire procedure takes about 10 to 15 minutes.

Make sure the patient has signed a consent form. Check the patient history for hypersensitivity to the local anesthetic. Make sure prothrombin time, partial thromboplastin time, and platelet counts have been performed and that the results are recorded on the patient's chart. A blood sample is usually drawn for baseline assessment of hematocrit.

Just before the biopsy, tell the patient to void. After he does, record vital signs. Inform him that he will receive a local anesthetic but may experience pain similar to that of a punch in his right shoulder as the biopsy needle passes the phrenic nerve.

Procedure

■ For aspiration biopsy using a Menghini needle, place the patient in the supine position, with his right hand under his head. Instruct him to maintain this position and remain as still as possible during the procedure.
■ The liver is palpated, the biopsy site is selected and marked, and the anesthetic is then injected.
■ The needle flange is set to control the depth of penetration, and 2 ml of sterile normal saline solution are

FAMILIAL HYPERLIPOPROTEINEMIAS

Type	Causes and incidence
I	■ Deficient lipoprotein lipase, resulting in increased chylomicrons ■ May be induced by alcoholismp ■ Incidence: rare
IIa	■ Deficient cell receptor, resulting in increased LDL levels and excessive cholesterol synthesis ■ May be induced by hypothyroidism ■ Incidence: common
IIb	■ Deficient cell receptor, resulting in increased LDL levels and excessive cholesterol synthesis ■ May be induced by dysgammaglobulinemia, hypothyroidism, uncontrolled diabetes mellitus, or nephrotic syndrome ■ Incidence: common
III	■ Unknown cause, resulting in deficient VLDL-to-LDL conversion ■ May be induced by hypothyroidism, uncontrolled diabetes mellitus, or paraproteinemia ■ Incidence: rare
IV	■ Unknown cause, resulting in decreased levels of lipoprotein lipase ■ May be induced by uncontrolled diabetes mellitus, alcoholism, pregnancy, steroid or estrogen therapy, dysgammaglobulinemia, or hyperthyroidism ■ Incidence: common
V	■ Unknown cause, resulting in defective triglyceride clearance ■ May be induced by alcoholism, dysgammaglobulinemia, uncontrolled diabetes mellitus, nephrotic syndrome, pancreatitis, or steroid therapy ■ Incidence: rare

drawn into the syringe. The syringe is attached to the biopsy needle, and the needle is introduced into the subcutaneous tissue, through the right eighth or ninth intercostal space, between the anterior and posterior axillary lines. One ml of normal saline solution is injected to clear the needle and the plunger; then the plunger is drawn back to the 4-ml mark to create negative pressure.

■ At this point in the procedure, ask the patient to take a deep breath, exhale, and hold his breath at the end of expiration to prevent any movement of the chest wall. As the patient holds his breath, the biopsy needle is quickly inserted into the liver and withdrawn in 1 second. After the needle is withdrawn, tell the patient to resume normal respirations.

Signs and symptoms	Laboratory findings
■ Eruptive xanthomas ■ Lipemia retinalis ■ Abdominal pain	■ Increased chylomicron, total cholesterol, and triglyceride levels ■ Normal or slightly increased very-low-density lipoprotein (VLDL) levels ■ Normal or decreased low-density lipoprotein (LDL) levels and high-density lipoprotein (HDL) levels ■ Cholesterol:triglyceride ratio under 0.2
■ Premature coronary artery disease (CAD) ■ Arcus cornea ■ Xanthelasma ■ Tendinous and tuberous xanthomas	■ Increased LDL levels ■ Normal VLDL levels ■ Cholesterol:triglyceride ratio over 2.0
■ Premature CAD ■ Obesity ■ Possible xanthelasmas	■ Increased LDL, VLDL, total cholesterol, and triglyceride levels
■ Premature CAD ■ Arcus cornea ■ Eruptive tuberous xanthomas	■ Increased total cholesterol, VLDL, and triglyceride levels ■ Normal or decreased LDL levels ■ Cholesterol:triglyceride ratio of VLDL over 0.4 ■ Broad beta band observe don electrophoresis
■ Possible premature CAD ■ Obesity ■ Hypertension ■ Peripheral neuropathy	■ Increased VLDL and triglyceride levels ■ Normal LDL ■ Cholesterol:triglyceride ratio of VLDL under 0.25
■ Premature CAD ■ Abdominal pain ■ Lipemia retinalis ■ Eruptive xanthomas ■ Hepatosplenomegaly	■ Increased VLDL, total cholesterol, and triglyceride levels ■ Chylomicrons present ■ Cholesterol:triglyceride ratio under 0.6

■ The tissue specimen is then placed in a properly labeled specimen cup containing 10% formalin solution. This is done by releasing negative pressure while the point of the needle is in the formalin solution.

■ Again, 1 ml of normal saline solution is injected to clear the needle of the tissue specimen. Apply pressure to the biopsy site to stop bleeding.

Precautions

■ Percutaneous liver biopsy is contraindicated in a patient with a platelet count below 100,000/µl, prothrombin time longer than 15 seconds, vascular tumor, hepatic angioma, hydatid cyst, tense ascites, or empyema of the lungs, pleurae, peritoneum, biliary tract, or liver. If extrahepatic obstruction is suspected, ultrasonography or subcutaneous transhepatic cholangiography should rule out this condition before the biopsy is considered.

■ Pain in the abdomen or dyspnea after the biopsy may indicate perforation of an abdominal organ or pneumothorax, respectively. In such cases, complete a thorough assessment and notify the doctor at once.

■ Send the specimen to the laboratory immediately.

Normal findings

Normal liver tissue consists of sheets of hepatocytes supported by a reticular framework.

Implications of results

Examination of the hepatic tissue may reveal diffuse hepatic disease, such as cirrhosis or hepatitis, or granulomatous infections, such as tuberculosis. Primary malignant tumors include hepatocellular carcinoma, cholangiocellular carcinoma, and angiosarcoma, but hepatic metastases are more common.

Nonmalignant findings with a known focal lesion require further studies, such as laparotomy or laparoscopy with biopsy.

Posttest care

■ Position the patient on his right side for 2 hours, with a small pillow or sandbag under the costal margin to provide extra pressure. Advise bed rest for 24 hours.

■ Check the patient's vital signs every 15 minutes for 1 hour, then every 30 minutes for 4 hours, and every 4 hours thereafter for 24 hours. Throughout, observe carefully for signs of shock.

■ Watch for bleeding or signs of bile peritonitis — tenderness and rigidity around the biopsy site. Be alert for symptoms of pneumothorax, rising respiratory rate, depressed breath sounds, dyspnea, persistent shoulder pain, and pleuritic chest pain. Report such complications promptly.

■ If the patient experiences pain, which may persist for several hours after the test, administer an analgesic.

■ Tell the patient he may resume his normal diet.

Interfering factors

■ Failure to obtain a representative specimen, to place the specimen in the proper preservative, or to transport the specimen to the laboratory immediately may affect the accuracy of test results.

Long-acting thyroid stimulator test

This test is used to determine whether a patient's serum contains long-acting thyroid stimulator (LATS), an abnormal immunoglobulin (also known as thyroid-stimu-

---

MEASURING LATS

In this test, samples of the patient's serum are mixed with cultured rat thyroid cells. The activation of the enzyme adenylate cyclase in the cells reflects the amount of long-acting thyroid stimulator (LATS).

---

lating immunoglobulin or 75 IgG) that mimics the action of thyroid-stimulating hormone (TSH), although its effects are more prolonged. LATS stimulates the thyroid gland to produce and secrete thyroid hormones in excessive amounts. Thus, through the normal negative feedback mechanism, it inhibits TSH secretion. LATS is often found in patients with Graves' disease (about 80%) and in neonates whose mothers have Graves' disease because LATS crosses the placenta.

Some authorities believe that the thyroid gland hyperplasia seen in Graves' disease may be caused by LATS or other circulating antibodies. Some consider the clinical significance of this test questionable.

Purpose

To confirm diagnosis of Graves' disease (not routinely done to diagnose thyroid disorders).

Patient preparation

Explain to the patient or his parents (if the patient is an infant or child) that this test helps evaluate thyroid function. Tell him this test requires a blood sample, who will perform the venipuncture and when, and that he may feel transient discomfort from the needle puncture and the tourniquet. Advise him that the laboratory requires several days to complete the analysis.

Procedure

Draw venous blood into a 5-ml clot-activator tube. (See *Measuring LATS.*)

Precautions

- Handle the sample gently to prevent hemolysis.
- Note on the laboratory request if the patient had a radioactive scan within 48 hours before the test.

Normal findings

Normally, LATS is not present in serum.

Implications of results

LATS in serum indicates Graves' disease, even without overt signs of hyperthyroidism. About 80% of patients with Graves' disease have detectable LATS in their sera.

Posttest care

If a hematoma develops at the venipuncture site, apply warm soaks.

Interfering factors

■ Radioactive iodine in the serum may affect test results.

■ Hemolysis caused by rough handling of the sample may interfere with accurate determination of test results.

Lung biopsy

In a lung biopsy, a specimen of pulmonary tissue is excised by closed or open technique for histologic examination. Closed technique, performed under local anesthesia, includes both needle and transbronchial biopsies; open technique, performed under general anesthesia in the operating room, includes both limited and standard thoracotomy.

Needle biopsy is appropriate when the lesion is readily accessible or when it originates in the lung parenchyma, is confined to it, or is affixed to the chest wall. This procedure provides a much smaller specimen than the open technique. Transbronchial biopsy, the removal of multiple tissue specimens through a fiber-optic bronchoscope, is appropriate for diffuse infiltrative pulmonary disease, tumors, or when severe debilitation contraindicates open biopsy. Open biopsy is appropriate for the study of a well-circumscribed lesion that may require resection.

Generally, a lung biopsy is recommended after chest X-rays, a computed tomography scan, and bronchoscopy have failed to identify the cause of diffuse parenchymal pulmonary disease or a pulmonary lesion. Possible complications of lung biopsy include bleeding, infection, and pneumothorax.

Purpose

To confirm a diagnosis of diffuse parenchymal pulmonary disease and pulmonary lesions.

Patient preparation

Describe the procedure to the patient, and answer any questions he may have. Explain that this test assesses the condition of the lungs. Instruct the patient to fast after midnight before the procedure. (Sometimes clear liquids are permitted the morning of the test.) Tell him who will perform the biopsy and where and that it takes 30 to 60 minutes. Also tell him that a chest X-ray and blood studies (prothrombin time, activated partial thromboplastin time, and platelet count) will be performed before the biopsy.

Make sure the patient has signed a consent form. Check the patient history for hypersensitivity to the local anesthetic. Administer a mild sedative 30 minutes before the biopsy to help the patient relax. Tell him he'll receive a local anesthetic but may experience a sharp, transient pain when the biopsy needle touches the lung.

Procedure

■ After the biopsy site is selected, lead markers are placed on the patient's skin and X-rays are used to verify their correct placement.

■ Place the patient in a sitting position, with arms folded on a table in front of him; instruct him to maintain this position, remaining as still as possible, and to refrain from coughing.

■ The skin over the biopsy site is prepared, and the area is draped. A local anesthetic is injected with a 25G needle just above the lower rib.

■ Using a 22G needle, the examiner anesthetizes the intercostal muscles and parietal pleura, makes a small incision (2 to 3 mm) with a scalpel, and introduces the biopsy needle through the incision, chest wall, and pleura, into the tumor or pulmonary tissue.

■ If the intercostal space at the incision site is wide, the needle is inserted at a 90-degree angle; if the ribs overlap and the intercostal space is narrow, at a 45-degree angle. When the needle is in the tumor or pulmonary tissue, the specimen is obtained and the needle is withdrawn. The specimen is divided immediately: The tissue for histologic examination is placed in a properly labeled bottle containing 10% neutral buffered formalin solution; the tissue for microbiologic culture is placed in a sterile container.

Precautions

■ Needle biopsy is contraindicated in patients with a lesion that has separated from the chest wall or that is accompanied by emphysematous bullae, cysts, or gross emphysema and in patients with coagulopathy, hypoxia, pulmonary hypertension, or cardiac disease with cor pulmonale.

CLINICAL ALERT During biopsy, observe for signs of respiratory distress — shortness of breath, elevated pulse rate, and cyanosis (late sign); if such signs develop, report them immediately.

■ Because coughing or movement during the biopsy can cause tearing of the lung by the biopsy needle, keep the patient calm and still.

Normal findings

Normal pulmonary tissue has uniform texture in alveolar ducts, alveolar walls, bronchioles, and small vessels.

Implications of results

Histologic examination of a pulmonary tissue specimen can reveal squamous cell carcinoma, oat cell carcinoma, or adenocarcinoma. Such examination supplements the results of microbiologic cultures, deep-cough sputum specimens, chest X-rays, bronchoscopy, and physical examination in confirming cancer or parenchymal pulmonary disease.

Posttest care

■ Exert pressure on the biopsy site to stop the bleeding, and then apply a small bandage.
■ Check vital signs every 15 minutes for 1 hour, every hour for 4 hours, then every 4 hours for 24 hours. Watch for bleeding, shortness of breath, elevated pulse rate, diminished breath sounds on the biopsy side, and eventually, cyanosis. Make sure the chest X-ray is repeated immediately after the biopsy is completed.
■ Tell the patient he may resume his normal diet.

Interfering factors

Failure to obtain a representative tissue specimen or to store the specimen in the appropriate containers may affect test results.

Lupus erythematosus cell preparation test

Lupus erythematosus (LE) cell preparation is an in vitro procedure used in diagnosing systemic lupus erythematosus (SLE). (See *All about SLE.*) Although this test is less sensitive and reliable than either the antinuclear antibody (ANA) or the antideoxyribonucleic acid (anti-DNA) antibody test, it's often used because it requires minimal equipment and reagents.

In this test, a blood sample is mixed with laboratory-treated nucleoprotein (the antigen). If cells in the sample contains ANA, the ANA reacts with the nucleoprotein, and the cells swell and rupture. Phagocytes in the sample engulf the extruded nuclei, forming LE cells, which are detected by microscopic examination of the sample.

Purpose

■ To aid diagnosis of SLE
■ To monitor treatment of SLE. (About 60% of successfully treated patients show no LE cells after 4 to 6 weeks of therapy.)

ALL ABOUT SLE	
Who gets it?	Systemic lupus erythematosus (SLE) is primarily a disease of young women; it affects five times as many women as men. In the United States, the incidence is higher in black and Hispanic than in white populations.
What is it?	SLE is a chronic inflammatory disease of the connective tissue that produces biochemical and structural changes in the skin, joints, and muscles, usually with multiple organ involvement. It may eventually cause death from failure of vital organs, especially the kidneys. The disease isn't always fatal and can be controlled in some patients. Presence of four or more of the following criteria help support the diagnosis: ■ facial erythema (butterfly rash) ■ alopecia ■ photosensitivity ■ Raynaud's phenomenon ■ pleuritis or pericarditis ■ hemolytic anemia, leukopenia, or thrombocytopenia ■ positive antinuclear antibody or LE cell test ■ chronic false-positive serologic test for syphilis ■ profuse proteinuria ■ cellular casts ■ discoid lupus erythematosus ■ nondeforming arthritis ■ oral or nasopharyngeal ulcerations ■ psychosis or seizures.
When does it first develop?	SLE typically first develops between ages 15 and 40, but it can occur at any age.
When does it occur?	The cause is unknown. SLE is believed to stem from an autoimmune malfunction triggered by a viral, drug, environmental, or genetic stimulus.

Patient preparation

Explain to the patient that this test helps detect antibodies to his own tissue. (See *Understanding autoantibodies in autoimmune disease,* pages 374 and 375.) If appropriate, inform him that the test will be repeated to monitor his response to therapy. Advise him that he needn't restrict food or fluids. Tell him the test requires a blood sample, who will perform the venipuncture and when, and that he may experience transient discomfort from the needle puncture and the pressure of the tourniquet.

Check the patient's medication history for drugs that may affect test results, such as isoniazid, hydralazine, and procainamide. If such drugs must be continued, be sure to note this on the laboratory request.

Procedure

Perform a venipuncture and collect the sample in a 7-ml clot-activator tube.

UNDERSTANDING AUTOANTIBODIES IN AUTOIMMUNE DISEASE

When the immune system produces autoantibodies against the antigens on and in cells, two types of autoimmune disease can result.

■ *Organ-specific diseases,* such as pernicious anemia, occur when the targeted antigenic determinants are specific to an organ or tissue, or to certain cells or cell types. Lymphocytes invade the target organ, tissue, or cell and destroy targeted cells.

■ *Non–organ-specific diseases,* such as myasthenia gravis, occur when the targeted antigenic determinants are shared with other cells (self-antigens). The

Disease	Affected site	Antigen
Hashimoto's thyroiditis	Thyroid gland	Thyroglobulin, second colloid antigen, cytoplasmic microsomes, cell surface antigens
Pernicious anemia	Hematopoietic system	Intrinsic factor
Pemphigus vulgaris	Skin	Desmosomes between prickle cells in the epidermis
Myasthenia gravis	Neuromuscular system	Acetylcholine receptors of skeletal and heart muscle
Autoimmune hemolytic anemia	Hematopoietic system	Red blood cells (RBCs)
Primary biliary cirrhosis	Small bile ducts in liver	Mitochondria
Rheumatoid arthritis	Joints, blood vessels, skin, muscles, lymph nodes	Immunoglobulin G (IgG)
Goodpasture's syndrome	Lungs and kidneys	Glomerular and lung basement membranes
Systemic lupus erythematosus	Skin, joints, muscles, lungs, heart, kidneys, brain, eyes	Deoxyribonucleic acid (DNA), nucleoprotein, blood cells, clotting factors, IgG, Wassermann antigen

Precautions

Handle the sample gently to prevent hemolysis.

Normal findings

No LE cells are normally present.

consequent formation and deposition of immune complexes (Type III hypersensitivity) can cause lesions anywhere in the body.

Various diagnostic techniques are used to detect antibodies in autoimmune disease, including radioimmunoassay, hemagglutination, complement fixation, and immunofluorescence. The chart below lists common test methods and findings in various autoimmune diseases.

Antibody	Diagnostic technique
Antibodies to thyroglobulin and microsomal antigens	Radioimmunoassay, hemagglutination, complement fixation, immunofluorescence
Antibodies to gastric parietal cells and vitamin B_{12}-binding site of intrinsic factor	Immunofluorescence, radioimmunoassay
Antibodies to intercellular substances of the skin and mucous membranes	Immunofluorescence
Anti-acetylcholine antibodies	Immunoprecipitation radioimmunoassay
Anti-RBC antibodies	Direct and indirect Coombs' test
Antimitochondrial antibodies	Immunofluorescence of mitochondrial-rich cells (kidney biopsy)
Anti-gamma-globulin antibodies	Sheep RBC agglutination, latex immunoglobulin agglutination, radioimmunoassay, immunofluorescence, immunodiffusion
Anti-basement membrane antibodies	Immunofluorescence of kidney biopsy sample, radioimmunoassay
Antinuclear antibodies, anti-DNA antibodies, anti-ds-DNA antibodies, anti-SS-DNA antibodies, anti-ribonucleoprotein antibodies, anti-gamma-globulin antibodies, anti-RBC antibodies, antilymphocyte antibodies, anti-platelet antibodies, antineuronal cell antibodies, anti-Sm antibodies	Counterelectrophoresis, hemagglutination, radioimmunoassay, immunofluorescence, Coombs' test

Implications of results

The presence of at least two LE cells per high power field suggests a diagnosis of SLE. Although these cells occur primarily in SLE, they may also appear in chronic active hepatitis, rheumatoid arthritis, scleroderma, and certain drug reactions. Also, up to 25% of patients with SLE demonstrate no LE cells.

In addition to supporting clinical signs, a definitive diagnosis of SLE may require a confirming ANA or anti-DNA test. The ANA test detects autoantibodies in the serum of many SLE patients with negative LE cell tests. Anti-DNA antibodies appear in two-thirds of all SLE patients but are rare in other conditions; thus, the presence of these antibodies is strong evidence of SLE.

Because many patients with SLE have compromised immune systems, keep a clean, dry bandage over the venipuncture site for at least 24 hours and check for infection.

If test results are positive, tell the patient further tests may be required to monitor treatment.

Posttest care

If a hematoma develops at the venipuncture site, apply warm soaks.

Interfering factors

■ Certain drugs—most commonly isoniazid, hydralazine, and procainamide—can cause a syndrome resembling SLE. Other such drugs include para-aminosalicylic acid, chlorpromazine, clofibrate, phenytoin, griseofulvin, ethosuximide, gold salts, methyldopa, oral contraceptives, penicillin, propylthiouracil, phenylbutazone, methysergide, streptomycin, sulfonamides, tetracyclines, mephenytoin, quinidine, primidone, reserpine, and trimethadione.
■ Hemolysis caused by rough handling of the sample may affect the accuracy of test results.

Luteinizing hormone test, plasma

This test (also known as the interstitial-cell-stimulating hormone test) is a quantitative analysis of serum luteinizing hormone (LH) levels. Performed most often on females, it's usually ordered for anovulation and infertility studies. For accurate diagnosis, results must be evaluated in light of findings obtained from related hormone tests (follicle-stimulating hormone [FSH], estrogen, and testosterone levels, for example).

LH is a glycoprotein secreted by basophilic cells of the anterior pituitary. In females, cyclic LH secretion (with FSH) causes ovulation and transforms the ovarian follicle into the corpus luteum, which, in turn, secretes progesterone. (See *LH secretion cycle.*) In males, continuous LH secretion stimulates the interstitial (Leydig) cells of the testes to release testosterone, which stimulates and maintains spermatogenesis (with FSH).

LH SECRETION CYCLE

The menstrual cycle is divided into three distinct phases: the menstrual phase (days 1 to 5); the proliferative, or follicular, phase (days 6 to 13); and after ovulation on day 14, the secretory, or luteal, phase (days 15 to 28).

In a normal cycle, the menstrual phase is characterized by endometrial sloughing, corpus luteum degeneration, and new follicle growth. During this stage, estrogen and progesterone levels are low, triggering increased secretion of follicle-stimulating hormone (FSH) and luteinizing hormone (LH).

During the follicular phase, the follicle stimulated by FSH reaches full size and increases its secretion of estrogen. Simultaneously, FSH decreases while LH increases slowly but steadily. During the late follicular phase, LH rises sharply and FSH rises slightly. At about the 14th day, within hours of this abrupt surge in LH, estrogen levels in the plasma drop and ovulation occurs. After ovulation, the concentration of both LH and FSH falls rapidly.

During the final, or luteal, phase, the follicle reorganizes as the corpus luteum and secretes progesterone and estrogen. Within 7 or 8 days after ovulation, if fertilization hasn't occurred, the corpus luteum regresses and progesterone and estrogen levels decrease. The endometrium sloughs, and the menstrual cycle begins again.

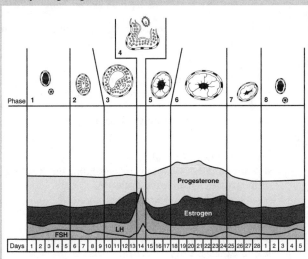

1. Menstrual phase
   (degeneration of corpus luteum)
2. Early follicular phase
   (development of follicle)
3. Late follicular phase
   (development of follicle)
4. Ovulation at midcycle
   (rupture of follicle)

5. Early luteal phase
   (development of corpus luteum)
6. Midluteal phase
   (development of corpus luteum)
7. Late luteal phase
   (development of corpus luteum)
8. Menstrual phase
   (degeneration of corpus luteum)

Purpose

- To detect ovulation
- To assess causes for infertility
- To evaluate amenorrhea
- To monitor therapy designed to induce ovulation.

Patient preparation

Explain to the patient that this test helps determine if her secretion of female hormones is normal. Because there is no evidence that LH levels are affected by fasting, eating, or exercise, such pretest restrictions may be unnecessary. Tell the patient that this test requires a blood sample, who will perform the venipuncture and when, and that she may experience discomfort from the needle puncture and the pressure of the tourniquet. Inform her that the laboratory requires at least 3 days to complete the analysis.

Withhold drugs that may interfere with plasma LH levels, such as steroids (including estrogens or progesterone), for 48 hours before the test. If these medications must be continued, note this on the laboratory request.

If the patient is trying to determine the optimal time to become pregnant, a home ovulation test may be useful as well.

Procedure

Perform a venipuncture and collect the sample in a 7-ml clot-activator tube.

Precautions

■ Handle the sample gently to prevent hemolysis.
■ If the patient is premenopausal, indicate the phase of her menstrual cycle on the laboratory request. If she is menopausal, note this on the laboratory request.

Reference values

Normal values vary widely:
■ Adult females — values vary, depending on the phase of the patient's menstrual cycle:
– follicular phase, to 15 mIU/ml
– ovulatory phase, 30 to 60 mIU/ml
– luteal phase, to 15 mIU/ml
■ Postmenopausal females: 50 to 100 mIU/ml
■ Adult males: 5 to 20 mIU/ml
■ Children: 4 to 20 mIU/ml.

Implications of results

In females, absence of a midcycle peak in LH secretion may indicate anovulation. Decreased or low-normal levels may indicate hypogonadism; these findings are commonly associated with amenorrhea. High LH levels may indicate congenital absence of ovaries or ovarian failure associated with Stein-Leventhal syndrome (polycystic ovary syndrome), Turner's syndrome (ovarian dysgenesis), menopause, or early-stage acromegaly. Infertility can result from either primary or secondary gonadal dysfunction.

In males, low values may indicate secondary gonadal dysfunction (of hypothalamic or pituitary origin); high values may indicate testicular failure (primary hypogonadism) or destruction or congenital absence of testes.

Posttest care

- If a hematoma develops at the venipuncture site, apply warm soaks.
- Resume administration of medications that were discontinued before the test.

Interfering factors

- Failure to observe medication restrictions may prevent accurate determination of test results. Steroids (including estrogens, progesterone, and testosterone) may decrease plasma LH levels.
- A radioactive scan performed within 1 week before the test may influence test results because plasma LH levels are determined by radioimmunoassay.
- Hemolysis caused by rough handling of the sample may interfere with accurate determination of test results.

Lyme disease serology test

Lyme disease is a multisystem disorder characterized by dermatologic, neurologic, cardiac, and rheumatic manifestations in various stages. Epidemiologic and serologic studies implicate a commonly tickborne spirochete, *Borrelia burgdorferi*, as the causative agent.

Serologic tests, both indirect immunofluorescent and enzyme-linked immunosorbent assays, measure antibody response to this spirochete and indicate current infection or past exposure. These assays can identify 50% of patients with early-stage Lyme disease; nearly 100% of patients with later complications of carditis, neuritis, or arthritis; and 100% of patients in remission.

In an indirect immunofluorescent assay, *Borrelia burgdorferi* is grown in culture, fixed to a microscope slide, and then incubated with a human serum sample. A fluorescein-labeled antiglobulin is then introduced into the antigen-antibody complex. Any human antibody that binds to the spirochete is detected by viewing (under an ultraviolet microscope) the fluorescent antiglobulin that attaches to it.

Purpose

To confirm or rule out diagnosis of Lyme disease.

Patient preparation

Explain to the patient that this test helps determine whether his symptoms are caused by Lyme disease. Tell him that this test requires a blood sample, who will perform the venipuncture and when, and that he may experience transient discomfort from the needle puncture and the pressure of the tourniquet.

Procedure

Perform a venipuncture and collect the sample in a 7-ml clot-activator tube.

Precautions

- Handle the specimen carefully to prevent hemolysis.
- Send the specimen to the laboratory immediately.

Normal findings

Normal serum is nonreactive.

Implications of results

A positive Lyme serologic test strongly suggests the diagnosis but isn't definitive.

Other treponemal diseases and high rheumatoid factor titers can cause false-positive results. Patients with other treponemal diseases demonstrate considerable cross-reactivity, and up to 20% of patients with high rheumatoid factor titers may have positive Lyme disease reactions.

In addition, a negative result doesn't rule out Lyme disease. More than 15% of patients with Lyme disease fail to develop antibodies.

Posttest care

If a hematoma develops at the venipuncture site, apply warm soaks.

Interfering factors

- Analysis of serum with high lipid levels may cause inaccurate test results and requires repetition of the test after a period of restricted fat intake.
- Blood samples contaminated with other bacteria can cause false-positive results.
- Hemolysis caused by excessive agitation of the sample can affect the accuracy of test results.

Lymph node biopsy

Lymph node biopsy is the surgical excision of an active lymph node or the needle aspiration of a nodal specimen for histologic examination. Both techniques usually use local anesthesia and sample the superficial nodes in the cervical, supraclavicular, axillary, or inguinal region. Excision is the preferred technique because it provides a larger specimen.

Usually flat and bean-shaped, lymph nodes swell during infection but return to normal size as infection clears. A biopsy is indicated when nodal enlargement is prolonged and accompanied by backache, leg edema, breathing and swallowing difficulties, and later, weight loss, weakness, severe itching, fever, night sweats, cough, hemoptysis, or hoarseness. Generalized or localized lymph node enlargement is typical of such diseases as chronic lymphocytic leukemia, Hodgkin's disease, malignant lymphoma, infectious mononucleosis, and rheumatoid arthritis.

A complete blood count, liver function studies, liver and spleen scans, and X-rays should precede this test.

Purpose

- To determine the cause of lymph node enlargement
- To distinguish between benign and malignant lymph node tumors
- To stage metastatic cancer.

Patient preparation

Describe the procedure to the patient, and ask if he has any questions. Explain that this test allows microscopic study of lymph node tissue.

If the biopsy will be excisional, instruct the patient to restrict food from midnight and to drink only clear liquids. (If a general anesthetic is needed for biopsy of deeper nodes, he must also restrict fluids.) For a needle biopsy, inform him that he needn't restrict food or fluids. Tell him who will perform the biopsy and where, that the procedure takes 15 to 30 minutes, and that the analysis takes 1 day to complete.

Make sure the patient has signed a consent form. Check the patient history for hypersensitivity to the anesthetic. If the patient will receive a local anesthetic, explain that he may experience discomfort during the injection. Just before the biopsy, record baseline vital signs.

Procedure

- *Excisional biopsy*: Prepare the skin over the biopsy site, and drape the area for privacy. The anesthetic is then administered. The surgeon makes an incision, removes an entire node, and places it in a properly labeled bottle containing normal saline solution. Then the wound is sutured, and a sterile dressing is applied.
- *Needle biopsy*: After preparing the biopsy site and administering a local anesthetic, the surgeon grasps the node between his thumb and forefinger, inserts the needle directly into the node, and obtains a small core spec-

imen. Then he removes the needle and places the specimen in a properly labeled bottle containing normal saline solution. Pressure is exerted on the biopsy site to control bleeding and an adhesive bandage is applied.

Precautions

Storing the tissue specimen in normal saline solution instead of in 10% formalin solution allows part of the specimen to be used for cytologic impression smears, which are studied along with the biopsy specimen.

Normal findings

The normal lymph node is encapsulated by collagenous connective tissue and is divided into smaller lobes by tissue strands called trabeculae. It has an outer cortex, composed of lymphoid cells and nodules or follicles containing lymphocytes, and an inner medulla, composed of reticular phagocytic cells that collect and drain fluid.

Implications of results

Histologic examination of the tissue specimen distinguishes between malignant and nonmalignant causes of lymph node enlargement. Lymphatic malignancy accounts for up to 5% of all cancers and is now thought to affect other tissues as well. Hodgkin's disease, a lymphoma affecting the entire lymph system, is the leading cancer affecting adolescents and young adults. Lymph node malignancy may also represent metastatic cancer.

When histologic results aren't clear or the nodes aren't involved, mediastinoscopy or laparotomy can provide another nodal specimen. Occasionally, lymphangiography can furnish additional diagnostic information.

Posttest care

■ Check vital signs and watch for bleeding, tenderness, and redness at the biopsy site.
■ Tell the patient that he may resume his usual diet.

Interfering factors

Improper specimen storage or failure to obtain a representative tissue specimen may alter test results.

Lymphocyte transformation test

Transformation tests permit evaluation of lymphocyte competence without injection of antigens into the patient's skin. These in vitro tests eliminate the risk of adverse effects, and they can accurately demonstrate the ability of lymphocytes to proliferate and to recognize and respond to antigens; this response is called transformation. Transformation tests include mitogen assays, antigen assays, and mixed lymphocyte culture (MLC) studies.

The mitogen assay, performed using nonspecific plant lectins, evaluates the mitotic response of T and B lymphocytes to a foreign antigen. Phytohemagglutinin (PHA) and concanavalin A (ConA) stimulate T lymphocytes preferentially, whereas pokeweed stimulates B lymphocytes primarily and T lymphocytes to a lesser extent.

In the mitogen assay, a purified culture of lymphocytes from the patient's blood is incubated with a nonspecific mitogen for 72 hours — the interval during which the mitogen's greatest effect on deoxyribonucleic acid (DNA) synthesis usually occurs. The culture is then pulse-labeled with radioactive thymidine, which is incorporated in the newly formed DNA of dividing cells.

The uptake of radioactive thymidine can be measured by a liquid scintillation spectrophotometer in counts per minute (cpm), which parallels the rate of mitosis. Lymphocyte responsiveness, or the extent of mitosis, is then reported as a stimulation index, determined by dividing the cpm of the stimulated culture by the cpm of a control culture.

The antigen assay uses specific antigens, such as purified protein derivative (PPD), Candida, mumps, tetanus toxoid, or streptokinase, to stimulate lymphocyte transformation. After incubation of 4-½ to 7 days, transformation is measured by the same method used in the mitogen assay.

The mixed lymphocyte culture (MLC) assay tests the response of lymphocytes to histocompatibility antigens determined by the D locus of the sixth chromosome. The MLC assay is useful in matching transplant recipients and donors and in testing immunocompetence. In this assay, lymphocytes from a recipient and potential donor are cultured together for 5 days to test compatibility. Recipient and potential donor lymphocytes (if viable and unaltered) will recognize any genetic differences and undergo transformation, demonstrating incompatibility. In the one-way MLC, one group of lymphocytes is pretreated with radiation or mitomycin C so that it can't divide but can still stimulate the other group of lymphocytes.

Lymphocyte transformation is identified by increased incorporation of radioactive thymidine labeling and is reported as the stimulation index. After the culture is labeled with radioactive thymidine, the MLC stimulation index is determined. Various lymphocyte marker assays

LYMPHOCYTE MARKER ASSAYS

A normal immune response requires a balance between the regulatory activities of several interacting cell types – primarily T-helper and T-suppressor cells. Highly specific monoclonal antibodies can define levels of lymphocyte differentiation in normal and malignant cell populations. Direct and indirect immunofluorescence, microcytotoxicity, and immunoperoxidase immunoassay techniques are used most frequently; these tests use an anticoagulated blood sample combined with monoclonal antibodies that react with specific T- and B-cell markers. The chart below lists some commonly ordered lymphocyte marker assays and their indications.

Lymphocyte marker assay	Indications
CD3	■ To measure mature T cells in immune dysfunction
CD4	■ To identify and characterize the proportion of T-helper cells in autoimmune or immunoregulatory disorders ■ To detect immunodeficiency disorders such as AIDS ■ To differentiate T-cell acute lymphoblastic leukemia from T-cell lymphomas and other lymphoproliferative disorders
CD8	■ To identify and characterize the proportion of T-suppressor cells in autoimmune and immunoregulatory disorders ■ To characterize lymphoproliferative disorders
CD20	■ To differentiate lymphoproliferative disorders of T-cell origin, such as T-cell lymphocytic leukemia and lymphoblastic lymphoma, from those of non-T-cell origin
CD19	■ To differentiate lymphoproliferative disorders of B-cell origin, such as B-cell chyronic lymphocytic leukemia
CALLA (common acute lymphocytic leukemia antigen) marker, CD10	■ To identify B-cell lymphoproliferative disorders, such as B-cell chronic lymphocytic leukemia ■ To identify bone marrow regeneration
Lymphocyte subset panel (CD3, CD4, CD8, CD19) Lymphocytic leukemia marker panel	■ To identify non-T-cell acute lymphocytic leukemia ■ To evaluate immunodeficiencies ■ To identify immunoregulation associated with autoimmune disorders
(CD3, CD4, CD8, CD19, CD10)	■ To characterize lymphoid malignancies ■ To characterize lymphocytic leukemias as T, B, or non-T/non-B, regardless of the stage of the malignant cells

can be performed to analyze malignant and normal cell populations. (See *Lymphocyte marker assays.*)

The neutrophils' ability to engulf and destroy bacteria and foreign particles can also be determined. (See *Neutrophil function tests.*)

Purpose

■ To assess and monitor genetic and acquired immunodeficiency states

NEUTROPHIL FUNCTION TESTS

Normal neutrophils—the body's primary defense against bacterial invasion—engulf and destroy bacteria and foreign particles by a process known as phagocytosis. In patients who have repeated bacterial infections, neutrophil function tests may show that the neutrophils cannot kill target bacteria or migrate to the infected site (chemotaxis).

Neutrophil killing activity can be evaluated by the *nitroblue tetrazolium (NBT) test,* which relies on neutrophil generation of bactericidal enzymes and toxins during killing. This action increases cellular oxygen consumption and glucose metabolism, which reduces colorless NBT to blue formazan. The reduced dye is extracted with pyridine and measured photometrically; the extent of reduction indicates phagocytic activity.

Neutrophil killing activity can also be evaluated by measuring the neutrophils' *chemiluminescence*—ability to emit light. After a neutrophil phagocytizes a microorganism, oxygen-containing substances form within phagocytic vacuoles. As the cell is stimulated, it emits light in proportion to the amount of oxygen-containing substances that are formed, providing an indirect measurement of phagocytosis.

Chemotaxis can be assessed in vitro by placing bacteria in the lower half of a two-part chamber and phagocytic neutrophils in the upper half. After incubation, migrating cells are counted microscopically and compared to standard values.

■ To provide histocompatibility typing of both tissue transplant recipients and donors

■ To detect if a patient has been exposed to various pathogens, such as those that cause malaria, hepatitis, and mycoplasmal pneumonia.

Patient preparation

Explain to the patient that this test evaluates lymphocyte function, which is the keystone of the immune system. If appropriate, inform him that the test monitors his response to therapy. For histocompatibility typing, explain that this test helps determine the best match for a transplant.

Advise the patient that he needn't restrict food or fluids. Tell him that this test requires a blood sample, who will perform the venipuncture and when, and that he may feel transient discomfort from the needle puncture and the pressure of the tourniquet. If a radioisotope scan is scheduled, make sure the serum sample for this test is drawn first.

Procedure

Perform a venipuncture. If the patient is an adult, collect the sample in a 7-ml heparinized tube; for a child, use a 5-ml heparinized tube.

Precautions

Fill the collection tube completely, and invert it gently several times to mix the sample and anticoagulant. Send the sample to the laboratory immediately. The specimen should be tested within 24 hours. Do not refrigerate or freeze the specimen.

Normal findings

Results depend on the mitogens used. Reference ranges accompany test results. In general, a positive test is normal; a negative test indicates deficiency.

Implications of results

■ Educate the patient about protection from unnecessary exposure to infectious agents.

■ In the mitogen and antigen assays, a low stimulation index or unresponsiveness indicates a depressed or defective immune system. Serial testing can be performed to monitor the effectiveness of therapy in a patient with an immunodeficiency disease.

In the MLC test, the stimulation index is a measure of compatibility. A high index indicates poor compatibility; conversely, a low stimulation index indicates good compatibility.

A high stimulation index in response to the relevant pathogen can also demonstrate exposure to malaria, hepatitis, mycoplasmal pneumonia, periodontal disease, and certain viral infections in patients who no longer have detectable serum antibodies.

Posttest care

■ Because many of these patients may have a compromised immune system, take special care to keep the venipuncture site clean and dry.

■ If a hematoma develops at the venipuncture site, apply warm soaks.

Interfering factors

■ Pregnancy or the use of oral contraceptives depresses lymphocyte response to PHA and thus causes a low stimulation index.

■ Chemotherapy may affect the accuracy of test results unless pretherapy baseline values are available for comparison.

■ A radioisotope scan performed within 1 week before the test or failure to send the sample to the laboratory immediately can affect the accuracy of test results.

Lysozyme test

Lysozyme, a low-molecular-weight enzyme, is present in mucus, saliva, tears, skin secretions, and various internal body cells and fluids. This enzyme (also known as muramidase) splits, or lyses, the cell walls of gram-positive bacteria and, with complement and other blood factors, acts to destroy them. Lysozyme seems to be synthesized in granulocytes and monocytes, and it first appears in serum after destruction of such cells. When serum lysozyme levels exceed three times the normal rate, the enzyme appears in the urine. However, because renal tissue also contains lysozyme, renal injury alone can cause measurable excretion of this enzyme.

This test measures urine lysozyme levels turbidimetrically. Serum lysozyme values, using the same method, confirm the results of urine testing.

Purpose

■ To aid diagnosis of acute monocytic or granulocytic leukemia and to monitor the progression of these diseases

■ To evaluate proximal tubular function and to diagnose renal impairment

■ To detect rejection or infarction of a kidney transplant.

Patient preparation

Explain to the patient that this test evaluates renal function and the immune system. Advise him that he need not restrict food or fluids before the test. Tell him the test requires collection of a 24-hour urine specimen, and instruct him how to collect the specimen correctly. Test results should be available in 1 day.

If a female patient is menstruating, the test may have to be rescheduled.

Procedure

Collect a 24-hour urine specimen.

Precautions

■ Tell the patient to avoid contaminating the urine specimen with toilet tissue or stool.

■ Cover and refrigerate the specimen during the collection period. If the patient is catheterized, keep the collection bag on ice.

■ Send the specimen to the laboratory as soon as the test is completed.

Reference values

Normally, urine lysozyme values are less than 3 mg/24 hours.

Implications of results

Elevated urine lysozyme levels are characteristic of impaired renal proximal tubular reabsorption, acute pyelonephritis, nephrotic syndrome, tuberculosis of the kidney, severe extrarenal infection, rejection or infarction of a kidney transplant, and polycythemia vera.

Urine levels rise markedly after acute onset or relapse of monocytic or myelomonocytic leukemia and rise moderately after acute onset or relapse of granulocytic (myeloid) leukemia.

Urine lysozyme levels remain normal or decrease in lymphocytic leukemia, and remain normal in myeloblastic and myelocytic leukemias.

Interfering factors

The presence of bacteria in the specimen decreases lysozyme levels; blood or saliva in the specimen raises lysozyme levels.

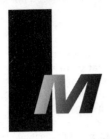

Magnesium test, serum

This quantitative test measures serum levels of magnesium, the most abundant intracellular cation after potassium. Magnesium helps regulate intracellular metabolism, activates many essential enzymes, and affects the metabolism of nucleic acids and proteins. Most important, it is essential to neuromuscular function; it helps transport sodium and potassium across cell membranes and, through its effect on the secretion of parathyroid hormone, influences intracellular calcium levels. Most magnesium is found in bone and in intracellular fluid; a small amount is found in extracellular fluid. Magnesium is absorbed by the small intestine and is excreted in the urine and feces.

Purpose

- To evaluate electrolyte status
- To assess neuromuscular or renal function.

Patient preparation

Explain to the patient that this test determines the magnesium content of the blood. Instruct him not to use magnesium salts (such as milk of magnesia or Epsom salts) for at least 3 days before the test but that he need not restrict food or fluids. Tell him that the test requires a blood sample, who will perform the venipuncture and when, and that he may feel transient discomfort from the needle puncture.

Procedure

Perform a venipuncture, without a tourniquet if possible, and collect the sample in a 7-ml clot-activator tube.

Precautions

Handle the sample gently to prevent hemolysis. This is crucial because 75% of the blood's magnesium is present in red blood cells.

Reference values

Normal serum magnesium levels range from 1.7 to 2.1 mg/dl or from 1.5 to 2.5 mEq/L.

Implications of results

High serum magnesium levels (hypermagnesemia) that aren't caused by magnesium administration or ingestion most commonly occur in renal failure, when the kidneys excrete inadequate amounts of magnesium. Adrenal insufficiency (Addison's disease) can also elevate serum magnesium levels.

CLINICAL ALERT In suspected or confirmed hypermagnesemia, observe the patient for lethargy; flushing; diaphoresis; decreased blood pressure; slow, weak pulse; nausea; vomiting; diminished deep tendon reflexes; muscle weakness; slow, shallow respirations; and cardiac arrhythmias.

Educate patients at risk for hypermagnesemia about antacids, laxatives, and mineral supplements that contain magnesium. Monitor and maintain airway and ventilation in patients who develop respiratory depression from hypermagnesemia. Patients with elevated magnesium levels require ECG monitoring for bradycardia, prolonged PR interval, wide QRS complex, prolonged QT interval, atrioventricular blocks, and asystole. Calcium I.V. may be administered to reverse respiratory depression and arrhythmias.

Abnormally low serum magnesium levels (hypomagnesemia) most commonly result from chronic alcoholism. Other causes include malabsorption syndrome, diarrhea, limited absorption after bowel resection, prolonged bowel or gastric aspiration, acute pancreatitis, primary aldosteronism, severe burns, conditions that cause hypercalcemia (including hyperparathyroidism), and use of certain diuretics.

CLINICAL ALERT In patients with hypomagnesemia, watch for leg and foot cramps, hyperactive deep tendon reflexes, mental status changes (disorientation, confusion, and hallucinations), cardiac arrhythmias, muscle weakness, seizures, twitching, tetany, and tremors.

For patients with hypomagnesemia, monitor ECG for tachycardia, widened QRS complex, prolonged QT interval, ST-segment depression, and T-wave inversion. These patients are highly susceptible to digitalis toxicity and must be monitored closely. Monitor and maintain the airway to prevent respiratory distress related to laryngeal spasm. Monitor for dysphagia. To prevent aspiration, assess swallowing before administering liquids or oral medications.

Posttest care

If a hematoma develops at the venipuncture site, ease discomfort by applying warm soaks.

Interfering factors

■ Obtaining a blood specimen above an I.V. site that's receiving a solution containing magnesium may cause a false-positive result.

■ Excessive use of antacids or cathartics or excessive infusion of magnesium sulfate raises magnesium levels.

■ Prolonged I.V. infusions that do not contain magnesium suppress levels.

■ Excessive use of diuretics decreases magnesium levels.

■ I.V. administration of calcium gluconate may falsely decrease serum magnesium levels determined by the Titan yellow method.

■ Using a tourniquet causes venous stasis and may alter test results.

■ Hemolysis causes falsely elevated serum magnesium levels.

Magnesium test, urine

This test measures the urine level of magnesium, an important electrolyte absorbed in the intestinal tract and excreted in the urine. Magnesium is found primarily in the bones and in intracellular fluid; a small amount is present in extracellular fluid. This element activates many enzyme systems, helps transport sodium and potassium across cell membranes, affects nucleic acid and protein metabolism, and influences intracellular calcium levels through its effect on parathyroid hormone secretion.

Measurement of urine magnesium was seldom used in the past, but it's becoming more widely used because magnesium deficiency is detectable earlier in urine than in serum. The test is used to rule out magnesium deficiency as the cause of neurologic symptoms and to help evaluate glomerular function in suspected renal disease.

Magnesium deficiency usually results from poor absorption, often caused by increased absorption of calcium; magnesium absorption increases as dietary intake of calcium increases.

Purpose

■ To rule out magnesium deficiency in patients with symptoms of central nervous system irritation

■ To detect excessive urinary excretion of magnesium

■ To help evaluate glomerular function in renal disease.

Patient preparation

Explain to the patient that this test determines urine magnesium levels. Advise him that no special restrictions are necessary and that the test requires a 24-hour urine specimen.

Inquire whether the patient is receiving magnesium-containing antacids, ethacrynic acid, thiazide diuretics (for example, spironolactone), or aldosterone. If he is, be sure to note this on the laboratory request.

Procedure

Collect a 24-hour urine specimen.

Precautions

Tell the patient not to contaminate the urine specimen with toilet tissue or stool and to avoid urinating directly into the container because it contains an acid preservative.

Reference values

Normal urinary excretion of magnesium is less than 150 mg/24 hours (atomic absorption).

Implications of results

Low urine magnesium levels may result from malabsorption, acute or chronic diarrhea, diabetic acidosis, dehydration, pancreatitis, advanced renal failure, primary aldosteronism, or decreased dietary intake of magnesium.

Elevated urine magnesium levels may result from early chronic renal disease, adrenocortical insufficiency (Addison's disease), chronic alcoholism, or chronic ingestion of magnesium-containing antacids.

Magnesium imbalances cause a variety of clinical effects. (See *Signs and symptoms of magnesium imbalance.*)

Interfering factors

■ Increased calcium intake reduces urinary excretion of magnesium.
■ Ethacrynic acid, thiazide diuretics, aldosterone, or excessive amounts of magnesium-containing antacids elevate urine magnesium levels.
■ Spironolactone lowers urine magnesium levels.
■ Failure to collect all urine during the test period may affect the accuracy of test results.

Manganese test

This test measures serum levels of the trace element manganese. Manganese is found throughout the body but concentrates mainly in the pituitary, pineal, and lactating mammary glands as well as in the liver and bones. Although the function of manganese in human physiology is only partially understood, it is known to activate several enzymes—including cholinesterase and arginase—that are essential to metabolism. Arginase,

SIGNS AND SYMPTOMS OF MAGNESIUM IMBALANCE

A deficiency or excess of magnesium can affect various body systems and cause numerous signs and symptoms, as shown below.

Body system	Hypomagnesemia	Hypermagnesemia
Neuromuscular system	■ Hyperirritability, tetany, leg and foot cramps, and Chvostek's sign (facial muscle spasms induced by tapping the area over the branches of the facial nerve)	■ Diminished reflexes, muscle weakness, flaccid paralysis, and respiratory muscle paralysis, which may cause respiratory distress
Central nervous system	■ Confusion, delusions, hallucinations, and seizures	■ Drowsiness, flushing, lethargy, confusion, and diminished sensorium
Cardiovascular system	■ Arrhythmias, vasomotor changes (vasodilation and hypotension) and, occasionally, hypertension	■ Bradycardia, weak pulse, hypotension, heart block, and cardiac arrest (common when serum levels reach 25 mEq/L)

for example, is necessary for the formation of urea during protein catabolism.

Because of poor intestinal absorption, the body retains only a fraction of the manganese supplied by such foods as unrefined cereals, green leafy vegetables, and nuts.

Industrial workers exposed to potentially dangerous levels of manganese may require testing for toxicity. Such toxicity can follow inhalation of manganese dust or fumes—a constant hazard in the steel and dry-cell battery industries—or ingestion of contaminated water.

Purpose

To detect manganese toxicity.

Patient preparation

Explain to the patient that this test determines the level of manganese in the blood. Inform him that he needn't restrict food or fluids. Tell him this test requires a blood sample, who will perform the venipuncture and when, and that he may feel some discomfort from the needle puncture and the pressure of the tourniquet.

Check the patient's medication history for use of drugs that may influence serum manganese levels and record them on the laboratory slip.

Procedure

Perform a venipuncture and collect the sample in a metal-free collection tube. Laboratories will supply a special kit for this test on request.

Precautions

Handle the sample gently to prevent hemolysis, and send it to the laboratory immediately.

Reference values

Normal serum manganese values range from 0.04 to 1.4 µg/dl.

Implications of results

Significantly elevated serum levels indicate manganese toxicity, which requires prompt medical attention to prevent central nervous system deterioration.

Depressed serum manganese levels may indicate deficient dietary intake, although deficiency hasn't been linked to human disease.

Posttest care

If a hematoma develops at the venipuncture site, apply warm soaks.

Interfering factors

■ High dietary intake of calcium and phosphorus can interfere with intestinal absorption of manganese and thus decrease serum levels.

■ Serum manganese levels are influenced by estrogen, which increases the circulating level. Glucocorticoids affect levels by altering the distribution of manganese in the body.

■ Hemolysis caused by rough handling of the sample may alter test results.

■ Failure to use a metal-free collection tube can affect test results.

Melanin test, urine

This relatively rare test measures urine levels of melanin, the brown-black pigment that colors the skin, hair, and eyes. An end product of tyrosine metabolism, melanin is produced by specialized cells called melanocytes.

Cutaneous melanomas—malignant tumors that produce excessive amounts of melanin—develop most often on the head and neck but may also originate in mucous membranes (as in the rectum), the retinas, or the central nervous system. Patients with these tumors may excrete melanin precursors—melanogens—in their urine. If the urine is left standing, exposure to air converts the melanogens to melanin in about 24 hours.

In Thormählen's test, sodium nitroprusside (sodium nitroferricyanide) causes characteristic color changes that reveal the presence of melanogens or melanin.

More specific tests, such as chromatography, isolate and measure the pigment.

Purpose

To aid in diagnosis of malignant melanomas.

Patient preparation

Explain to the patient what melanin is, and tell him this test detects its presence in urine. Inform him that he needn't restrict food or fluids before the test. Tell him the test requires a random urine specimen, and teach him the correct collection technique.

Procedure

Collect a random urine specimen.

Precautions

Send the specimen to the laboratory immediately.

Normal findings

A negative test for melanogens or melanin is normal.

Implications of results

In the presence of a visible skin tumor, large quantities of melanin or melanogens in urine indicate advanced metastasis. Because primary melanomas may develop in internal organs, large quantities of melanin or melanogens in a urine specimen from a patient who does not have a visible skin tumor indicate an internal melanoma.

Posttest care

Offer emotional support if a malignancy is diagnosed.

Interfering factors

Failure to send the urine specimen to the laboratory immediately may interfere with test results.

Methemoglobin test

Methemoglobin (MetHb, Hb M) is a structural hemoglobin (Hb) variant, which is formed when the heme portion of deoxygenated Hb is oxidized from the normal ferrous state to the abnormal ferric state. When this occurs, the heme is incapable of combining with oxygen and transporting it to the tissues, and the patient becomes cyanotic. Exposure to nitrites, such as aniline dyes, in the workplace or in certain drugs, such as acetanilid, nitroglycerin, benzocaine, chlorates, lidocaine, dietary nitrates and nitrites, phenacetin, sulfonamides, primaquine, and resorcinol; carbon monoxide poisoning; or excessive radiation create a high risk of methemoglobinemia.

Purpose
- To detect acquired methemoglobinemia from excessive radiation or the toxic effects of chemicals or drugs
- To detect congenital methemoglobinemia.

Patient preparation
Obtain a history of the patient's hematologic status and hemoglobin disorder, conditions that produce nitrite, and exposure to drugs that are nitrite sources. Explain to the patient that this test is used to detect abnormal Hb in the blood. Tell him that a blood sample will be taken, who will perform the venipuncture and when, and that he may feel slight discomfort from the tourniquet pressure and the needle puncture. Tell the patient to avoid medications that can interfere with test results, such as benzocaine, nitrates, and sulfonamides.

Procedure
Perform a venipuncture and collect a sample in a 7-ml heparinized tube.

Precautions
- Completely fill the collection tube, and invert it gently several times.
- To avoid hemolysis, do not shake the tube vigorously.
- Place the collection tube on ice and send it to the laboratory immediately.

Reference values
Normal MetHb levels are 0% to 1.5% of total Hb.

Implications of results
High MetHb levels may reflect acquired or hereditary methemoglobinemia, carbon monoxide poisoning, use of certain drugs, or exposure to certain substances.

MetHb levels may be low in patients with pancreatitis.

Posttest care
If a hematoma develops at the venipuncture site, apply warm soaks.

Interfering factors
- Inorganic nitrate consumed by the mother can be converted to the nitrite ion in breast-feeding infants, causing nitrite toxicity and increased MetHb levels.
- Acetanilid, aniline dyes, nitroglycerin, benzocaine, chlorates, lidocaine, nitrates, nitrites, phenacetin, sulfonamides, radiation, primaquine, and resorcinol may increase MetHb levels.

Monoclonal test for cytomegalovirus, rapid

Cytomegalovirus (CMV), a member of the herpesvirus group, can cause systemic infection in congenitally infected infants and in immunocompromised patients, such as transplant recipients, patients receiving chemotherapy for neoplastic disease, and those with acquired immunodeficiency syndrome.

In the past, CMV infections were detected in the laboratory by recognizing the distinctive cytopathic effects (CPEs) that the virus produced in conventional tube cell cultures. In this slow method of detecting CMV, CPE cultures grow in about 9 days. The faster shell vial assay (rapid monoclonal test) is based on the availability of a monoclonal antibody specific for the 72-kd protein of CMV synthesized during the immediate early stage of viral replication.

Through indirect immunofluorescence, CMV-infected fibroblasts are recognized by their dense, homogeneous staining confined to the nucleus. The smooth, regular shape of the nucleus and the surrounding nuclear membrane readily differentiate infected cells from nonspecific background fluorescence that may be present in some specimens.

Purpose

To obtain rapid laboratory diagnosis of CMV infection, especially in immunocompromised patients who are at risk for developing systemic CMV infection.

Patient preparation

Explain the purpose of the test, and describe the procedure for collecting the specimen, which will depend on the laboratory used.

Procedure

Specimens should be collected during the prodromal and acute stages of clinical infection to maximize the chances of detecting CMV. Each type of specimen requires a specific collection device, as follows:

- throat: microbiologic transport swab
- urine or cerebrospinal fluid: sterile screw-capped tube or vial
- bronchoalveolar lavage tissue fluid: sterile screw-capped jar
- blood: sterile tube with anticoagulant (heparin).

Precautions

- Transport the specimen to the laboratory as soon as possible after collection. If the anticipated time between

collection and inoculation into shell vial cell cultures is longer than 3 hours, store the specimen at 39.2° F (4° C). Don't freeze the specimen or allow it to become dry.
■ Use gloves when obtaining and handling all specimens.

Normal findings

Normally, CMV isn't present in a culture specimen.

Implications of results

The test can detect CMV in urine or throat specimens from patients who are asymptomatic. Detection from these sites indicates active, asymptomatic infection, which may herald symptomatic involvement, especially in immunocompromised patients. Detection of CMV in blood samples, tissue specimens, and specimens from bronchoalveolar lavage generally reflects the presence of systemic infection and disease.

Posttest care

No specific posttest care is necessary.

Interfering factors

Administration of antiviral drugs before collection of the specimen may interfere with detection of CMV.

Myoglobin test, serum

Myoglobin, which is normally present in skeletal and cardiac muscle, functions as an oxygen-binding muscle protein. Ischemia, trauma, or inflammation of the muscle release it into the bloodstream.

Purpose

■ As a nonspecific test, to estimate damage to skeletal or cardiac muscle tissue
■ To predict flare-ups of polymyositis
■ Specifically, to determine if myocardial infarction (MI) has occurred.

Patient preparation

Explain the purpose of the test to the patient. Obtain a patient history, including disorders that may be associated with increased myoglobin levels. Tell the patient who will perform the venipuncture and when, and explain that he may experience slight discomfort from the needle puncture and the pressure of the tourniquet. Inform the patient that the results need to be correlated with other tests for a definitive diagnosis.

Procedure

Perform a venipuncture and collect the sample in a 5-ml tube with no additives.

Precautions

- Expect to collect blood samples 4 to 8 hours after the onset of an acute MI.
- Handle the sample gently to avoid hemolysis.
- Send the sample to the laboratory immediately.

Reference values

Normal myoglobin values are 0 to 0.09 µg/ml.

Implications of results

Besides MI, increased myoglobin levels may reflect acute alcohol intoxication, dermatomyositis, hypothermia (with prolonged shivering), muscular dystrophy, polymyositis, severe burn injuries, trauma, severe renal failure, or systemic lupus erythematosus.

Posttest care

If a hematoma develops at the venipuncture site, apply warm soaks.

Interfering factors

- Radioactive scans performed within 1 week before the test or hemolysis may interfere with test results.
- Recent angina or cardioversion may increase myoglobin levels.
- Poor timing of the test or I.M. injection may cause a false-positive result.

Myoglobin test, urine

This test detects the presence of myoglobin—a red pigment found in the cytoplasm of cardiac and skeletal muscle cells—in the urine. Extensive damage to muscle cells, as by disease or severe crushing trauma, releases myoglobin into the blood. The myoglobin is quickly cleared by renal glomerular filtration and eliminated in the urine (myoglobinuria). For example, myoglobin appears in the urine within 24 hours after myocardial infarction. Because urine myoglobin and urine hemoglobin are structurally similar, qualitative assays can't satisfactorily differentiate them.

The test method most commonly used to detect myoglobinuria is the differential precipitation test. Hemoglobin—bound to haptoglobin—precipitates when urine is mixed with ammonium sulfate, but myoglobin remains soluble and can be measured.

Purpose

- To aid diagnosis of muscle disease
- To detect extensive infarction of muscle tissue
- To assess the extent of muscular damage from crushing trauma.

Patient preparation

Explain to the patient that this test detects a red pigment found in muscle cells and helps evaluate muscle injury or disease. Inform him that he needn't restrict food or fluids before the test. Tell him that this test requires a random urine specimen, and teach him the proper collection technique.

Procedure

Collect a random urine specimen.

Precautions

Send the specimen to the laboratory immediately.

Normal findings

Normally, myoglobin isn't present in the urine.

Implications of results

Myoglobinuria occurs in acute or chronic muscular disease, alcoholic polymyopathy, familial myoglobinuria, and extensive myocardial infarction. It also results from severe trauma to the skeletal muscles (as in a crushing injury, extreme hyperthermia, or severe burns). Transient myoglobinuria ("march" myoglobinuria) may follow strenuous or prolonged exercise but disappears after rest.

Interfering factors

■ If this test is performed with Chemstrip or other reagent strips, recent ingestion of large amounts of vitamin C can inhibit the reaction, thereby causing false-negative results.
■ Contamination of urine with iodine applied during surgery may produce false-positive results.
■ Extremely dilute urine can reduce test sensitivity.

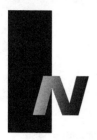

Nasopharyngeal culture

This test evaluates nasopharyngeal secretions for the presence of pathogenic organisms. Direct microscopic inspection of a Gram-stained smear of the specimen provides preliminary identification of organisms, which may guide clinical management and determine the need for additional testing. Streaking a culture plate with the swab and allowing any organisms present to grow permits isolation and identification of pathogens. Cultured pathogens may then require susceptibility testing to determine appropriate antimicrobial therapy.

Nasopharyngeal cultures are often useful for identifying *Bordetella pertussis* and *Neisseria meningitidis*, especially in very young, elderly, or debilitated patients. They can also be used to isolate viruses, especially carriers of influenza virus A and B. A new point-of-care diagnostic test called QuickVue enables an immediate diagnosis of influenza A and B. The conventional laboratory procedure required for such testing is complex, time-consuming, and costly, and it's performed infrequently.

Purpose

- To identify pathogens causing upper respiratory tract symptoms
- To identify proliferation of normal nasopharyngeal flora, which may be pathogenic in debilitated and other immunocompromised persons
- To detect asymptomatic carriers of infectious organisms, such as *N. meningitidis* and *B. pertussis*.

Patient preparation

Describe the procedure to the patient, and explain that this test isolates the cause of nasopharyngeal infection and allows identification of the organism and testing for antimicrobial susceptibility. Tell him that a cotton-tipped swab will be used to obtain secretions from the back of the nose and the throat and who will perform this procedure. Warn him that he may experience slight discomfort and may gag, but reassure him that obtaining the specimen takes less than 15 seconds. Inform him that initial test results are available in 48 to 72 hours but that viral test results take longer.

Equipment

- gloves
- penlight
- sterile, flexible wire swab
- small, sterile, open-ended glass tube or sterile nasal speculum
- tongue blade
- culture tube
- transport medium (broth)
- sterile water or saline.

Procedure

- Put on gloves. Moisten the swab with sterile water or saline. Ask the patient to cough before you begin collecting the specimen, and then position the patient with his head tilted back.
- Using a penlight and a tongue blade, inspect the nasopharyngeal area. Next, gently pass the swab through the nostril and into the nasopharynx, keeping the swab near the septum and floor of the nose, or place the glass tube in the patient's nostril and carefully pass the swab through the tube into the nasopharynx. Rotate the swab for 5 seconds, and then place it in the culture tube with the transport medium. Remove the glass tube. Label the specimen appropriately, including date and time of collection, origin of the material, and suspected organism.
- Ideally, a fresh culture medium should be inoculated with specimens for *B. pertussis* at the patient's bedside because of this organism's susceptibility to environmental changes.
- If the specimen is for isolation of a virus, verify the laboratory's recommended collection techniques.
- Keep the specimen cold to avoid virus deterioration.

Precautions

- Use gloves when performing the procedure and handling the specimen.
- To avoid specimen contamination, don't let the swab touch the sides of the patient's nostril or his tongue.
- Note recent antimicrobial therapy or chemotherapy on the laboratory request.
- Keep the container upright.
- Tell the laboratory if *Corynebacterium diphtheriae* or *B. pertussis* is suspected; these organisms need special growth media.
- Refrigerate a viral specimen according to your laboratory's procedure.

■ If *B. pertussis* is suspected, use Dacron or calcium alginate minitipped swabs.

■ When specimens can't be directly plated onto growth medium, the best transport medium is one supplemented with antibiotics to reduce the growth of normal flora.

Normal findings

Flora commonly found in the nasopharynx include nonhemolytic streptococci, alpha-hemolytic streptococci, *Neisseria* species (except *N. meningitidis* and *N. gonorrhoeae*), coagulase-negative staphylococci such as *Staphylococcus epidermidis* and, occasionally, coagulase-positive *S. aureus*.

Implications of results

Pathogens may include group A beta-hemolytic streptococci; occasionally groups B, C, and G beta-hemolytic streptococci; *B. pertussis*; *C. diphtheriae*; *S. aureus*; large numbers of pneumococci; *Haemophilus influenzae*; *M. influenza*; *M. parainfluenza*; *Candida albicans*; *Mycoplasma* sp.; and *Mycobacterium tuberculosis*.

Posttest care

None reported.

Interfering factors

■ Recent antimicrobial therapy decreases bacterial growth.

■ Improper collection technique may contaminate the specimen.

■ Failure to place the specimen in transport medium allows the specimen to dry out and the organisms die.

■ Failure to send the specimen to the laboratory immediately after collection permits proliferation of organisms.

■ Failure to keep a viral specimen cold causes the viruses to deteriorate.

5'-Nucleotidase assay

The enzyme 5'-nucleotidase (5'NT) is a phosphatase formed almost entirely in the hepatobiliary tract. Unlike alkaline phosphatase (ALP), which is a nonspecific enzyme, 5'-NT only hydrolyzes nucleoside 5'-phosphate groups. Although serum 5'NT, ALP, and leucine aminopeptidase (LAP) levels all rise in hepatic metastases, hepatocarcinoma, and biliary tract obstruction, only 5'NT remains normal in skeletal disease and pregnancy; thus, 5'NT is more specific for hepatic dysfunction than ALP or LAP.

The serum 5'NT assay is technically more difficult than the ALP assay. It hasn't been widely used as a liver function study, although some authorities consider it more sensitive than ALP in revealing cholangitis, biliary cirrhosis, and malignant infiltrations of the liver. It is used most often to determine whether ALP elevation is caused by skeletal or hepatic disease.

Purpose

■ To distinguish between hepatobiliary and skeletal disease when the source of elevated ALP levels is uncertain
■ To help differentiate biliary obstruction from acute hepatocellular damage
■ To detect hepatic metastasis in the absence of jaundice.

Patient preparation

Explain to the patient that this test evaluates liver function. Inform him that he needn't restrict food or fluids. Tell him that the test requires a blood sample, who will perform the venipuncture and when, and that he may experience discomfort from the needle puncture and the pressure of the tourniquet.

Procedure

Perform a venipuncture and collect the sample in a 7-ml tube without additives.

Precautions

Handle the sample gently.

Reference values

Serum 5'NT values in adults range from 2 to 17 U/L; values in children may be lower.

Implications of results

Marked 5'NT elevations occur in common bile duct obstruction caused by calculi or tumors in diseases that cause severe intrahepatic cholestasis, such as neoplastic infiltrations of the liver. Slight to moderate increases may reflect acute hepatocellular damage or active cirrhosis.

Posttest care

If a hematoma develops at the venipuncture site, apply warm soaks.

Interfering factors

■ Cholestatic drugs, such as phenothiazines, morphine, meperidine, and codeine as well as aspirin, acetaminophen, and phenytoin, elevate 5'NT levels.
■ Hemolysis may interfere with results.

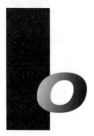

Occult blood test, fecal

Fecal occult blood, invisible because of its minute quantity, can be detected by microscopic analysis or by chemical tests for hemoglobin, such as the guaiac or orthotoluidine test. Because small amounts of blood (2 to 2.5 ml/day) normally appear in the feces, tests for occult blood are designed to detect quantities larger than this. These tests are indicated for patients whose clinical symptoms and preliminary blood studies suggest GI bleeding. If a test is positive, additional tests are required to pinpoint the origin of the bleeding.

Stool color correlates roughly with the site of bleeding — for example, melena usually results from hemorrhage in the esophagus or stomach, where gastric juices digest this blood, thereby blackening it. Melena may also result from hemorrhage in the jejunum or ileum, if the blood passes through the intestine slowly. Dark maroon stools result from hemorrhage beyond the ligament of Treitz. Stool color can also be affected by ingestion of certain foods. (See *Nonpathologic causes of variant stool color*, page 406.)

Purpose

- To detect GI bleeding
- To aid early diagnosis of colorectal cancer.

Patient preparation

Explain to the patient that this test helps detect abnormal GI bleeding. Instruct him to maintain a high-fiber diet and to refrain from eating red meat, poultry, fish, turnips, and horseradish for 48 to 72 hours before the test and throughout the collection period. Tell him the test requires collection of three stool specimens. Occasionally, only a random specimen is collected.

As ordered, withhold iron preparations, bromides, iodides, rauwolfia derivatives, indomethacin, colchicine, salicylates, phenylbutazone, steroids, and ascorbic acid for 48 hours before the test and during the collection period. If these medications must be continued, note this on the laboratory request. Up to 325 mg of aspirin may be ingested daily without affecting test results.

NONPATHOLOGIC CAUSES OF VARIANT STOOL COLOR

Changes in stool color are not always the result of a disease or disorder. Some benign causes are listed below.

Stool color	Food or fluid	Drug
Red	Carrots, beets, tomatoes, red peppers	Pyrvinium
Black	Licorice, grape juice	Iron salts, phenylbutazone
Brown	Cocoa, high intake of meat protein (dark brown)	Anthraquinone
Green-blue or black	Spinach	Bismuth preparations
Yellow	Rhubarb; high intake of milk (yellow-brown)	Senna
White discoloration or speckling	None known	Antacids containing aluminum hydroxide

Procedure

■ Collect three stool specimens or a random specimen, as ordered. Be sure to obtain specimens from two different areas of each stool to allow for variation in distribution of blood.

■ Two of the most commonly used screening tests are Hematest and Hemoccult. Hematest uses orthotoluidine to detect hemoglobin, and Hemoccult uses guaiac.

HEMATEST

■ Use a wooden applicator to smear a bit of the stool specimen on the filter paper supplied with the kit, or, after performing a digital rectal examination, wipe the finger you used for examination on a square of the filter paper. Place the filter paper with the stool smear on a glass plate.

■ Remove a reagent tablet from the bottle, and immediately replace the cap tightly. Then place the tablet in the center of the stool smear on the filter paper. Add one drop of water to the tablet, and allow it to soak in for 5 to 10 seconds. Add a second drop, letting it run from the tablet onto the specimen and filter paper. If necessary, tap the plate gently to dislodge any water from the top of the tablet.

■ After 2 minutes, the filter paper will turn blue if the test is positive. Don't read the color that appears on the tablet itself or develops on the filter paper after the 2-minute period. Note the results, and discard the filter paper. Remove and discard your gloves, and wash your hands thoroughly.

HEMOCCULT

■ Open the flap on the slide packet, and use a wooden applicator to apply a thin smear of the stool specimen to the guaiac-impregnated filter paper exposed in box A or, after performing a digital rectal examination, wipe the finger you used for examination on a square of the filter paper. Apply a second smear from another part of the specimen to the filter paper exposed in box B because some parts of the specimen may not contain blood.

■ Allow the specimen to dry for 3 to 5 minutes. Open the flap at the rear of the slide package, and place 2 drops of Hemoccult developing solution on the paper over each smear. A blue reaction will appear in 30 to 60 seconds if the test is positive. Record the results and discard the slide package. Remove and discard your gloves and wash your hands thoroughly.

INSTANT-VIEW TEST

■ Add a stool sample to the collection tube. Shake it to mix the sample with the extraction buffer, and then dispense four drops into the sample well of the cassette. Results will appear on both the test region and the control region of the cassette in 5 to 10 minutes, indicating whether the level of hemoglobin is greater than 0.05 µg/ml of stool. Results will also indicate if the device is performing properly.

Precautions

■ Instruct the patient to avoid contaminating the stool specimen with toilet tissue or urine.

■ Send the specimen to the laboratory or perform the test immediately.

Reference values

Less than 2.5 ml of blood, which causes a green reaction, is normal.

Implications of results

A positive test indicates GI bleeding, which may result from many disorders, such as varices, peptic ulcer, carcinoma, ulcerative colitis, dysentery, and hemorrhagic disease. This test is particularly important for early diagnosis of colorectal cancer because it is positive in 80% of persons with this type of cancer. Further tests, such as barium swallow, analyses of gastric contents, and endoscopic procedures, are necessary to define the site and extent of bleeding.

Posttest care

As ordered, the patient may resume his usual diet and medications after testing is completed.

Interfering factors

■ Bleeding may result from use of iron preparations, bromides, rauwolfia derivatives, indomethacin, colchicine, phenylbutazone, or steroids.

■ Ascorbic acid (vitamin C) can cause false-negative results even in the presence of significant bleeding.

■ Failure to adhere to dietary or medication restrictions, to test the specimen immediately, or to send it to the laboratory immediately may affect test results.

■ Ingestion of 2 to 5 ml of blood (for example, from bleeding gums) can cause false-positive results.

■ Active bleeding from hemorrhoids may cause false-positive results.

One-stage factor assay: Extrinsic coagulation system

When prothrombin time (PT) and activated partial thromboplastin time (APTT) are prolonged, a one-stage assay helps detect a deficiency of factor II, V, or X. If PT is abnormal but APTT is normal, factor VII may be deficient.

In this test, diluted samples of the patient's plasma are added to a substrate plasma that is deficient in a single factor. The activity of this mixture is compared with normal activity plotted on a predetermined standard curve for each factor. If the clotting time for these patient-substrate mixtures is longer than normal, the patient may be deficient in the factor being tested.

Purpose

■ To identify a specific factor deficiency in persons with prolonged PT or APTT

■ To study patients with congenital or acquired coagulation defects

■ To monitor the effects of blood component therapy in factor-deficient patients.

Patient preparation

Explain that this test assesses the function of the blood coagulation mechanism. Tell the patient that he needn't restrict food or fluids. Inform him that the test requires a blood sample, who will perform the venipuncture and when, and that he may experience discomfort from the puncture and the tourniquet.

Withhold oral anticoagulants before the test, as ordered. If they must be continued, note that on the laboratory request. If the patient is factor-deficient and receiving blood component therapy, tell him that he may need a series of tests. (See *Factor XIII assay: The missing link.*)

FACTOR XIII ASSAY: THE MISSING LINK

When a patient has poor wound healing and other symptoms of a bleeding disorder and coagulation test results are normal, a factor XIII assay is recommended. In this test, a plasma sample is incubated with either chloracetic acid or urea after normal clotting takes place. The clot is observed for 24 hours; if it dissolves, a severe factor XIII deficiency exists.

Factor XIII stabilizes the fibrin clot, the final step in the clotting process. An unstable clot breaks loose, resulting in scarring and poor wound healing. Deficiency of this factor is usually transmitted as an autosomal recessive trait but may result from hepatic disease or from tumors.

Effects of deficiency

The clinical effects of factor XIII deficiency include umbilical bleeding in neonates, prolonged bleeding after trauma, hemarthrosis, spontaneous abortion (rarely), intraovarian bleeding (more common in factor XIII deficiency than in other bleeding disorders), and recurrent ecchymoses, hematomas, and poor wound healing. Bleeding after trauma may begin immediately or as long as 36 hours later.

Prognosis improving

Treatment with infusions of plasma or cryoprecipitate has improved the prognosis of patients with factor XIII deficiency; some patients may live normal lives. However, before appropriate treatment can begin, diagnostic evaluation must rule out other bleeding disorders. Dysfibrinogenemia, hyperfibrinogenemia, and disseminated intravascular coagulation cause rapid clot dissolution in this assay, but unlike factor XIII deficiency, they also cause an abnormal fibrinogen level and thrombin time.

Procedure

Perform a venipuncture and collect the sample in a 7-ml silicon-coated tube.

Precautions

■ If the patient has a suspected coagulation defect, avoid excessive probing during venipuncture, don't leave the tourniquet on too long (it will cause bruising), and apply pressure to the puncture site for 5 minutes or until the bleeding stops.

■ Completely fill the collection tube and invert it gently several times to mix the sample and the anticoagulant.

■ Handle the sample gently to prevent hemolysis and send it to the laboratory immediately.

Reference values

The reference range for most factors is approximately 50% to 150% of normal activity.

Implications of results

Deficiency of factor II, VII, or X may indicate hepatic disease or vitamin K deficiency; deficiency of factor X may also indicate disseminated intravascular coagulation (DIC). Factor V deficiency suggests severe hepatic disease, DIC, or fibrinogenolysis. Deficiencies of all four factors may be congenital, although absence of factor II is lethal.

Posttest care

■ If a hematoma develops at the venipuncture site, apply warm soaks.
■ A patient with a bleeding disorder may require a pressure bandage to stop bleeding at the venipuncture site.

Interfering factors

■ Oral anticoagulant therapy may increase bleeding time by inhibiting vitamin K-dependent synthesis and activation of clotting factors II, VII, and X, which are formed in the liver.
■ Hemolysis caused by rough handling of the sample may affect test results.
■ Failure to mix the sample and the anticoagulant adequately or to send the sample to the laboratory immediately may affect test results.

One-stage factor assay: Intrinsic coagulation system

When prothrombin time is normal but activated partial thromboplastin time is abnormal, a one-stage assay helps identify a deficiency in the intrinsic coagulation system — factor VIII, IX, XI, or XII.

In this test, diluted samples of the patient's plasma are added to a substrate plasma that is deficient in a single factor. The activity of this mixture is compared with normal activity plotted on a predetermined standard curve for each factor. If the clotting time of these patient-substrate mixtures is longer than normal, the patient may be deficient in the factor being tested.

Purpose

■ To identify a specific factor deficiency
■ To study patients with congenital or acquired coagulation defects
■ To monitor the effects of blood component therapy in factor-deficient patients.

Patient preparation

Explain to the patient that this test assesses the function of the blood coagulation mechanism. Inform him that he needn't restrict food or fluids. Tell him that the test requires a blood sample, who will perform the venipuncture and when, and that he may experience discomfort from the needle puncture and the pressure of the tourniquet.

Withhold oral anticoagulants before the test, as ordered. If such medications must be continued, note this on the laboratory request.

If the patient is factor-deficient and is receiving blood component therapy, tell him that a series of tests may be needed to monitor therapeutic progress.

Procedure

Perform a venipuncture and collect the sample in a 7-ml silicon-coated tube.

Precautions

■ If a coagulation defect is suspected, avoid excessive probing during venipuncture, don't leave the tourniquet on too long (it will cause bruising), and apply pressure to the puncture site for 5 minutes or until the bleeding stops.

■ Completely fill the collection tube, and invert it gently several times to mix the sample and anticoagulant adequately.

■ Handle the sample gently to prevent hemolysis, and send it to the laboratory immediately.

Reference values

The reference range for most factors is approximately 50% to 150% of normal activity.

Implications of results

Factor VIII deficiency may indicate hemophilia A, von Willebrand's disease, or factor VIII inhibitor. An acquired deficiency of factor VIII may result from disseminated intravascular coagulation or fibrinolysis. The factor VIII antigen and ristocetin cofactor tests distinguish between hemophilia A (and its carrier state) and von Willebrand's disease. (See *Factor VIII-related antigen test*, page 412.)

Factor IX deficiency may suggest hemophilia B, or it may be acquired as a result of hepatic disease, factor IX inhibitor, vitamin K deficiency, or coumarin therapy. (Factors VIII and IX inhibitors are antibodies specific to each factor that occur after transfusions in patients deficient in either factor.)

Factor XI deficiency may appear after the stress of trauma or surgery or transiently in neonates. Factor XII deficiency may be inherited or acquired (as in nephrosis) and may also appear transiently in neonates.

FACTOR VIII-RELATED ANTIGEN TEST

Bleeding time tests and patient history can usually distinguish between classic hemophilia and von Willebrand's disease. However, when bleeding time tests are inconclusive and the patient has no family history of bleeding, the factor VIII-related antigen test can provide helpful diagnostic information.

In this test, a sample of the patient's plasma is compared with a control sample after both are placed in an agarose gel impregnated with factor VIII antibody. Electrophoresis is performed; the gel is then examined for the rocket-shaped immunoprecipitates that indicate a factor VIII antigen response.

In people with hemophilia and carriers of hemophilia, normal activity is 45% to 185% of the number of immunoprecipitates of the control sample. Plasma from patients with von Willebrand's disease is nonreactive or produces few immunoprecipitates.

Posttest care

■ If a hematoma develops at the venipuncture site, apply warm soaks.
■ A patient with a bleeding disorder may require a pressure bandage to stop bleeding at the venipuncture site.
■ As ordered, resume administration of medications discontinued before the test.

Interfering factors

■ Oral anticoagulants decrease factor IX levels.
■ Pregnancy elevates factor VIII levels.
■ Hemolysis caused by rough handling of the sample may alter test results.
■ Failure to mix the sample and the anticoagulant adequately or to send the sample to the laboratory immediately may alter test results.

Osmolality test, urine

The kidneys normally concentrate or dilute urine according to fluid intake. When intake is excessive, the kidneys excrete more water in the urine; when intake is limited, they excrete less. To make such variation possible, the distal segment of the renal tubule varies its permeability to water in response to antidiuretic hormone, which, with renal blood flow, determines urine concentration or dilution.

This test measures the concentrating ability of the kidneys in acute and chronic renal failure. Osmolality is a more sensitive index of renal function than dilution techniques that measure specific gravity. It measures the number of osmotically active ions or particles present per kilogram of water. Osmolality is high in concentrated urine and low in dilute urine. It is determined by the effect of solute particles on the freezing point of the fluid.

Purpose

- To evaluate renal tubular function
- To detect renal impairment.

Patient preparation

Explain to the patient that this test evaluates kidney function. Tell him the test requires a urine specimen and collection of blood within 1 hour before or after the urine is collected. Withhold diuretics, as ordered.

Emphasize to the patient that his cooperation is necessary to obtain accurate results.

Procedure

- Collect a random urine specimen. If a 24-hour urine collection is ordered, record the total urine volume on the laboratory request. (Preservatives in the 24-hour urine container aren't required.)
- After collecting the first urine specimen, discard it. Record the time you discard it as the beginning of the 24-hour test. The next day, ask the patient to void at the same time, and add this last specimen to the container.

Precautions

- Send each specimen to the laboratory immediately after collection.
- If the patient is unable to urinate into the specimen containers, provide him with a clean bedpan, urinal, or toilet specimen pan. Rinse the collection device after each use.
- If the patient is catheterized, empty the drainage bag before the test. Obtain the specimens from the catheter.

Reference values

In a random urine specimen, osmolality normally ranges from 50 to 1,400 mOsm/kg; in a 24-hour urine specimen, normal osmolality ranges from 300 to 900 mOsm/kg.

Implications of results

Decreased renal capacity to concentrate urine in response to fluid deprivation, or to dilute urine in response to fluid overload, may indicate tubular epithelial damage, decreased renal blood flow, loss of functional nephrons, or pituitary or cardiac dysfunction.

Monitor the patient's electrolyte levels. Also monitor for signs of dehydration or overhydration. Provide adequate hydration, as indicated.

Posttest care
■ After collecting the final specimen, provide the patient with a balanced meal or a snack.
■ Make sure the patient voids within 10 hours after the catheter has been removed.

Interfering factors
■ Diuretics increase urine volume and dilution, thereby lowering specific gravity.
■ Nephrotoxic drugs cause tubular epithelial damage, thereby decreasing renal concentrating ability.
■ Patients who have been markedly overhydrated for several days before the test may have abnormally low osmolality.
■ Patients who are dehydrated or have electrolyte imbalances (either abnormally high or low, depending upon hydration) may retain fluids, leading to inaccurate results.
■ Incomplete collection of 24-hour urine sample will invalidate results.

Osmotic fragility test

Osmotic fragility measures red blood cell (RBC) resistance to hemolysis when exposed to a series of increasingly dilute saline solutions. The test is based on osmosis, which is movement of water across a semipermeable membrane from a less concentrated solution to a more concentrated one in a natural tendency to correct the imbalance.

RBCs suspended in an isotonic saline solution — one with the same salt concentration (osmotic pressure) as normal plasma (0.85 g/dl) — keep their shape. If RBCs are added to a hypotonic (less concentrated) solution, they swell until they rupture (hemolysis); if placed in a hypertonic solution, they shrink.

The degree of hypotonicity needed to cause hemolysis varies inversely with the RBC's osmotic fragility; the closer tonicity is to normal physiologic values when hemolysis occurs, the more fragile the cells. Sometimes, RBCs don't hemolyze immediately, and their incubation in solution for 24 hours improves test sensitivity.

This test provides quantitative confirmation of abnormal RBC morphology and should supplement the stained cell examination.

Purpose
■ To aid diagnosis of hereditary spherocytosis
■ To confirm morphologic RBC abnormalities.

Patient preparation

Explain to the patient that this test helps identify the cause of anemia. Inform him that he needn't restrict food or fluids. Tell the patient the test requires a blood sample, who will perform the venipuncture and when, and that he may experience transient discomfort from the needle puncture and the pressure of the tourniquet.

Procedure

- Perform a venipuncture and collect the sample in a 7-ml heparinized tube.
- Make sure that bleeding has stopped before removing pressure.

Precautions

- Because this isn't a routine test, notify the outside laboratory before drawing the sample if the test is not being performed by the facility's laboratory. Reference laboratories have certain guidelines and testing dates that you'll need to follow.
- Completely fill the tube, and invert it gently several times to mix the sample and anticoagulant adequately.
- Handle the sample gently to prevent hemolysis.

Normal findings

Osmotic fragility values (percent of RBCs hemolyzed) that have been obtained photometrically are plotted against decreasing saline tonicities to produce an S-shaped curve with a slope characteristic of the disorder.

Implications of results

Low osmotic fragility (increased resistance to hemolysis) is characteristic of thalassemia, iron deficiency anemia, sickle cell anemia, and other RBC disorders in which target cells are found. Low osmotic fragility also occurs after splenectomy.

High osmotic fragility (increased tendency to hemolysis) is characteristic in patients with hemolytic disease of the newborn (erythroblastosis fetalis), hereditary spherocytosis, or spherocytosis associated with autoimmune hemolytic anemia, severe burns, or chemical poisoning.

Posttest care

If a hematoma develops at the venipuncture site, apply warm soaks.

Interfering factors

■ Failure to use the proper anticoagulant in the collection tube, to fill the tube completely, or to mix the sample and anticoagulant adequately may affect test results.
■ Hemolysis caused by rough handling of the sample may affect test results.
■ Presence of hemolytic organisms in the sample may affect test results.
■ Conditions such as severe anemia will provide fewer RBCs for testing.
■ Recent transfusion may affect test results.

Oxalate test, urine

This test measures urine levels of oxalate, a salt of oxalic acid. Oxalate is an end product of metabolism and is excreted almost exclusively in the urine. The test detects hyperoxaluria, a disorder in which oxalate accumulates in the soft and connective tissues, especially in the kidneys and bladder, causing chronic inflammation and fibrosis. Calcium oxalate deposits are the most common cause of renal calculi, which may damage the kidneys.

Purpose

■ To detect primary hyperoxaluria in infants
■ To rule out hyperoxaluria in patients with renal insufficiency.

Patient preparation

Explain to the patient (or to the parents if the patient is a child) that this test determines if the urine contains excess oxalate. Instruct him to restrict intake of tomatoes, strawberries, rhubarb, spinach, and vitamin C supplements for about 1 week before the test. Tell him the test requires a 24-hour urine specimen and that the laboratory requires at least 2 days to complete the analysis.

Procedure

Collect a 24-hour urine specimen in a light-resistant container with 30-ml of 6 N HCl.

CLINICAL ALERT The strong acid may cause skin burns, so handle the container carefully.

Precautions

■ Tell the patient not to urinate directly into the 24-hour specimen container and not to contaminate the urine specimen with toilet tissue or stool.
■ Oxalate in acidified urine is stable for up to 7 days at room temperature or when refrigerated at 35.6° to 46.4° F (2° to 8° C).

Reference values

Urine oxalate levels up to 40 mg/24 hours are considered normal.

Implications of results

Elevated urine oxalate levels (hyperoxaluria) result from excessive metabolic production of oxalate or increased oxalate intake. Levels as high as 400 mg/24 hours can occur.

Primary hyperoxaluria, a rare inborn metabolic disorder, causes excessive production and urinary excretion of oxalate. In this type of hyperoxaluria, elevated urine oxalate levels typically precede elevated serum levels.

Secondary hyperoxaluria can result from pancreatic insufficiency, diabetes mellitus, cirrhosis, pyridoxine deficiency, Crohn's disease, ileal resection, ingestion of antifreeze (ethylene glycol) or stain remover, or a reaction to a methoxyflurane anesthetic.

Interfering factors

■ Ingestion of strawberries, tomatoes, rhubarb, or spinach increases urine oxalate levels.
■ Vitamin C increases oxalate excretion and may be a risk factor for calcium oxalate nephrolithiasis in individuals consuming megadoses of this vitamin.
■ Failure to collect all urine during the test period or to store the specimen properly may alter test results.

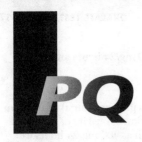

Papanicolaou test

The Papanicolaou (Pap) cytologic test is widely used for early detection of cervical cancer. To perform this test, a doctor or a specially trained nurse scrapes cells from the patient's cervix and spreads them on a slide. After the slide is immersed in a fixative, it's sent to the laboratory for cytologic analysis. This test relies on the ready exfoliation of malignant cells from the cervix.

Although cervical scrapings are the most common test specimen, the Pap test also permits cytologic evaluation of the vaginal pool, prostatic secretions, urine, gastric secretions, cavity fluids, bronchial aspirates, sputum, and solid tumor cells obtained by fine-needle aspiration. It also shows cell maturity, metabolic activity, and morphologic variations. The Pap test can also detect atypical cells that suggest the presence of vaginitis. (See *Vaginal smears.*)

Most gynecologists recommend a Pap test every year. The American Cancer Society recommends a Pap test every 3 years for women between ages 20 and 40 who aren't in a high-risk category and who have had negative results from three previous Pap tests. Yearly tests (or tests at doctor-recommended intervals) are advised for women over age 40, for those in a high-risk category, and for those who have had a positive test. If a Pap test is positive or suggests malignancy, a cervical biopsy can confirm the diagnosis.

Purpose

- To detect malignant cells
- To evaluate estrogen effects
- To detect inflammatory changes in tissue
- To assess response to chemotherapy and radiation therapy
- To detect viral, fungal and, occasionally, parasitic invasion.

Patient preparation

Explain to the patient that the test allows the study of cervical cells. Stress its importance as an aid for detecting cancer at a stage when the disease is often asympto-

VAGINAL SMEARS

Although the Papanicolaou (Pap) test wasn't developed to detect vaginitis, a cytologist can usually identify cells associated with vaginitis while examining the stained cells for cancer. The most reliably detected changes are those associated with *Trichomonas vaginalis, Candida,* and herpes simplex type 2. If such cells are present, the Pap test indicates atypical cells with no evidence of malignancy.

The conventional way to detect vaginitis is the vaginal smear. The examiner uses a cotton-tipped applicator or wooden spatula to collect vaginal secretions and places them at opposite ends of a slide. After adding a drop of normal saline solution to one end of the slide and a drop of 10% to 20% potassium hydroxide (KOH) to the other end (wet-mount preparation), he examines the slide immediately. Trichomonads, white cells, epithelial cells, "clue" cells, and bacteria readily appear at the saline-treated end; *Candida,* at the KOH-treated end.

In the vaginal pool smear, secretions are aspirated through a pipette that's attached to a bulb for suction. Part of the secretion is smeared on a slide and fixed.

Scrapings for cytohormonal evaluation can also be taken from the vagina. In this procedure, the lateral vaginal wall is gently scraped, and the scrapings are spread on a glass slide and fixed. The cytologist assesses the estrogenic effect by determining the percentage of superficial and intermediate squamous cells with a fatty pyknotic nucleus.

---

matic and still curable. The test shouldn't be scheduled during the menstrual period: The best time is midcycle. Instruct the patient to avoid having intercourse for 24 hours, douching for 48 hours, and using vaginal creams or medications for 1 week because these activities can wash away cellular deposits and change the vaginal pH.

Tell her the test requires that the cervix be scraped, who will perform the procedure and when, and that she may experience slight discomfort but no pain from the speculum (but that she may feel some pain when the cervix is scraped). Reassure her that the procedure takes only 5 to 10 minutes to perform (slightly longer if the vagina, pelvic cavity, and rectum are examined bimanually).

Obtain an accurate patient history, and ask the following questions: When did you last have a Pap test? Have you ever had an abnormal Pap test? When was your last menstrual period? Are your periods regular? How many days do they last? Is bleeding heavy or light? Have you taken or are you presently taking hormones or oral contraceptives? Do you use an intrauterine device? Do you have any vaginal discharge, pain, or itching? What, if any, gynecologic disorders have occurred in your family? Have you ever had gynecologic surgery, chemotherapy, or radiation therapy? If so, describe it fully.

Note any pertinent history information on the laboratory request. If the patient is anxious, be supportive and tell her approximately when test results should be available.

Just before the test, ask the patient to empty her bladder.

Equipment

- gloves, drape, and vaginal speculum
- collection device, such as a Pap stick (wooden spatula) and endocervical brush
- saline solution, glass microscopic slides, and fixative (commercial spray or 95% ethyl alcohol solution in a jar).

Procedure

- After the patient has disrobed from the waist down and draped herself, ask her to lie on the examining table and to place her heels in the stirrups. She may be more comfortable if she keeps her shoes on. Tell her to slide her buttocks to the edge of the table. Adjust the drape to minimize exposure. To avoid startling the patient, tell her when the examiner will begin the examination.
- The examiner puts on gloves and inserts an unlubricated speculum into the vagina. To make insertion easier, he may moisten the speculum with saline solution or warm water.
- After locating the cervix, the examiner collects secretions from the cervix and material from the endocervical canal. He places the endocervical brush inside the endocervix and rolls it firmly inside the canal. If he's using a Pap stick (wooden spatula), he places it against the cervix with the longest protrusion in the cervical canal and then rotates the stick clockwise 360 degrees firmly against the cervix. Then he spreads the specimen on the slide, according to laboratory policy, and immediately immerses the slide in a fixative or sprays it with fixative held 9″ to 12″ (23 to 30 cm) from the slide.
- Alternatively, the examiner may collect posterior vaginal pool secretions and pancervical material and smear it on a single slide and then fix it immediately according to laboratory instructions.
- Label the specimen appropriately, including the date, patient's name and age, date of her last menstrual period, and the collection site and method. A bimanual examination may follow removal of the speculum. When the examination is completed, help the patient up and instruct her to dress.

Precautions

■ Make sure the cervical specimen is aspirated and scraped from the cervix.

■ Examine the consistency of the specimen. It should be just thick enough that it's not transparent. A specimen that is too thin will dry and leave too few cells for adequate screening; if it's too thick, the stain won't penetrate.

■ A vaginal pool sample isn't recommended for cervical or endometrial cancer screening.

■ If vaginal or vulval lesions are present, scrapings taken directly from the lesion are preferred.

■ In a patient whose uterus is involuting or atrophying from age, use a small pipette, if necessary, to aspirate cells from the squamocolumnar junction and the cervical canal. Use two slides to reduce air-drying artifact.

■ Preserve the slides immediately.

Normal findings

No malignant cells or abnormalities are present in a normal specimen.

Implications of results

Usually, malignant cells have relatively large nuclei and only small amounts of cytoplasm. They show abnormal nuclear chromatin patterns and marked variation in size, shape, and staining properties, and they may have prominent nucleoli.

A Pap smear may be graded in different ways, so check your laboratory's reporting format. In the Bethesda system, the current standardized method, potentially premalignant squamous lesions fall into three categories: atypical squamous cells of undetermined significance, low-grade squamous intraepithelial lesions, and high-grade squamous intraepithelial lesions. The low-grade squamous intraepithelial lesion category includes mild dysplasia and the changes of the human papillomavirus. The high-grade squamous intraepithelial lesion category includes moderate to severe dysplasia and carcinoma in situ.

To confirm a suggestive or positive cytology report, the test may be repeated, followed by a biopsy, or both. (See *ThinPrep*, page 422.)

Posttest care

■ If cervical bleeding occurs, supply the patient with a sanitary napkin.

■ Tell the patient when to return for her next Pap test.

THINPREP

A new tool for analyzing cervical cells, ThinPrep is collected in the same manner as a Pap test using a cytobrush and plastic spatula. Specimens are deposited in a bottle that contains a fixative and sent to a specialized laboratory. A filter is then inserted into the bottle, and excess mucus, blood, and inflammatory cells are filtered out by centrifuge. Remaining cells are then placed on a slide in a uniform, thin layer and read as a Pap test. This causes fewer slides to be classified as unreadable, significantly reducing the incidence of false-negatives and the need for repeat tests.

Further prospective trials and cost-effectiveness studies are needed before groups such as the American College of Obstetrics and Gynecology can recommend the test for routine use. Most insurance companies are now reimbursing for this test as more laboratories are being certified to perform it. Patients should be aware that they might have to pay the difference in cost, which could be prohibitive.

Interfering factors

- Delay in fixing a specimen allows the cells to dry, destroys the effectiveness of the nuclear stain, and makes cytologic interpretation difficult.
- Use of any lubricating jelly on the speculum can damage the specimen.
- Douching within 48 hours or having intercourse within 24 hours before a Pap test can wash away cellular deposits.
- Use of a specimen collected from the vaginal fornix alone, without an endocervical specimen, may yield false-negative test results.
- Collection of the specimen during menstruation may affect the accuracy of test results.

Parathyroid hormone test

Parathyroid hormone (PTH), also known as parathormone, is a polypeptide secreted by the parathyroid glands that regulates plasma concentrations of calcium and phosphorus. Normally, PTH release is regulated by a negative feedback mechanism. Normal or elevated levels of circulating calcium (especially the ionized form) inhibit PTH release; decreased levels stimulate PTH release. The overall effect of PTH is to raise plasma levels of calcium and lower phosphorus levels by stimulating osteoclasts and osteocytes to mobilize both calcium and phosphorus from bone, acting on renal tubular cells to promote calcium reabsorption and phosphorus excretion (phosphaturia), and (with biological vitamin D [1,25-dihydroxycholecalciferol]) promoting intestinal absorption of calcium.

Circulating PTH exists in three distinct molecular forms: the intact molecule, which originates in the parathyroids, and two smaller circulating forms — N-terminal fragments and C-terminal fragments — that are cleaved from the intact molecule by the kidney and liver; to a lesser extent the parathyroid glands cleave the C-fragment from the intact molecule.

Currently, two radioimmunoassays are available to detect intact PTH and the N- and C-terminal fragments. Both tests can be used to confirm a diagnosis of hyperparathyroidism and hypoparathyroidism, but they have other specific applications as well. The C-terminal PTH assay is more useful for diagnosing chronic disturbances in PTH metabolism, such as secondary and tertiary hyperparathyroidism; it's also better for differentiating ectopic from primary hyperparathyroidism. The assay for intact PTH and the N-terminal fragment (measured concomitantly) more accurately reflects acute changes in PTH metabolism and thus is useful in monitoring a patient's response to PTH therapy.

An inappropriate deficiency or excess of PTH has clinical and diagnostic consequences directly related to the effects of PTH on bone and renal tubules and to the interaction of PTH with ionized calcium and biologically active vitamin D. Consequently, measuring serum calcium, phosphorus, and creatinine levels with serum PTH is useful in identifying states of pathologic parathyroid function. Suppression or stimulation tests may be of confirming value.

Purpose

To aid in the differential diagnosis of parathyroid disorders.

Patient preparation

Explain to the patient that this test helps evaluate parathyroid function. Instruct him to fast overnight because food may affect PTH levels and interfere with the test results. Tell him that this test requires a blood sample, who will perform the venipuncture and when, and that he may experience transient discomfort from the needle puncture. Advise him that the laboratory will need several days to complete the analysis.

Procedure

Draw 3 ml of venous blood into two separate 7-ml clot-activator tubes.

CLINICAL IMPLICATIONS OF ABNORMAL PARATHYROID HORMONE SECRETION

Conditions	Causes	PTH levels	Calcium (ionized) levels
Primary hyperparathyroidism	■ Parathyroid adenoma or carcinoma ■ Parathyroid hyperplasia	● High	● to ● High to Normal
Secondary hyperparathyroidism	■ Chronic renal disease ■ Severe vitamin D deficiency ■ Calcium malabsorption ■ Pregnancy and lactation	● High	○ Low
Tertiary hyperparathyroidism	■ Progressive secondary hyperparathyroidism leading to autonomous hyperparathyroidism	● High	● to ● High to Normal
Hypoparathyroidism	■ Usually, accidental removal of the parathyroid glands during surgery ■ Occasionally associated with autoimmune disease	○ Low	○ Low
Malignant tumors	■ Squamous cell carcinoma of the lung ■ Renal, pancreatic, or ovarian carcinoma	● to ● High to Normal	● High

KEY: High ●   Normal ●   Low ○

Precautions

Handle the sample gently to prevent hemolysis. Send it to the laboratory immediately so the serum can be separated and frozen for assay.

Reference values

Normal serum PTH levels vary, depending on the laboratory, and must be interpreted in relation to serum calcium levels. Typical values are as follows:
■ intact PTH: 210 to 310 pg/ml
■ N-terminal fraction: 230 to 630 pg/ml
■ C-terminal fraction: 410 to 1760 pg/ml.

Implications of results

Measured concomitantly with serum calcium levels, abnormally elevated PTH values may indicate primary, secondary, or tertiary hyperparathyroidism. Abnormally low PTH levels may result from hypoparathyroidism and from certain malignant diseases. (See *Clinical implications of abnormal parathyroid hormone secretion.*)

Posttest care

■ If a hematoma develops at the venipuncture site, apply warm soaks.
■ As ordered, resume the patient's normal diet after the test.

Interfering factors

■ Failure to observe an overnight fast may interfere with accurate determination of test results.
■ Hemolysis caused by rough handling of the sample may interfere with accurate determination of test results.

Parvovirus B-19 antibody test

Parvovirus B-19 is a small, single-stranded deoxyribonucleic acid virus belonging to the family Parvoviridae. It destroys red blood cell (RBC) precursors and interferes with normal RBC production. It's also associated with erythema infectiosum (a self-limiting, low-grade fever and rash in young children) and aplastic crisis (in patients with chronic hemolytic anemia and immunodeficient patients with bone marrow failure). Enzyme-linked immunosorbent assay (ELISA) and immunofluorescence tests can detect immunoglobulin G (IgG) and IgM antibodies to the virus.

Purpose

■ To detect parvovirus B-19 antibody, especially in prospective organ donors
■ To diagnosis erythema infectiosum, parvovirus B-19 aplastic crisis, and related parvovirus B-19 diseases.

Patient preparation

Explain to the patient the test purpose and procedure. To a potential organ donor, explain that the test is part of a panel of tests performed before organ donation to protect the organ recipient from potential infection. Tell the patient that the test requires a blood sample and who will perform the venipuncture and when. Reassure the patient that, although he may experience transient discomfort from the needle puncture and the tourniquet, collection of the sample takes less than 3 minutes.

Procedure

Perform a venipuncture, collect the blood sample in a 5-ml clot-activator tube, and store it on ice.

Precautions

Handle the sample gently to prevent hemolysis.

Normal findings

Normal results are negative for IgM- and IgG-specific antibodies to parvovirus B-19.

Implications of results

About 50% of all adults lack immunity to parvovirus B-19; as many as 20% of susceptible adults become infected after exposure. Infection may manifest as joint arthralgia, hydrops fetalis, fetal loss, transient aplastic anemia, chronic anemia in immunocompromised patients, and bone marrow failure.

Abnormal findings for parvovirus B-19 should be confirmed by the Western blot test.

Posttest care

■ If a hematoma develops at the venipuncture site, apply warm soaks.
■ As ordered, resume the patient's normal diet after the test.

Interfering factors

■ Failure to send the sample on ice may alter test results.
■ Hemolysis caused by rough handling of the sample may alter test results.

Pericardial fluid analysis

Pericardial fluid analysis begins with needle aspiration (pericardiocentesis) of pericardial fluid. This procedure has both therapeutic and diagnostic purposes. It's most useful as an emergency measure to relieve cardiac tamponade, but it also provides a fluid sample than can confirm and identify the cause of pericardial effusion (excess pericardial fluid).

Normally, small amounts of plasma-derived fluid in the pericardium reduce friction between heart and pericardial tissues during expansions and contractions. Pericardial fluid may accumulate after inflammation, rupture, or penetrating trauma (gunshot or stab wounds) of the pericardium. Rapidly forming effusions such as those that develop after penetrating trauma may induce cardiac tamponade, a potentially lethal syndrome — marked by increased intrapericardial pressure — that prevents complete ventricular filling and thus restricts cardiac output. Slowly forming effusions, such as those of pericarditis, typically pose less immediate danger because they allow the pericardium more time to adapt to the accumulating fluid.

Pericardiocentesis should be performed cautiously. It carries the risks of potentially fatal complications —

such as laceration of a coronary artery or of the myocardium — as well as ventricular fibrillation or vasovagal arrest, pleural infection, and accidental puncture of the lung, liver, or stomach. To minimize the risk of complications, echocardiography should be performed before pericardiocentesis to determine the effusion site. Generally, surgical drainage and biopsy are safer than pericardiocentesis.

Purpose

To help identify the cause of pericardial effusion and to help determine appropriate therapy.

Patient preparation

Explain to the patient that this test detects the presence and cause of excessive fluid around the heart and helps determine appropriate therapy. Inform him that he need not restrict food or fluids before the test. Tell him who will perform the test and where and that it takes 10 to 20 minutes.

Inform the patient that a local anesthetic will be injected before the aspiration needle is inserted. Although fluid aspiration isn't painful, warn him that he may experience pressure when the needle is inserted into the pericardial sac. Advise him that he may be asked to briefly hold his breath to aid needle insertion and placement.

Tell the patient that an I.V. line will be started just before the procedure and that he'll receive I.V. sedation as ordered. Assure him that someone will remain with him during the test and that his pulse and blood pressure will be monitored after the procedure.

Check the patient's history for current use of antimicrobial drugs, and record such use on the laboratory request. Make sure that the patient or a responsible family member has signed a consent form. If pericardiocentesis is performed to relieve cardiac tamponade and the patient is in shock, explain the test to the family.

Equipment

Prepackaged pericardiocentesis tray. If such a tray isn't available, have ready the following:
- 70% alcohol or povidone-iodine solution
- 1% procaine or 1% lidocaine for local anesthetic
- sterile needles (25G for anesthetic and 14G, 16G, and 18G 4″ or 5″ cardiac needles) and 50-ml syringe with luer-lok tip
- 7-ml sterile test tubes (one red-top with clot-activator, one green-top with heparin, and one lavender-top with EDTA)

- sterile specimen container for culture
- 4" x 4" gauze pads, vial of heparin 1:1000, bandage, three-way stopcock, Kelly clamp, alligator clips
- electrocardiograph or bedside monitor
- defibrillator and emergency drugs.

Procedure

- The patient is placed in the supine position with the thorax elevated 60 degrees. When he's positioned comfortably and well supported, instruct him to remain still during the procedure. After preparing the skin with povidone-iodine solution from the left costal margin to the xiphoid process, administer the local anesthetic at the insertion site.
- With the three-way stopcock open, aseptically attach a 50-ml syringe to one end and the cardiac needle to the other. The patient is connected to a bedside monitor, which is set to read lead V. (Make sure a crash cart is nearby.)
- The needle is inserted through the chest wall into the pericardial sac, maintaining gentle aspiration until fluid appears in the syringe. The needle is angled 35 to 45 degrees toward the tip of the right scapula between the left costal margin and the xiphoid process; this subxiphoid approach minimizes the risk of lacerating the coronary vessels or the pleura.
- Once the needle is properly positioned, a Kelly clamp is attached to it at the skin surface so it won't advance further. While the fluid is being aspirated, the specimen tubes are labeled and numbered. When the needle is withdrawn, pressure is applied to the site immediately with sterile gauze pads for 3 to 5 minutes. Then a bandage is applied.

Precautions

CLINICAL ALERT Carefully observe the ECG tracing when the cardiac needle is being inserted; ST-segment elevation indicates that the needle has reached the epicardial surface and should be retracted slightly; an abnormally shaped QRS complex may indicate perforation of the myocardium. Premature ventricular contractions usually indicate that the needle has touched the ventricular wall.

CLINICAL ALERT Watch for grossly bloody aspirate — a sign of inadvertent puncture of a cardiac chamber.

- Be sure to use specimen tubes with the proper additives. Although fibrin isn't a normal component of pericardial fluid, it is present in some pericardial diseases and in carcinoma, and clotting is possible.

■ Clean the top of the culture and sensitivity tube with povidone-iodine solution to reduce the risk of extrinsic contamination.

■ If bacterial culture and sensitivity tests are scheduled, record on the laboratory request any antimicrobial drugs that the patient is receiving. If anaerobic organisms are suspected, consult the laboratory about the proper collection technique to avoid exposing the aspirate to air. The aspirate may be placed in an anaerobic collection tube or the syringe may be filled completely, displacing all air, and the collection tube capped tightly with a sterile rubber tip.

■ Send all specimens to the laboratory immediately.

CLINICAL ALERT Have resuscitation equipment on hand.

Normal findings

The pericardium normally contains 10 to 50 ml of sterile fluid. Pericardial fluid is clear and straw-colored, without evidence of pathogens, blood, or malignant cells. The white blood cell (WBC) count in the fluid is usually less than $1,000/\mu l$. Its glucose concentration should approximate the glucose levels in whole blood.

Implications of results

Pericardial effusions are typically classified as transudates or exudates. Transudates are protein-poor effusions that usually arise from mechanical factors that alter fluid formation or resorption, such as increased hydrostatic pressure, decreased plasma oncotic pressure, or obstruction of the pericardial lymphatic drainage system by a tumor.

Most exudates result from inflammation that damages the capillary membrane and contain large amounts of plasma proteins that have leaked into the pericardial fluid. Both types of effusion are characteristic of pericarditis, neoplasms, acute myocardial infarction, tuberculosis, rheumatoid disease, and systemic lupus erythematosus.

An elevated WBC count or neutrophil fraction may accompany inflammatory conditions such as bacterial pericarditis; a high lymphocyte fraction suggests fungal or tuberculous pericarditis.

Turbid or milky effusions may result from the accumulation of lymph or pus in the pericardial sac or from tuberculosis or rheumatoid disease.

Bloody pericardial fluid suggests hemopericardium, hemorrhagic pericarditis, or a traumatic tap. Hemopericardium, the accumulation of blood in the pericardium, may result from myocardial rupture after infarction or from aortic rupture secondary to dissecting aortic aneurysm or thoracic trauma. In hemopericardium, the fluid hematocrit (HCT) is similar to that of whole blood; in hemorrhagic pericarditis, it has a relatively low HCT and doesn't clot on standing. Hemorrhagic effusions may indicate cancer, Dressler's syndrome, closed chest trauma, or postcardiotomy syndrome. A traumatic tap is easily distinguished from hemopericardium or hemorrhagic pericarditis because the fluid becomes progressively clearer.

Glucose concentrations below whole blood levels may reflect increased local metabolism caused by cancer, inflammation, or infection. Bacterial pericarditis may be caused by *Staphylococcus aureus*, *Haemophilus influenzae*, and various gram-negative organisms; granulomatous pericarditis, by *Mycobacterium tuberculosis* and various fungal agents; and viral pericarditis, by coxsackieviruses, echoviruses, and others.

Posttest care

Check blood pressure readings, pulse and respiratory rates, and heart sounds every 15 minutes until stable, then every half hour for 2 hours, every hour for 4 hours, and every 4 hours thereafter. Reassure the patient that such monitoring is routine.

CLINICAL ALERT Be alert for respiratory or cardiac distress. Watch especially for signs of cardiac tamponade, including muffled and distant heart sounds, distended neck veins, paradoxical pulse, and shock. Cardiac tamponade may result from rapid reaccumulation of pericardial fluid or puncture of a coronary vessel, causing bleeding into the pericardial sac.

Interfering factors

- Antimicrobial therapy can prevent isolation of the causative organism.
- Failure to use aseptic technique can impair microbiological analysis of the sample because skin contaminants may be isolated and mistaken for the causative organisms.
- Failure to use the proper additives in test tubes affects the accuracy of test results.

Peritoneal fluid analysis

The peritoneum is a tough, semipermeable membrane that lines the abdominal and visceral cavities and encloses, supports, and lubricates the organs within these cavities. It also serves an important osmoregulatory function; passive diffusion of water and solute particles (up to a certain size) occurs across this membrane to maintain osmotic and chemical equilibrium with associated blood and lymphatic systems. Accumulation of fluid in the peritoneal space — ascites — can result from such conditions as hepatic, renal, or cardiovascular disorders; inflammation; infection; or neoplasm.

This test assesses a sample of peritoneal fluid obtained by paracentesis, a procedure that entails inserting a trocar and cannula through the abdominal wall. If the sample of fluid is being removed for therapeutic purposes, the trocar can be connected to a drainage system. If only a small amount of fluid is being removed for diagnostic purposes, an 18G needle can be substituted for the trocar and cannula. In a four-quadrant tap, fluid is aspirated from each quadrant of the abdomen to verify abdominal trauma and confirm the need for surgery.

Peritoneal fluid analysis includes examination of gross appearance, red blood cell (RBC) and white blood cell (WBC) counts, cytologic studies, microbiological studies for bacteria and fungi, and determinations of protein, glucose, amylase, ammonia, and alkaline phosphatase levels. Complications associated with this test include shock and hypovolemia, perforation of abdominal organs, hemorrhage, and hepatic coma.

Purpose

- To determine the cause of ascites
- To detect abdominal trauma.

Patient preparation

Explain to the patient that this procedure helps determine the case of ascites or detects abdominal trauma. Inform him that he needn't restrict food or fluids before the test. Tell him that the test requires a peritoneal fluid sample, that he'll receive a local anesthetic to minimize discomfort, and that the procedure may take up to 45 minutes to perform.

Provide psychological support to decrease the patient's anxiety, and assure him that complications are rare. If the patient has severe ascites, inform him that the procedure will relieve his discomfort and allow him to breathe more easily.

Make sure the patient or responsible family member has signed a consent form. Record baseline vital signs and weight for comparison with post-test readings; abdominal girth measurements may also be ordered. Tell the patient a blood sample may be taken for laboratory analysis (hemoglobin level, hematocrit, prothrombin time, activated partial thromboplastin time, and platelet count).

Just before the test, tell the patient to urinate. This helps prevent accidental bladder injury during needle insertion.

Procedure

■ Position the patient on a bed or in a chair, as ordered, with his feet flat on the floor and his back well supported. If he can't tolerate being out of bed, place him in high Fowler's position. Make him as comfortable as you can. Except for the puncture site, keep him covered to prevent him from becoming too chilly. Provide a plastic sheet or absorbent pad to collect spillage and to protect the patient and bed linens.

■ The puncture site is then shaved, the skin prepared, and the area draped. A local anesthetic is injected, and the needle or trocar and cannula are inserted, usually 1" to 2" (2.5 to 5 cm) below the umbilicus. (However, insertion may also be through the flank, the iliac fossa, the border of the rectus abdominis, or at each quadrant of the abdomen.) If a trocar and cannula are used, a small incision is made to facilitate insertion. When the needle pierces the peritoneum, it "gives" with an audible sound. The trocar is removed, and a sample of fluid is aspirated with a 50-ml luer-lok syringe.

■ The paracentesis tray contains specimen tubes for the various tests. If fluid is to be drained, assist in attaching one end of an I.V. tube to the cannula and the other end to a collection bag. The fluid is then aspirated (no more than 1,500 ml). If fluid aspiration is difficult, reposition the patient as ordered. After aspiration, the trocar or needle is removed, and a pressure dressing is applied. Occasionally, the wound may be sutured first. Label the specimens in the order that they were drawn. If the patient has received antibiotic therapy, note this on the laboratory request.

■ Carefully and properly dispose of needles and contaminated articles according to Centers for Disease Control and Prevention guidelines; incinerate disposable items and return reusable ones to the central supply area.

■ Apply a gauze dressing to the puncture site; make sure it's thick enough to absorb all drainage.

Precautions

Peritoneal fluid analysis should be used cautiously in patients who are pregnant and in those with bleeding tendencies or unstable vital signs.

CLINICAL ALERT Check vital signs every 15 minutes during the procedure. Watch for deviations from baseline findings. Observe for dizziness, pallor, perspiration, and increased anxiety.

NORMAL FINDINGS IN PERITONEAL FLUID ANALYSIS

Element	Normal findings
Gross appearance	Sterile, odorless, clear to pale yellow color; scant amount (< 50 ml)
Red blood cells	None
White blood cells	< 300/μl
Protein	0.3 to 4.1 g/dl (albumin, 50% to 70%; globulin, 30% to 45%; fibrinogen, 0.3% to 4.5%)
Glucose	70 to 100 mg/dl
Amylase	138 to 404 amylase U/L
Ammonia	< 50 μg/dl
Alkaline phosphatase	Males over age 18: 90 to 239 U/L Females under age 45: 76 to 196 U/L Females over age 45: 87 to 250 U/L
Lactate dehydrogenase	Equal to serum level
Cytology	No malignant cells present
Bacteria	None
Fungi	None

CLINICAL ALERT If rapid fluid aspiration induces hypovolemia and shock, reduce the distance between the trocar and the collection bag to slow the drainage rate. If necessary, stop drainage by turning the stopcock off or by clamping the tubing.

■ To ensure the reliability of abdominal X-rays, perform any needed X-rays before peritoneal fluid analysis, since this test may interfere with the integrity of the X-ray.

■ Avoid contaminating the specimens. Send them to the laboratory immediately.

Normal findings

Peritoneal fluid is normally odorless and clear to pale yellow in color. (See *Normal findings in peritoneal fluid analysis.*)

Implications of results

Milk-colored peritoneal fluid may result from chyle escaping from a thoracic duct that is damaged or blocked by a malignant tumor, lymphoma, tuberculosis, a parasitic infection, an adhesion, or hepatic cirrhosis; pseudochylous fluid may result from the presence of WBCs or tumor cells.

Differential diagnosis of true chylous ascites depends on the presence of elevated triglyceride levels (> 400 mg/dl) and microscopic fat globules. Cloudy or turbid fluid may indicate peritonitis associated with primary bacterial infection, ruptured bowel (after trauma), pancreatitis, strangulated or infarcted intestine, or appendicitis. Bloody fluid may result from a benign or malignant tumor, hemorrhagic pancreatitis, or perforated intestine or duodenal ulcer.

An RBC count over 100/μl suggests neoplasm or tuberculosis; over 100,000/μl, intra-abdominal trauma. A WBC count over 300/μl, with more than 25% neutrophils, occurs in 90% of patients with spontaneous bacterial peritonitis and in 50% of those with cirrhosis. A high percentage of lymphocytes suggests tuberculous peritonitis or chylous ascites. Numerous mesothelial cells reflect tuberculous peritonitis.

Protein levels rise above 3 g/dl in cancer and above 4 g/dl in tuberculous peritonitis. Peritoneal fluid glucose levels fall below 60 mg/dl in 30% to 50% of patients with tuberculous peritonitis or peritoneal carcinomatosis. Amylase levels rise in about 90% of patients with pancreatic trauma, pancreatic pseudocyst, or acute pancreatitis and may also rise in intestinal necrosis or strangulation. Peritoneal alkaline phosphatase levels rise to more than twice the normal serum levels in about 90% of patients with a ruptured or strangulated small intestine. Peritoneal ammonia levels also exceed twice the normal serum levels in patients with ruptured or strangulated large and small intestines and in a ruptured ulcer or appendix.

A protein ascitic fluid/serum ratio of 0.5 or greater, a lactate dehydrogenase (LD) ascitic fluid/serum ratio over 0.6, and an LD ascitic fluid level over 400 μ/ml suggest malignant, tuberculous, or pancreatic ascites. Any two of these findings indicates a nonhepatic cause; absence of all three usually suggests uncomplicated hepatic disease. An albumin gradient between ascitic fluid and serum over 1 g/dl indicates chronic hepatic disease; a lesser value suggests malignancy.

Cytologic examination of peritoneal fluid accurately detects malignant cells. Microbiological examination can reveal coliforms, anaerobes, and enterococci, which can enter the peritoneum from a ruptured organ or from infections accompanying appendicitis, pancreatitis, tuberculosis, or ovarian disease. Gram-positive cocci commonly reflect primary peritonitis; gram-negative organisms, secondary peritonitis. Fungi may indicate histoplasmosis, candidiasis, or coccidioidomycosis.

Posttest care

■ Check the dressing frequently, whenever you check vital signs; reinforce or apply a pressure dressing if needed. Observe CDC standard precautions.

■ Position the patient in bed, and monitor his vital signs. Maintain bed rest until vital signs are stable and return to baseline values. If the patient's recovery is poor, check vital signs every 15 minutes, as ordered. Weigh the patient and measure abdominal girth; compare these with baseline measurements.

■ Monitor urine output for at least 24 hours, and watch for hematuria, which may indicate bladder trauma.

■ If a large amount of fluid was aspirated, watch for signs of vascular collapse (skin-color change, elevated pulse rate and respirations, decreased blood pressure and central venous pressure, mental status changes, and dizziness). Administer fluids orally if the patient is alert and can accept them.

CLINICAL ALERT Watch for signs of hemorrhage and shock and for increasing pain and abdominal tenderness. These may indicate a perforated intestine or, depending on the site of the tap, puncture of the inferior epigastric artery, hematoma of the anterior cecal wall, or rupture of the iliac vein or bladder.

CLINICAL ALERT Observe the patient with severe hepatic disease for signs of hepatic coma, which may result from loss of sodium and potassium and accompanying hypovolemia. Watch for mental status changes, drowsiness, and stupor. Such a patient is also prone to uremia, infection, hemorrhage, and protein depletion.

■ Administer I.V. infusions and albumin as ordered. Check the laboratory report for electrolyte (especially sodium) and serum protein levels.

Interfering factors

■ Failure to send the sample to the laboratory immediately or unsterile collection technique will affect the accuracy of test results.

■ Injury to underlying structures during paracentesis may contaminate the sample with bile, blood, urine, or feces.

Phenolsulfonphthalein excretion test

The phenolsulfonphthalein (PSP) excretion test evaluates kidney function. This test is indicated in patients with abnormal results in the urine concentration test, one of the earliest signs of renal dysfunction.

Purpose

- To determine renal plasma flow
- To evaluate renal tubular function.

Patient preparation

Explain to the patient that this test evaluates kidney function. Inform him that he needn't restrict food before the test. Encourage him to drink fluids before and during the test to maintain adequate urine flow. Tell him the test requires an I.V. injection and collection of urine specimens 15 minutes, 30 minutes, 1 hour and, if ordered, 2 hours after the I.V. injection. Inform him who will administer the I.V. injection and when. Advise him that he may feel transient discomfort from the needle puncture and the pressure of the tourniquet and that the dye temporarily turns the urine red. If the patient is unable to void and requires catheterization, tell him that he may have the urge to void when the catheter is in place.

Withhold drugs that may affect test results, such as chlorothiazide, aspirin, phenylbutazone, sulfonamides, penicillin, and probenecid. If they must be continued, note this on the laboratory request.

Equipment

- 6 mg of PSP dye in 1 ml of solution
- equipment for indwelling urinary catheterization
- four urine specimen containers.

Procedure

- Instruct the patient to empty his bladder and discard the urine.
- The doctor will administer 1 ml of PSP, which equals 6 mg of dye, I.V.
- Collect a urine specimen at 15 minutes, 30 minutes, 1 hour and, if ordered, 2 hours after the injection.
- Because 40 ml of urine is required for each specimen, encourage fluid intake.
- If the patient is catheterized, make sure to clamp the catheter between collections.
- Record the PSP dosage on the laboratory request.
- Properly label each specimen, including the collection time.

Precautions

- Use this test cautiously in a patient with cardiac dysfunction or renal insufficiency because the increased fluid intake necessary for proper hydration may precipitate heart failure.

CLINICAL ALERT Keep epinephrine available because allergic reactions to PSP occasionally occur.

■ Don't use the urine in the drainage bag if the patient already has a catheter in place. Empty the bag and clamp the catheter for 1 hour before the test.
■ Send specimen to the laboratory immediately after each collection.
■ Refrigerate the specimen if more than 10 minutes will elapse before transport.

Reference values

Normally, 25% of the PSP dose is excreted in 15 minutes, 50% to 60% in 30 minutes, 60% to 70% in 1 hour, and 70% to 80% in 2 hours. Normal excretion by children (excluding infants) is 5% to 10% higher than by adults.

Implications of results

The 15-minute value is the most sensitive indicator of both renal tubular function and renal plasma flow. Depressed excretion at this interval but normal excretion later suggests relatively mild or early-stage bilateral renal disease. A depressed 2-hour value may reveal moderate-to-severe renal impairment. Depressed PSP excretion is also characteristic in renal vascular disease, urinary tract obstruction, heart failure, and gout.

Elevated PSP excretion is characteristic of hypoalbuminemia, hepatic disease, and multiple myeloma.

Posttest care

■ Elevate the arm and apply warm soaks if phlebitis develops at the I.V. site.
■ If the patient is catheterized, make sure he voids within 8 to 10 hours after the catheter is removed.
■ Resume administration of medications withheld during the test.

Interfering factors

■ Beets, carrots, and rhubarb may increase or decrease PSP excretion.
■ Radiographic contrast agents, chlorothiazide, salicylates, sulfonamides, penicillin, cascara sagrada, ethanol, indomethacin, nitrofurantoin, phenylbutazone, probenecid, and vitamins can increase or decrease PSP excretion.
■ Incorrect PSP dosage will result in increased or decreased PSP excretion.
■ Failure to collect an adequate specimen at required times will alter test results.
■ High serum protein levels will decrease PSP excretion.
■ Severe hypoalbuminemia, excessive albuminuria, or severe liver disease may have an effect on excretion.

Phenylalanine test

This test (also known as the Guthrie screening test) is a screening method used to detect elevated levels of serum phenylalanine, a naturally occurring amino acid essential to growth and nitrogen balance. Such an elevation may indicate phenylketonuria (PKU), a metabolic disorder inherited as an autosomal recessive trait. An infant with PKU usually has normal phenylalanine levels at birth, but after he begins feeding with breast milk or formula (both contain phenylalanine), levels gradually rise because of a deficiency of the liver enzyme that converts phenylalanine to tyrosine. The resulting accumulation of phenylalanine, phenylpyruvic acid, and other metabolites hinders normal development of central nervous system cells, causing mental retardation.

Dietary restriction of foods that contain phenylalanine prevents accumulation of toxic compounds and hence prevents mental retardation. As the child matures, other metabolic pathways develop to metabolize phenylalanine.

The serum phenylalanine screening test detects abnormal phenylalanine levels through the growth rate of *Bacillus subtilis*, an organism that needs phenylalanine to thrive. To ensure accurate results, the test must be performed after 3 full days (preferably 4 days) of breast milk or formula feeding. (In some states a preliminary test is done 25 hours after birth.)

Purpose

To screen infants for PKU.

Patient preparation

Explain to the parents of the infant that the test is a routine screening measure for PKU and is required in many states. Tell them that a small amount of blood will be drawn from the infant's heel.

Procedure

■ Perform a heelstick, and collect three drops of blood — one in each circle — on the filter paper.
■ Reassure the parents of a child who may have PKU that early detection and continuous treatment with a low-phenylalanine diet can prevent permanent mental retardation.

Precautions

Note the infant's name and birth date and the date of the first breast milk or formula feeding on the laboratory request and send the sample to the laboratory immediately.

CONFIRMING PKU

After the Guthrie screening test detects the possible presence of phenylketonuria (PKU), serum phenylalanine and tyrosine levels are measured to confirm the diagnosis. Phenylalanine hydroxylase is the enzyme that converts phenylalanine to tyrosine. If this enzyme is absent, phenylalanine levels rise and tyrosine levels fall concomitantly.

Samples are obtained by venipuncture (femoral or external jugular) and measured by fluorometry. Serum phenylalanine levels greater than 4 mg/dl and tyrosine levels less than 0.6 mg/dl — with urinary excretion of phenylpyruvic acid — confirm PKU.

Normal findings

In the laboratory, the sample is added to a culture medium containing a phenylalanine-dependent strain of *B. subtilis* and an antagonist to phenylalanine. A negative test, in which the presence of the phenylalanine antagonist inhibits growth of *B. subtilis* around the blood on the filter paper, indicates normal phenylalanine levels (less than 2 mg/dl) and no appreciable danger of PKU.

Implications of results

Growth of *B. subtilis* on the filter paper indicates that serum phenylalanine levels are high enough to overcome the antagonist. Such a positive test suggests the possibility of PKU. Diagnosis requires exact serum phenylalanine measurement and urine testing. (See *Confirming PKU*.) A positive Guthrie test may also result from hepatic disease, galactosemia, or delayed development of certain enzyme systems.

Interfering factors

Performing the test before the infant has received at least 3 full days of breast milk or formula feeding can yield a false-negative finding.

Phosphates test, serum

This test measures serum levels of phosphates, the dominant cellular anions. Phosphates are essential in the storage and utilization of energy, calcium regulation, red blood cell function, acid-base balance, formation of bone, and the metabolism of carbohydrates, protein, and fat.

When vitamin D levels are adequate, the intestine absorbs a considerable amount of phosphates from dietary sources. The kidneys regulate phosphate excretion and retention. Because calcium and phosphates interact in a reciprocal relationship, urinary excretion of phosphates increases or decreases in inverse proportion to serum calcium levels.

Abnormal phosphate levels result more often from abnormal excretion than from abnormal ingestion or absorption from dietary sources.

Purpose

■ To aid diagnosis of renal disorders and acid-base imbalance

■ To detect endocrine, skeletal, and calcium disorders.

Patient preparation

Explain to the patient that this test measures the blood levels of phosphate. Inform him that he needn't restrict food or fluids before the test. Tell him that this test requires a blood sample, who will perform the venipuncture and when, and that he may feel discomfort from the needle puncture. Check the patient history for use of drugs that alter phosphate levels.

Procedure

Perform a venipuncture (if possible, without using a tourniquet) and collect the sample in a 7-ml clot-activator tube.

Precautions

Handle the sample gently to prevent hemolysis.

Reference values

Normal serum phosphate levels in adults range are 2.5 to 4.5 mg/dl (when measured by atomic absorption) or 1.8 to 2.6 mEq/L. In children, the normal range is 4.5 to 7 mg/dl or 2.6 to 4.1 mEq/L.

Implications of results

Depressed phosphate levels (hypophosphatemia) may result from malnutrition, malabsorption syndromes, hyperparathyroidism, renal tubular acidosis, or treatment of diabetic acidosis. In children, hypophosphatemia can suppress normal growth.

Elevated levels (hyperphosphatemia) may result from skeletal disease, healing fractures, hypoparathyroidism, acromegaly, diabetic acidosis, high intestinal obstruction, and renal failure. Hyperphosphatemia is rarely clinically significant; however, if prolonged, it can alter bone metabolism by causing abnormal calcium phosphate deposits.

Treat the underlying cause of hyperphosphatemia. Hemodialysis may be required in patients with renal failure.

Posttest care

If a hematoma develops at the venipuncture site, apply warm soaks.

Interfering factors

■ Low phosphate levels may result from excessive excretion associated with prolonged vomiting and diarrhea or from vitamin D deficiency.

■ Obtaining a specimen above an I.V. site receiving a solution containing phosphate may cause falsely high results.

■ Excessive vitamin D intake and therapy with anabolic corticosteroids or androgens may elevate serum phosphate levels.

■ Extended I.V. infusion of dextrose 5% in water, use of phosphate-binding antacids, and use of acetazolamide, insulin, and epinephrine may alter test results in either direction.

■ Using a tourniquet causes venous stasis and may alter phosphate levels.

■ Hemolysis of the sample falsely increases serum phosphate levels.

Phospholipid test

The phospholipid assay was formerly an important test because of the lack of more specific tests and the relative unreliability of other lipid assays. Today, however, this quantitative analysis of phospholipid levels adds minimal information to that provided by cholesterol levels. Phospholipids aren't associated with coronary artery disease and are seldom included in routine lipid evaluation.

Phospholipids, the largest and most soluble of the lipid elements, contain glycerol, fatty acids, and phosphate. In human plasma, the main phospholipids are lecithins, cephalins, and sphingomyelins. Dietary phospholipids are partially broken down by pancreatic enzymes before absorption by the mucosal cells.

Phospholipids fulfill various functions in the body, including involvement in cellular membrane composition and permeability and some control of enzyme activity within the membrane. They have a tendency to concentrate at cell membranes and aid the transport of fatty acids and lipids across the intestinal barrier and from the liver and other fat deposits to other body tissues.

Phospholipids, especially saturated lecithin, are essential for pulmonary gas exchange, as evidenced by neonatal respiratory distress syndrome in premature infants who lack them.

Lecithin and sphingomyelin comprise the basis of the L/S ratio. A test to determine this ratio is performed on amniotic fluid to estimate the maturity level of a fetus.

Purpose

■ To aid in the evaluation of fat metabolism
■ To aid diagnosis of hypothyroidism, diabetes mellitus, nephrotic syndrome, chronic pancreatitis, obstructive jaundice, and hypolipoproteinemia.

Patient preparation

Explain to the patient that this test helps determine how the body metabolizes fats. Instruct him to abstain from ingestion of alcohol for 24 hours before the test. Fasting isn't necessary unless this test is part of a lipid panel; if it is, the patient shouldn't have any food and fluids after midnight before the test. Tell him the test requires a blood sample, who will perform the venipuncture and when, and that he may experience transient discomfort from the needle puncture and the pressure of the tourniquet. Withhold antilipemic drugs, as ordered.

Procedure

Perform a venipuncture and collect the sample in a 10- to 15-ml tube without additives.

Precautions

Send the sample to the laboratory immediately because spontaneous redistribution may occur among plasma lipids.

Reference values

Normal phospholipid levels range from 180 to 320 mg/dl. Although males usually have higher levels than females, values in pregnant females exceed those of males.

Implications of results

Elevated levels may indicate hypothyroidism, diabetes mellitus, nephrotic syndrome, chronic pancreatitis, or obstructive jaundice. Decreased levels may indicate primary hypolipoproteinemia.

Posttest care

■ If a hematoma develops at the venipuncture site, apply warm soaks.
■ Resume diet and administration of medications that were discontinued before the test, as ordered.

Interfering factors

■ Failure to follow dietary restrictions may interfere with test results.

■ Clofibrate and other antilipemics may lower phospholipid levels.
■ Estrogens, epinephrine, and some phenothiazines increase phospholipid levels.

Placental estriol test, urine

This test monitors fetal viability by measuring urine levels of placental estriol, the predominant estrogen excreted in urine during pregnancy. Toward the end of the first trimester, placental constituents combine with estriol precursors from the fetal adrenal cortex and liver to steadily increase estriol production. This steady rise in estriol reflects a properly functioning placenta and, in most cases, a healthy, growing fetus. Normally, estriol is secreted in much smaller amounts by the ovaries in nonpregnant females, by the testes in males, and by the adrenal cortex in both sexes.

The usual clinical indication for this test is high-risk pregnancy, such as one complicated by maternal hypertension, diabetes mellitus, pregnancy-induced hypertension (preeclampsia), eclampsia, or a history of stillbirth. Serial testing is necessary to plot the expected rise in estriol levels or to show the absence of such a rise.

A 24-hour urine specimen is preferred for this test because estriol levels fluctuate diurnally. Radioimmunoassay is the usual test method. Generally, serum estriol levels are more reliable than urine levels. Serum levels aren't influenced by maternal glomerular filtration rate (GFR) nor are they as readily affected by drugs, some of which actually destroy urinary estriol.

Purpose

To assess fetoplacental status, especially in high-risk pregnancy.

Patient preparation

Explain to the patient that this test helps determine if the placenta is functioning properly, which is essential to the health of the fetus. Tell her she needn't restrict food or fluids. Advise her that a 24-hour urine specimen is required for this test, and teach her how to collect it. Emphasize that proper collection technique is necessary for test results to be valid. Check the patient's medication history for use of drugs that may affect urine estriol levels.

Procedure

■ Collect a 24-hour urine specimen in a bottle containing a preservative to keep the specimen at a pH of 3.0 to

5.0. Note the week of gestation on the laboratory request and send the specimen to the laboratory.

■ As ordered, resume administration of medications discontinued before the test.

Precautions

Refrigerate the specimen or keep it on ice during the collection period.

Normal findings

Normal values vary considerably, but a series of urine estriol levels plotted on a graph should show a steadily rising curve. (See *Urine estriol levels in a typical pregnancy.*)

Implications of results

A 40% drop from baseline values occurring over 2 consecutive days strongly suggests placental insufficiency and impending fetal distress. A 20% drop over 2 weeks or failure of consecutive estriol levels to rise in a normal curve similarly indicates inadequate placental function and undesirable fetal status. These developments may necessitate cesarean section, depending on the patient's condition and on other apparent signs of fetal distress.

A chronically low urine estriol curve may result from fetal adrenal insufficiency, congenital anomalies (such as anencephaly), Rh isoimmunization, or placental sulfatase deficiency. A high-risk pregnancy in which maternal GFR decreases, as in hypertension or diabetes mellitus, may cause a low-normal estriol curve. In such a case, the pregnancy may continue as long as no complications develop and estriol levels continue to rise. However, falling estriol levels or a sudden drop from baseline values indicates severe fetal distress.

Because levels may vary daily, false-positive or false-negative results are possible. Some doctors use an average of three previous values as a control and use nonstress fetal monitoring to determine fetoplacental health.

High urine estriol levels are possible in multiple pregnancy.

Explain measures needed to maintain pregnancy. Prepare for cesarean section if tests indicate fetal distress. Monitor for preeclampsia. Discuss activity modification, if needed. Refer to community resources, if applicable.

Interfering factors

■ Maternal hemoglobinopathy, anemia, malnutrition, and hepatic or intestinal disease characteristically decrease estriol levels.

URINE ESTRIOL LEVELS IN A TYPICAL PREGNANCY

Because urine estriol levels rise as normal gestation proceeds (as shown below), any significant changes in serial urine determinations suggest abnormal conditions that may require prompt medical intervention.

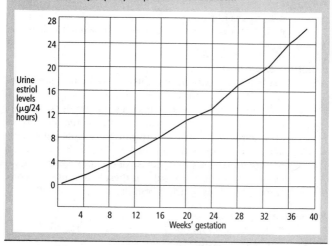

Urine estriol levels (μg/24 hours) vs. Weeks' gestation

■ Administration of the following drugs may influence urine estriol levels: steroid hormones (including estrogens, progesterone, and corticosteroids), methenamine mandelate, phenothiazines, ampicillin, phenazopyridine, tetracyclines, cascara sagrada, senna, phenolphthalein, hydrochlorothiazide, and meprobamate.
■ Failure to collect all urine during the 24-hour period may affect the accuracy of test results.
■ Failure to refrigerate the specimen or keep it on ice may alter test results.
■ Failure to maintain the prescribed pH level in the specimen may alter test results.

Plasminogen test, plasma

Measurement of plasminogen, the precursor of plasmin, is one way to evaluate the fibrinolytic system. During fibrinolysis, plasmin dissolves fibrin clots to prevent excessive coagulation and resultant impairment of blood flow. Plasmin doesn't circulate in active form, and therefore it can't be measured directly; instead, measurement of its circulating precursor, plasminogen, reflects how well this system is functioning.

In this test, streptokinase, a plasminogen activator, is added to a plasma sample. Streptokinase converts plasminogen to active plasmin; the plasmin then converts a substrate, a colored substance that's measured spectrophotometrically or fluorometrically. The intensity of color is proportional to the functional plasminogen in the sample. Plasminogen may also be measured immunologically.

Purpose

- To assess fibrinolysis
- To detect congenital and acquired fibrinolytic disorders.

Patient preparation

Explain to the patient that this test evaluates blood clotting. Inform him that he needn't restrict food or fluids. Tell him that the test requires a blood sample, who will perform the venipuncture and when, and that he may experience minor discomfort from the needle puncture and the pressure of the tourniquet. Check the patient history for use of streptokinase or other drugs that may cause inaccurate test results. If these drugs must be continued, note this on the laboratory request.

Procedure

- Perform a venipuncture and collect the sample in a 7-ml silicon coated tube.
- Make sure that bleeding has stopped before removing pressure.
- If a hematoma develops at the venipuncture site, apply warm soaks.
- If the hematoma is large, monitor pulses distal to the venipuncture site.
- Resume medications withheld before the test, as ordered.

Precautions

- Collect the sample as quickly as possible to prevent stasis, which can slow blood flow, causing coagulation and plasminogen activation.
- To prevent hemolysis, avoid excessive probing during venipuncture and handle the specimen gently.
- Invert the tube gently several times and send the sample to the laboratory immediately. If testing must be delayed, plasma must be separated and frozen at –94° F (–70° C).

Reference values

Normal plasminogen levels are 10 to 20 mg/dl by immunologic methods and 80 to 120 U/dl by other methods.

Implications of results

Low plasminogen levels can result from disseminated intravascular coagulation, tumors, preeclampsia, and eclampsia, which accelerate plasminogen conversion to plasmin and increase fibrinolysis. Some liver diseases prevent formation of sufficient plasminogen and thereby inhibit fibrinolysis.

Interfering factors

■ Oral contraceptives may slightly increase plasminogen levels. Thrombolytic drugs, such as streptokinase or urokinase, may decrease levels also.

■ Failure to use the proper tube, to mix the sample and citrate adequately, to send the sample to the laboratory immediately, or to have it separated and frozen may alter results.

■ Hemolysis caused by excessive probing during venipuncture or rough handling of the sample may alter results.

■ Prolonged tourniquet use before venipuncture may cause stasis, falsely decreasing plasminogen levels.

Platelet aggregation test

After vascular injury, platelets gather at the injury site and clump together (aggregate) to form a plug that helps maintain hemostasis and promotes healing. The platelet aggregation test, an in vitro procedure, measures the rate at which the platelets in a sample of citrated platelet-rich plasma form a clump after the addition of an aggregating reagent (adenosine diphosphate, epinephrine, thrombin, arachidonic acid, collagen, or ristocetin).

This test is a major diagnostic tool for detecting von Willebrand's disease; people with this disorder lack the ristocetin cofactor that enables platelets to aggregate in the presence of ristocetin.

Purpose

■ To assess platelet aggregation
■ To detect congenital and acquired platelet bleeding disorders.

Patient preparation

Explain to the patient that this test helps determine if his blood clots properly. Instruct him to fast or to maintain a nonfat diet for 8 hours before the test because lipemia can affect test findings. Tell him that the test requires a blood sample, who will perform the venipuncture and when, and that he may experience transient discomfort from the needle puncture and the pressure of the tourniquet.

Withhold aspirin and aspirin compounds for 14 days, and phenylbutazone, sulfinpyrazone, phenothiazines, antihistamines, anti-inflammatory drugs, and tricyclic antidepressants for 48 hours, as ordered. If these medications must be continued, note this on the laboratory request. Because the list of medications known to alter the results of this test is long and continually growing, the patient should be as free of drugs as possible before the test. (See *Aspirin and platelet aggregation*.) In addition, certain herbal preparations — such as large amounts of dietary garlic or garlic tablets — can alter results.

Procedure

Perform a venipuncture and collect the sample in a 7-ml siliconized tube.

Precautions

■ Be careful to avoid excessive probing at the venipuncture site. Don't leave the tourniquet on too long because it can cause bruising. Apply pressure to the venipuncture site for 5 minutes or until the bleeding stops.
■ Completely fill the collection tube, and invert it gently several times to mix the sample and anticoagulant adequately.
■ Handle the sample gently to prevent hemolysis and keep it between 71.6°F (22° C) and 98.6° F (37° C) to prevent aggregation.
■ If the patient has taken aspirin within the past 14 days and the test can't be postponed, notify the laboratory. The technician will then use arachidonic acid as the reagent to verify the presence of aspirin in the plasma. If test results are abnormal for such a sample, aspirin use must be discontinued and the test repeated in 2 weeks.

Reference values

Normal aggregation occurs in 3 to 5 minutes, but findings depend on the temperature and vary with the laboratory. Aggregation curves obtained by using different reagents help to distinguish various qualitative platelet defects.

Implications of results

Abnormal findings may indicate von Willebrand's disease, Bernard-Soulier syndrome, storage pool disease, polycythemia vera, severe liver disease, uremia, or Glanzmann's thrombasthenia.

ASPIRIN AND PLATELET AGGREGATION

Unlike other salicylates, aspirin inhibits platelet aggregation. The inhibition occurs in the second phase of platelet aggregation, when the aspirin prevents the release of adenosine diphosphate from platelets. Mean bleeding time may double after a healthy person ingests aspirin. In children or in patients with bleeding disorders such as hemophilia, bleeding time may be even more prolonged.

Effect on platelets

The effect of aspirin on platelets seems to result from the inhibition of prostaglandin synthesis. A single 325-mg oral dose results in about 90% inhibition of the enzyme cyclooxygenase in circulating platelets, preventing the synthesis of compounds that induce platelet aggregation. The inhibition of cyclooxygenase is irreversible; thus, its effect lasts for 4 to 6 days — the life span of platelets. Bleeding time peaks within 12 hours. Altered hemostasis persists about 36 hours after the last dose of aspirin, sometimes longer for patients receiving long-term therapy.

Effect on blood vessels

Aspirin's effect on blood vessels may oppose its effect on platelets because cyclooxygenase plays a different role in the vascular endothelium. Here, the enzyme produces prostacyclin, which inhibits platelet aggregation and causes vasodilation. Inhibition of cyclooxygenase in the vascular endothelium, in effect, counteracts aspirin's antithrombotic effect on platelets. However, studies suggest that platelet cyclooxygenase is more sensitive than the vascular-endothelial form; therefore, a low aspirin dosage (for example, 80 mg daily or 325 mg every other day) may prove more effective in preventing thrombosis than higher dosages.

Researchers are continuing to investigate whether antithrombotic therapy with aspirin is beneficial to women.

Posttest care

■ If a hematoma develops at the venipuncture site, apply warm soaks; prolonged pressure to the venipuncture site (up to 5 minutes) may be needed.

■ As ordered, resume diet and administration of medications withheld before the test.

Interfering factors

■ Hemolysis caused by rough handling of the sample or by trauma at the venipuncture site may alter test results.

■ Failure to use the proper anticoagulant or to mix the sample and anticoagulant adequately may alter test results.

■ Failure to observe restrictions of diet and medications may affect test results. Platelet aggregation is inhibited by aspirin and aspirin compounds, phenylbutazone, sulfinpyrazone, phenothiazines, antihistamines, anti-inflammatory drugs, tricyclic antidepressants, and ingestion of large amounts of garlic.

Platelet count

Platelets, or thrombocytes, are the smallest formed elements in the blood. Vital to the formation of the hemostatic plug in vascular injury, they promote coagulation by supplying phospholipids to the intrinsic coagulation pathway.

The platelet count is one of the most important screening tests of platelet function. Accurate counts are vital for monitoring severe thrombocytosis or the thrombocytopenia associated with chemotherapy and radiation therapy. A platelet count that falls below 50,000/µl can cause spontaneous bleeding; when the count drops below 5,000/µl, fatal central nervous system bleeding or massive GI hemorrhage is possible.

Properly prepared and stained, peripheral blood films provide a reliable estimate of platelet number. A more accurate visual method involves use of a hemocytometer counting chamber and a phase microscope. Automated systems use the voltage pulse or electrooptical counting system. Results from such automated systems should always be checked against a visual estimate from a stained blood film.

Purpose

- To evaluate platelet production
- To assess effects of chemotherapy or radiation therapy on platelet production
- To aid diagnosis of thrombocytopenia and thrombocytosis
- To confirm visual estimate of platelet number and morphology from a stained blood film.

Patient preparation

Explain to the patient that this test helps determine if his blood clots normally. Inform him that he needn't restrict food or fluids before the test. Tell him the test requires a blood sample, who will perform the venipuncture and when, and that he may experience transient discomfort from the needle puncture and the pressure of the tourniquet.

Check the patient history for use of medications that may affect test results. Notify the laboratory if such drugs have been used.

Procedure

Perform a venipuncture and collect the sample in a 7-ml EDTA tube.

Precautions
- To prevent hemolysis, handle the sample gently and avoid excessive probing at the venipuncture site.
- Fill the collection tube, and invert it gently several times to mix the sample and anticoagulant adequately.

Reference values
A normal platelet count is 140,000 to 400,000/µl in adults and 150,000 to 450,000/µl in children.

Implications of results
A low platelet count (thrombocytopenia) can result from aplastic or hypoplastic bone marrow; infiltrative bone marrow disease, such as leukemia or disseminated infection; megakaryocytic hypoplasia; ineffective thrombopoiesis associated with folic acid or vitamin B12 deficiency; pooling of platelets in an enlarged spleen; increased platelet destruction caused by drugs or immune disorders; disseminated intravascular coagulation; Bernard-Soulier syndrome; or mechanical injury to platelets.

If the platelet count falls below 20,000/µl, a platelet transfusion may be given. One unit of platelets should increase the count by at least 5,000/µl. Invasive procedures and I.M. injections may need to be postponed.

A high platelet count (thrombocytosis) can result from hemorrhage, infectious disorders, cancers, iron deficiency anemia, or inflammatory disease or from recent surgery, pregnancy, or splenectomy. In such cases, the platelet count returns to normal after the patient recovers from the primary disorder. However, the count remains elevated in primary thrombocythemia, myelofibrosis with myeloid metaplasia, polycythemia vera, and chronic myelogenous leukemia.

When the platelet count is abnormal, diagnosis usually requires further studies, such as a complete blood count, bone marrow biopsy, direct antiglobulin test (direct Coombs' test), and serum protein electrophoresis.

Posttest care
- Make sure bleeding has stopped before removing pressure.
- If a hematoma develops at the venipuncture site, apply warm soaks.
- If the hematoma is large, monitor pulses distal to the phlebotomy site.

Interfering factors
- Medications that may decrease the platelet count include acetazolamide, acetohexamide, antineoplastics, brompheniramine maleate, carbamazepine, chloram-

phenicol, ethacrynic acid, furosemide, gold salts, hydroxychloroquine, indomethacin, isoniazid, mephenytoin, mefenamic acid, methazolamide, methimazole, methyldopa, oral diazoxide, oxyphenbutazone, penicillamine, penicillin, phenylbutazone, phenytoin, pyrimethamine, quinidine sulfate, quinine, salicylates, streptomycin, sulfonamides, thiazide and thiazide-like diuretics, and tricyclic antidepressants. Heparin causes transient, reversible thrombocytopenia.

■ Failure to use the proper anticoagulant or to mix the sample and anticoagulant promptly and adequately may affect test results.

■ Hemolysis caused by rough handling of the sample or excessive probing at the venipuncture site may alter test results.

■ The platelet count normally increases at high altitudes, with persistent cold temperature, and during strenuous exercise and excitement; the count may decrease just before menstruation.

Pleural biopsy

Pleural biopsy is the removal of pleural tissue, by needle biopsy or open biopsy, for histologic examination. Needle pleural biopsy is performed under local anesthesia. It usually follows thoracentesis — aspiration of pleural fluid — which is performed when the cause of the effusion is unknown, but it can be performed separately.

Open pleural biopsy permits direct visualization of the pleura and the underlying lung. It's done only when pleural effusion is absent and is performed in the operating room.

Purpose

■ To differentiate between nonmalignant and malignant disease
■ To diagnose viral, fungal, or parasitic disease and collagen vascular disease of the pleura.

Patient preparation

Describe the procedure to the patient and answer his questions. Explain that this test permits microscopic examination of pleural tissue. Tell him who will perform the biopsy and where, that it takes 30 to 45 minutes to perform, and that the needle remains in the pleura less than 1 minute. Also tell him that blood studies will precede the biopsy and that chest X-rays will be taken before and after the biopsy.

Make sure the patient has signed a consent form. Check the patient history for hypersensitivity to the local anesthetic. Tell him that he'll receive an anesthetic and should experience little pain. Just before the procedure, record vital signs.

Procedure

- Seat the patient on the side of the bed, with his feet resting on a stool and his arms supported by the overbed table or upper body. Tell him to hold this position and to remain still during the procedure. If he's unable to sit up, position him in a side-lying position with the side to be biopsied up. Prepare the skin and drape the area. The local anesthetic is then administered.
- For Vim-Silverman needle biopsy: The needle is inserted through the appropriate intercostal space into the biopsy site. When the outer tip is distal to the pleura, the central portion is pushed in deeper and held in place; the outer case is inserted about 3/8″ (1 cm), the entire assembly rotated 360 degrees, and the needle and tissue specimen are withdrawn.
- For Cope's needle biopsy: The trocar is introduced through the appropriate intercostal space into the biopsy site. The sharp obturator is then removed and a hooked stylet is inserted through the trocar. The opened notch is directed against the pleura, along the intercostal space, and is slowly withdrawn. While the outer tube is held stationary, the inner tube is twisted to cut off the tissue specimen, and the assembly is withdrawn.
- The specimen is immediately put in 10% neutral buffered formalin solution in a labeled specimen bottle. Then the skin around the biopsy site is cleaned and an adhesive bandage is applied.

Precautions

- Pleural biopsy is contraindicated in patients with severe bleeding disorders.
- Send the specimen to the laboratory immediately.

Normal findings

The normal pleura consists primarily of mesothelial cells, flattened in a uniform layer. Layers of areolar connective tissue — containing blood vessels, nerves, and lymphatics — lie below.

Implications of results

Histologic examination of the tissue specimen can reveal malignant disease, tuberculosis, or viral, fungal, parasitic, or collagen vascular disease. Primary neoplasms of the pleura are generally fibrous and epithelial.

Posttest care

- Check the patient's vital signs every 15 minutes for 1 hour and then every hour for 4 hours or until stable.

■ Make sure the chest X-ray is repeated immediately after the biopsy.

■ Instruct the patient to lie on his unaffected side to promote healing of the biopsy site.

CLINICAL ALERT Watch for signs of respiratory distress (shortness of breath), shoulder pain, and other complications, such as pneumothorax (immediate) and pneumonia (delayed).

Interfering factors

Failure to use the proper fixative or to obtain an adequate specimen may alter results.

Pleural fluid analysis

The pleura, a two-layer membrane covering the lungs and lining the thoracic cavity, contains a small amount of lubricating fluid between its layers to minimize friction during respiration. Excessive fluid in this space — the result of diseases such as cancer and tuberculosis or of blood or lymphatic disorders — can cause respiratory difficulty.

In pleural fluid aspiration (also known as thoracentesis), the thoracic wall is punctured to obtain a specimen of pleural fluid for analysis or to relieve pulmonary compression and resultant respiratory distress. The specimen is examined for color, consistency, pH, glucose and protein content, cellular composition, and the enzymes lactate dehydrogenase (LD) and amylase; it's also examined cytologically for malignant cells and cultured for pathogens. Locating the fluid before thoracentesis — by physical examination and chest X-ray or ultrasonography — reduces the risk of puncturing the lung, liver, or spleen.

Purpose

■ To provide a fluid specimen to determine the cause and nature of pleural effusion

■ To permit better radiographic visualization of a lung with large effusions.

Patient preparation

Explain to the patient that this test assesses the space around the lungs for fluid. Inform him who will perform the test and where and that he needn't restrict food or fluids.

Inform the patient that a chest X-ray or ultrasound study may precede the test to help locate the fluid. Check the patient's history for hypersensitivity to local anesthetics. Warn him that he may feel a stinging sensation on injection of the anesthetic and some pressure during withdrawal of the fluid. Advise him not to cough, breathe deeply, or move during the test to minimize the risk of injury to the lung.

Equipment

- Sterile collection bottles, sterile gloves, adhesive tape
- Sterile thoracentesis tray: a prepackaged, disposable tray with 70% alcohol or povidone-iodine solution, drapes, local anesthetic (usually 1% lidocaine), sterile 5-ml syringe for local anesthetic and 25G needle, 50-ml syringe for removing fluid and 17G aspiration needle, sterile specimen bottle or tube (ideally, a negative-pressure bottle), three-way stopcock or sterile tubing to prevent air from entering the pleural cavity, and a small sterile dressing.

Procedure

- Record baseline vital signs. Shave the area around the needle insertion site, if necessary. Position the patient to widen the intercostal spaces and provide easier access to the pleural cavity; make sure he's well supported and comfortable. If possible, seat him at the edge of the bed with a chair or stool supporting his feet and his head and arms resting on a padded overbed table. If he can't sit up, position him on his unaffected side with the arm on the affected side elevated above his head. Remind him not to cough, breathe deeply, or move suddenly during the procedure.
- After the patient is properly positioned, the doctor disinfects the skin, drapes the area, injects a local anesthetic into the subcutaneous tissue, and inserts the thoracentesis needle above the rib to avoid lacerating intercostal vessels. When the needle reaches the pocket of fluid, he attaches the 50-ml syringe and the stopcock and opens the clamps on the tubing to aspirate fluid into the container. During aspiration, check the patient for signs of respiratory distress, such as weakness, dyspnea, pallor, cyanosis, changes in heart rate, tachypnea, diaphoresis, blood-tinged frothy mucus, and hypotension.
- After the needle is withdrawn, apply slight pressure and a small adhesive bandage to the puncture site. Label the specimen, and record the date and time of the test and the amount, color, and character of the fluid (clear, frothy, purulent, bloody) on the laboratory request. Note any signs of distress the patient exhibited during the procedure. Document the exact location from which fluid was removed because this information may aid diagnosis.

CHARACTERISTICS OF PULMONARY TRANSUDATE AND EXUDATE

The following characteristics help classify pleural fluid as either a transudate or an exudate.

Characteristic	Transudate	Exudate
Appearance	Clear	Cloudy, turbid
Specific gravity	<1.016	>1.016
Clot (fibrinogen)	Absent	Present
Protein	<3 g/dl	>3 g/dl
White blood cells	Few lymphocytes	Many lymphocytes; may be purulent
Red blood cells	Few	Variable
Glucose level	Equal to serum level	May be less than serum level
Lactate dehydrogenase	Low	High

Precautions

CLINICAL ALERT Thoracentesis is contraindicated in patients with a history of bleeding disorders or anticoagulant therapy. The benefits of the procedure should outweigh the risks. Generally, the procedure can be performed on a patient taking an anticoagulant who has an INR of 1.5 to 2.5.

■ Use strict aseptic technique.
■ Note the patient's temperature and use of antimicrobial therapy, if applicable, on the laboratory request.
■ Send the specimen to the laboratory immediately.

Normal findings

The pleural cavity normally maintains negative pressure and contains less than 20 ml of serous fluid.

Implications of results

Pleural effusion results from the abnormal formation or reabsorption of pleural fluid. Pleural fluid is either a transudate (a low-protein fluid that has leaked from normal blood vessels) or an exudate (a protein-rich fluid that has leaked from blood vessels with increased permeability). (See *Characteristics of pulmonary transudate and exudate.*)

Pleural fluid may contain blood (hemothorax), chyle (chylothorax), or pus and necrotic tissue. Blood-tinged fluid may indicate a traumatic tap; if so, the fluid should clear as aspiration progresses.

Transudative effusion usually results from diminished colloidal pressure, increased negative pressure within the pleural cavity, ascites, systemic and pulmonary venous hypertension, heart failure, hepatic cirrhosis, and nephritis.

Exudative effusion results from disorders that increase pleural capillary permeability (possibly with changes in hydrostatic or colloid osmotic pressures), lymphatic drainage interference, infections, pulmonary infarctions, and neoplasms. Exudative effusion in association with depressed glucose levels, elevated LD levels, rheumatoid arthritis cells, and negative smears, cultures, and cytologic examination may indicate pleurisy associated with rheumatoid arthritis.

The most common pathogens that appear in culture studies of pleural fluid include *Mycobacterium tuberculosis, Staphylococcus aureus, Streptococcus pneumoniae* and other streptococci, *Haemophilus influenzae* and, in the case of a ruptured pulmonary abscess, anaerobes such as *Bacteroides*. Cultures are usually positive during the early stages of infection; however, antibiotic therapy may produce a negative culture despite a positive Gram stain and grossly purulent fluid. Empyema may result from complications of pneumonia, pulmonary abscess, perforation of the esophagus, and penetration from mediastinitis. A high percentage of neutrophils suggests septic inflammation; predominating lymphocytes suggest tuberculosis or fungal or viral effusions.

Serosanguineous fluid may indicate metastasis of a malignant tumor into the pleura. Elevated LD levels in a nonpurulent, nonhemolyzed, nonbloody effusion also suggest a malignant tumor. Pleural fluid glucose levels that are 30 to 40 mg/dl lower than blood glucose levels suggest cancer, bacterial infection, nonseptic inflammation, or metastasis. Amylase levels are elevated in pleural effusions associated with pancreatitis.

Posttest care

■ Reposition the patient comfortably on the affected side or as ordered by the doctor. Tell him to remain on this side for at least 1 hour to seal the puncture site. Elevate the head of the bed to facilitate breathing.

■ Monitor vital signs every 30 minutes for 2 hours and then every 4 hours until they're stable.

CLINICAL ALERT Tell the patient to call a nurse immediately if he experiences difficulty breathing.

CLINICAL ALERT Watch for signs of pneumothorax, tension pneumothorax, fluid reaccumulation and, if a large amount of fluid was withdrawn, pulmonary edema or cardiac distress associated with mediastinal shift. Usually, a post-test X-ray is ordered to detect these com-

---

RECOGNIZING COMPLICATIONS OF THORACENTESIS

You can identify the following potential complications of thoracentesis by watching for their characteristic signs and symptoms:

■ *pneumothorax:* apprehension, increased restlessness, cyanosis, sudden breathlessness, tachycardia, chest pain
■ *tension pneumothorax:* dyspnea, chest pain, tachycardia, hypotension, absent or diminished breath sounds on affected side
■ *subcutaneous emphysema:* local tissue swelling, crackling on palpation of site
■ *infection:* fever, rapid pulse rate, pain
■ *mediastinal shift:* labored breathing, cardiac arrhythmias, cardiac distress, pulmonary edema (pink, frothy sputum; paradoxical pulse).

---

plications before clinical symptoms appear. (See *Recognizing complications of thoracentesis.*)
■ Check the puncture site for fluid leakage. A large amount of leakage is abnormal. Also check the site and surrounding area for subcutaneous emphysema.

Interfering factors

■ Antimicrobial therapy before aspiration of fluid for culture may decrease the number of bacteria, making isolation of the infecting organism difficult.
■ Failure to use aseptic technique may contaminate the specimen.
■ Failure to send the specimen to the laboratory immediately may affect the accuracy of test results.

Porphyrin test, urine

This test is a quantitative analysis of urine porphyrins (most notably, uroporphyrins and coproporphyrins) and their precursors (porphyrinogens, such as porphobilinogen [PBG]). Porphyrins are red-orange fluorescent molecules that are produced during heme biosynthesis. They are present in RBCs, participate in energy storage and utilization, and are normally excreted in urine in small amounts. Elevated urine levels of porphyrins or porphyrinogens, therefore, reflect impaired heme biosynthesis. Such impairment may result from inherited enzyme deficiencies (congenital porphyrias) or from defects caused by such disorders as hemolytic anemias and hepatic disease (acquired porphyrias).

Determining the specific porphyrins and porphyrinogens found in a urine specimen can help identify the impaired metabolic step in heme biosynthesis. Occasionally, a preliminary qualitative screening is performed on a random specimen; a positive finding on the screening test must be confirmed by the quantitative analysis of a 24-hour specimen. For correct diagnosis of a specific porphyria, urine porphyrin levels should be correlated with plasma and fecal porphyrin levels.

Purpose

To aid diagnosis of congenital or acquired porphyrias.

Patient preparation

Explain to the patient that this test detects abnormal hemoglobin formation. Inform him that he needn't restrict food or fluids before the test. Tell him the test requires a 24-hour urine specimen, and teach him the proper collection technique.

Check the patient's history for current pregnancy, menstruation, or drug use; such conditions may affect test results. Inform the laboratory and the doctor, who may reschedule the test or restrict drugs before the test.

Procedure

Collect a 24-hour urine specimen in a light-resistant specimen bottle containing a preservative to prevent degradation of the light-sensitive porphyrins and their precursors.

Precautions

■ Refrigerate the specimen or keep it on ice during the collection period. Send it to the laboratory as soon as the collection is completed.

■ If a light-resistant container isn't available, protect the specimen from light exposure. If an indwelling urinary catheter is in place, put the collection bag in a dark plastic bag.

Reference values

Normal urine porphyrin and precursor values are as follows:

■ uroporphyrins: in women, 1 to 22 µg/24 hours; in men, undetectable to 42 µg/24 hours

■ coproporphyrins: in women, 1 to 57 µg/24 hours; in men, undetectable to 96 µg/24 hours

■ PBG: in both sexes, undetectable to 1.5 mg/24 hours.

Implications of results

Levels of most porphyrins and their precursors increase in patients with porphyria. Because heme synthesis occurs primarily in bone marrow and the liver, porphyrias are classified as erythropoietic or hepatic. (See *Urine porphyrin levels in porphyria*, pages 460 and 461.)

Infectious hepatitis, Hodgkin's disease, central nervous system disorders, cirrhosis, and heavy metal, benzene, or carbon tetrachloride toxicity can also increase porphyrin levels.

URINE PORPHYRIN LEVELS IN PORPHYRIA

Defective heme biosynthesis increases levels of most urinary porphyrins and their corresponding precursors, as shown below.

Porphyria	Porphyrins	
	Uroporphyrins	Coproporphyrins
Erythropoietic porphyria	Highly increased	Increased
Erythropoietic protoporphyria	Normal	Normal
Acute intermittent porphyria	Variable	Variable
Variegate porphyria	Normal or slightly increased; may be highly increased during acute attack	Normal or slightly increased; may be highly increased during acute attack
Coproporphyria	Not applicable	May be highly increased during acute attack
Porphyria cutanea tarda (assumed to be acquired in association with other hepatic diseases; genetic causes possible)	Highly increased	Increased

Posttest care

As ordered, resume medications that were discontinued before the test.

Interfering factors

■ Oral contraceptives and griseofulvin can elevate urine porphyrin levels; rifampin turns urine red-orange, interfering with results.
■ Barbiturates, chloral hydrate, chlorpropamide, sulfonamides, meprobamate, and chlordiazepoxide generally induce porphyria or porphyrinuria; they should be discontinued 10 to 12 days before the test, if possible.
■ Elevated urine urobilinogen levels can interfere with test results by affecting the reagent used in the PBG screening test.
■ Pregnancy and menstruation may increase porphyrin levels.
■ If the urine specimen is left standing for a few hours, PBG levels decline.

Potassium test, serum

Potassium is the major intracellular cation. The intracellular concentration of potassium is 150 to 160 mEq/L,

Porphyrin precursors	
Delta-aminolevulinic acid	**Porphobilinogen**
Normal	Normal
Normal	Normal
Highly increased	Highly increased
Highly increased during acute attack	Normal or slightly increased; highly increased during acute attack
Increased during acute attack	Increased during acute attack
Variable	Variable

and the extracellular concentration is 3.5 to 4.5 mEq/L. Serum potassium assays measure extracellular levels.

Potassium is important in maintaining cellular electrical neutrality. The sodium-potassium active transport pump maintains the ratio of intracellular potassium to extracellular potassium that determines the resting membrane potential necessary for nerve impulse transmission. Disturbances in this ratio change cardiac rhythms, transmission and conduction of nerve impulses, and muscle contraction.

Aldosterone and acid-base balance regulate serum potassium concentration. Aldosterone release stimulates the distal tubules of the kidney to excrete excess potassium in the urine. The kidneys reabsorb sodium and excrete potassium to maintain balance. Changes in pH (acid-base balance) cause shifts in the concentration of potassium. Alkalosis increases renal excretion of potassium; acidosis inhibits its excretion.

Because the kidneys excrete nearly all ingested potassium daily, a dietary intake of at least 40 mEq/day is essential. A normal diet usually includes 60 to 100 mEq of potassium. (See *Dietary sources of potassium*, page 462.)

DIETARY SOURCES OF POTASSIUM

A healthy person needs to consume at least 40 mEq of potassium daily. Foods and beverages that contain plentiful amounts of potassium are listed below.

Foods and beverages	Serving size	Amount of potassium (mEq)
Meats		
Beef	4 oz (112 g)	11.2
Chicken	4 oz	12.0
Scallops	5 large	30.0
Veal	4 oz	15.2
Vegetables		
Artichokes	1 large bud	7.7
Asparagus, fresh, frozen, cooked	½ cup	5.5
Asparagus, raw	6 spears	7.7
Beans, dried, cooked	½ cup	10.0
Beans, lima	½ cup	9.5
Broccoli, cooked	½ cup	7.0
Carrots, cooked	½ cup	5.7
Carrots, raw	1 large	8.8
Mushrooms, raw	4 large	10.6
Potato, baked	1 small	15.4
Spinach, fresh, cooked	½ cup	8.5
Squash, winter, baked	½ cup	12.0
Tomato, raw	1 medium	10.4
Fruits		
Apricots, dried	4 halves	5.0
Apricots, fresh	3 small	8.0
Banana	1 medium	12.8
Cantaloupe	small	13.0
Figs, dried	7 small	17.5
Peach, fresh	1 medium	6.2
Pear, fresh	1 medium	6.2
Beverages		
Apricot nectar	1 cup (240 ml)	9.0
Grapefruit juice	1 cup	8.2
Orange juice	1 cup	11.4
Pineapple juice	1 cup	9.0
Prune juice	1 cup	14.4
Tomato juice	1 cup	11.6
Milk, whole, skim	1 cup	8.8

Purpose

■ To evaluate clinical signs of potassium excess (hyperkalemia) or potassium depletion (hypokalemia)
■ To monitor renal function, acid-base balance, and glucose metabolism
■ To evaluate neuromuscular and endocrine disorders
■ To detect the origin of arrhythmias.

Patient preparation

Explain to the patient that this test determines the potassium content of blood. Inform him he needn't restrict food or fluids. Tell him the test requires a blood sample, who will perform the venipuncture and when, and that he may feel some transient discomfort from the needle puncture and the pressure of the tourniquet.

Check the patient history for use of drugs that may influence test results. If these medications must be continued, note this on the laboratory request.

Procedure

Perform a venipuncture and collect the sample in a 7-ml clot-activator tube.

Precautions

■ Draw the sample immediately after applying the tourniquet because a delay may elevate the potassium level by allowing intracellular potassium to leak into the serum.

■ Handle the sample gently to avoid hemolysis.

Reference values

Normal serum potassium levels are 3.8 to 5.5 mEq/L.

Implications of results

Hyperkalemia reflects increased potassium intake, a shift in the concentration from intracellular to extracellular fluid, or decreased renal excretion. An increase in dietary intake doesn't usually cause hyperkalemia unless renal impairment is present.

Patients with hyperkalemia require ECG monitoring to detect prolonged PR interval, wide QRS complex, ST-segment depression, tall and peaked T waves, bradycardia, and ventricular arrhythmias, tachycardia, or fibrillation. Educate patients at risk for hyperkalemia about dietary intake of potassium and foods to avoid, if indicated.

Hypokalemia reflects depletion of total body potassium caused by shifts from extracellular fluid to intracellular fluid. Metabolic causes include diabetic ketoacidosis and insulin administration without potassium supplements and respiratory alkalosis. Other causes include gastrointestinal and renal disorders, and excessive licorice ingestion causes hypokalemia resulting from the aldosterone-like effect of glycyrrhizii.

CLINICAL ALERT Observe a patient with hypokalemia for decreased reflexes, mental confusion, hypotension, anorexia, muscle weakness, paresthesia, and rapid, weak, irregular pulse.

Observe for digitalis toxicity. Hypokalemia potentiates digoxin and causes toxicity at lower drug levels.

Posttest care

If a hematoma develops at the venipuncture site, apply warm soaks.

Interfering factors

■ Repeated clenching of the fist before venipuncture may cause elevated potassium levels.

■ Excessive or rapid potassium infusion, spironolactone or penicillin G potassium therapy, or renal toxicity from administration of amphotericin B, methicillin, or tetracycline elevates serum potassium levels.

■ Insulin and glucose administration, diuretic therapy (especially with thiazides, but not with triamterene, amiloride, or spironolactone), or I.V. infusions without potassium suppress serum potassium levels.

■ Excessive hemolysis of the sample or delay in drawing blood after application of a tourniquet elevates potassium levels.

Potassium test, urine

This quantitative test measures urine levels of potassium, a major intracellular cation that helps regulate acid-base balance and neuromuscular function. Potassium imbalance may cause such signs and symptoms as muscle weakness, nausea, diarrhea, confusion, hypotension, and electrocardiogram (ECG) changes; a severe imbalance may lead to cardiac arrest.

A serum potassium test is usually performed to detect hyperkalemia or hypokalemia. A urine potassium test may be performed to evaluate hypokalemia when a history and physical examination fail to uncover the cause. Because kidneys regulate potassium balance through potassium excretion in the urine, measuring urine potassium levels can determine whether hypokalemia results from a renal disorder, such as renal tubular acidosis, or an extrarenal disorder, such as malabsorption syndrome. If results suggest a renal disorder, additional renal function tests may be ordered.

Purpose

To determine whether hypokalemia is caused by renal or extrarenal disorders.

Patient preparation

Explain to the patient that this test evaluates his kidney function. Advise him that no special dietary restrictions are necessary and that the test requires a 24-hour urine specimen. If the specimen is to be collected at home, teach him the correct collection technique. Check his medication history for drugs that may alter test results.

If they must be continued, note this on the laboratory request.

Procedure

Collect a 24-hour urine specimen.

Precautions

■ Tell the patient not to contaminate the specimen with toilet tissue or stool.
■ Refrigerate the specimen or place it on ice during the collection period.
■ After collection, send the specimen to the laboratory immediately or refrigerate it.

Reference values

Normal potassium excretion is 25 to 125 mEq/24 hours, with an average potassium concentration of 25 to 100 mEq/L. In a patient with hypokalemia and normal kidney function, potassium concentration will be less than 10 mEq/L, indicating that potassium loss is most likely the result of a GI disorder such as malabsorption syndrome.

Implications of results

In a patient with hypokalemia lasting more than 3 days, urine potassium levels above 10 mEq/L indicate renal losses that may result from such disorders as aldosteronism, renal tubular acidosis, or chronic renal failure. However, extrarenal disorders, such as dehydration, starvation, Cushing's disease, or salicylate intoxication, may also elevate urine potassium levels.

Posttest care

■ Monitor the hypokalemic patient for diminished reflexes, confusion, hypotension, anorexia, muscle weakness, paresthesias, and rapid, weak, irregular pulse. Watch for ECG alterations, especially a flattened T wave, ST-segment depression, and U-wave elevation. Severe potassium imbalance may lead to ventricular fibrillation, respiratory paralysis, and cardiac arrest.
■ Administer potassium supplements and monitor serum levels, as ordered.
■ Provide dietary supplements and nutritional counseling, as ordered.
■ Replace volume loss with I.V. or oral fluids, as ordered.
■ Resume medications withheld before the test, as ordered.

Interfering factors

■ Excess dietary potassium raises urine potassium levels.

- Potassium-wasting medications, such as ammonium chloride, thiazide diuretics, and acetazolamide, raise potassium levels.
- Excessive vomiting or stomach suctioning produces test results that don't reflect actual potassium depletion.
- Failure to collect all urine during the test period or to store the specimen properly may alter test results.

Pregnanediol test, urine

Using gas chromatography or radioimmunoassay, this test measures urine levels of pregnanediol, the chief metabolite of progesterone. Although biologically inert, pregnanediol has diagnostic significance because it reflects about 10% of the endogenous production of its parent hormone.

In nonpregnant females the corpus luteum produces progesterone during the latter half of each menstrual cycle to prepare the uterus for implantation of a fertilized ovum. If implantation doesn't occur, progesterone secretion drops sharply; if implantation does occur, the corpus luteum secretes more progesterone to further prepare the uterus for pregnancy and to begin development of the placenta. Toward the end of the first trimester, the placenta becomes the primary source of progesterone secretion, producing the progressively larger amounts needed to maintain pregnancy.

Normally, urine levels of pregnanediol reflect variations in progesterone secretion during the menstrual cycle and during pregnancy. Direct measurement of plasma progesterone levels by radioimmunoassay may also be done. Pregnanediol is present in the urine as a metabolite of progesterone and is produced in small amounts by the adrenal cortex, the principal site of secretion in males, postmenopausal women, and menstruating females before ovulation.

Purpose

- To evaluate placental function in pregnant females
- To evaluate ovarian function in nonpregnant females.

Patient preparation

Explain to the patient that this test evaluates placental or ovarian function. Inform her that she needn't restrict food or fluids. Tell her the test requires a 24-hour urine specimen, and teach her the proper collection technique.

Check the patient's medication history for recent use of drugs that may affect pregnanediol levels.

Procedure

Collect a 24-hour urine specimen.

Precautions

- Refrigerate the specimen or keep it on ice during the collection period.
- If the patient is pregnant, note the approximate week of gestation on the laboratory request. For other pre-menopausal females, note the stage of the menstrual cycle.

Reference values

In nonpregnant females, the normal range of urine pregnanediol values is 0.5 to 1.5 mg/24 hours during the proliferative phase of the menstrual cycle. Pregnanediol levels begin to rise within 24 hours after ovulation and continue to rise for 3 to 10 days as the corpus luteum develops. During this luteal phase, the normal range is 2 to 7 mg/24 hours. If fertilization doesn't occur, levels drop sharply as the corpus luteum degenerates, and menstruation begins.

During pregnancy, urine pregnanediol levels rise markedly, peaking around the 36th week of gestation and returning to prepregnancy levels by day 5 to day 10 postpartum. (See *Urine pregnanediol values in pregnancy*, page 468.)

Normal postmenopausal values in the range of 0.2 to 1 mg/24 hours. In males, levels rarely rise above 1.5 mg/24 hours.

Implications of results

During pregnancy, a marked decrease in urine pregnanediol in a single 24-hour urine specimen or a steady decrease in serial measurements may indicate placental insufficiency and requires immediate investigation. A precipitous drop in pregnanediol values may suggest fetal distress, as in threatened abortion or preeclampsia, or fetal death. However, pregnanediol levels aren't reliable indicators of fetal viability because they can remain normal even after fetal death as long as maternal circulation to the placenta remains adequate.

In nonpregnant females, abnormally low urine pregnanediol levels may reflect anovulation, amenorrhea, and other menstrual abnormalities. Low to normal levels may be associated with hydatidiform mole. Elevated levels may indicate luteinized granulosa or theca cell tumors, diffuse thecal luteinization, or metastatic ovarian cancer.

Adrenal hyperplasia or biliary tract obstruction may elevate urine pregnanediol values in males or females. Some forms of primary hepatic disease produce very low levels in both sexes.

URINE PREGNANEDIOL VALUES IN PREGNANCY

Serial determinations of average pregnanediol levels (middle line on chart) rise steadily until about 32 weeks' gestation and then level off. Excretion decreases 24 hours postpartum and drops to prepregnancy levels within 5 to 10 days. Normal values cover a wide range, including high-normal, low-normal, and average levels, as shown below.

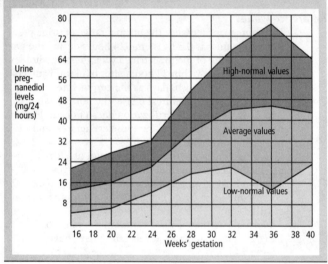

Posttest care

■ As ordered, resume administration of drugs withheld before the test.

■ Advise the pregnant patient that this test may be repeated several times to obtain serial measurements.

■ If pregnanediol level is low and supplementation is ordered, explain the use of progesterone. Provide support and prepare for further testing if results indicate neoplasm or threatened abortion.

Interfering factors

■ Methenamine mandelate, methenamine hippurate, and drugs containing corticotropin elevate urine pregnanediol levels. Progestogens and combination oral contraceptives characteristically lower them.

■ Failure to collect all urine during the collection period may alter test results.

■ Failure to refrigerate the specimen or to keep it on ice during the collection period may alter test results.

Pregnanetriol test, urine

Using spectrophotometry, this test determines urine levels of pregnanetriol, the metabolite of the cortisol precursor 17-hydroxyprogesterone. Minute amounts of pregnanetriol are normally excreted in the urine. However, when cortisol biosynthesis is impaired at the point of 17-hydroxyprogesterone conversion, urinary excretion of pregnanetriol increases significantly. Such impairment results from the absence or deficiency of particular biosynthetic enzymes that convert 17-hydroxyprogesterone to cortisol; in turn, low plasma cortisol levels interfere with the negative feedback mechanism that inhibits secretion of corticotropin. Consequently, excessive 17-hydroxyprogesterone accumulates in the plasma, leading to increased formation and excretion of pregnanetriol in urine.

Urine pregnanetriol levels may be measured concomitantly with urine 17-ketosteroids and urine 17-ketogenic steroids to assess androgen levels, which also rise with impaired cortisol biosynthesis. Elevated androgen levels, which occur in adrenogenital syndrome (congenital adrenal hyperplasia), result from conversion of excessive 17-hydroxyprogesterone to androgens and from hypersecretion of adrenal androgens in response to excessive corticotropin stimulation.

Purpose

- To aid diagnosis of adrenogenital syndrome
- To monitor cortisol replacement.

Patient preparation

Explain to the patient (or to his parents if the patient is a child) that this test evaluates hormone secretion. Inform him that he needn't restrict food or fluids before the test. Tell him the test requires collection of a 24-hour urine specimen, and teach him the proper collection technique.

Procedure

Collect a 24-hour urine specimen in a bottle containing a preservative to keep the specimen at a pH of 4.0 to 4.5.

Precautions

Refrigerate the specimen or keep it on ice during the collection period. Send the specimen to the laboratory as soon as the collection is completed.

Reference values

The normal urine pregnanetriol values for males age 16 and over are 0.2 to 2 mg/24 hours; for females age 16 and over, 0 to 1.4 mg/24 hours.

Implications of results

Elevated urine pregnanetriol levels suggest adrenogenital syndrome, marked by excessive adrenal androgen secretion and resulting virilization. Females with this condition fail to develop normal secondary sex characteristics and show marked masculinization of external genitalia at birth.

Males usually appear normal at birth but later develop signs of somatic and sexual precocity.

In monitoring treatment with cortisol replacement, elevated urine pregnanetriol levels indicate insufficient dosage of cortisol. When cortisol replacement adequately inhibits hypersecretion of corticotropin and subsequent overproduction of 17-hydroxyprogesterone, pregnanetriol levels fall to normal.

Assess for changes in genitalia, breasts, and hairline (receding) caused by adrenogenital syndrome. Support the patient with body-image changes. Explain reasons for virilization caused by adrenal gland problem. Monitor pregnanetriol levels in patients receiving cortisol replacement.

Interfering factors

- Corticotropin administration may increase levels.
- Oral contraceptives and progesterone may decrease levels.
- Failure to collect all urine during the test period or to store the specimen properly may interfere with test results.

Progesterone test, plasma

Progesterone, an ovarian steroid hormone secreted by the corpus luteum, causes thickening and secretory development of the endometrium in preparation for implantation of the fertilized ovum. Progesterone levels, therefore, peak during the midluteal phase of the menstrual cycle. Progesterone may prolong the surge of luteinizing hormone after ovulation. If implantation doesn't occur, progesterone (and estrogen) levels drop sharply and menstruation begins about 2 days later. During pregnancy, the placenta releases about 10 times the normal monthly amount of progesterone to maintain the pregnancy. Increased secretion begins toward the end of the first trimester and continues until delivery. Progesterone causes thickening of the endometrium, which contains large amounts of stored nutrients for the developing ovum (blastocyst). In addition, progesterone prevents abortion by decreasing uterine contractions and, with estrogen, prepares the breasts for lactation.

This radioimmunoassay is a quantitative analysis of plasma progesterone levels. It provides reliable information about corpus luteum function in fertility studies or placental function in pregnancy. Serial determinations are recommended. Although plasma levels provide accurate information, progesterone can also be monitored by measuring urine pregnanediol, a catabolite of progesterone.

Purpose

■ To assess corpus luteum function as part of infertility studies
■ To evaluate placental function during pregnancy
■ To aid in confirming ovulation; test results support basal body temperature readings.

Patient preparation

Explain to the patient that this test helps determine if her female sex hormone secretion is normal. Inform her that she needn't restrict food or fluids. Tell her the test requires a blood sample, who will perform the venipuncture and when, and that she may experience transient discomfort from the needle puncture. Inform her that the test may be repeated at specific times coinciding with phases of her menstrual cycle or at each prenatal visit.

Procedure

Perform a venipuncture and collect the sample in a 7-ml heparinized tube.

Precautions

■ Handle the sample gently to prevent hemolysis.
■ Completely fill the collection tube; then invert it gently at least 10 times to mix sample and anticoagulant adequately.
■ Indicate the date of the patient's last menstrual period and the phase of her cycle on the laboratory request. If the patient is pregnant, indicate the month of gestation.
■ Send the sample to the laboratory immediately.

Reference values

Normal values during menstruation:
■ follicular phase: < 150 ng/dl
■ luteal phase: about 300 ng/dl (rises daily during periovulation)

■ midluteal phase: 2,000 ng/dl.
Normal values during pregnancy:
■ first trimester: 1,500 to 5,000 ng/dl
■ second and third trimesters: 8,000 to 20,000 ng/dl.

Implications of results

Elevated progesterone levels may indicate ovulation, luteinizing tumors, ovarian cysts that produce progesterone, or adrenocortical hyperplasia and tumors that produce progesterone along with other steroid hormones.

Low progesterone levels are associated with amenorrhea associated with several causes (such as panhypopituitarism or gonadal dysfunction), toxemia of pregnancy, threatened abortion, and fetal death.

Posttest care

If a hematoma develops at the venipuncture site, apply warm soaks.

Interfering factors

■ Progesterone or estrogen therapy may interfere with test results.
■ Use of radioisotopes or radionuclide scans within 1 week before the test may affect test results.
■ Hemolysis caused by rough handling of the sample may affect test results.

Prolactin test, serum

Similar in molecular structure and biological activity to human growth hormone (hGH), prolactin is a polypeptide hormone secreted by the anterior pituitary. It's essential for the development of the mammary glands for lactation during pregnancy and for stimulating and maintaining lactation postpartum. Prolactin (also known as lactogenic hormone or lactogen) is also secreted in males and nonpregnant females, but its function in these groups is unknown. Like hGH, prolactin acts directly on tissues, and its levels rise in response to sleep and to physical or emotional stress.

This radioimmunoassay is a quantitative analysis of serum prolactin levels, which normally rise 10- to 20-fold during pregnancy, corresponding to concomitant elevations in human placental lactogen levels. After delivery, prolactin secretion falls to basal levels in mothers who don't breast-feed. Prolactin secretion increases during breast-feeding, apparently as a result of a stimulus triggered by suckling that curtails the release of prolactin-inhibiting factor by the hypothalamus. This, in turn, allows transient elevations of prolactin secretion

TRH STIMULATION TEST

This test evaluates hypothalamic dysfunction and pituitary tumors by stimulating the release of prolactin. The procedure is as follows: perform a venipuncture to obtain a baseline prolactin level, and then help the patient into the supine position. Administer an I.V. bolus of synthetic thyrotropin-releasing hormone (TRH) in a dose of 500 µg/ml over 15 to 30 seconds. Blood samples are taken at 15- and 30-minute intervals to measure prolactin.

A baseline prolactin reading greater than 200 ng/ml indicates a pituitary tumor, although levels between 30 and 200 ng/ml are also consistent with this condition. Normally, patients show at least a twofold increase in prolactin after injection of TRH. If the prolactin level doesn't rise, hypothalamic dysfunction or adenoma of the pituitary gland is likely.

by the pituitary. This test is considered useful in patients suspected of having pituitary tumors, which are known to secrete prolactin in excessive amounts.

Another test used to evaluate hypothalamic dysfunction is the thyrotropin-releasing hormone (TRH) stimulation test. (See *TRH stimulation test.*)

Purpose

■ To facilitate diagnosis of pituitary dysfunction that may be caused by pituitary adenoma
■ To aid in the diagnosis of hypothalamic dysfunction regardless of cause
■ To evaluate secondary amenorrhea and galactorrhea.

Patient preparation

Tell the patient that this test helps evaluate hormonal secretion. Advise her to restrict food and fluids and limit physical activity for 12 hours before the test. Encourage her to relax for about 30 minutes before the test. Tell her who will draw the blood sample and when and that she may experience some discomfort from the needle puncture. Advise her that the laboratory requires at least 4 days to complete the analysis. As ordered, withhold drugs that may influence serum prolactin levels, such as chlorpromazine and methyldopa. If they must be continued, note this on the laboratory request.

Procedure

Perform a venipuncture at least 3 hours after the patient wakes; samples drawn earlier are likely to show sleep-induced peak levels. Collect the sample in a 7-ml clot-activator tube.

Precautions

■ Handle the sample gently to prevent hemolysis.

■ Confirm slight elevations with repeat measurements on two other occasions.

Reference values

Normal values range from undetectable to 23 ng/ml in nonlactating females.

Implications of results

Abnormally high prolactin levels (100 to 300 ng/ml) suggest autonomous prolactin production by a pituitary adenoma, especially when amenorrhea or galactorrhea is present (Forbes-Albright syndrome). Rarely, hyperprolactinemia may also result from severe endocrine disorders, such as hypothyroidism. Idiopathic hyperprolactinemia may be associated with anovulatory infertility.

Decreased prolactin levels in a lactating mother cause failure of lactation and may be associated with postpartum pituitary infarction (Sheehan's syndrome). Abnormally low prolactin levels have also been found in a few patients with empty-sella syndrome. In these patients, a flattened pituitary gland makes the pituitary fossa appear empty.

Posttest care

■ If a hematoma develops at the venipuncture site, apply warm soaks.
■ As ordered, resume administration of discontinued medications.

Interfering factors

■ Failure to take into account physiologic variations related to sleep or stress may invalidate test results.
■ Pretest use of drugs that raise prolactin levels (such as ethanol, morphine, methyldopa, and estrogens) may interfere with test results.
■ Pretest use of apomorphine, ergot alkaloids, and levodopa lowers prolactin levels.
■ Radioactive scan performed within 1 week before the test or recent surgery may interfere with test results.
■ Breast stimulation may alter results.
■ Hemolysis caused by rough handling of the sample may affect test results.

Prostate gland biopsy

Prostate gland biopsy is the needle excision of a prostate tissue specimen for histologic examination. A perineal, transrectal, or transurethral approach may be used; the transrectal approach is usually used for high prostatic lesions. Indications include potentially malignant prostatic hypertrophy and prostatic nodules.

Purpose

- To confirm prostate cancer
- To determine the cause of prostatic hypertrophy.

Patient preparation

Describe the procedure to the patient, answer his questions, and tell him the test provides a tissue specimen for microscopic study. Tell him who will perform the biopsy and where, that he'll receive a local anesthetic, and that the procedure takes less than 30 minutes.

Make sure the patient has signed a consent form. Check the patient history for hypersensitivity to the anesthetic or to other drugs. For a transrectal approach, prepare the bowel by administering enemas until the return is clear. As ordered, administer an antibacterial to minimize the risk of infection. Just before the biopsy, check vital signs and administer a sedative, as ordered. Instruct the patient to remain still during the procedure and to follow instructions.

Procedure

- For perineal approach: Place the patient in the proper position (left lateral, knee-chest, or lithotomy), and clean the perineal skin. After the local anesthetic is administered, a 2-mm incision may be made into the perineum. The examiner immobilizes the prostate by inserting a finger into the rectum and introduces the biopsy needle into a prostate lobe. The needle is rotated gently, pulled out about 5 mm, and reinserted at another angle. The procedure is repeated at several areas. Specimens are placed immediately in a labeled specimen bottle containing 10% formalin solution. Pressure is exerted on the puncture site, which is then bandaged.
- For transrectal approach: This approach may be performed on outpatients without an anesthetic. Place the patient in a left lateral position. A curved needle guide is attached to the finger palpating the rectum. The biopsy needle is pushed along the guide, into the prostate. As the needle enters the prostate, the patient may experience pain. The needle is rotated to cut off the tissue and then is withdrawn.
- An alternative method of transrectal detection is the automated cone biopsy, in which the doctor uses a spring-powered device with an inner trocar needle to cut through prostatic tissue. This relatively new technique is quick and reportedly painless. With both transrectal methods, the specimen is placed immediately in a labeled specimen bottle containing 10% formalin solution.

■ For transurethral approach: An endoscopic instrument is passed through the urethra, permitting direct viewing of the prostate and passage of a cutting loop. The loop is rotated to chip away pieces of tissue and is then withdrawn. The specimen is placed immediately in a labeled specimen bottle containing 10% formalin solution.

Precautions

Complications may include transient, painless hematuria and bleeding into the prostatic urethra and bladder.

Normal findings

The prostate gland normally consists of a thin, fibrous capsule surrounding the stroma, which is made up of elastic and connective tissues and smooth-muscle fibers. The epithelial glands, found in these tissues and muscle fibers, drain into the chief excreting ducts.

Implications of results

Histologic examination can confirm cancer. Bone scans, bone marrow biopsy, and measurement of prostate-specific antigen (PSA) and serum acid phosphatase values determine its extent. Acid phosphatase levels usually rise in metastatic prostate cancer and tend to be low in cancer that is confined to the prostatic capsule.

Histologic examination can also detect benign prostatic hyperplasia, prostatitis, tuberculosis, lymphomas, and rectal or bladder cancers.

Posttest care

■ Check vital signs immediately after the procedure, every 2 hours for 4 hours, and then every 4 hours.
■ Observe the biopsy site for a hematoma and for signs of infection, such as redness, swelling, and pain.
■ Watch for urine retention or urinary frequency and for hematuria.

Interfering factors

Failure to obtain an adequate tissue specimen or to place the specimen in formalin solution may affect the accuracy of test results.

Prostate-specific antigen test

Until recently, digital rectal examination and measurement of prostatic acid phosphatase were the primary methods of monitoring the progression of prostate cancer. Now measurement of PSA helps track the course of this disease and evaluates response to treatment.

Biochemically and immunologically distinct from prostatic acid phosphatase, PSA appears in varying concentrations in normal, benign hyperplastic, and malig-

CONTROVERSY OVER PSA SCREENING

Measurement of prostate-specific antigen (PSA) allows earlier detection of prostate cancer than digital rectal examination (DRE) alone. Accordingly, the American Cancer Society and the American Urological Association currently recommend that PSA screening begin at age 40 (in combination with DRE) in black men and any man who has a father or brother with prostate cancer and at age 50 in all other men.

But does this test actually reduce mortality from prostate cancer? The answer to that question remains unknown. Some specialists question the value of all prostate cancer screening tests because of the costs involved, the uncertain benefits, and the known risks associated with current treatments.

Before undergoing a PSA test, the patient should understand that controversy surrounds nearly every aspect of prostate cancer screening and treatment. Among the issues he'll face are the following:

■ Even if cancer is detected, treatment may not be advisable, either because of the patient's advanced age or because the doctor believes the tumor is so slow-growing that it won't cause death.

■ The current treatments for prostate cancer — surgery and radiation therapy — may not be as effective as experts formerly believed, and no effective chemotherapy protocol is currently available.

■ Surgery and radiation therapy carry a high risk of impotence, incontinence, and other problems, which the patient must weigh against the uncertain benefits of therapy.

■ Screening tests sometimes yield false-positive results, requiring transrectal ultrasonography or a biopsy to confirm the diagnosis.

■ A mildly elevated PSA level may be the result of normal age-related increases. Data from a study of more than 9,000 men showed that PSA levels increase about 30% a year in men under age 70 and more than 40% a year in men over age 70.

In summary, the value of prostate cancer screening in general and PSA testing in particular won't be clearly established until studies show a definitive link between early treatment and reduced mortality.

nant prostatic tissue as well as in metastatic prostate cancer. For this reason, measurement of serum PSA levels along with a digital rectal examination is now recommended as a screening test for prostate cancer in men over age 50. (See *Controversy over PSA screening.*) It's also useful in assessing response to treatment in patients with stage B3 to D1 prostate cancer and in detecting tumor spread or recurrence.

Purpose

■ To screen for prostate cancer in men over age 50
■ To monitor the course of prostate cancer and help evaluate the effectiveness of treatment.

Patient preparation

Explain to the patient that this test is used to screen for prostate cancer or, if appropriate, to monitor the course of treatment. Inform him that he needn't restrict food or fluids. Tell him that this test requires a blood sample, who will perform the venipuncture and when, and that he may experience discomfort from the needle puncture.

Procedure

Perform a venipuncture, and collect the sample in a 7-ml clot-activator tube.

Precautions

■ Collect the sample either before a digital rectal examination or at least 48 hours after it to avoid falsely elevated PSA levels.
■ Send the sample, on ice, to the laboratory immediately.
■ Handle the sample gently to prevent hemolysis.

Reference values

■ Age 40 to 50: 2 to 2.8 ng/ml
■ Age 51 to 60: 2.9 to 3.8 ng/ml
■ Age 61 to 70: 4 to 5.3 ng/ml
■ Age 71 or older: 5.6 to 7.2 ng/ml.

Implications of results

About 80% of patients with prostate cancer have pretreatment PSA values greater than 4 ng/ml. This percentage is higher in advanced stages and lower in early stages.

However, PSA results alone shouldn't be considered diagnostic for prostate cancer because approximately 20% of patients with benign prostatic hyperplasia also have levels over 4 ng/ml. Further testing, including tissue biopsy and digital rectal examination, is needed to confirm a diagnosis of cancer.

Posttest care

If a hematoma develops at the venipuncture site, apply warm soaks.

Interfering factors

■ Excessive doses of chemotherapeutic drugs, such as cyclophosphamide, diethylstilbestrol, and methotrexate, may alter test results.
■ Hemolysis caused by rough handling of the sample may alter test results.

Protein C test

A vitamin K-dependent protein, protein C is produced in the liver and circulates in the plasma. After activation by thrombin in the presence of a capillary endothelial cofactor, it acts as a potent anticoagulant that suppresses the procoagulation activity of activated factors V and VIII. Both acquired and congenital deficiencies of protein C have been identified.

Homozygous deficiency of protein C, which is rare, is characterized by rapidly fatal thrombosis in the perinatal period, a syndrome known as purpura fulminans. The more common heterozygous deficiency is associated with familial susceptibility to venous thromboembolism before age 30 and continuing throughout life.

Measurement of protein C should include a functional assay and an immunologic study to determine the type of deficiency. Protein C values are used to investigate the cause of otherwise unexplained thrombosis and to establish patterns of inheritance. A positive finding for heterozygous deficiency suggests the possible need for long-term treatment with warfarin therapy or protein C supplements from plasma fractions.

Purpose

To investigate the mechanism of idiopathic venous thrombosis.

Patient preparation

Explain to the patient that this test evaluates the blood clotting mechanism. Tell him that the test requires a blood sample, who will perform the venipuncture and when, and that he may have some discomfort from the needle puncture and the tourniquet pressure. If the patient is receiving anticoagulant therapy, note this on the laboratory request.

Procedure

Perform a venipuncture. Collect a 3-ml sample in a silicon-coated vacuum specimen tube or in a special syringe with anticoagulant provided by the laboratory.

Precautions

■ Avoid excessive probing during venipuncture; handle the sample gently.
■ Completely fill the collection tube, and invert it several times to mix the sample and anticoagulant adequately.
■ Send the sample to the laboratory immediately.

Reference values

The normal range is 70% to 140% of the population mean, depending on the test method.

Implications of results

Identifying the role of protein C deficiency in idiopathic venous thrombosis may help prevent thromboembolism. Low protein C values are associated with disseminated intravascular coagulation, especially when it occurs in patients with cancer. Protein C deficiency is also seen in patients with liver cirrhosis and vitamin K deficiency and in those taking warfarin.

Posttest care

If a hematoma develops at the venipuncture site, apply warm soaks.

Interfering factors

■ Anticoagulant therapy may alter test results.
■ Hemolysis caused by excessive probing during venipuncture or rough handling of the sample may alter test results.

Protein electrophoresis test

This test separates serum albumin and globulins by using an electric field to differentiate the proteins — according to their size, shape, and electric charge at pH 8.6 — into five distinct fractions: albumin and alpha$_1$, alpha$_2$, beta, and gamma globulins. Each fraction has a recognizable, measurable pattern.

Albumin, which constitutes more than 50% of total serum protein, maintains oncotic pressure (preventing leakage of capillary plasma) and transports substances that are insoluble in water alone, such as bilirubin, fatty acids, hormones, and drugs. Of the four types of globulins, alpha$_1$, alpha$_2$, and beta act primarily as carrier proteins that transport lipids, hormones, and metals through the blood, and gamma globulin is an important component in the body's immune system.

Chemical analysis of total and individual proteins is a common laboratory procedure, and electrophoresis yields meaningful data about the five major fractions. Multiplying the relative percentage of each component protein fraction by the total protein concentration converts the proportions to absolute values. Regardless of test method used, a single protein fraction value is rarely significant by itself. The usual clinical indication for this test is suspected hepatic disease or protein deficiency. (See *How hepatic diseases affect protein fractions.*)

HOW HEPATIC DISEASES AFFECT PROTEIN FRACTIONS

Because the liver synthesizes albumin and alpha and beta globulins, changes in the concentration of these major plasma proteins suggest hepatic malfunction or hepatocellular damage. Although total protein levels — the sum of albumin and globulin fractions — may remain normal, hepatic disease will alter one, several, or all of the protein fractions.

	Normal	Hepatitis	Cirrhosis	Obstructive jaundice	Metastatic liver cancer
Total protein	100%	0	–	0	0
Albumin	53%	0	–	0/–	–
Alpha₁-globulin	14%	–	0	0	+
Alpha₂-globulin	14%	–	0	0/+	+
Beta globulin	12%	+	+	0/+	0/+
Gamma globulin	20%	+	+	0	0/+

KEY: 0 = normal + = increased – = decreased

Purpose

To aid diagnosis of hepatic disease, protein deficiency, and renal disorders as well as GI and neoplastic diseases.

Patient preparation

Explain to the patient that this test determines the protein content of blood. Inform him that he needn't restrict food or fluids. Tell him that the test requires a blood sample, who will perform the venipuncture and when, and that he may feel some discomfort from the needle puncture and the pressure of the tourniquet.

Review the patient's medication history for drugs that may influence serum protein levels. If they must be continued, note this on the laboratory request.

Procedure

Perform a venipuncture and collect the sample in a 7-ml clot-activator tube.

Precautions

This test must be performed on a serum sample to avoid measuring the fibrinogen fraction. (The fibrinogen fraction, if present, would be indistinguishable from certain abnormal monoclonal gamma globulins.)

Reference values

- total serum protein: 6.6 to 7.9 g/dl
- albumin: 3.3 to 4.5 g/dl
- alpha₁-globulin: 0.1 to 0.4 g/dl
- alpha₂-globulin: 0.5 to 1.0 g/dl

ALPHA₁-ANTITRYPSIN TEST

Using radioimmunoassay or isoelectric focusing, this test measures fasting serum levels of alpha₁-antitrypsin (AAT), a major component of alpha₁-globulin. AAT is believed to inhibit release of protease into body fluids by dying cells.

Congenital absence or deficiency of AAT increases susceptibility to emphysema. As a result, the serum AAT test provides a useful screening tool for high-risk patients. Such patients must be instructed to avoid smoking because irritants in tobacco stimulate leukocytes in the lungs to release protease.

The AAT test also is a nonspecific method of detecting inflammation, severe infection, and necrosis.

- beta globulin: 0.7 to 1.2 g/dl
- gamma globulin: 0.5 to 1.6 g/dl.

For information on another test involving alpha₁-globulin, see *Alpha₁-antitrypsin test.*

Implications of results

See *Clinical implications of abnormal protein levels.*

Posttest care

If a hematoma develops at the venipuncture site, apply warm soaks.

Interfering factors

- Pretest administration of a contrast agent (such as sulfobromophthalein) falsely elevates total protein test results.
- Pregnancy or cytotoxic drug use may lower serum albumin levels.
- Use of plasma instead of serum alters test results.
- Pregnancy may lower serum albumin levels.

Protein test, urine

This is a quantitative test for proteinuria. Normally, the glomerular membrane allows only proteins of low molecular weight to enter the filtrate. The renal tubules then reabsorb most of these proteins, normally excreting a small amount that's undetectable by a screening test. A damaged glomerular capillary membrane and impaired tubular reabsorption allow excretion of proteins in the urine.

A qualitative screening often precedes this test. (See *Random specimen screening for protein*, page 484.) A positive result requires quantitative analysis of a 24-hour urine specimen by acid precipitation tests. Electrophoresis can detect Bence Jones protein, hemoglobins, myoglobins, and albumin.

CLINICAL IMPLICATIONS OF ABNORMAL PROTEIN LEVELS

Abnormal levels of albumin or globulins are characteristic in many pathologic states such as those listed below.

INCREASED LEVELS

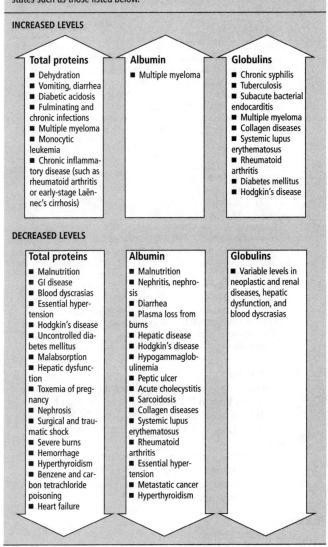

Total proteins
- Dehydration
- Vomiting, diarrhea
- Diabetic acidosis
- Fulminating and chronic infections
- Multiple myeloma
- Monocytic leukemia
- Chronic inflammatory disease (such as rheumatoid arthritis or early-stage Laënnec's cirrhosis)

Albumin
- Multiple myeloma

Globulins
- Chronic syphilis
- Tuberculosis
- Subacute bacterial endocarditis
- Multiple myeloma
- Collagen diseases
- Systemic lupus erythematosus
- Rheumatoid arthritis
- Diabetes mellitus
- Hodgkin's disease

DECREASED LEVELS

Total proteins
- Malnutrition
- GI disease
- Blood dyscrasias
- Essential hypertension
- Hodgkin's disease
- Uncontrolled diabetes mellitus
- Malabsorption
- Hepatic dysfunction
- Toxemia of pregnancy
- Nephrosis
- Surgical and traumatic shock
- Severe burns
- Hemorrhage
- Hyperthyroidism
- Benzene and carbon tetrachloride poisoning
- Heart failure

Albumin
- Malnutrition
- Nephritis, nephrosis
- Diarrhea
- Plasma loss from burns
- Hepatic disease
- Hodgkin's disease
- Hypogammaglobulinemia
- Peptic ulcer
- Acute cholecystitis
- Sarcoidosis
- Collagen diseases
- Systemic lupus erythematosus
- Rheumatoid arthritis
- Essential hypertension
- Metastatic cancer
- Hyperthyroidism

Globulins
- Variable levels in neoplastic and renal diseases, hepatic dysfunction, and blood dyscrasias

Purpose

To aid diagnosis of pathologic states characterized by proteinuria, primarily renal disease.

RANDOM SPECIMEN SCREENING FOR PROTEIN

Qualitative screening tests for proteinuria include reagent strips (dipsticks) and acids that precipitate proteins (sulfosalicylic acid or acetic acid with heat).

To perform such a test, collect a clean-catch urine specimen, preferably in the morning, when the urine is most concentrated and yields the most reliable information. A reagent strip (such as Chemstrips) is usually used. Dip the strip into the urine; remove excess urine by tapping the strip against a clean surface or the edge of the container. Hold the strip in a horizontal position to prevent mixing of chemicals from adjacent areas. Immediately place the strip close to the color block on the bottle and carefully compare colors.

The results correspond to the number of milligrams per deciliter of protein (usually albumin, as strips are most sensitive to this protein).

Negative = 0 to 5 mg/dl
Trace = 5 to 20 mg/dl
1+ = 30 mg/dl
2+ = 100 mg/dl
3+ = 300 mg/dl
4+ = 1,000 mg/dl.

Normally, no detectable protein is present in a random specimen, although normal kidneys do excrete a minute amount. A positive result requires quantitative analysis of a 24-hour urine specimen.

Phenazopyridine (pyridium), a dye sometimes used to treat the discomfort associated with urinary tract infections, can alter the color reaction of certain brands of reagent strips due to its local anesthetic properties; so can high salt or alkaline content of the urine specimen. Acetazolamide and sodium bicarbonate can cause false-positive results with some reagent strips.

Patient preparation

Explain to the patient that this test detects proteins in the urine. Inform him that he needn't restrict food or fluids. Tell him that the test requires a 24-hour urine specimen, and teach him the correct collection technique.

Check the patient's medication history for drugs that may affect test results. Review your findings with the laboratory, and notify the doctor; he may want to restrict medications before the test.

Procedure

Collect a 24-hour urine specimen. A special specimen container can be obtained from the laboratory.

Precautions

■ Tell the patient not to contaminate the urine with toilet tissue or stool.

■ Refrigerate the specimen or place it on ice during the collection period.

Reference values

Normally, less than 150 mg of protein is excreted in 24 hours.

Implications of results

Proteinuria is characteristic of renal disease. When proteinuria is present in a single specimen, a 24-hour urine collection is required to identify specific renal abnormalities.

Proteinuria can result from glomerular leakage of plasma proteins (a major cause of protein excretion), from overflow of filtered proteins of low molecular weight (when they are present in excessive concentrations), from impaired tubular reabsorption of filtered proteins, and from the presence of renal proteins derived from the breakdown of kidney tissue.

Persistent proteinuria indicates renal disease resulting from increased glomerular permeability. Minimal proteinuria (less than 0.5 g/24 hours), however, is most often associated with renal disease in which glomerular involvement isn't a major factor, such as chronic pyelonephritis.

Moderate proteinuria (0.5 to 4 g/24 hours) occurs in several types of renal disease — acute or chronic glomerulonephritis, amyloidosis, and toxic nephropathies — and in diseases in which renal failure often develops as a late complication (such as diabetes and heart failure). Heavy proteinuria (more than 4 g/24 hours) is commonly associated with nephrotic syndrome.

When accompanied by an elevated white blood cell (WBC) count, proteinuria reflects urinary tract infection; with hematuria, proteinuria reflects local or diffuse urinary tract disorders. Other pathologic states (such as infections and lesions of the central nervous system) can also result in detectable amounts of proteins in the urine.

Many drugs (such as amphotericin B, gold preparations, aminoglycosides, polymyxins, or trimethadione) inflict renal damage, causing true proteinuria. Therefore, routine evaluation of urine proteins is essential during treatment with these drugs.

In all forms of proteinuria, fractionation results obtained by electrophoresis provide more precise information than the screening test. For example, excessive hemoglobin in the urine indicates intravascular hemolysis; elevated myoglobin suggests muscle damage; albumin,

---

POSTURAL PROTEINURIA

A benign form of proteinuria, postural (orthostatic) proteinuria oc- curs when a patient stands but not when he's recumbent. It can also happen when he assumes a lordotic position — from bending backward over a chair, for example. Generally, this condition is found in healthy children or young adults and has no pathologic significance, although it causes extensive proteinuria.

Postural proteinuria probably results from obstruction of renal venous outflow, which causes renal congestion and ischemia. To confirm this condition, diagnostic tests must rule out renal disease and clearly establish the absence of proteinuria when the patient is recumbent. In one test, the patient voids before retiring and re- mains recumbent for 12 hours. A urine specimen is collected as soon as he awakens and, for comparison, at specific times during the next 12 hours while he is ambulatory. In postural proteinuria, the specimen collected at the end of recumbency is free of proteins, but those collected during the ambulatory period contain proteins.

---

increased glomerular permeability; and Bence Jones pro- tein, multiple myeloma.

Not all forms of proteinuria have pathologic signifi- cance. Benign proteinuria can result from changes in body position. (See *Postural proteinuria*.) Functional pro- teinuria is associated with exercise, as well as emotional or physiologic stress, and is usually transient.

Posttest care

As ordered, resume administration of medications with- held before the test.

Interfering factors

■ Administration of tolbutamide, para-aminosalicylic acid, acetazolamide, sodium bicarbonate, penicillin, sul- fonamides, iodine contrast media, or cephalosporins may cause false-positive results in acid precipitation tests.

■ Contamination of the urine specimen with heavy mu- cus, vaginal or prostatic secretions, or the presence of numerous WBCs can alter test results, regardless of lab- oratory method used.

■ Very dilute urine (which may result from forcing flu- ids) may depress protein values and cause false-negative results.

Prothrombin time test

Prothrombin, or factor II, is a plasma protein produced by the liver. This test (commonly known as pro time, or PT) measures the time required for a fibrin clot to form in a citrated plasma sample after addition of calcium ions and tissue thromboplastin (factor III). It is an excellent screening procedure for overall evaluation of extrinsic coagulation factors V, VII, and X and of prothrombin and fibrinogen. PT is the test of choice for monitoring oral anticoagulant therapy.

Purpose

- To evaluate the extrinsic coagulation system
- To monitor response to oral anticoagulant therapy.

Patient preparation

Explain to the patient that this test helps determine if his blood clots normally or evaluates the effects of his anticoagulant therapy. Advise him that he needn't restrict food or fluids. Tell him that the test requires a blood sample, who will perform the venipuncture and when, and that he may experience discomfort from the needle puncture and the pressure of the tourniquet. Check the patient history for use of medications that may affect test results, such as vitamin K or antibiotics.

When appropriate, explain to the patient that this test monitors the effects of medications (oral anticoagulants). Tell him that the test will be performed daily when therapy begins and will be repeated at longer intervals when medication levels stabilize.

Procedure

Perform a venipuncture and collect the sample in a 7-ml silicon-coated tube.

Precautions

- To prevent hemolysis, avoid excessive probing during venipuncture and handle the sample gently.
- Completely fill the collection tube, and invert it gently several times to mix the sample and the anticoagulant adequately. If the tube isn't filled to the correct volume, an excess of citrate appears in the sample.

Reference values

Normally, PT ranges from 10 to 14 seconds. In a patient receiving warfarin therapy, PT is usually maintained between one and two times the normal control value. (See *International Normalized Ratio*, page 488.)

Implications of results

Prolonged PT may indicate hepatic disease or deficiencies in fibrinogen, prothrombin, vitamin K, or factors V, VII, or X (specific assays can pinpoint such deficiencies), or it may result from ongoing oral anticoagulant therapy. Prolonged PT that exceeds two times the control value is commonly associated with abnormal bleeding.

INTERNATIONAL NORMALIZED RATIO

The international normalized ratio (INR) system is generally viewed as the best means of standardizing measurement of prothrombin time (PT) to monitor oral anticoagulant therapy. However, the INR should never be used to screen patients for coagulopathies. Because PT testing is performed using different thromboplastin reagents and different instruments, each laboratory may have different "normal values."

Many types of thromboplastin are used in PT testing (rabbit brain, human brain, recombinant). Each type of reagent has a different sensitivity. The greater the reagent's sensitivity, the longer the PT will be. For example, using the same patient plasma, a sensitive thromboplastin will result in a PT of approximately 30 seconds, but a less sensitive thromboplastin will result in a PT of approximately 20 seconds.

The INR helps to standardize oral anticoagulant therapy so that a patient's therapeutic outcomes can be easily evaluated by various institutions that may use different instruments and thromboplastin reagents. Recent guidelines for patients receiving warfarin therapy recommend an INR of 2.0 to 3.0, except for those with mechanical prosthetic heart valves. For these patients, an INR of 2.5 to 3.5 is suggested.

The doctor may order AquaMEPHYTON (vitamin K) or fresh frozen plasma to reverse the anticoagulant effects.

Posttest care
- Make sure bleeding has stopped before removing pressure.
- If a hematoma develops at the venipuncture site, apply warm soaks.
- If the hematoma is large, monitor pulses distal to the venipuncture site.

Interfering factors
- Shortened PT can result from the use of antihistamines, chloral hydrate, corticosteroids, cardiac glycosides, diuretics, glutethimide, griseofulvin, progestin-estrogen combinations, pyrazinamide, vitamin K, or xanthines (caffeine or theophylline).
- Prolonged PT can result from overuse of alcohol or from the use of corticotropin, anabolic steroids, cholestyramine resin, I.V. heparin (within 5 hours of collection), indomethacin, mefenamic acid, para-aminosalicylic acid, methimazole, oxyphenbutazone, phenylbutazone, phenytoin, propylthiouracil, quinidine, quinine, thyroid hormones, or vitamin A.
- Prolonged or shortened PT can follow ingestion of antibiotics, barbiturates, hydroxyzine, sulfonamides, sali-

cylates (more than 1 g/day prolongs PT), mineral oil, or clofibrate.

■ Hemolysis may interfere with the accuracy of test results.

■ Failure to mix the sample and anticoagulant adequately or to send the sample to the laboratory promptly may alter test results.

■ Fibrin or fibrin split products in the sample or plasma fibrinogen levels less than 100 mg/dl can prolong PT.

■ Falsely prolonged PT may occur if the collection tube isn't filled to capacity with blood; this results in too much anticoagulant for the blood sample.

Pyruvate kinase test

The erythrocyte enzyme pyruvate kinase (PK) takes part in the anaerobic metabolism of glucose (Embden-Meyerhof pathway). Abnormally low PK levels, revealed in a serum sample by erythrocyte enzyme assay, are inherited as an autosomal recessive trait and may cause a nonspherocytic erythrocyte membrane defect associated with congenital hemolytic anemia.

Although PK deficiency is fairly uncommon, it's the most prevalent congenital nonspherocytic hemolytic anemia after glucose-6-phosphate dehydrogenase (G6PD) deficiency. PK assay confirms PK deficiency when red cell enzyme deficiency is the suspected cause of anemia.

Purpose

■ To differentiate PK-deficient hemolytic anemia from other congenital hemolytic anemias (such as G6PD deficiency) and from acquired hemolytic anemia (when the patient history or laboratory tests do not reveal a genetic red cell defect)

■ To detect PK deficiency in asymptomatic, heterozygous inheritance.

Patient preparation

Explain to the patient that this test is used to detect inherited enzyme deficiencies. Inform him that he needn't restrict food or fluids. Tell him that this test requires a blood sample, who will perform the venipuncture and when, and that he may experience transient discomfort from the needle puncture and the pressure of the tourniquet.

Check the patient history for a recent blood transfusion, and note it on the laboratory request.

Procedure

Perform a venipuncture and collect the sample in a 7-ml EDTA tube.

Precautions

- Completely fill the collection tube, and invert it gently several times to mix the sample and the anticoagulant.
- Handle the sample gently.
- Refrigerate the sample if you can't send it to the laboratory immediately.

Reference values

In a routine assay (ultraviolet), serum PK levels range from 9 to 22 U/g of hemoglobin; in the low substrate assay, from 1.7 to 6.8 U/g of hemoglobin.

Implications of results

Low serum PK levels confirm a diagnosis of PK deficiency and allow differentiation between PK-deficient hemolytic anemia and other inherited disorders.

Posttest care

If a hematoma develops at the venipuncture site, apply warm soaks.

Interfering factors

- Failure to use a collection tube with the proper anticoagulant or to adequately mix the sample and anticoagulant may affect test results.
- Hemolysis caused by rough handling of the sample may affect test results.
- Because PK levels in white blood cells remain normal in hemolytic anemia, the laboratory removes white cells from the sample to prevent false results.

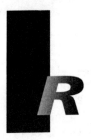

Radioactive iodine uptake test

The radioactive iodine uptake (RAIU) test evaluates thyroid function by measuring the amount of orally ingested ^{123}I or ^{131}I that accumulates in the thyroid gland after 2, 6, and 24 hours. An external single-counting probe measures the radioactivity in the thyroid as a percentage of the original dose, thus indicating the capacity of the gland to trap and retain iodine.

This test accurately diagnoses hyperthyroidism (about 90%) but is less accurate for hypothyroidism. When performed concurrently with radionuclide thyroid imaging and the T3 resin uptake test, the RAIU test helps differentiate Graves' disease from toxic adenoma. Indications for this test include abnormal results of chemical tests used to evaluate thyroid function.

Patients with suspected Hashimoto's disease or an enzyme defect may undergo the perchlorate suppression test in addition to the RAIU. (See *Perchlorate suppression test*, page 492.)

Purpose

- To evaluate thyroid function
- To aid diagnosis of hyperthyroidism or hypothyroidism
- To help distinguish between primary and secondary thyroid disorders (in combination with other tests).

Patient preparation

Explain to the patient that this test assesses thyroid function. Instruct him to fast from midnight before the test. Tell him that he'll ingest a radioactive iodine capsule or liquid and will be scanned 6 and 24 hours later to determine the amount of radioactive substance present in the thyroid gland—an indicator of thyroid function. Assure him that the test is painless and that the small amount of radiation used for the procedure is harmless.

Check the patient history for past or present iodine exposure, which may interfere with test results. If the patient previously had radiologic tests using contrast media or nuclear medicine procedures, or if he's current-

PERCHLORATE SUPPRESSION TEST

This test is used to evaluate patients with suspected Hashimoto's disease or to demonstrate an enzyme deficiency in the thyroid gland. Because potassium perchlorate competes with and displaces the iodide ions that aren't organified, this study can identify defects in the iodide organification process within the thyroid.

In this procedure, a small dose of radioactive iodine is administered orally. A radioactive iodine uptake test is performed 1 and 2 hours afterward. After the 2-hour uptake test, the patient receives 400 mg to 1 g of potassium perchlorate orally. Uptake tests are performed every 15 minutes for the first hour after the dose and then every 30 minutes for the next 2 to 3 hours.

The results of the uptake tests performed after administration of potassium perchlorate are compared with those of the 2-hour uptake test before perchlorate was administered. In a normal person, the uptake of radioactive iodine won't change significantly after administration of perchlorate. Patients with either Hashimoto's disease or an enzyme deficiency will experience a decrease in uptake. Those with an enzyme deficiency will experience a drop in their uptake by more than 15% after administration of perchlorate.

ly receiving iodine preparations or thyroid medications, note this on the request.

Equipment

- oral dose of ^{123}I or ^{131}I (radiologist determines the exact dosage)
- external single counting probe.

Procedure

- At 2, 6, and 24 hours after an oral dose of radioactive iodine is administered, the patient's thyroid is scanned by placing the anterior portion of his neck in front of an external single counting probe.
- The amount of radioactivity that the probe detects is compared with the amount in the original dose to determine the percentage of radioactive iodine retained by the thyroid.

Precautions

This test is contraindicated during pregnancy and lactation because of possible teratogenic effects. It is also contraindicated in patients who are allergic to iodine and shellfish.

Reference values

After 2 hours, 4% to 12% of the radioactive iodine has accumulated in the normal thyroid; after 6 hours, 5% to 20%; after 24 hours, 8% to 29%. The remaining radioactive iodine is excreted in the urine.

Local variations in the normal range of iodine uptake may stem from regional differences in dietary iodine intake or procedural differences among individual laboratories.

Implications of results

Below-normal percentages of iodine uptake suggest hypothyroidism, subacute thyroiditis, or iodine overload. Above-normal percentages suggest hyperthyroidism, early Hashimoto's disease, hypoalbuminemia, ingestion of lithium, or iodine-deficient goiter. In hyperthyroidism, the rate of turnover may be so rapid that the 24-hour measurement appears falsely normal.

Posttest care

■ As ordered, instruct the patient to resume a light diet 2 hours after taking the oral dose of ^{123}I or ^{131}I.

■ After the study is complete, tell the patient to resume his normal diet.

Interfering factors

■ Renal failure, diuresis, severe diarrhea, radiographic contrast media studies, ingesting iodine preparations (including iodized salt, cough syrups, and some multivitamins), or using other drugs (thyroid hormones, thyroid hormone antagonists, salicylates, penicillins, antihistamines, anticoagulants, corticosteroids, and phenylbutazone) can decrease iodine uptake, thereby affecting the accuracy of test results.

■ An iodine-deficient diet or ingestion of phenothiazines can increase iodine uptake, affecting the accuracy of test results.

Radioallergosorbent test

The radioallergosorbent test (RAST) measures immunoglobulin E (IgE) antibodies in serum by radioimmunoassay and identifies specific allergens that cause rashes, asthma, hay fever, drug reactions, or other atopic complaints. Before RAST was developed, skin testing was the only reliable method of identifying allergens. RAST is easier to perform and more specific than skin testing; it is also less painful for and less dangerous to the patient. However, careful selection of specific allergens, based on the patient's clinical history, is crucial for effective testing.

Although skin testing is still the preferred means of diagnosing IgE-mediated hypersensitivity, RAST may be more useful when a skin disorder makes accurate reading of skin tests difficult, when a patient requires continual antihistamine therapy, or when skin tests are negative but the patient's clinical history supports IgE-mediated hypersensitivity.

In RAST, a sample of the patient's serum is exposed to a panel of allergen particle complexes (APCs) on cellulose disks. The patient's IgE binds only to the APCs to which it is sensitive. Radiolabeled anti-IgE antibody is then added, and this binds to the IgE-APC complexes. After centrifugation, the amount of radioactivity in the particulate material is directly proportional to the amount of IgE antibodies present. Test results are compared with control values and represent the patient's reactivity to a specific allergen.

Purpose
■ To identify allergens to which the patient has an immediate (IgE-mediated) hypersensitivity
■ To monitor response to therapy.

Patient preparation
Explain to the patient that this test may detect the cause of an allergy or, as appropriate, that it monitors the effectiveness of treatment. Inform him that he needn't restrict food or fluids. Tell him that the test requires a blood sample, who will perform the venipuncture and when, and that he may experience transient discomfort from the needle puncture and the pressure of the tourniquet. If the patient is scheduled for a radioactive scan, make sure the sample is collected before the scan.

Procedure
Perform a venipuncture and collect the sample in a 7-ml clot-activator tube. Generally, 1 ml of serum is sufficient for five allergen assays. Be sure to note on the laboratory request the specific allergens tested.

Precautions
None.

Normal findings
RAST results are interpreted in relation to a control or reference serum, which differs among laboratories.

Implications of results
Elevated serum IgE levels suggest hypersensitivity to the specific allergen or allergens used.

Posttest care
If a hematoma develops at the venipuncture site, apply warm soaks.

Interfering factors

A radioactive scan within 1 week before sample collection may affect the accuracy of test results.

Raji cell assay

This assay, which is performed to detect the presence of circulating immune complexes, studies the Raji lymphoblastic cell line. Identifying these cells, which have receptors for immunoglobulin G (IgG) complement, is helpful in evaluating autoimmune disease.

Purpose

- To detect circulating immune complexes
- To aid the study of autoimmune disease.

Patient preparation

Explain the purpose of the test and tell the patient that it requires a blood sample, who will perform the venipuncture and when, and that he may experience transient discomfort from the needle puncture and the pressure of the tourniquet.

Procedure

Perform a venipuncture and collect the sample in a clot-activator tube. Send the sample to the laboratory promptly.

Precautions

Handle the specimen gently to avoid hemolysis.

Normal findings

No Raji cells are present in the sample.

Implications of results

The Raji cell assay can detect immune complexes formed in viral, microbial, and parasitic infections; metastasis; autoimmune disorders; or drug reactions. It also may also detect immune complexes associated with celiac disease, cirrhosis, Crohn's disease, cryoglobulinemia, dermatitis herpetiformis, sickle cell anemia, or ulcerative colitis.

Posttest care

If a hematoma develops at the venipuncture site, apply warm soaks.

Interfering factors

Hemolysis of the sample can cause misinterpretation of results.

Red blood cell count

This test, also known as an erythrocyte count, reports the number of red blood cells (RBCs) found in a microliter (cubic milliliter) of whole blood and is included in the complete blood count. Traditionally counted by hand with a hemacytometer, RBCs are now commonly counted with electronic devices such as the Coulter counter, which provide faster, more accurate results. The RBC count itself provides no qualitative information regarding the size or shape of the cells or the concentration of intracellular hemoglobin, but it may be used to calculate two erythrocyte indices: mean corpuscular volume (MCV) and mean corpuscular hemoglobin (MCH).

Purpose

■ To supply figures for computing the erythrocyte indices, which reveal RBC size and hemoglobin content
■ To support other hematologic tests in diagnosis of anemia and polycythemia.

Patient preparation

Explain to the patient that this test evaluates the number of RBCs to detect suspected blood disorders. Inform him that he needn't restrict food or fluids. Tell him this test requires a blood sample, who will perform the venipuncture and when, and that he may experience transient discomfort from the needle puncture and the pressure of the tourniquet. If the patient is an infant or child, explain to the parents (and to the child if he is old enough to understand) that a small amount of blood will be drawn from his finger or earlobe.

Procedure

For adults and older children, draw venous blood into a 7-ml EDTA tube. For younger children, collect capillary blood in a microcollection device.

Precautions

■ Completely fill the collection tube, and invert it gently several times to mix the sample and the anticoagulant.
■ Handle the sample gently to prevent hemolysis.

Reference values

Normal RBC values vary, depending on age, sex, sample, and geographic location. In adult males, the normal RBC count in venous blood is 4.5 to 6.2 million/μl; in adult females, 4.2 to 5.4 million/μl; and in children, 4.6 to 4.8 million/μl. In full-term neonates, normal values are 4.4 to 5.8 million/μl of capillary blood at birth, 3 to

3.8 million/µl at age 2 months; the RBC count rises slowly thereafter. Values are generally higher in persons living at high altitudes.

Implications of results

An elevated RBC count may reflect absolute or relative polycythemia. A depressed count suggests anemia, fluid overload, or hemorrhage lasting more than 24 hours. Further tests, such as stained-cell examination, hematocrit, hemoglobin, red-cell indices, and white-cell studies, are needed to confirm diagnosis.

Posttest care

- Make sure that subdermal bleeding has stopped before removing pressure.
- If a hematoma develops at the venipuncture site, apply warm soaks to ease discomfort.
- If the hematoma is large, monitor pulses distal to the phlebotomy site.

Interfering factors

- Hemodilution caused by drawing the sample from the same arm that is being used for I.V. infusion of fluids may alter test results.
- Failure to use the proper anticoagulant in the collection tube or to adequately mix the sample and anticoagulant may alter test results.
- Hemolysis caused by rough handling of the sample or use of a small-gauge needle for blood aspiration may alter test results.
- Hemoconcentration caused by prolonged tourniquet constriction may alter test results.
- High WBC count, which falsely elevates the RBC count in semiautomated and automated counters, may alter test results.
- Diseases that cause RBCs to agglutinate or form rouleaux, leading to a falsely decreased RBC count, may alter test results.

Red blood cell survival time test

Normally, red blood cells (RBCs) are destroyed only when they reach senility. However, in hemolytic diseases, RBCs of all ages are randomly destroyed, resulting in anemia. This test measures the survival time of circulating RBCs and detects sites of abnormal RBC sequestration and destruction, aiding evaluation of unexplained anemia.

Survival time is measured by labeling a random sample of RBCs with radioactive sodium chromate-51 (^{51}Cr). The ^{51}Cr quickly crosses RBC membranes, reduces to chromium ion, and binds to hemoglobin. This labeled group of RBCs is then injected back into the patient. Serial blood samples measure the percentage of labeled cells per unit volume over 3 to 4 weeks, until 50% of the cells disappear (disappearance rate corresponds to destruction of a random cell population).

A normal RBC survives about 120 days (half-life of 60 days); the ^{51}Cr-labeled RBCs have a shorter half-life (25 to 30 days) because about 1% of senescent RBCs are removed from the circulation each day, and about 1% of ^{51}Cr is spontaneously eluted from the labeled RBCs each day.

During the test period, a gamma camera scans the body for sites of abnormally high radioactivity, which indicate sites of excessive RBC sequestration and destruction. Other tests performed with the RBC survival time test may include spot checks of the stool to detect GI blood loss, hematocrit, blood volume studies, and radionuclide iron uptake and clearance tests to aid differential diagnosis of anemia.

Purpose
■ To help evaluate unexplained anemia, particularly hemolytic anemia
■ To identify sites of abnormal RBC sequestration and destruction.

Patient preparation
Explain to the patient that this test helps identify the cause of his anemia. Advise him that he needn't restrict food or fluids. Inform him that the test involves labeling a blood sample with a radioactive substance and requires regular blood samples at 3-day intervals for 3 to 4 weeks.

Tell him who will perform the procedures and when and that he may experience slight discomfort from the needle punctures. Reassure him that collecting each sample takes less than 3 minutes and that the small amount of radioactive substance used is harmless. If the doctor orders a stool collection to test for GI bleeding, teach the patient the proper collection technique.

Procedure
■ A 30-ml blood sample is drawn and mixed with 100 microcuries of ^{51}Cr for an adult (less for a child). After an incubation period, the mixture is injected I.V. into the patient. A blood sample is drawn 30 minutes after injection to determine blood and RBC volumes.
■ A 6-ml sample is collected in a heparinized tube after 24 hours; follow-up samples are collected at 3-day inter-

vals for 3 to 4 weeks. (The interval between samples may vary, depending on the laboratory.) To avoid error from physical decay of the ^{51}Cr, each sample is measured with a scintillation-well counter on the day it's drawn. Radioactivity per milliliter of RBCs is calculated, and the results are plotted to determine mean RBC survival time. Simultaneous gamma camera scans of the precordium, sacrum, liver, and spleen detect radioactivity at sites of excess RBC sequestration. A hematocrit is done on a small portion of each blood sample to check for blood loss.

■ At the end of the study, a sample is drawn to compare ending blood and RBC volumes with beginning volumes.

Precautions

■ This test is contraindicated during pregnancy because it exposes the fetus to radiation.

■ Because excess blood loss can invalidate test results, this test is usually contraindicated in patients with active bleeding or poor clotting function. However, if the test is necessary for a patient with poor clotting function, observe the venipuncture sites carefully for signs of hemorrhage.

■ The patient shouldn't receive blood transfusions during the test period and shouldn't have blood samples drawn for other tests.

Normal findings

The normal half-life for RBCs labeled with ^{51}Cr is 25 to 35 days. Normal gamma camera scans reveal slight radioactivity in the spleen, liver, and sometimes the bone marrow.

Implications of results

Decreased RBC survival time indicates a hemolytic disease, such as chronic lymphocytic leukemia, congenital nonspherocytic hemolytic anemia, hemoglobin C–thalassemia disease, hereditary spherocytosis, idiopathic acquired hemolytic anemia, paroxysmal nocturnal hemoglobinuria, elliptocytosis, pernicious anemia, sickle cell anemia, sickle cell–hemoglobin C disease, or hemolytic-uremic syndrome.

If hemolytic anemia is diagnosed, additional tests using cross-transfusion of labeled RBCs can determine whether anemia results from an intrinsic RBC defect or an extrinsic factor.

A gamma camera scan that detects a site of excess RBC sequestration provides a direction for treatment.

For example, abnormally high RBC sequestration in the spleen may require a splenectomy.

Posttest care
If a hematoma develops at the venipuncture site, apply warm soaks.

Interfering factors
■ Dehydration, overhydration, or blood loss (from hemorrhage or taking other blood samples) can alter the circulating RBC volume and invalidate test results.
■ Blood transfusions during the test period alter the proportion of labeled RBCs to total RBCs, thus affecting the accuracy of test results.

Red cell indices

Using the results of the red blood cell (RBC) count, hematocrit, and total hemoglobin tests, the red cell indices (also known as erythrocyte indices) provide important information about the size, hemoglobin concentration, and hemoglobin weight of an average RBC. The indices include mean corpuscular volume (MCV), mean corpuscular hemoglobin (MCH), and mean corpuscular hemoglobin concentration (MCHC).

MCV, the ratio of hematocrit (packed cell volume) to the RBC count, expresses the average size of the erythrocytes and indicates whether they are undersized (microcytic), oversized (macrocytic), or normal (normocytic). MCH, the ratio of hemoglobin weight to the RBC count, gives the weight of hemoglobin in an average red cell. MCHC, the ratio of hemoglobin weight to hematocrit, defines the concentration of hemoglobin in 100 ml of packed red cells. It helps distinguish normally colored (normochromic) red cells from paler (hypochromic) red cells.

Purpose
To aid diagnosis and classification of anemias.

Patient preparation
Explain to the patient that this test helps determine if he has anemia. Tell him the test requires a blood sample, who will perform the venipuncture and when, and that he may experience transient discomfort from the needle puncture and the pressure of the tourniquet.

Procedure
Perform a venipuncture and collect the sample in a 7-ml EDTA tube.

COMPARING RED CELL INDICES IN ANEMIAS

Decreased or increased red cell indices suggest various types of anemia, as shown below.

Index	Normal (normocytic, normochromic)	Iron deficiency anemia (microcytic, hypochromic)	Pernicious anemia (macrocytic, normochromic)
MCV	84 to 99 fl	60 to 80 fl	96 to 150 fl
MCH	26 to 32 pg	5 to 25 pg	33 to 53 pg
MCHC	30 to 36 g/dl	20 to 30 g/dl	33 to 38 g/dl

Precautions
■ Completely fill the collection tube, and invert it gently several times to adequately mix the sample and anticoagulant.
■ Handle the sample gently to prevent hemolysis.

Reference values
The range of normal red cell indices is as follows:
■ MCV: 84 to 99 fl
■ MCH: 26 to 32 pg
■ MCHC: 30 to 36 g/dl.

Implications of results
The red cell indices help to classify anemias. Low MCV and MCHC indicate microcytic, hypochromic anemias caused by iron deficiency anemia, pyridoxine-responsive anemia, or thalassemia. A high MCV suggests macrocytic anemias caused by megaloblastic anemias caused by folic acid or vitamin B12 deficiency, inherited disorders of DNA synthesis, or reticulocytosis. (See *Comparing red cell indices in anemias.*) Because MCV reflects the average volume of many cells, a value within normal range can encompass RBCs of varying size, from microcytic to macrocytic.

Posttest care
■ Make sure that subdermal bleeding has stopped before removing pressure.
■ If a hematoma develops at the venipuncture site, apply warm soaks.
■ If the hematoma is large, monitor pulses distal to the phlebotomy site.

Interfering factors
■ Failure to use the proper anticoagulant in the collection tube or to adequately mix the sample and anticoag-

ulant may interfere with accurate determination of test results.

■ Hemolysis caused by rough handling of the sample or use of a small-gauge needle for blood aspiration may interfere with test results.

■ Hemoconcentration caused by prolonged tourniquet constriction may interfere with accurate determination of test results.

■ High white cell count falsely elevates the RBC count in semiautomated and automated counters and thereby invalidates MCV and MCH results.

■ Falsely elevated hemoglobin values invalidate MCH and MCHC results.

■ Diseases that cause RBCs to agglutinate or form rouleaux, leading to a falsely decreased RBC count, may invalidate test results.

Renal biopsy, percutaneous

Percutaneous renal biopsy is the needle excision of a core of kidney tissue. The biopsy specimen is examined by light, electron, or immunofluorescent microscopy. Such examination provides valuable information about glomerular and tubular function. Acute and chronic glomerulonephritis, pyelonephritis, renal vein thrombosis, amyloid infiltration, and systemic lupus erythematosus produce characteristic histologic changes in the kidneys.

Complications of percutaneous renal biopsy may include bleeding, hematoma, arteriovenous fistula, and infection. Despite the risk of these complications, this procedure is considered safer than open biopsy, which is usually the preferred method for removing a tissue specimen from a solid lesion. However, more recent noninvasive procedures, especially renal ultrasonography and computed tomography scans, have replaced percutaneous renal biopsy in many hospitals.

In some cases, a renal tissue specimen is obtained by a brush biopsy of the urinary tract.

Purpose

■ To aid diagnosis of renal parenchymal disease
■ To monitor progression of renal disease and to assess the effectiveness of treatment.

Patient preparation

Describe the procedure to the patient, and ask him if he has any questions. Explain that this test helps diagnose kidney disorders. Instruct the patient to restrict food and fluids for 8 hours before the test. Tell him who will perform the biopsy and where, that the procedure takes only 15 minutes, and that the needle is in the kidney for only a few seconds.

Tell the patient that blood and urine specimens are collected and tested before the biopsy and that other tests, such as excretory urography, ultrasonography, or an erect film of the abdomen, may be ordered to help identify the biopsy site.

Make sure the patient has signed a consent form. Check the patient history for hemorrhagic tendencies and hypersensitivity to the local anesthetic. As ordered, 30 minutes to 1 hour before the biopsy administer a mild sedative to help the patient relax. Inform him that he'll receive a local anesthetic but may experience a pinching pain when the needle is inserted through the back into the kidney. Check vital signs, and tell the patient to void just before the test.

Procedure

■ Place the patient in a prone position on a firm surface, with a sandbag beneath his abdomen. Tell him to take a deep breath while his kidney is being palpated. A 7″ 20G needle is used to inject the local anesthetic at the biopsy site. Instruct the patient to hold his breath and remain immobile as the needle is inserted just below the angle formed by the intersection of the lowest palpable rib and the lateral border of the sacrospinal muscle. The needle is directed through the back muscles, the deep lumbar fascia, the perinephric fat, and the kidney capsule.

■ After the needle is inserted, tell the patient to take several deep breaths. If the needle swings smoothly during deep breathing, it has penetrated the kidney capsule. After the penetration depth is marked on the needle shaft, instruct the patient to hold his breath and remain as still as possible while the needle is withdrawn and the local anesthetic is injected into the back tissues and skin.

■ After a small incision is made in the anesthetized skin, instruct the patient to hold his breath and remain immobile while the Vim-Silverman needle with stylet is inserted through the incision and down the tract of the infiltrating needle to the measured depth. Then tell the patient to breathe deeply. If the characteristic needle swing occurs, instruct him to hold his breath and remain still while the tissue specimen is obtained. The specimen is examined immediately under a hand lens to ensure that it contains tissue from both the cortex and the medulla; then the tissue is placed on a saline-soaked gauze pad and placed in a properly labeled container.

■ If an adequate tissue specimen hasn't been obtained, the procedure is repeated immediately. After an adequate specimen is secured, apply pressure to the biopsy site for 3 to 5 minutes to stop superficial bleeding. Then apply a pressure dressing.

Precautions

■ Percutaneous renal biopsy is contraindicated in a patient with a renal tumor, a severe bleeding disorder, markedly reduced plasma or blood volume, severe hypertension, hydronephrosis, perinephric abscess, advanced renal failure with uremia, or only one kidney. **CLINICAL ALERT** Instruct the patient to hold his breath and remain still whenever the needle is advanced into or retracted from the kidney.

■ Send the tissue specimen to the laboratory immediately.

Normal findings

A section of normal kidney tissue shows Bowman's capsule (the area between two layers of flat epithelial cells), the glomerular tuft, and the capillary lumen. The tubule sections differ, depending on the area of tubule involved. The proximal tubule is one layer of epithelial cells with microvilli that form a brush border; the descending loop of Henle has flat, squamous epithelial cells; and the ascending, distal convoluted, and collecting tubules are lined with squamous epithelial cells.

Implications of results

Histologic examination of renal tissue can reveal malignancy or renal disease. Malignant tumors include Wilms' tumor, usually present in early childhood, and renal cell carcinoma, most prevalent in persons over age 40. Characteristic histologic changes can indicate disseminated lupus erythematosus, amyloid infiltration, acute and chronic glomerulonephritis, renal vein thrombosis, and pyelonephritis.

Posttest care

■ Instruct the patient to lie flat on his back without moving for at least 12 hours to prevent bleeding. Check vital signs every 15 minutes for 4 hours, then every 30 minutes for 4 hours, then every hour for 4 hours, and finally every 4 hours. Report any changes.

■ Examine all urine for blood; small amounts may be present after biopsy but should disappear within 8 hours. Hematocrit may be monitored after the procedure to screen for internal bleeding.

■ Encourage the patient to drink fluids to initiate mild diuresis, which minimizes colic and obstruction from blood clotting in the renal pelvis.

■ Tell the patient he may resume his normal diet.

■ Discourage the patient from engaging in strenuous activities for several days after the procedure to prevent possible bleeding.

Interfering factors

Failure to obtain an adequate tissue specimen, to store the specimen properly, or to send the specimen to the laboratory immediately may affect test results.

Renin activity test, plasma

Renin secretion from the kidneys is the first stage of the renin-angiotensin-aldosterone cycle, which controls the body's sodium-potassium balance, fluid volume, and blood pressure. Renin is released into the renal veins in response to sodium depletion and blood loss. This test is a screening procedure for renovascular hypertension but doesn't unequivocally confirm it.

Purpose

■ To screen for renal origin of hypertension
■ To help plan treatment of essential hypertension, a genetic disease often aggravated by excessive sodium intake
■ To help identify hypertension linked to unilateral (sometimes bilateral) renovascular disease by renal vein catheterization
■ To help identify primary aldosteronism (Conn's syndrome) resulting from aldosterone-secreting adrenal adenoma
■ To confirm primary aldosteronism (sodium-depleted plasma renin test).

Patient preparation

Explain to the patient that this test is used to help determine the cause of hypertension.

Tell the patient to discontinue or hold the use of diuretics, antihypertensives, vasodilators, oral contraceptives, and licorice as ordered by the doctor and to maintain a normal sodium diet (3 g/day) during this period.

For the sodium-depleted plasma renin test, tell the patient that he'll receive furosemide (or, if he has angina or cerebrovascular insufficiency, chlorthiazide) and will follow a specific low-sodium diet for 3 days. (See *Low-sodium diet for renin testing*, page 506.)

Make sure the patient hasn't received radioactive treatments for several days before the test.

Tell him that the test requires a blood sample. Explain who will perform the venipuncture and when. Explain that he may experience slight discomfort from the needle puncture and the tourniquet but that collecting the

LOW-SODIUM DIET FOR RENIN TESTING

Before undergoing renin testing, the patient must drastically restrict his intake of sodium for 3 days to ensure accurate test results. If he is following this diet at home, make certain he understands these precautions:
- Eat only the foods included in the meal plan provided by the doctor. He may choose not to eat some foods on this diet, but he may not add foods.
- Measure all portions using standard measuring cups and spoons.
- Use 4 oz (112 g) *unsalted* beefsteak or ground beef for lunch and 4 oz *unsalted* chicken for dinner. (Amount refers to weight before cooking.)
- Eat only the following *unsalted* (fresh or frozen) vegetables: asparagus, green or wax beans, cabbage, cauliflower, lettuce, tomatoes.
- Drink only the specified amount of coffee or tea.
- If thirsty between meals, drink distilled water but not other beverages.
- Prepare all foods without salt and don't use salt at the table.
  Below is a sample meal plan for a day.

Breakfast
1 egg, poached or boiled or fried in *unsalted* fat
2 slices *unsalted* toast
1 shredded wheat biscuit or ⅔ cup *unsalted* cooked cereal
4 oz (120 ml) milk
8 oz (240 ml) coffee
8 oz (240 ml) orange juice
Sugar, jam or jelly, and *unsalted* butter, as desired

Lunch
4 oz (120 ml) *unsalted* tomato juice
4 oz (112 g) *unsalted* beefsteak or ground beef; may be broiled or fried in *unsalted* fat
½ cup *unsalted* potato
½ cup *unsalted* green beans or other allowed vegetable
1 serving fruit
8 oz (240 ml) coffee
1 slice *unsalted* bread
Sugar, jam or jelly, and *unsalted* butter, as desired

Dinner
4 oz (112 g) *unsalted* chicken; may be baked or broiled, or fried in *unsalted* fat
½ cup *unsalted* potato
Lettuce salad (vinegar and oil dressing)
½ cup *unsalted* green beans or other allowed vegetable
1 serving fruit
8 oz (240 ml) coffee
1 slice *unsalted* bread
Sugar, jam or jelly, and *unsalted* butter, as desired

sample usually takes less than 3 minutes. Collect a morning sample, if possible.

If a recumbent sample is ordered, instruct the patient to remain in bed at least 2 hours before the sample is obtained because posture influences renin secretion. If an upright sample is ordered, instruct him to stand or sit upright for 2 hours before the test is performed.

If renal vein catheterization is ordered, make sure the patient has signed an informed consent form. Tell him that the procedure will be done in the radiography department and that he'll receive a local anesthetic.

Procedure

PERIPHERAL VEIN SAMPLE
■ Perform a venipuncture, collect the sample in a chilled 7-ml EDTA tube, and put it on ice immediately.
■ Note on the laboratory slip if the patient was fasting and whether he was upright or supine during sample collection.

RENAL VEIN CATHETERIZATION
A catheter is advanced to the kidneys through the femoral vein under fluoroscopic control, and samples are obtained from both renal veins and the vena cava.

Precautions

■ Because renin is unstable, the sample must be drawn into a chilled syringe and collection tube, placed on ice, and sent to the laboratory immediately.
■ Completely fill the collection tube, and invert it gently several times to mix the sample and the anticoagulant.

Reference values

Levels of plasma renin activity and aldosterone decrease with advancing age, as follows:
■ Sodium-depleted, upright, peripheral vein
– Ages 18 to 39, 2.9 to 24 ng/ml/hour; mean, 10.8 ng/ml/hour.
– Age 40 and over, 2.9 to 10.8 ng/ml/hour; mean, 5.9 ng/ml/hour.
■ Sodium-replete, upright, peripheral vein
– Ages 18 to 39, 0.6 to 4.3 ng/ml/hour; mean, 1.9 ng/ml/hour.
– Age 40 and over, 0.6 to 3 ng/ml/hour; mean, 1 ng/ml/hour.

Implications of results

Elevated renin levels may occur in essential hypertension (uncommon), malignant and renovascular hypertension, cirrhosis, hypokalemia, hypovolemia caused by hemorrhage, renin-producing renal tumors (Bartter's syndrome), and adrenal hypofunction (Addison's disease). High renin levels may also occur in chronic renal failure with parenchymal disease, end-stage renal disease, and transplant rejection.

Subnormal renin levels may indicate hypervolemia associated with a high-sodium diet, salt-retaining steroids, primary aldosteronism, Cushing's syndrome, licorice ingestion syndrome, or essential hypertension with low renin levels.

High serum and urine aldosterone levels with low plasma renin activity help identify primary aldosteronism. In the sodium-depleted renin test, low plasma renin confirms this and differentiates it from secondary aldosteronism (characterized by increased renin).

Posttest care

PERIPHERAL VEIN SAMPLE
If a hematoma develops at the peripheral venipuncture site, apply warm soaks.

RENAL VEIN CATHETERIZATION
■ After renal vein catheterization, apply pressure to the catheterization site for 10 to 20 minutes to prevent extravasation.

■ Monitor vital signs, and check the catheterization site every 30 minutes for 2 hours and then every hour for 4 hours to ensure that the bleeding has stopped. Check distal pulse for signs of thrombus formation and arterial occlusion (cyanosis, loss of pulse, coolness of skin).

BOTH METHODS
■ Tell the patient he may resume his usual diet.
■ Resume administration of medications that were discontinued before the test.

Interfering factors

■ Salt-retaining corticosteroid therapy and antidiuretic therapy may decrease plasma renin activity.
■ Use of oral contraceptives and therapy with diuretics, antihypertensives, or vasodilators may increase plasma renin activity.
■ Radioisotope use within several days before the test may interfere with test results.
■ Failure to observe pretest restrictions may alter test results.
■ Improper patient positioning during test may affect test results.
■ Failure to use the proper anticoagulant in the collection tube (EDTA helps preserve angiotensin I; heparin does not), to completely fill it, or to adequately mix the sample and the anticoagulant can affect test results.
■ Failure to chill the collection tube, syringe, and sample or to send the sample to the laboratory immediately may affect test results.

■ High salt intake, severe blood loss, ingestion of licorice, and pregnancy may increase plasma renin activity.

Respiratory syncytial virus antibody test

Respiratory syncytial virus (RSV), a member of the paramyxovirus group, is the major viral cause of severe lower respiratory tract disease in infants, but it may cause infections in persons of any age. RSV infections are most common and produce the most severe disease during the first 6 months of life. Initial infection involves viral replication in epithelial cells of the upper respiratory tract, but in younger children especially the infection spreads to the bronchi, bronchioli, and even to the parenchyma of the lungs.

Immunoglobulin G (IgG) and IgM antibodies can be easily quantified using the indirect immunofluorescence test. Specific results for IgM are obtained only after separating this class of antibody from IgG. In the general population, prevalence of IgG antibodies to RSV is extremely high (greater than 95%), especially in adults.

Purpose

To diagnose infections caused by RSV.

Patient preparation

Explain the purpose of the test, and inform the patient that the test requires a blood sample, who will perform the venipuncture and when, and that he may experience transient discomfort from the needle puncture and the pressure of the tourniquet.

Procedure

■ Perform a venipuncture and collect 5 ml of sterile blood in a clot-activator tube. Allow the blood to clot for at least 1 hour at room temperature.
■ Transfer the serum to a sterile tube or vial and send it to the laboratory at once.
■ If transfer must be delayed, store the serum at 39.2° F (4° C) for 1 to 2 days or at –4° F (–20° C) for longer periods to avoid bacterial contamination.

Precautions

Handle the sample gently to prevent hemolysis.

Normal findings

Serum from patients who have never been infected with RSV will have no detectable antibodies to the virus (less than 1:5). In infants, serologic diagnosis of RSV infections is difficult because of the presence of maternal IgG antibodies; thus, the presence of IgM antibodies is most significant.

Implications of results

RSV infection can be ruled out in patients whose serum samples have no detectable antibodies to the virus. The qualitative presence of IgM or a fourfold or greater increase in IgG antibodies indicates active RSV infection.

Posttest care

If a hematoma develops at the venipuncture site, apply warm soaks.

Interfering factors

Hemolysis of the sample may alter test results.

Reticulocyte count

Reticulocytes are nonnucleated, immature red blood cells (RBCs) that remain in the peripheral blood for 24 to 48 hours while they mature. They are generally larger than mature RBCs and contain ribosomes, the centriole, particles of Golgi vesicles, and mitochondria that produce hemoglobin. Because reticulocytes retain remnants of normoblasts (their precursors) that absorb supravital stains, such as new methylene blue or brilliant cresyl blue, they sometimes can be distinguished from other blood cells in a peripheral blood smear.

In this test, reticulocytes in a whole blood sample are counted and expressed as a percentage of the total RBC count. The reticulocyte count is useful for evaluating anemia and is an index of effective erythropoiesis and bone marrow response to anemia. Because the manual method for counting reticulocytes uses a relatively small sample size, values may be imprecise and should be compared with the RBC count or hematocrit.

Purpose

- To aid in distinguishing between hypoproliferative and hyperproliferative anemias
- To help assess blood loss, bone marrow response to anemia, and therapy for anemia.

Patient preparation

Tell the patient this test helps detect anemia and monitor its treatment. Advise him that he needn't restrict food or fluids. Tell him that the test requires a blood sample, who will perform the venipuncture and when, and that he may experience transient discomfort from the needle puncture and the pressure of the tourniquet. If the patient is an infant or child, explain to the parents (and to the child if he's old enough to understand) that a small amount of blood will be drawn from his finger or earlobe.

Withhold corticotropin, antimalarials, antipyretics, azathioprine, chloramphenicol, dactinomycin, furazolidone (from infants), levodopa, methotrexate, phenacetin, and sulfonamides, as ordered. If such medications must be continued, note this on the laboratory request.

Procedure

Perform a venipuncture and collect the sample in a 7-ml EDTA tube.

Precautions

■ Completely fill the collection tube, and invert it gently several times to mix the sample and the anticoagulant.
■ Handle the sample gently.

Reference values

Reticulocytes constitute 0.5% to 2% of the total RBC count. In infants, the percentage is normally higher at birth (2% to 6%) but decreases to adult levels in 1 to 2 weeks.

Implications of results

A low reticulocyte count indicates hypoproliferative bone marrow (hypoplastic anemia) or ineffective erythropoiesis (pernicious anemia). A high reticulocyte count indicates a bone marrow response to anemia caused by hemolysis or blood loss. The reticulocyte count may also rise after effective therapy for iron deficiency anemia or pernicious anemia.

Assess the patient's nutritional status and consult a dietitian, if appropriate.

Monitor patient for manifestations of anemia: fatigue, tachycardia, and dyspnea. Adjust nursing care to minimize symptoms, such as spacing activities and ensuring adequate rest.

Prepare the patient for transfusion therapy, if indicated.

Arrange for genetic counseling if the anemia is a hereditary disorder.

If intramuscular iron is prescribed in iron-deficiency anemia, use the Z-track injection technique to minimize discomfort and prevent skin staining.

Posttest care

■ Ensure subdermal bleeding has stopped before removing pressure.
■ If a hematoma develops at the venipuncture site, apply warm soaks.

■ If the hematoma is large, monitor pulses distal to the phlebotomy site.

■ As ordered, resume administration of any medications that were withheld before the test.

■ When following a patient with an abnormal reticulocyte count, look for trends in repeated tests or very gross changes in the numeric value.

Interfering factors

■ False-low test results can be caused by azathioprine, chloramphenicol, dactinomycin, and methotrexate. False-high results can be caused by corticotropin, antimalarials, antipyretics, furazolidone (in infants), and levodopa. Sulfonamides can cause false-low or false-high results.

■ Failure to use the proper anticoagulant in the collection tube or to adequately mix the sample and anticoagulant may affect the accuracy of test results.

■ Prolonged tourniquet constriction may alter test results.

■ Hemolysis caused by rough handling of the sample or use of a small-gauged needle for blood aspiration may affect test results.

■ Recent transfusions may affect results.

Rh typing

The Rh system classifies blood by the presence or absence of the $Rh_o(D)$ antigen on the surface of red blood cells (RBCs). In this test, a patient's RBCs are mixed with serum containing anti-$Rh_o(D)$ antibodies and are observed for agglutination. If agglutination occurs, the $Rh_o(D)$ antigen is present, and the patient's blood is typed Rh-positive; if agglutination doesn't occur, the antigen is absent, and the patient's blood is typed Rh-negative.

Rh typing is performed routinely on prospective blood donors and on blood recipients before a transfusion. Only prospective blood donors are fully tested to exclude the D^u variant of the $Rh_o(D)$ antigen before being classified as having Rh-negative blood. Persons who have this antigen are considered Rh-positive donors but are generally transfused as Rh-negative recipients.

Purpose

■ To establish blood type according to the Rh system

■ To help determine the compatibility of the donor before transfusion

■ To determine if the patient will require $Rh_o(D)$ immune globulin injection.

Patient preparation

Explain to the patient that this test determines or verifies his blood group—an important step in ensuring a safe transfusion. Inform him that he needn't fast before the test. Tell him the test requires a blood sample, who will perform the venipuncture and when, and that he may experience transient discomfort from the needle puncture and the pressure of the tourniquet.

Check the patient history for recent administration of dextran, I.V. contrast media, or drugs that may alter results.

Procedure

Perform a venipuncture and collect the sample in a 7-ml EDTA tube, as ordered.

Precautions

■ Label the sample with the patient's name, the hospital or blood bank number, the date, and the initials of the phlebotomist.
■ Handle the sample gently and send it to the laboratory immediately.
■ If a transfusion is ordered, a transfusion request form must accompany the sample to the laboratory.

Normal findings

Classified as Rh-positive, Rh-negative, or Rh-positive D^u, donor blood may be transfused only if it's compatible with the recipient's blood.

Implications of results

If an Rh-negative woman delivers an Rh-positive baby or aborts a fetus whose Rh-type is unknown, she should receive an injection of $Rh_o(D)$ immune globulin within 72 hours to prevent hemolytic disease of the newborn in future births. (See *Implications of $Rh_o(D)$ typing test results*, page 514.)

Posttest care

■ If a hematoma develops at the venipuncture site, apply warm soaks to ease discomfort.
■ If available, give the pregnant patient a card identifying that she may need to receive $Rh_o(D)$ immune globulin.

Interfering factors

■ Recent administration of dextran or I.V. contrast media results in cellular aggregation, which resembles antibody-mediated agglutination.
■ Methyldopa, cephalosporins, and levodopa may cause a false-positive result for the D^u antigen because these

IMPLICATIONS OF RH$_O$(D) TYPING TEST RESULTS		
Classified as Rh$_O$(D)-positive, Rh$_O$(D)-negative, or Rh(D^u)-positive, donor blood may be transfused only if it's compatible with the recipient's blood, as shown below.		
Rh$_O$(D) recipient types	**Compatible Rh$_O$(D) donor types**	**Incompatible Rh$_O$(D) donor types**
Rh$_O$(D)-positive	Rh$_O$(D)-positive or Rh$_O$(D)-negative	None
Rh$_O$(D)-negative	Rh$_O$(D)-negative	Rh$_O$(D)-positive
Rh(D^u)-positive	Rh(D^u)-positive, Rh$_O$(D)-negative, or Rh$_O$(D)-positive (the least desirable choice as it may cause a mild hemolytic reaction)	None

drugs may produce a positive direct antiglobulin (Coombs') test.

Rheumatoid factor test

The rheumatoid factor (RF) test is the most useful immunologic test for confirming rheumatoid arthritis (RA). In this disease, "renegade" immunoglobulin G (IgG) antibodies, produced by lymphocytes in the synovial joints, react with other IgG or IgM molecules to produce immune complexes, activate complement, and destroy tissues. How IgG molecules become antigenic is still unknown, but they may be altered by aggregating with viruses or other antigens. The immune complexes can migrate from the synovial fluid to other areas of the body, causing vasculitis, subcutaneous nodules, or lymphadenopathy. The IgG or IgM molecules that react with IgG-antigen are called rheumatoid factors.

The sheep cell agglutination test and the latex fixation test can detect RF. In the sheep cell test, rabbit IgG adsorbed onto sheep red blood cells (RBCs) is mixed with the patient's serum in serial dilutions; in the latex fixation test, human IgG adsorbed onto latex particles is mixed with the patient's serum. Visible agglutination indicates the presence of RF. The last tube dilution to show visible agglutination is used as the titer. The sheep cell agglutination test is the better diagnostic method for confirming RA; the latex fixation test is the better screening method.

Purpose

To confirm diagnosis of RA, especially when clinical diagnosis is doubtful.

Patient preparation

Explain to the patient that this test helps confirm the diagnosis of RA. Advise him that he needn't restrict food or fluids before the test. Tell him that the test requires a blood sample, who will perform the venipuncture and when, and that he may experience transient discomfort from the needle puncture and the pressure of the tourniquet.

Procedure

Perform a venipuncture and collect the sample in a 7-ml clot-activator tube.

CLINICAL ALERT Monitor the patient for signs of thrombosis related to the vasculitis.

Precautions

None.

Reference values

Normal RF titer is less than 1:20; normal rheumatoid screening test is nonreactive.

Implications of results

Positive RF titers are found in 80% of patients with RA. Titers above 1:80 strongly suggest a diagnosis of RA; titers between 1:20 and 1:80 are difficult to interpret because they occur in many other diseases, such as systemic lupus erythematosus, scleroderma, polymyositis, tuberculosis, infectious mononucleosis, leprosy, syphilis, sarcoidosis, chronic hepatic disease, subacute bacterial endocarditis, and chronic pulmonary interstitial fibrosis. In addition, 5% of the general population, including as many as 25% of the elderly, have positive RF titers.

Conversely, a negative RF titer doesn't rule out RA; 20% to 25% of patients with RA lack reactive RF titers, and RF itself isn't reactive until 6 months after the onset of active disease. Repeating the test is sometimes useful. However, a correlation between RF and RA is inconclusive, and positive diagnosis always requires correlation with clinical status.

Posttest care

■ Because a patient with RA may be immunocompromised from the disease or from corticosteroid therapy, keep the venipuncture site covered with a clean, dry bandage for 24 hours. Check regularly for signs of infection.

■ If a hematoma develops at the venipuncture site, apply warm soaks.

Interfering factors
■ Inadequately activated complement may cause false-positive results.
■ High lipid or cryoglobulin levels in serum may cause false-positive test results and require repetition of the test after restriction of fat intake.
■ Serum with high IgG levels may cause false-negative results through competition with IgG-antigen on the surface of latex particles or sheep RBCs used as substrate.

Rubella antibody test

Although rubella (German measles) is generally a mild viral infection in children and young adults, it can produce severe infection in a fetus, resulting in spontaneous abortion, stillbirth, or congenital rubella syndrome. Because rubella infection normally induces immunoglobulin G (IgG) and IgM antibody production, measuring rubella antibodies can determine present infection and immunity resulting from past infection.

Various methods of detecting rubella antibodies are available, including hemagglutination inhibition, passive hemagglutination, latex agglutination, enzyme immunoassay, fluorescence immunoassay, and radioimmunoassay. Suspected cases of congenital rubella may be confirmed if rubella-specific IgM antibodies are present in the infant's serum. Immune status in adults can be confirmed by an IgG-specific titer.

Exposure risk (when the immunity status is unknown) may be evaluated by using two serum samples. The first sample should be drawn in the acute phase of clinical symptoms. If clinical symptoms aren't apparent, the sample should be drawn as soon as possible after the suspected exposure. The second sample should be drawn 3 to 4 weeks later during the convalescent phase.

Purpose
■ To diagnose rubella infection, especially congenital infection
■ To determine susceptibility to rubella in women of childbearing age and in children.

Patient preparation
Explain that this test diagnoses or evaluates susceptibility to German measles. Inform the patient that she needn't restrict food or fluids before the test and that this test requires a blood sample (if a current infection is suspected, a second blood sample will be needed in 3 to 4 weeks to identify a rise in the titer). Explain who will perform the venipuncture and when and that she may experience

transient discomfort from the needle puncture and the pressure of the tourniquet.

Procedure

Perform a venipuncture and collect the sample in a 7-ml clot-activator tube.

Precautions

Handle the specimen gently to prevent hemolysis.

Reference values

Titer of 1:8 or less indicates little or no immunity against rubella; titer greater than 1:10 indicates adequate protection against rubella.

Implications of results

Demonstrable antibody levels normally appear 2 to 4 days after the onset of the rash, peak in 3 to 4 weeks, and then slowly decline but remain detectable for life. In rubella infection, acute serum titers range from 1:8 to 1:16; convalescent serum titers, from 1:64 to 1:1,024+. A fourfold rise or greater from the acute to the convalescent titer indicates a recent rubella infection.

The presence of rubella-specific IgM antibodies indicates recent infection in an adult and congenital rubella in an infant.

When appropriate, instruct the patient to return for another blood test.

If a woman of childbearing age is found susceptible to rubella, explain that vaccination can prevent rubella and that she must wait at least 3 months after the vaccination before becoming pregnant or risk permanent damage or death to the fetus.

If a pregnant patient is found susceptible to rubella, instruct her to return for follow-up rubella antibody tests to detect possible subsequent infection.

Posttest care

■ If a hematoma develops at the venipuncture site, apply warm soaks.
■ If the test confirms rubella in a pregnant woman, be supportive and refer her for counseling, as needed.

Interfering factors

Hemolysis caused by excessive agitation of the specimen may alter test results.

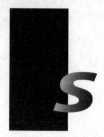

Semen analysis

Inexpensive, technically simple, and reasonably definitive, semen analysis is usually the first test performed on a male to evaluate fertility. The procedure usually includes measuring the volume of seminal fluid, assessing the sperm count, and examining a stained specimen for motility and morphology.

Abnormal findings suggest the need for further testing (such as liver, thyroid, pituitary, and adrenal function tests) to identify the underlying cause and to screen for metabolic abnormalities (such as diabetes mellitus). Significantly abnormal semen—such as greatly decreased sperm count or motility or a marked increase in morphologically abnormal forms—may indicate a testicular biopsy.

Semen analysis is also used to detect semen on a rape victim, to identify the blood group of an alleged rapist, or to prove sterility in a paternity suit. (See *Identifying semen for medicolegal purposes.*) Some laboratories offer specialized semen tests, such as screening for antibodies to spermatozoa.

Purpose

- To evaluate male fertility (most common use)
- To determine the effectiveness of vasectomy
- To detect semen on the body or clothing of a suspected rape or homicide victim or elsewhere at the crime scene
- To identify blood group substances that may exonerate or incriminate a criminal suspect (rare)
- To rule out paternity on grounds of complete sterility (rare).

Patient preparation

Patient preparation depends on the purpose of the study.

EVALUATION OF FERTILITY

Provide written instructions, and inform the patient that the most desirable specimen requires masturbation, ideally in a doctor's office or a laboratory. Instruct him to follow the doctor's orders regarding the period of continence before the test because it may increase his sperm count. Some doctors specify a fixed number of

IDENTIFYING SEMEN FOR MEDICOLEGAL PURPOSES

Semen analysis can demonstrate that the semen of a suspect in a rape or homicide investigation is different from or consistent with semen found in or on the victim's body. Forensic laboratories can detect and positively identify semen from vaginal aspirates or smears or from stains on clothing, other fabrics, skin, or hair.

Spermatozoa or their fragments persist in the vagina for more than 72 hours after sexual intercourse. Spermatozoa taken from the vagina of an exhumed body that has been properly embalmed and remains reasonably intact can also be identified.

To determine which stains or fluids require further investigation, clothing or other fabrics can be scanned with ultraviolet light to detect the typical green-white fluorescence of semen. Soaking appropriate samples of clothing, fabric, or hair in physiologic saline solution elutes the semen and spermatozoa. Deposits of dried semen can be gently sponged from the victim's skin.

The two most common tests to identify semen are the determination of acid phosphatase concentration (the more sensitive test) and microscopic examination for the presence of spermatozoa. Concentrations of acid phosphatase are significantly higher in semen than in any other body fluid. Microscopic examination can identify spermatozoa or head fragments in stained smears prepared directly from vaginal scrapings or aspirates or in the concentrated sediment of eluates or lavages.

Like other body fluids, semen contains the soluble A, B, and H blood group substances in the approximately 80% of males who are genetically determined secretors (that is, who are homozygous or heterozygous for the dominant secretor gene). Thus, the male who has group A blood and is a secretor has soluble blood group A antigen in his seminal fluid. This fact can be of considerable medicolegal importance.

days, usually 2 to 5; others advise a period of continence equal to the usual interval between episodes of intercourse.

If the patient prefers to collect the specimen at home, emphasize the importance of delivering the specimen to the laboratory within 1 hour after collection. Warn him not to expose the specimen to extreme temperatures or to direct sunlight (which can increase its temperature). Ideally, it should remain at body temperature until liquefaction is complete (about 20 minutes). If the weather is cold, suggest that the patient keep the specimen container in a coat pocket on the way to the laboratory.

Alternatives to collection by masturbation include coitus interruptus or the use of a condom or special sheath. For collection by coitus interruptus, instruct the patient to withdraw immediately before ejaculation and to deposit the ejaculate in a suitable specimen container. Prior to collection by condom, tell the patient to wash the condom with soap and water, rinse it thoroughly, and allow it to dry completely. (Powders or lubricants applied to the condom may be spermicidal.) Instruct the patient to tie the condom, place it in a glass jar, and deliver it to the laboratory promptly, observing the same precautions as for a masturbation sample. Special sheaths that don't contain spermicides are also available for semen collection.

Inform a patient who is undergoing infertility studies that test results should be available in 24 hours.

POSTCOITAL EXAMINATION

Fertility may also be determined by collecting semen postcoitally from the female to assess the ability of the spermatozoa to penetrate the cervical mucus and remain active. The postcoital cervical mucus test should be performed 1 or 2 days before ovulation. After reviewing several months of basal body temperature, the provider will be able to advise the patient when to schedule testing.

A urine luteinizing hormone test may help predict ovulation in patients with irregular cycles. Instruct the couple to abstain from intercourse for 2 days and then to have sex 2 to 8 hours before the examination. Remind them to avoid using lubricants. Explain to the patient scheduled for this test that it takes only a few minutes. Tell her she'll be placed in the lithotomy position and the doctor will insert a speculum in the vagina to collect the specimen. She may feel some pressure but no pain during this procedure.

COLLECTION FROM A RAPE VICTIM

Explain to the patient that the doctor will try to obtain a semen specimen from her vagina. Prepare her for insertion of the speculum as you would the patient scheduled for postcoital examination. Handle the patient's clothes as little as possible. If her clothes are moist, put them in a paper bag—not a plastic bag (which causes seminal stains and secretions to mold). Label the bag properly and send it to the laboratory immediately.

Provide emotional support by speaking to the patient calmly and reassuringly. Encourage her to express her fears and anxieties. Listen sympathetically. If the patient is scheduled for vaginal lavage, tell her to expect a cold sensation when saline solution is instilled to wash out the specimen. To help her relax during this procedure, instruct her to breathe deeply and slowly through her mouth. Just before the test, instruct the patient to urinate, but warn her not to wipe the vulva afterward, because this may remove semen.

Equipment

For collection by masturbation, by coitus interruptus, or with a condom: clean plastic specimen container (for example, disposable urine or sputum container) with a lid.

For collection from a rape victim: clean plastic specimen container ■ vaginal speculum ■ rubber gloves ■ cotton-tipped applicators ■ glass microscopic slides with frosted ends ■ physiologic (0.85%) saline solution ■ Pap sticks ■ Coplin jars containing 95% ethanol ■ large syringe, rubber bulb, or other device suitable for vaginal lavage.

For postcoital collection: clean plastic specimen container ■ vaginal speculum ■ rubber gloves ■ cotton-tipped applicators ■ glass microscopic slides with frosted ends ■ 1-ml tuberculin syringe without a cannula or needle.

Procedure

■ To obtain a semen specimen for a fertility study, ask the patient to collect semen in a clean, plastic specimen container.

■ The doctor obtains a specimen from the vagina of a rape victim by direct aspiration, saline lavage, or a direct smear of vaginal contents, using a Pap stick or, less desirably, a cotton-tipped applicator. Dried smears are usually collected from the suspected rape victim's skin by gently washing the skin with a small piece of gauze, moistened with physiologic saline solution. Prepare direct smears on glass microscopic slides after labeling the frosted end. Immediately place the smeared slides in Coplin jars containing 95% ethanol.

■ Before a postcoital examination, the examiner wipes any excess mucus from the external cervix and collects the specimen by direct aspiration of the cervical canal with a 1-ml tuberculin syringe without a cannula or needle.

Precautions

■ Instruct the male patient who wants to collect a specimen during coitus interruptus to avoid any loss of semen during ejaculation.

■ Deliver all specimens, regardless of source or collection method, to the laboratory within 1 hour.

■ Protect semen specimens for fertility studies from extreme temperatures and direct sunlight during delivery to the laboratory.

■ Don't lubricate the vaginal speculum. Oil and grease hinder examination of spermatozoa by interfering with smear preparation and staining and by inhibiting sperm motility through toxic ingredients. Instead, moisten the speculum with water or physiologic saline solution.

■ Use extreme caution in securing, labeling, and delivering all specimens to be used for medicolegal purposes. You may be asked to testify as to when, where, and from whom the specimen was obtained; the specimen's general appearance and identifying features; steps taken to ensure the specimen's integrity; and when, where, and to whom the specimen was delivered for analysis. If your facility uses routing slips for such specimens, fill them out carefully, and deposit them in the permanent medicolegal file.

Reference values

Semen volume normally ranges from 0.7 to 6.5 ml. Paradoxically, many males in infertile marriages have increased semen volume. Abstinence for 1 week or more results in progressively increased semen volume. (With abstinence up to 10 days, the sperm count increases, sperm motility progressively decreases, and sperm morphology stays the same.) Liquefied semen is generally highly viscid, translucent, and gray-white, with a musty or acrid odor. After liquefaction, specimens of normal viscosity can be poured in drops. Normally, semen is slightly alkaline, with a pH of 7.3 to 7.9.

Other normal characteristics of semen: It coagulates immediately and liquefies within 20 minutes. The sperm count is 20 to 150 million/ml. At least 40% of spermatozoa have normal morphology, and at least 20% of spermatozoa show progressive motility within 4 hours of collection. (A reference value for the number of motile sperm per high power field hasn't been established. Some suggest that virtually any number of motile sperm is normal; others maintain that 10 to 20 sperm per high power field is normal.)

A spinnbarkeit (a measurement of the tenacity of the mucus) of at least 4" (10 cm) indicates that cervical mucus has adequate receptivity. Dead sperm suggest the presence of antisperm antibodies.

Implications of results

Abnormal semen is not synonymous with infertility. Only one viable spermatozoon is needed to fertilize an ovum. Although a normal sperm count is more than 20 million/ml, many males with sperm counts below 1 million/ml have fathered normal children. Only males who can't deliver any viable spermatozoa in their ejaculate during sexual intercourse are absolutely sterile. Nevertheless, subnormal sperm counts, decreased sperm motility, and abnormal morphology are usually associated with decreased fertility.

Adding to the difficulty of diagnosing male infertility is the variability in count and motility among successive semen specimens from the same man. A complete evaluation may require other tests to evaluate the patient's general health and metabolic status or the function of specific endocrine systems (pituitary, thyroid, adrenal, or gonadal).

Refer a suspected rape victim to appropriate specialists for counseling: a gynecologist, psychiatrist, clinical psychologist, nursing specialist, member of the clergy, or representative of a community rape victim support group.

Interfering factors

■ Delayed delivery of the specimen, exposure of the specimen to extreme temperatures or direct sunlight, or the presence of toxic chemicals in the specimen container or the condom can decrease the number of viable sperm.

■ An incomplete specimen—from incomplete collection by coitus interruptus, for example—diminishes the volume of the specimen.

■ The most common cause of an abnormal postcoital test is miscalculation of timing within the menstrual cycle.

■ Prior cervical conization or cryotherapy as well as some medications, such as clomiphene citrate, may adversely affect cervical mucus and yield abnormal postcoital test results.

Sentinel lymph node biopsy

Sentinel lymph node biopsy is considered experimental for breast cancer patients but has become part of the standard of care for melanoma patients. A sentinel lymph node is defined as the first node in the lymphatic basin into which a primary tumor site drains. Hypothetically, the histology of the sentinel node reflects the histology of the rest of the nodes in that basin. Hence, if that sentinel node is identified and is negative for tumor invasion, the rest of the nodes are also negative. If the hypothesis is proven true in breast cancer, axillary lymph node dissections and their resulting morbidity will no longer be necessary.

Two techniques can identify the sentinel node: lymphoscintigraphy, performed in nuclear medicine with injected technetium-99 (^{99}Tc), and injection of blue dye. Both are commonly used, but either may be used alone.

Purpose

To identify the sentinel lymph node and evaluate it for the presence or absence of tumor cells indicating nodal metastasis.

Patient preparation

Explain to the patient that this test evaluates a particular lymph node to determine if cancer has spread into the lymph system.

Tell the patient that a radioactive substance will be injected under the skin. Assure her that she won't be radioactive and that the amount of radiation exposure will be less than that of a routine chest radiograph.

Procedure

■ The patient is positioned on the table in the nuclear medicine suite. A standard dose of ^{99}Tc is injected circumferentially around the margins of a palpable mass, using a 25G needle. For a nonpalpable mass, injections are guided by ultrasound. If the tumor has already been excised, the injections are made around the tumor bed. Images of the axilla are taken with a gamma camera. The location of the sentinel node is marked on the skin in indelible ink and noted on a data sheet.

■ The patient is then transported to the operating room and placed under appropriate anesthesia. Blue dye is injected circumferentially in the tissue immediately surrounding the biopsy site. Within 10 to 15 minutes of the dye injection, a small incision is made in the axilla over the suspected location of the sentinel lymph node. The surgeon follows the trail of stained lymphatics to the sentinel lymph node. The node is identified by the blue dye and by using an intraoperative gamma probe that measures radioactivity; the node having the highest radioactivity is deemed the sentinel node and removed. The axilla is then checked for remaining radioactivity; if none is noted, the surgical procedure concludes. Before it's processed, the sentinel lymph node is stored in formalin until the isotope is no longer radioactive (24 to 48 hours).

Precautions

■ Because ^{99}Tc is radioactive, all radiation precautions must be implemented. Staff members need to be monitored for radiation exposure. After the procedure, radiation levels must be determined in the nuclear medicine suite and the operating room.

■ Allergy to the ^{99}Tc or blue dye is a rare occurrence, but all patients should be observed for signs of allergic reaction (skin changes and respiratory difficulties).

Normal findings

Normal findings are the same as for a normal lymph node biopsy.

Implications of results

Sentinel lymph node biopsy is performed only in breast cancer and melanoma, so abnormal findings mean the identification of melanoma or breast cancer cells. Their presence indicates lymph node metastasis and guides the prognosis and treatment.

Interfering factors

■ Inability to raise the arm to allow access to the axilla can hinder biopsy.
■ Allergy to the radioactive substance will prevent the test from being performed.
■ Inability to obtain an adequate specimen will interfere with test results.
■ Improper specimen storage may affect test results.

Sex chromatin tests

Although sex chromatin tests can screen for abnormalities in the number of sex chromosomes, they've been widely replaced by the full karyotype (chromosome analysis) test, which is faster, simpler, and more accurate. Sex chromatin tests are usually indicated in abnormal sexual development, ambiguous genitalia, amenorrhea, and suspected chromosomal abnormalities.

After fluorescent-staining techniques, the Y chromosome is the most fluorescent chromosome in a karyotype. The fluorescence is confined to the long arm of the chromosome, which is tightly condensed during interphase (that is, between cycles of cell division). When cells are stained with quinacrine, a bright dot (the Y chromatin mass) appears in the nuclei of cells containing a Y chromosome. The number of such masses is identical to the number of Y chromosomes in the cell. Barr bodies (the X chromatin mass) can be stained with any nuclear stain, usually carbolfuchsin, to reveal the number of X chromatin bodies. (See *Understanding sex chromosome anomalies*, pages 526 and 527.)

Purpose

■ To quickly screen for abnormal sexual development (X and Y chromatin tests)
■ To aid assessment of an infant with ambiguous genitalia (X chromatin test only)
■ To determine the number of Y chromosomes in an individual (Y chromatin test only).

UNDERSTANDING SEX CHROMOSOME ANOMALIES

Variations from the normal XX or XY karyotype are called aneuploidies. Each aneuploidy is associated with a specific clinical disorder. Some are incompatible with life. The following table summarizes the clinical implications of the known variants.

Disorder and aneuploidy	Causes and incidence	Phenotypic features
Klinefelter's syndrome		
■ 47, XXY ■ 48, XXXY ■ 49, XXXXY ■ 48, XXYY ■ 49, XXXYY ■ Mosaics: XXY, XXXY, or XXXXY with XX or XY	Nondisjunction or improper chromatid separation during anaphase I or II of oogenesis or spermatogenesis results in abnormal gamete. 1 in 1,000 male births	■ Syndrome usually inapparent until puberty ■ Small penis and testes ■ Sparse facial and abdominal hair; feminine distribution of pubic hair ■ Somewhat enlarged breasts (gynecomastia) ■ Sexual dysfunction ■ Truncal obesity ■ Sterility ■ Possible mental retardation (incidence greater with increasing number of X chromosomes)
Polysomy Y		
■ 47, XYY	Nondisjunction during anaphase II of spermatogenesis causes both Y chromosomes to pass to the same pole and results in Y sperm. 1 in 1,000 male births	■ Above-average stature (often over 72″ [183 cm]) ■ Increased incidence of severe acne ■ Displays of aggressive, psychopathic, or criminal behavior ■ Normal fertility ■ Learning disabilities
Turner's syndrome (ovarian dysgenesis)		
■ XO or 45, X ■ Mosaics: XO/XX or XO/XXX ■ Aberrations of X chromosomes, including deletion of short arm of one X chromosome, presence of a ring chromosome, or presence of an isochromosome (a chromosome in which the arms on either side of the centromere are identical) on the long arm of an X chromosome.	Nondisjunction during anaphase I or II of spermatogenesis results in sperm with no sex chromosomes. 1 in 3,500 female births (most common chromosome complement in first-trimester spontaneous abortions)	■ Short stature (usually under 57″ [145 cm]) ■ Webbed neck ■ Low posterior hairline ■ Broad chest with widely spaced nipples ■ Underdeveloped breasts ■ Juvenile external genitalia ■ Primary amenorrhea (common) ■ Congenital heart disease (30% with coarctation of the aorta) ■ Renal abnormalities ■ Sterility caused by undeveloped internal reproductive organs (ovaries are merely strands of connective tissue) ■ No mental retardation, but possible problems with space perception and orientation

UNDERSTANDING SEX CHROMOSOME ANOMALIES *(continued)*		
Disorder and aneuploidy	**Causes and incidence**	**Phenotypic features**
Other X polysomes	Nondisjunction at anaphase I or II of oogenesis	
■ 47, XXX	1 in 1,400 female births	■ In many cases, no obvious anatomic abnormalities ■ Normal fertility
■ 48, XXXX	Rare	■ Mental retardation ■ Ocular hypertelorism ■ Reduced fertility
■ 49, XXXXX	Rare	■ Severe mental retardation ■ Ocular hypertelorism with unco-ordinated eye movement ■ Abnormal development of sexual organs ■ Various skeletal anomalies

Patient preparation

Explain to the patient or to his parents, if appropriate, why the test is being performed. Tell him the test requires that the inside of his cheek be scraped to obtain a specimen and who will perform the test. Inform the patient that the test takes only a few minutes but may require a follow-up chromosome analysis. Tell him that the laboratory generally requires as long as 4 weeks to complete the analysis.

Equipment

Wooden or metal spatula ■ clean glass slide ■ cell fixative.

Procedure

Scrape the buccal mucosa firmly with a wooden or metal spatula at least twice to obtain a specimen of healthy cells (vaginal mucosa is occasionally used in young women). Rub the spatula over the glass slide, making sure the cells are evenly distributed. Spray the slide with cell fixative and send it to the laboratory with a brief patient history and indications for the test.

Precautions

Make sure the buccal mucosa is scraped firmly to ensure a sufficient number of cells. Check that the specimen isn't saliva, which contains no cells.

Normal findings

A normal female (XX) has only one X chromatin mass (the number of X chromatin masses discernible is one less than the number of X chromosomes in the cells examined). An X chromatin mass is ordinarily discernible in only 20% to 50% of the buccal mucosal cells of a normal female.

A normal male (XY) has only one Y chromatin mass (the number of Y chromatin masses equals the number of Y chromosomes in the cells examined).

Implications of results

In most laboratories, if less than 20% of the cells in a buccal smear contain an X chromatin mass, some cells are presumed to contain only one X chromosome, necessitating full karyotyping. Persons with female phenotype and Y chromatin masses run a high risk of developing malignant tumors in their intra-abdominal gonads. In such persons, removal of these gonads is indicated and should generally be performed before age 5.

After the cause of a chromosomal abnormality has been identified, the patient or his parents require genetic counseling. If a child is phenotypically of one sex and genotypically of the other, a medical team of knowledgeable doctors, psychologists, psychiatrists and, possibly, the child's parents and educators must decide the child's sex. This careful evaluation should be made early to prevent developmental problems related to incorrect gender identification.

Interfering factors

■ Obtaining saliva instead of buccal cells provides a false specimen.
■ Failure to apply cell fixative to the slide allows cells to deteriorate.
■ The presence of bacteria or wrinkles in the cell membrane, analysis of degenerative cells, or use of an outdated stain can produce misleading results.

Sickle cell test

Sickle cells are severely deformed erythrocytes. The sickling phenomenon is caused by hemoglobinopathy—most commonly, the polymerization of hemoglobin S (Hb S) in the presence of low pH, low oxygen tension, elevated osmolarity, and elevated temperature, to form elongated structures (tactoids) that deform red blood cells (RBCs). Reversing these conditions depolymerizes Hb S and lets the RBCs resume their normal shape. However, repeated sickling leads to permanent RBC deformity. Sickle cell trait (Hb S) is found almost exclu-

INHERITANCE PATTERNS IN SICKLE CELL ANEMIA

When both parents have sickle cell anemia (left), childbearing, if possible at all, is dangerous for the mother, and all offspring will have sickle cell anemia. When one parent has sickle cell anemia and one is normal (right), all offspring will be carriers of sickle cell anemia.

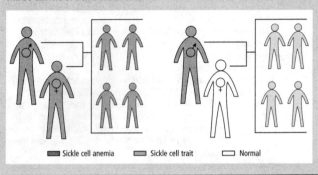

■ Sickle cell anemia   ■ Sickle cell trait   □ Normal

sively in blacks: 0.2% of the blacks born in the United States have sickle cell disease. (See *Inheritance patterns in sickle cell anemia.*)

People who are homozygous for Hb S usually show abundant spontaneously sickled RBCs on a peripheral blood smear. People who are heterozygous for Hb S alone or with another hemoglobinopathy (that is, double heterozygous, sickle cell) may have normal RBCs that can be easily changed to sickled forms by lowering oxygen tension. This sickling tendency can be identified by sealing a drop of blood between a glass slide and coverslip and adding a reducing agent, such as sodium metabisulfate. The RBC can then be observed under a microscope and compared to a central slide containing blood and saline solution. The concentration of Hb S governs the prevalence and rapidity of the sickling.

Although this test (also known as the hemoglobin S test) is useful as a rapid screening procedure, it may produce erroneous results; consequently, hemoglobin electrophoresis should be performed if sickle cell trait is strongly suspected.

Fetuses can also be tested for sickle cell disease or trait. (See *Fetal sickle cell test,* page 530.)

Purpose

To identify sickle cell disease and sickle cell trait. (See *Sickle cell trait,* page 531.)

FETAL SICKLE CELL TEST

When both parents of a developing fetus are suspected carriers of sickle cell trait, a reliable test can detect whether the fetus has the sickle cell trait or the disease.

The fetal sickle cell test, developed in 1970 at the University of California at San Francisco, was the first diagnostic tool to result from recombinant deoxyribonucleic acid (DNA) research. Many major medical centers throughout the United States now perform the test. Any doctor can request the test if he suspects that both parents are carriers. The appropriate samples can be mailed to the nearest test center.

The test requires a venous blood sample from both parents and an amniotic fluid specimen. Diagnosis is based on analysis of the genes and DNA in the fetal cell and the DNA in parental leukocytes. About 1 week is required to complete the test, which is generally performed between the 14th and 18th weeks of pregnancy. This timing provides a sufficient opportunity for the couple to seek genetic counseling.

Patient preparation

Explain to the patient that this test helps detect sickle cell disease. Inform him that he needn't restrict food or fluids. Tell him that the test requires a blood sample, who will perform the venipuncture and when, and that he may experience discomfort from the needle puncture and the pressure of the tourniquet. If the patient is an infant or child, explain to the parents (and to the child if he's old enough to understand) that a small amount of blood will be drawn from his finger.

Check the patient history for a blood transfusion within the past 3 months.

Procedure

Perform a venipuncture and collect the sample in a 7-ml EDTA tube. For younger children, collect capillary blood in a microcollection device.

Precautions

Completely fill the collection tube, and invert it gently several times to adequately mix the sample and the anticoagulant. Don't shake the tube vigorously.

Normal findings

Results of this test are reported as positive or negative. A normal, or negative, test suggests the absence of Hb S.

Implications of results

A positive test may indicate the presence of sickle cells, but hemoglobin electrophoresis is needed to distinguish between homozygous and heterozygous forms. Rarely,

SICKLE CELL TRAIT

This relatively benign condition results from heterozygous inheritance of the abnormal hemoglobin S (Hb S) gene. Like sickle cell anemia, it's most common in blacks.

In persons with sickle cell trait, 20% to 40% of their total hemoglobin is Hb S; the rest is normal. Such persons, called carriers, usually have no symptoms. They have normal hemoglobin and hematocrit values and can expect a normal life span. Nevertheless, they must avoid situations that provoke hypoxia, which occasionally causes a sickling crisis similar to that in sickle cell anemia.

Genetic counseling is essential for sickle cell carriers. Every child of two sickle cell carriers has a 25% chance of inheriting sickle cell anemia and a 50% chance of being a carrier.

other abnormal hemoglobins cause sickling in the absence of Hb S.

Posttest care
■ Make sure subdermal bleeding has stopped before removing pressure.
■ If a hematoma develops at the venipuncture site, apply warm soaks.
■ If the hematoma is large, monitor pulses distal to the phlebotomy site.

Interfering factors
■ Hemoglobin concentration under 10%, elevated Hb S levels in infants under age 6 months, or a blood transfusion within the past 3 months may produce false-negative test results.
■ Failure to use the proper anticoagulant in the collection tube, to completely fill the tube, or to adequately mix the sample and the anticoagulant may affect the accuracy of test results.
■ Hemolysis caused by rough handling of the sample or use of a small-gauge needle for blood aspiration may affect test results.

Skin biopsy

Skin biopsy is the removal of a small piece of tissue from a lesion suspected of being malignant. A specimen for histologic examination may be obtained by one of three techniques — shave, punch, or excision. A shave biopsy cuts the lesion at the skin line and leaves the lower layers of dermis intact, permitting further biopsy at the site. A punch biopsy removes an oval core from the center of a lesion. An excision biopsy, the procedure of choice, removes the entire lesion; it's indicated for rapidly expanding lesions; for sclerotic, bullous, or atrophic lesions; and for examination of a lesion's border and surrounding normal skin.

Lesions suspected of being malignant usually have changed color, size, or appearance or have failed to heal properly after injury. Fully developed lesions should be selected for biopsy whenever possible because they provide more diagnostic information than those that are resolving or in early developing stages. For example, if blisters are present, the biopsy should include the most mature ones.

Purpose

■ To provide differential diagnosis of basal cell carcinoma, squamous cell carcinoma, malignant melanoma, and benign growths
■ To diagnose chronic bacterial or fungal skin infections.

Patient preparation

Describe the procedure to the patient and answer any questions he may have. Explain that the biopsy provides a sample of skin for microscopic study. Inform him that he needn't restrict food or fluids. Tell him who will perform the procedure and where, that he'll receive a local anesthetic to minimize pain during the procedure, and that the biopsy takes approximately 15 minutes.

Make sure the patient has signed a consent form. Check the patient history for hypersensitivity to the local anesthetic.

Procedure

■ Position the patient comfortably and clean the biopsy site. A local anesthetic is administered.
■ For shave biopsy: The protruding growth is cut off above the skin line with a #15 scalpel, and the tissue is placed immediately in a properly labeled specimen bottle containing 10% formalin solution. Pressure is applied to the area to stop the bleeding.
■ For punch biopsy: The skin surrounding the lesion is pulled taut, and the punch is firmly introduced into the lesion and rotated to obtain a tissue specimen. The plug is lifted with forceps or a needle and is severed as deeply into the fat layer as possible. The specimen is placed in a properly labeled specimen bottle containing 10% formalin solution or, if indicated, in a sterile container. The method used to close the wound depends on the size of the punch. A 3-mm punch biopsy requires only an adhesive bandage, a 4-mm punch biopsy requires one suture, and a 6-mm punch biopsy requires two sutures.
■ For excision biopsy: A #15 scalpel is used to excise the lesion completely; the incision is made as wide and as

deep as necessary. The examiner removes the tissue specimen and places it immediately in a properly labeled specimen bottle containing 10% formalin solution. Pressure is applied to the site to stop the bleeding. The wound is closed using 4-0 sutures. If the incision is large, skin graft may be required.

Precautions

Send the specimen to the laboratory immediately.

Normal findings

Normal skin consists of squamous epithelium (epidermis) and fibrous connective tissue (dermis).

Implications of results

Histologic examination of the tissue specimen may reveal a benign or malignant lesion. Benign growths include cysts, seborrheic keratoses, warts, pigmented nevi (moles), keloids, dermatofibromas, and multiple neurofibromas. Malignant skin cancers include basal cell carcinoma, squamous cell carcinoma, and malignant melanoma. Basal cell carcinoma occurs on hair-bearing skin, the most common location being the face—including the nose and its folds. Squamous cell carcinoma most often appears on the lips, mouth, and genitalia. Malignant melanoma, the most deadly skin cancer, can spread throughout the body by way of the lymphatic system and the blood vessels.

Cultures can detect chronic bacterial and fungal infections in which flora are relatively sparse.

Posttest care

■ Check the biopsy site for bleeding.
■ If the patient experiences pain at the biopsy site, administer medication, as ordered.
■ Advise the patient with sutures to keep the area clean and as dry as possible. Tell him the facial sutures will be removed in 3 to 5 days; trunk sutures, in 7 to 14 days. Instruct the patient with adhesive strips to leave them in place for 14 to 21 days or until they fall off.

Interfering factors

■ Improper selection of the biopsy site may affect test results.
■ Failure to use the appropriate fixative or to use a sterile container when it's indicated may alter test results.

Small-bowel biopsy

Small-bowel biopsy helps evaluate diseases of the intestinal mucosa, which may cause malabsorption or diarrhea. Use of a capsule provides larger specimens than

ENDOSCOPIC BIOPSY OF THE GI TRACT

Endoscopy provides direct visualization of the GI tract and allows biopsy of tissue samples for histologic analysis. This relatively painless procedure can:

■ detect cancer, lymphoma, amyloidosis, candidiasis, or gastric ulcers

■ confirm a diagnosis of Crohn's disease, chronic ulcerative colitis, gastritis, esophagitis, or melanosis coli in laxative abuse

■ monitor progression of Barrett's esophagus, multiple gastric polyps, colon cancer and polyps, or chronic ulcerative colitis.

Its complications, notably hemorrhage, perforation, and aspiration, are rare.

Preparation

Careful patient preparation is vital for this procedure. Describe the procedure to the patient and reassure him that he'll be able to breathe with the endoscope in place. Instruct him to fast for at least 8 hours before the procedure. For lower GI biopsy, instruct the patient to clean the bowel, as ordered. Make sure the patient has signed a consent form.

Just before the procedure, sedate the patient, as ordered. He should be relaxed but not asleep because his cooperation promotes smooth passage of the endoscope. Spray the back of his throat with a local anesthetic to suppress his gag reflex. Have suction equipment and bipolar cauterizing electrodes available to prevent aspiration and excessive bleeding.

Procedure

After the doctor passes the endoscope into the upper or lower GI tract and visualizes a lesion, node, or other abnormal area, he pushes a biopsy forceps through a channel in the endoscope until he can see the forceps. Then he opens the forceps, positions it at the biopsy site, and closes it on the tissue. The closed forceps and tissue specimen are removed through the endoscope, and the tissue is taken from the forceps.

The specimen is placed mucosal side up on fine-mesh gauze or filter paper and put into a labeled specimen bottle containing fixative. When all specimens have been collected, the endoscope is removed. Specimens are sent to the laboratory immediately.

does endoscopic biopsy and allows removal of tissue from areas beyond an endoscope's reach. (See *Endoscopic biopsy of the GI tract.*)

Several types of capsules are available, all similar in design and use. The Carey capsule, for example, is a spring-loaded, two-piece capsule that's 8 mm in diameter and 1″ (2.5 cm) long. A mercury-weighted bag is attached to one end of the capsule and a thin polyethylene tube about 4′ (150 cm) long to the other end. Once the bag, capsule, and tube are in place in the small bowel, suction applied to the tube causes the mucosa to enter the capsule. Continued suction closes the capsule, cutting off the piece of tissue within.

This test verifies the diagnosis of some diseases, such as Whipple's disease, and may help confirm others, such as tropical sprue. Capsule biopsy is an invasive procedure, but it causes little pain and complications are rare.

Purpose

To help diagnose diseases of the intestinal mucosa.

Patient preparation

Describe the procedure to the patient, and ask if he has any questions. Explain that this test helps identify intestinal disorders. Instruct him to restrict food and fluids for at least 8 hours before the test. Tell him who will perform the biopsy and where and that the procedure takes 45 to 60 minutes but causes little discomfort.

Make sure the patient has signed a consent form. Ensure that coagulation tests have been performed and that the results are recorded on the patient's chart. Withhold aspirin and anticoagulants, as ordered. If these must be continued, note this on the laboratory request.

Procedure

■ Check the tubing and the mercury bag for leaks. Lightly lubricate the tube and the capsule with a water-soluble lubricant, and moisten the mercury bag with water. Spray the back of the patient's throat with a local anesthetic, as ordered, to decrease gagging during passage of the tube. Ask the patient to sit upright. The capsule is placed in his pharynx, and he is asked to flex his neck and swallow as the doctor advances the tube about 20″ (50 cm). (If a local anesthetic is used to control the gag reflex, the patient must not receive any fluids to help him swallow the capsule.) Place the patient on his right side; the doctor then advances the tube another 20″. The tube's position must be checked by fluoroscopy or by instilling air through the tube and listening with a stethoscope for air to enter the stomach.

■ Next, the tube is advanced 2″ to 4″ (5 to 10 cm) at a time to pass the capsule through the pylorus. Talk to the patient about food to stimulate the pylorus and help the capsule pass. When fluoroscopy confirms that the capsule has passed the pylorus, keep the patient on his right side to allow the capsule to move into the second and third portions of the small bowel. Tell the patient that he may hold the tube loosely to one side of his mouth if it makes him more comfortable. Capsule position is checked again by fluoroscopy.

■ When the capsule is at or beyond the ligament of Treitz, the biopsy sample can be taken. The doctor will determine the biopsy site. Place the patient in the supine position so the capsule's position can be verified fluoroscopically. A 100-ml glass syringe is placed on the end of the tube, and steady suction is applied to close the capsule and cut off a tissue specimen. Suction is maintained on the syringe as the tube and capsule are removed; then the suction is released. This opens the capsule and exposes the specimen, mucosal side down. The specimen is gently removed with forceps, placed mucosal side up on a piece of mesh, and placed in a biopsy bottle with required fixative. Send the specimen to the laboratory at once.

Precautions

- Keep suction equipment nearby to prevent aspiration if the patient vomits.
- Don't allow the patient to bite the tubing.
- Handle the tissue specimen carefully and place it correctly on the slide, as ordered.
- Biopsy is contraindicated in uncooperative patients, those taking aspirin or anticoagulants, and those with uncontrolled coagulation disorders.

Normal findings

A normal small-bowel biopsy specimen consists of fingerlike villi, crypts, columnar epithelial cells, and round cells.

Implications of results

Histologic changes in cell structure may be diagnostic of Whipple's disease, abetalipoproteinemia, lymphoma, lymphangiectasia, eosinophilic enteritis, and such parasitic infections as giardiasis and coccidiosis. Histologic abnormalities may also suggest celiac disease, tropical sprue, infectious gastroenteritis, intraluminal bacterial overgrowth, folate and B12 deficiency, radiation enteritis, and malnutrition, but these disorders require further studies.

Posttest care

- As ordered, resume diet after confirming return of the gag reflex.
- Complications are rare. However, watch for signs of hemorrhage, bacteremia with transient fever and pain, and bowel perforation. Tell the patient to report abdominal pain or bleeding.

Interfering factors

- Failure to fast before the biopsy may yield a poor specimen or cause vomiting and aspiration.
- Mechanical failure of the biopsy capsule or any hole in the tubing can prevent removal of a tissue specimen.

FLUID IMBALANCES

This chart lists the causes, signs and symptoms, and diagnostic test findings associated with hypervolemia (increased fluid volume) and hypovolemia (decreased fluid volume).

Causes	Signs and symptoms	Laboratory findings
Hypervolemia ■ Increased water intake ■ Decreased water output caused by renal disease ■ Congestive heart failure ■ Excessive ingestion or infusion of sodium chloride ■ Long-term administration of adrenocortical hormones ■ Excessive infusion of isotonic solutions	■ Increased blood pressure, pulse rate, body weight, and respiratory rate ■ Bounding peripheral pulses ■ Moist pulmonary crackles ■ Moist mucous membranes ■ Moist respiratory secretions ■ Edema ■ Weakness ■ Seizure and coma caused by swelling of brain cells	■ Decreased red blood cell (RBC) count, hemoglobin concentration, packed cell volume, serum sodium concentration (dilutional decrease), and urine specific gravity
Hypovolemia ■ Decreased water intake ■ Fluid loss caused by fever, diarrhea, and vomiting ■ Systemic infection ■ Impaired renal concentrating ability ■ Fistulous drainage ■ Severe burns ■ Hidden fluid in body cavities	■ Increased pulse and respiratory rates ■ Decreased blood pressure and body weight ■ Weak and thready peripheral pulses ■ Thick, slurred speech ■ Thirst ■ Oliguria ■ Anuria ■ Dry skin	■ Increased RBC count, hemoglobin concentration, packed cell volume, serum sodium concentration, and urine specific gravity

■ Incorrect handling or positioning of the specimen may alter test results.

■ Failure to place the specimen in a fixative or a delay in transport to the laboratory may alter test results.

Sodium test, serum

This test measures serum levels of sodium, the major extracellular cation. Sodium affects body water distribution, maintains osmotic pressure of extracellular fluid, and helps promote neuromuscular function; it also helps maintain acid-base balance and influences chloride and potassium levels. Sodium is absorbed by the kidneys; a small amount is lost through the skin.

Because extracellular sodium concentration in the kidneys regulates body water (low sodium levels promote water excretion and high levels promote retention), serum levels of sodium are evaluated in relation to the amount of water in the body. For example, a sodium deficit (hyponatremia) refers to a serum sodium that is low in relation to body water. (See *Fluid imbalances.*) Aldosterone normally acts to regulate sodium-water balance by inhibiting sodium excretion and promoting its resorption (with water) by the renal tubules. Low sodium levels stimulate aldosterone secretion; high sodium levels depress aldosterone secretion.

Purpose

To evaluate fluid-electrolyte and acid-base balance and related neuromuscular, renal, and adrenal functions.

Patient preparation

Explain to the patient that this test determines the sodium content of blood. Inform him that he needn't restrict food or fluids. Tell him this test requires a blood sample, who will perform the venipuncture and when, and that he may feel some discomfort from the needle puncture and the pressure of the tourniquet.

Check the patient's medication history for use of drugs that influence sodium levels. If these medications must be continued, note this on the laboratory request.

Procedure

Perform a venipuncture and collect the sample in a 7-ml clot-activator tube.

Precautions

Handle the sample gently to prevent hemolysis.

Reference values

Normal serum sodium levels are 135 to 145 mEq/L.

Implications of results

Sodium imbalance can result from a loss or gain of sodium or from a change in water volume. Remember, serum sodium results must be interpreted in light of the patient's state of hydration.

Elevated serum sodium (hypernatremia) may be caused by inadequate water intake, water loss that exceeds sodium loss (as in diabetes insipidus, impaired renal function, prolonged hyperventilation and, occasionally, severe vomiting or diarrhea), or sodium retention (as in aldosteronism). Hypernatremia can also result from excessive sodium intake.

CLINICAL ALERT In a patient with hypernatremia and associated loss of water, observe for signs of thirst, restlessness, dry and sticky mucous membranes, flushed skin, oliguria, and diminished reflexes.

If increased total body sodium causes water retention, observe for hypertension, dyspnea, and edema.

Treatment of hypernatremia should include a gradual lowering of the serum sodium level over 48 hours or more to prevent fluid shifts causing cerebral edema.

Abnormally low serum sodium (hyponatremia) may result from inadequate sodium intake or excessive sodium loss caused by profuse sweating, GI suctioning, diuretic therapy, diarrhea, vomiting, adrenal insufficiency, burns, or chronic renal insufficiency with acidosis. Urine sodium determinations are frequently more sensitive to early changes in sodium balance and should always be evaluated simultaneously with serum sodium findings. The underlying cause must be treated. Monitor fluid balance and restrict water intake.

CLINICAL ALERT In a patient with hyponatremia, watch for apprehension, lassitude, headache, decreased skin turgor, abdominal cramps, and tremors that may progress to seizures.

Posttest care

If a hematoma develops at the venipuncture site, apply warm soaks.

Interfering factors

■ Most diuretics suppress serum sodium levels by promoting sodium excretion; lithium, chlorpropamide, and vasopressin suppress sodium levels by inhibiting water excretion.

■ Corticosteroids elevate serum sodium levels by promoting sodium retention. Antihypertensives, such as methyldopa, hydralazine, and reserpine, may cause sodium and water retention.

■ Hemolysis caused by rough handling of the sample may interfere with accurate determination of test results.

Sodium and chloride test, urine

This test determines urine levels of sodium, the major extracellular cation, and of chloride, the major extracellular anion. Less sensitive than serum assay (and, consequently, performed less frequently), urine sodium and chloride measurement is used to evaluate renal conservation of these two electrolytes and to confirm serum sodium and chloride values.

Sodium and chloride help maintain osmotic pressure and water and acid-base balance. After these ions are absorbed by the intestinal tract, they're regulated by the kidneys and rise and fall in tandem. The kidneys conserve constant serum levels of sodium and chloride — even at the risk of dehydration or edema — or excrete excessive amounts.

Purpose

■ To help evaluate fluid and electrolyte imbalance

■ To monitor the effects of a low-salt diet
■ To help evaluate renal and adrenal disorders.

Patient preparation

Explain to the patient that this test helps determine the balance of salt and water in his body. Advise him that no special restrictions are necessary and that the test requires a 24-hour urine specimen. If the specimen is to be collected at home, teach the patient the proper collection technique. Check the patient's medication history for drugs that may influence test results.

Procedure

Collect a 24-hour urine specimen.

Precautions

Tell the patient not to contaminate the specimen with toilet tissue or stool.

Reference values

Although levels of sodium and chloride in the urine vary greatly with dietary salt intake and perspiration, the normal range for urine sodium excretion is 30 to 280 mEq/24 hours; for urine chloride excretion, 110 to 250 mEq/24 hours; and for urine sodium-chloride excretion, 5 to 20 g/24 hours.

Implications of results

Usually, urine sodium and chloride levels are parallel, rising and falling in tandem. Isolated urine chloride, without urine sodium and potassium, or without serum electrolytes, can provide misleading information. Abnormal sodium and chloride levels may indicate the need for more specific tests. Elevated urine sodium levels may reflect increased salt intake, adrenal failure, salicylate toxicity, diabetic acidosis, salt-losing nephritis, or water-deficient dehydration. Decreased urine sodium levels suggest decreased salt intake, primary aldosteronism, acute renal failure, or congestive heart failure.

Elevated urine chloride levels may result from water-deficient dehydration, salicylate toxicity, diabetic acidosis, adrenocortical insufficiency (Addison's disease), or salt-losing renal disease. Decreased levels may result from excessive diaphoresis, congestive heart failure, or hypochloremic metabolic alkalosis caused by prolonged vomiting or gastric suctioning.

To evaluate fluid-electrolyte imbalance, results must be correlated with serum electrolyte findings.

Interfering factors

- Ammonium chloride and potassium chloride elevate urine chloride levels.
- Sodium bicarbonate and thiazide diuretics raise urine sodium levels; steroids suppress them.
- Failure to collect all urine during the test period may alter test results.

Soluble amyloid beta protein precursor test

The presence of the amyloid beta protein in the senile plaques of the brain is a hallmark of Alzheimer's disease, leading researchers to believe that this protein may be responsible for the disease's neurotoxic effects. Although amyloid is found in the cerebrospinal fluid (CSF) of healthy people, it's found in smaller amounts in some patients with dementia, making it a useful diagnostic tool.

Purpose

To assist in the diagnosis of Alzheimer's disease. (See *Two tests for Alzheimer's disease*, page 542.)

Patient preparation

Explain to the patient that a specimen of CSF is collected by lumbar puncture, and a small portion is tested using the enzyme-linked immunosorbent assay (ELISA) test. Tell the patient who will perform the procedure and where. Inform him that he needn't restrict food or fluids. Advise him that a headache is the most common adverse effect of lumbar puncture, but reassure him that his cooperation during the test helps minimize this effect. Make sure that a signed consent form has been obtained.

Equipment

Lumbar puncture tray ■ sterile gloves ■ local anesthetic (1% lidocaine) ■ povidone-iodine solution ■ small adhesive bandage.

Procedure

- Position the patient on his side at the edge of the bed, with his knees drawn up to his abdomen and his chin on his chest. Provide pillows to support the spine on a horizontal plane. This position allows full flexion of the spine and easy access to the lumbar subarachnoid space. Help the patient maintain this position by placing one arm around his knees and the other arm around his neck. If the sitting position is preferred, have the patient sit up and bend his chest and head toward his knees.

TWO TESTS FOR ALZHEIMER'S DISEASE

Two relatively new tests can be useful in evaluating patients with symptoms of dementia. One test determines the level of tau protein in conjunction with beta amyloid in the cerebrospinal fluid and requires a lumbar puncture. Elevated levels of tau and reduced levels of beta amyloid are associated with Alzheimer's disease. The manufacturer claims that this test is 95% accurate in ruling out or confirming Alzheimer's disease in about 60% of symptomatic patients over age 60.

The second test determines the person's apolipoprotein E (ApoE) genotype, which is statistically significant in determining the probability of Alzheimer's disease. The presence of two copies of the ApoE4 allele may increase the probability to over 90%.

Although these tests may prove helpful in diagnosing Alzheimer's disease, experts caution that further studies are necessary to confirm their reliability.

Help him maintain this position throughout the procedure.

■ After the skin is prepared for injection, the area is draped. Warn the patient that he'll probably experience a transient burning sensation when the local anesthetic is injected. Tell the patient that, when the spinal needle is inserted, he may feel some transient local pain as the needle transverses the dura mater. Ask him to report any pain or other sensations that differ from or continue after this expected discomfort because such sensations could indicate irritation or puncture of a nerve root, requiring repositioning of the needle. Instruct the patient to remain still and breathe normally during the procedure; movement and hyperventilation can alter pressure readings or cause injury.

■ The anesthetic is injected and the spinal needle is inserted in the midline between the spinous processes of the vertebrae, usually between the third and fourth lumbar vertebrae. At this point, initial (or opening) CSF pressure is measured and a specimen is obtained.

■ After the specimen is collected, label the containers in the order in which they were filled, and determine if there are any specific instructions for the laboratory. Next, a final pressure reading is taken, and the needle is removed. Clean the puncture site with a local antiseptic, such as povidone-iodine solution, and apply a small adhesive bandage.

Precautions

CLINICAL ALERT Infection at the puncture site contraindicates removal of CSF; in a patient with increased intracranial pressure, CSF should be removed with extreme caution because the rapid reduction in pressure that follows withdrawal of fluid can cause cerebellar tonsillar herniation and medullary compression.

During the procedure, observe closely for adverse reactions, such as elevated pulse rate, pallor, or clammy skin. Report any significant changes immediately.

Record the collection time on the test request form. Send the form and labeled specimens to the laboratory immediately.

Reference values

Normal amyloid beta protein levels in CSF are greater than 450 units/L, based on age-matched controls using the ELISA test.

Implications of findings

Soluble amyloid beta protein precursor is found in the CSF of healthy people. Low CSF levels suggest a change in processing of the amyloid beta-protein precursor to form amyloid beta protein. Low precursor levels correlate with clinically diagnosed and autopsy-confirmed Alzheimer's disease.

Posttest care

■ Check whether the patient must lie flat or if the head of his bed may be slightly elevated. In most cases, you'll be instructed to keep the patient lying flat for 8 hours after lumbar puncture. Some doctors permit a 30-degree elevation at the head of the bed. Remind the patient that, although he shouldn't raise his head, he can turn from side to side.

■ Encourage the patient to drink fluids. Provide a flexible straw.

■ Check the puncture site for redness, swelling, and drainage every hour for the first 4 hours and then every 4 hours the first 24 hours.

■ If CSF pressure is elevated, assess neurologic status every 15 minutes for 4 hours. If the patient is stable, assess him every hour for 2 hours and then every 4 hours or according to the pretest schedule.

Interfering factors

■ Patient positioning and activity may increase or decrease CSF pressure.

■ Crying, coughing, or straining may increase CSF pressure.

■ Delay in collection time and laboratory testing may interfere with test results.

Sputum culture

Bacteriologic examination of sputum—material raised from the lungs and bronchi during deep coughing—is an important aid in managing lung disease. During passage through the throat and oropharynx, sputum specimens are commonly contaminated with indigenous bacterial flora, such as alpha-hemolytic streptococci, *Neisseria* species, diphtheroids, some *Haemophilus* species, pneumococci, staphylococci, and yeasts such as *Candida*.

Pathogenic organisms most often found in sputum include *Streptococcus pneumoniae*, *Mycobacterium tuberculosis*, *Klebsiella pneumoniae* (and other Enterobacteriaceae), *H. influenzae*, *Staphylococcus aureus*, and *Pseudomonas aeruginosa*. Other pathogens, such as *Pneumocystis carinii*, *Legionella* species, *Mycoplasma pneumoniae*, and respiratory viruses, may exist in the sputum and can cause lung disease, but they usually require serologic or histologic diagnosis rather than diagnosis by sputum culture.

The usual method of specimen collection is expectoration (which may require ultrasonic nebulization, hydration, physiotherapy, or postural drainage); other methods include tracheal suctioning and bronchoscopy.

A Gram stain of expectorated sputum must be examined to ensure that it's a representative specimen of secretions from the lower respiratory tract (many white blood cells [WBCs], few epithelial cells) rather than one contaminated by oral flora (few WBCs, many epithelial cells). Careful examination of an acid-fast smear of sputum may provide presumptive evidence of a mycobacterial infection, such as tuberculosis.

Purpose

To isolate and identify the cause of a pulmonary infection, thus aiding diagnosis of respiratory diseases (most frequently bronchitis, tuberculosis, lung abscess, and pneumonia).

Patient preparation

Explain to the patient that this test helps to identify the organism causing respiratory tract infection. Tell him the test requires a sputum specimen and who will perform the procedure. If the suspected organism is *M. tuberculosis*, tell him that specimens may need to be collected on at least three consecutive mornings.

Test results are usually available in 48 to 72 hours. However, because cultures for tuberculosis take up to 2 months, diagnosis of this disorder is usually based on clinical symptoms, a smear for acid-fast bacilli, a chest radiograph, and response to a purified protein derivative skin test.

If the specimen is to be collected by expectoration, encourage fluid intake the night before collection to help sputum production. Have the patient brush his teeth and gargle with water immediately before obtaining the specimen to reduce the number of contaminating oropharyngeal bacteria. Teach the patient how to expectorate by taking three deep breaths and forcing a deep cough. Emphasize that sputum isn't the same as saliva, which will be rejected for culturing.

If the specimen is to be collected by tracheal suctioning, tell the patient he'll experience discomfort as the catheter passes into the trachea.

If the specimen is to be collected by bronchoscopy, instruct the patient to fast for 6 hours before the procedure. Make sure he or a responsible member of the family has signed a consent form. Tell him he'll receive a local anesthetic just before the test to minimize discomfort during passage of the tube.

Equipment

For expectoration: ■ clean gloves ■ sterile, disposable, impermeable container with a tight-fitting cap ■ 10% sodium chloride, acetylcysteine, propylene glycol, or sterile or distilled water aerosol, to induce cough, as ordered ■ leakproof bag.

For tracheal suctioning: ■ size 16 or 18 French suction catheter ■ water-soluble lubricant ■ sterile gloves ■ sterile specimen container or in-line specimen trap ■ normal saline solution.

For bronchoscopy: ■ bronchoscope ■ local anesthetic ■ sterile needle and syringe ■ sterile specimen container ■ normal saline solution ■ bronchial brush ■ sterile gloves.

Procedure

■ For expectoration: Put on gloves. Instruct the patient to cough deeply and expectorate into the container. If the cough is nonproductive, use chest physiotherapy or nebulization to induce sputum, as ordered. Using aseptic technique, close the container securely. Dispose of equipment properly; seal the container in a leakproof bag before sending it to the laboratory.

■ For tracheal suctioning: Administer oxygen to the patient before and after the procedure, as necessary. Attach the sputum trap to the suction catheter. Using sterile gloves, lubricate the catheter with normal saline solution, and pass the catheter through the patient's nostril, without suction. (The patient will cough when the catheter passes through the larynx.) Advance the catheter into the trachea. Apply suction for no longer than 15 seconds to obtain the specimen. Stop suction, and gently remove the catheter. Discard the catheter and gloves in the proper receptacle. Then detach the in-line sputum trap from the suction apparatus and cap the opening.

■ For bronchoscopy: After a local anesthetic is sprayed into the patient's throat or the patient gargles with a local anesthetic, the bronchoscope is inserted through the pharynx and trachea into the bronchus. Secretions are then collected with a bronchial brush or aspirated through the inner channel of the scope, using an irrigating solution (such as normal saline solution) if necessary. After the specimen is obtained, the bronchoscope is removed.

■ Label the container with the patient's name. Include on the laboratory request the nature and origin of the specimen, the date and time of collection, the initial diagnosis, and any current antimicrobial therapy.

Precautions

■ Tracheal suctioning is contraindicated in patients with esophageal varices or cardiac disease.

CLINICAL ALERT In a patient with asthma or chronic bronchitis, watch for aggravated bronchospasms with use of more than 10% concentration of sodium chloride or acetylcysteine in an aerosol.

■ During tracheal suctioning, suction for only 5 to 10 seconds at a time. Never suction longer than 15 seconds. If the patient becomes hypoxic or cyanotic, remove the catheter immediately and administer oxygen.

■ Use gloves when performing the procedure and handling specimens.

■ Because the patient may cough violently during suctioning, wear gloves and a mask to avoid exposure to pathogens.

■ Do not use more than 20% propylene glycol with water as an inducer for a specimen scheduled for tuberculosis culturing; higher concentrations inhibit the growth of *M. tuberculosis*. (If propylene glycol isn't available, use 10% to 20% acetylcysteine with water or sodium chloride.)

■ Send the specimen to the laboratory immediately after collection.

Normal findings

Flora commonly found in the respiratory tract include alpha-hemolytic streptococci, *Neisseria* species, and diphtheroids. However, the presence of normal flora doesn't rule out infection.

Implications of results

Because sputum is invariably contaminated with normal oropharyngeal flora, a culture isolate must be interpreted in light of the patient's overall clinical condition. Isolation of *M. tuberculosis* is always a significant finding.

Posttest care

- Provide good mouth care.
- After tracheal suctioning, offer the patient a drink of water.

CLINICAL ALERT After bronchoscopy, observe the patient carefully for signs of hypoxemia (cyanosis), laryngospasm (laryngeal stridor), bronchospasm (paroxysms of coughing or wheezing), pneumothorax (dyspnea, cyanosis, pleural pain, tachycardia), perforation of the trachea or bronchus (subcutaneous crepitus), or trauma to respiratory structures (bleeding). Also, check for difficulty breathing or swallowing. Don't give liquids until the gag reflex returns.

Interfering factors

- Improper collection or handling of the specimen may alter test results.
- Failure to report current or recent antimicrobial therapy may cause false-negative results.
- An extended sputum collection time may cause pathogens to deteriorate or become overgrown by commensals and won't be accepted as a valid specimen by most laboratories.

Sputum examination

This test evaluates a sputum specimen for parasites. Such infestation is rare in the United States but may result from exposure to *Entamoeba histolytica, Ascaris lumbricoides, Echinococcus granulosus, Strongyloides stercoralis, Paragonimus westermani,* or *Necator americanus.* The specimen is obtained by expectoration or tracheal suctioning.

Purpose

To identify pulmonary parasites.

Patient preparation

Explain to the patient that this test helps identify parasitic pulmonary infection. Tell him the test requires a sputum specimen or, if necessary, tracheal suctioning.

Inform him that early morning collection is preferred because secretions accumulate overnight.

For expectoration, encourage fluid intake the night before collection to increase sputum production. Teach the patient how to expectorate by taking three deep breaths and forcing a deep cough. For tracheal suctioning, tell him he'll experience discomfort from the catheter.

Equipment

For expectoration: ■ sterile, disposable, impermeable container with screw cap or tight-fitting cap ■ nebulizer, intermittent positive-pressure breathing ventilator, and 10% sodium chloride, acetylcysteine, or sterile or distilled water aerosols to induce cough, as ordered.

For tracheal suctioning: ■ size 16 or 18 French suction catheter ■ sterile gloves ■ sterile specimen container or sputum trap ■ sterile normal saline solution.

Procedure

■ For expectoration: Instruct the patient to breathe deeply a few times and then to cough deeply and expectorate into the container. If the cough is nonproductive, use chest physiotherapy or heated aerosol spray (nebulization), as ordered. Close the container securely and clean the outside of it. Dispose of equipment properly, and take proper precautions in sending the specimen to the laboratory.

■ For tracheal suctioning: Administer oxygen before and after the procedure, if necessary. Attach a sputum trap to the suction catheter. While wearing a sterile glove, lubricate the tip of the catheter, and pass it through the patient's nostril, without suction. (The patient will cough when the catheter passes into the larynx.) Advance the catheter into the trachea. Apply suction for no longer than 15 seconds to obtain the specimen. Stop suction, and gently remove the catheter. Discard the catheter and glove in a proper receptacle. Then detach the sputum trap from the suction apparatus and cap the opening. Label all specimens carefully.

Precautions

■ Use gloves when performing procedures and handling specimens.

■ Tracheal suctioning is contraindicated in patients with esophageal varices or cardiac disease.

CLINICAL ALERT In a patient with asthma or chronic bronchitis, watch for aggravated bronchospasms with use of more than 10% concentration of sodium chloride or acetylcysteine in an aerosol.

■ During tracheal suctioning, suction for only 5 to 10 seconds at a time. Never suction for more than 15 seconds. If the patient becomes hypoxic or cyanotic, remove the catheter immediately, and administer oxygen.
■ Send the specimen to the laboratory immediately, or place it in preservative.

Normal findings

No parasites or ova should be present.

Implications of results

The parasite identified indicates the type of pulmonary infection and the presence of adult-stage intestinal infection:

■ *E. histolytica* trophozoites: pulmonary amebiasis
■ *A. lumbricoides* larvae and adults: pneumonitis
■ *E. granulosus* cysts of larval stage: hydatid disease
■ *S. stercoralis* larvae: strongyloidiasis
■ *P. westermani* ova: paragonimiasis
■ *N. americanus* larvae: hookworm disease.

Posttest care

■ After suctioning, offer the patient water and monitor vital signs every hour until stable.
■ Provide good mouth care.

Interfering factors

■ Recent therapy with anthelmintics or amebicides may alter test results.
■ Improper collection may produce a nonrepresentative specimen, thereby affecting test results.
■ Delay in sending the specimen to the laboratory may alter test results.

Stool culture

Bacteriologic examination of the feces is valuable for identifying pathogens that cause overt GI disease — such as typhus and dysentery — and carrier states. Normally, feces contains many species of bacterial flora and several potentially pathogenic organisms. The most common pathogenic organisms of the GI tract are *Shigella*, *Salmonella*, and *Campylobacter jejuni*. Less common pathogenic organisms include *Candida albicans*, *Vibrio cholerae*, *Clostridium botulinum*, *Clostridium difficile*, *Clostridium perfringens*, *Staphylococcus aureus*, enterotoxicogenic *Escherichia coli*, *Bacillus cereus*, *Yersinia enterocolitica*, *Aeromonas hydrophila*, and *Vibrio parahaemolyticus*. (See *Pathogens of the GI tract*, page 550.) Identifying these organisms is vital to treat the patient, to prevent possibly fatal complications (especially in a debilitated patient), and to confine these severe infec-

PATHOGENS OF THE GI TRACT

The presence of the following pathogens in a stool culture may indicate the cause of certain disorders:

- *Aeromonas hydrophila:* gastroenteritis, which causes diarrhea, especially in children
- *Bacillus cereus:* food poisoning, acute gastroenteritis (rare)
- *Campylobacter jejuni:* gastroenteritis
- *Clostridium botulinum:* food poisoning and infant botulism (a possible cause of sudden infant death syndrome)
- Toxin-producing *Clostridium difficile:* pseudomembranous enterocolitis
- *Clostridium perfringens:* food poisoning
- Enterotoxicogenic *Escherichia coli:* gastroenteritis (resembles cholera or shigellosis)
- *Salmonella:* gastroenteritis, typhoid fever, nontyphoidal salmonellosis, paratyphoid fever, enteric fever
- *Shigella:* shigellosis, bacillary dysentery
- *Staphylococcus aureus:* food poisoning, suppression of normal bowel flora from antimicrobial therapy
- *Vibrio cholerae:* cholera
- *Vibrio parahaemolyticus:* food poisoning, especially seafood
- *Yersinia enterocolitica:* gastroenteritis, enterocolitis (resembles appendicitis), mesenteric lymphadenitis, ileitis.

tious diseases. A sensitivity test may follow isolation of the pathogen.

Some viruses, such as rotavirus and parvovirus, may also cause GI symptoms. However, these viruses can be detected only by immunoassay or electron microscopy. Stool culture may detect other viruses, such as enterovirus, which can cause aseptic meningitis.

Purpose

- To identify pathogenic organisms causing GI disease
- To identify carrier states.

Patient preparation

Explain to the patient that this test helps determine the cause of GI distress and may establish whether he is a carrier of infectious organisms. Inform him that he needn't restrict food or fluids. Tell him the test may require the collection of a stool specimen on 3 consecutive days.

Check the patient history for dietary patterns, recent antimicrobial therapy, and recent travel that might suggest an endemic infection or infestation.

Specimens should be collected before antimicrobial therapy is started.

Equipment

Gloves ∎ half-pint, waterproof container with tight-fitting lid, or sterile swab and commercial sterile collection and transport system ∎ tongue blade ∎ bedpan (if needed).

Procedure

∎ Collect a stool specimen directly in the container. If the patient isn't ambulatory, collect it in a clean, dry bedpan; then, using a tongue blade, transfer the specimen to the container. If you must collect the specimen by rectal swab, insert the swab past the anal sphincter, rotate it gently, and withdraw it. Then place the swab in the appropriate container.

∎ Check with the laboratory for the proper collection procedure before obtaining a specimen for a virus test.

∎ Label the specimen with the patient's name, doctor's name, hospital number, and date and time of collection.

Precautions

∎ If specimens can't be transported to the laboratory within 1 hour, the specimen should be refrigerated or placed in transport media.

∎ If the patient uses a bedpan or a diaper, avoid contaminating the stool specimen with urine.

∎ Send the specimen to the laboratory immediately; be sure to include mucoid and bloody portions. The specimen must always represent the first, middle, and last portion of the feces passed.

∎ Use gloves when performing the procedure and handling the specimen. Be sure to put the specimen container in a leakproof bag before sending it to the laboratory.

∎ Indicate the suspected cause of the patient's GI disorder and include current antimicrobial therapy on the laboratory request.

Normal findings

More than 95% of normal fecal flora consist of anaerobes, including non-spore-forming bacilli, clostridia, and anaerobic streptococci. The remainder consist of aerobes, including gram-negative bacilli (predominantly *E. coli* and other *Enterobacteriaceae*, plus small amounts of *Pseudomonas*), gram-positive cocci (mostly enterococci), and a few yeasts.

Implications of results

Isolation of some pathogens (such as *Salmonella*, *Shigella*, *Campylobacter*, *Yersinia*, and *Vibrio*) reflects bacterial infection in patients with acute diarrhea and may require antimicrobial sensitivity tests. Because normal fecal flora may include *C. difficile, E. coli,* and other organisms, isolation of these may require further tests to demonstrate invasiveness or toxin production.

Isolation of pathogens such as *C. botulinum* indicates food poisoning, although the pathogens must also be isolated from the contaminated food. In patients undergoing long-term antimicrobial therapy as well as those with acquired immunodeficiency disease or who are taking immunosuppressant drugs, isolation of large numbers of *S. aureus* or such yeasts as *Candida* may indicate infection. Asymptomatic carrier states are also indicated by these enteric pathogens. Isolation of enteroviruses may indicate aseptic meningitis.

If a stool culture shows no unusual growth, detection of viruses by immunoassay or electron microscopy may diagnose nonbacterial gastroenteritis. A highly increased polymorphonuclear leukocyte count in fecal material suggests an invasive pathogen.

Interfering factors

■ Improper collection technique or contamination of the specimen by urine may injure or destroy some enteric pathogens.

■ Antimicrobial therapy may inhibit bacterial growth in the specimen.

■ Failure to transport the specimen promptly or, if delivery is delayed, to use a transport medium that stabilizes pH (such as a buffered glycerol medium) may result in loss of some enteric pathogens or overgrowth of nonpathogenic organisms.

Stool examination for ova and parasites

Examination of a stool specimen can detect several types of intestinal parasites. Some of these parasites live in nonpathogenic symbiosis; others cause intestinal disease. In the United States, the most common parasites include the roundworms *Ascaris lumbricoides* and *Necator americanus* (commonly called hookworm); the tapeworms *Diphyllobothrium latum, Taenia saginata* and, rarely, *T. solium;* the amoeba *Entamoeba histolytica;* and the flagellate *Giardia lamblia.* Cyclospora can also be detected in stool examination for ova and parasites.

Detection of pinworm requires a different collection method. (See *Collection procedure for pinworm.*)

Purpose

To confirm or rule out intestinal parasitic infection and disease.

COLLECTION PROCEDURE FOR PINWORM

The ova of the pinworm *Enterobius vermicularis* seldom appear in feces because the female migrates to the anus and deposits her ova there. To collect them, place a piece of cellophane tape, sticky side out, on the end of a tongue blade, and press it firmly on the anal area. Then transfer the tape, sticky side down, to a slide (kits with tape or a sticky paddle and a slide are available). Because the female usually deposits her ova at night, collect the specimen early in the morning, before the patient bathes or defecates. Pinworm infection shouldn't be ruled out until five consecutive negative specimens have been obtained.

Patient preparation

Explain to the patient that this test detects intestinal parasitic infection. Instruct him to avoid treatments with castor or mineral oil, bismuth, magnesium or antidiarrheal compounds, barium enemas, and antibiotics for 7 to 10 days before the test. Tell him the test requires three stool specimens — one every other day or every third day. Up to six specimens may be required to confirm the presence of *E. histolytica*.

If the patient has diarrhea, record recent dietary and travel history. Check the patient history for use of antiparasitic drugs, such as tetracycline, paromomycin, metronidazole, and iodoquinol, within 2 weeks before the test.

Equipment

Gloves ■ waterproof container with tight-fitting lid ■ bedpan (if necessary) ■ tongue blade.

Procedure

■ Put on gloves and collect a stool specimen directly in the container. If the patient is bedridden, collect the specimen in a clean, dry bedpan; then, using a tongue blade, transfer it into a properly labeled container. Note on the laboratory request the date and time of collection and the specimen consistency. Also record recent or current antimicrobial therapy and any pertinent travel or dietary history.

■ Commercial stool collection and preservation kits for detection of ova and parasites are available. In the commercial two-vial transport system, one vial contains 8 to 10 ml of 10% formalin and the other contains 8 to 10 ml of polyvinyl alcohol. To each vial, add 2 to 3 ml of feces. Thoroughly mix the specimen and fluid. Cap each vial tightly.

■ As ordered, resume administration of medications discontinued before the test.

Precautions

- Don't contaminate the stool specimen with urine, which can destroy trophozoites.
- Don't collect stool from a toilet bowl because water is toxic to trophozoites and may contain organisms that interfere with test results.
- Send the specimen to the laboratory immediately. If a liquid or soft stool specimen can't be examined within 30 minutes of passage, place some of it in a preservative; if a formed stool specimen can't be examined immediately, refrigerate it or place it in preservative.
- If the entire stool can't be sent to the laboratory, include macroscopic worms or worm segments as well as bloody and mucoid portions of the specimen.
- Use gloves when performing the procedure and handling the specimen, disposing of equipment, sealing the container, and transporting the specimen. Dispose of gloves after specimen collection and transport.

Normal findings

No parasites or ova should appear in stool.

Implications of results

The presence of *E. histolytica* confirms amebiasis; *G. lamblia*, giardiasis. However, the extent of infection depends on the degree of tissue invasion. If amebiasis is suspected but stool examinations are negative, specimen collection after saline catharsis using buffered sodium biphosphate or during sigmoidoscopy may be necessary. If giardiasis is suspected but stool examinations are negative, examination of duodenal contents may be necessary.

Because injury to the host is difficult to detect — even when helminth ova or larvae appear — the number of worms is usually correlated with the patient's clinical symptoms to distinguish between infestation and disease. Eosinophilia also suggests parasitic infection.

Helminths may migrate from the intestinal tract and cause pathologic changes in other parts of the body. For example, the roundworm *Ascaris* may perforate the bowel wall, causing peritonitis, or may migrate to the lungs, causing pneumonitis. Hookworms can cause hypochromic microcytic anemia secondary to blood-sucking and hemorrhage, especially in patients with iron-deficient diets. The tapeworm *D. latum* may cause megaloblastic anemia by removing vitamin B_{12}.

Interfering factors

■ Failure to observe pretest drug restrictions may interfere with microscopic analysis or reduce the number of parasites.

■ Any radiographic contrast media given to the patient within 5 to 10 days prior to specimen collection will alter test results.

■ Improper collection technique or the presence of urine may cause false-negative results.

■ Collection of too few specimens may cause false-negative results.

■ Failure to transport the specimen promptly or to refrigerate or preserve it if transport is delayed may influence test results.

■ Excessive heat or excessive cold can destroy parasites.

Stool examination for rotavirus antigen

Rotavirus (previously referred to as orbivirus, reovirus-like agent, duovirus, and gastroenteritis virus) is the most frequent cause of infectious diarrhea in infants and young children, associated with approximately 50% of pediatric hospitalizations for gastroenteritis.

Clinical features of rotavirus infection include diarrhea, vomiting, fever, and abdominal pain leading to dehydration. This infection is most prevalent in children ages 3 months to 2 years during the winter months. In contrast to the severe clinical illness it causes in hospitalized infants, rotavirus may cause only mild symptoms in adults.

Human rotaviruses don't replicate efficiently in the usual laboratory cell cultures. Therefore, detection of the typical virus particles in stool specimens by electron microscopy has been replaced by sensitive, specific enzyme immunoassays that can provide results within minutes or a few hours (depending on the assay) after the specimen is received in the laboratory.

Purpose

To obtain a laboratory diagnosis of rotavirus gastroenteritis.

Patient preparation

Explain the purpose of the test to the patient or to the parents if the patient is a child. Inform him that the test requires a stool specimen. The specimens should be collected during the prodromal and acute stages of clinical infection to ensure detection of the viral antigens by enzyme immunoassay.

Procedure
- A stool specimen (1 g in a screw-capped tube or vial) is preferred for detecting rotaviruses. If a microbiologic transport swab is used, it must be heavily stained with feces to be diagnostically productive for rotavirus.
- Monitor the patient's intake and output to avoid dehydration caused by vomiting and diarrhea.

Precautions
- Avoid using collection containers with preservatives, metal ions, detergents, or serum, which may interfere with the assay.
- Store stool specimens for up to 24 hours at 35.6° F to 46.4° F (2° C to 8° C). If a longer period of storage or shipment is necessary, freeze the specimens at –4° F (–20° C) or colder. Repeated freezing and thawing will cause the specimen to deteriorate and yield misleading results.
- Don't store the specimen in a self-defrosting freezer.
- Use gloves when obtaining or handling all specimens.

Normal findings
The detection of rotavirus by enzyme immunoassay is evidence of current infection with the organism.

Implications of results
Rotavirus can infect all age-groups, but the disease is generally more severe in young children than in adults.

Rotavirus infections are easily transmitted in group settings, such as day-care centers and nursing homes. Transmission is presumed to occur from person to person by the fecal-oral route. Nosocomial spread of this viral infection can have significant medical and economic effects in a hospital setting.

Interfering factors
Collecting the specimen in containers with preservatives, metal ions, detergents, or serum may interfere with detection of the virus.

Sweat test
The sweat test quantitatively measures electrolyte concentrations (primarily sodium and chloride) in sweat, usually through pilocarpine iontophoresis (pilocarpine is a sweat inducer). This test is used almost exclusively in children to confirm cystic fibrosis, a congenital condition that raises the sodium and chloride electrolyte levels in sweat.

Purpose
- To confirm cystic fibrosis

■ To exclude the diagnosis in siblings of children with cystic fibrosis.

Patient preparation

Because the patient is generally a child, explain the test to him as simply as possible (if he's old enough to understand). Inform the patient and his parents that there are no restrictions of diet, medications, or activity before the test. Tell the patient who will perform the test and where and that it takes 20 to 45 minutes (depending on the equipment used).

Tell the child he may feel a slight tickling sensation during the procedure but won't feel any pain. Instruct him to tell the examiner immediately if he feels a burning sensation. If he becomes nervous or frightened during the test, try to distract him with a book, television, or another appropriate diversion.

Encourage the parents to assist with preparations and to stay with their child during the test. Their presence will minimize the child's anxiety.

Equipment

Analyzer ■ two skin chloride electrodes (positive and negative) ■ distilled water ■ two standardizing solutions (chloride concentrations) ■ sterile 2″ x 2″ gauze pads (kept in airtight container) ■ pilocarpine pads ■ forceps (for handling pads) ■ straps (for securing electrodes) ■ gram scale ■ normal saline solution.

Procedure

■ With distilled water, wash the area to be tested, and dry it. The flexor surface of the right forearm is commonly used or, when the patient's arm is too small to secure electrodes, as in an infant, the right thigh. Place a gauze pad saturated with premeasured pilocarpine solution on the positive electrode; place a gauze pad saturated with normal saline solution on the negative electrode. Apply both electrodes to the area to be tested, and secure them with straps.

■ Lead wires to the analyzer — which are attached in a manner similar to that used for ECG electrodes — are given a current of 4 mA in 15 to 20 seconds. This process (iontophoresis) is continued at 15- to 20-second intervals for 5 minutes. After iontophoresis, remove both electrodes. Discard the pads, clean the patient's skin with distilled water, and then dry it.

■ Using forceps, place a dry gauze pad or filter paper (previously weighed on a gram scale) on the area where the pilocarpine was used. Cover the pad or filter paper with a slightly larger piece of plastic, and seal the edges of the plastic with waterproof adhesive tape. Leave the gauze pad or filter paper in place for about 45 minutes. (The appearance of droplets on the plastic usually indicates induction of an adequate amount of sweat.)

■ Remove the pad or filter paper with the forceps, place it immediately in the weighing bottle, and insert the stopper in the bottle. The difference between the first and second weights indicates the weight of the sweat specimen collected.

Precautions

CLINICAL ALERT Always perform iontophoresis on the right arm (or right thigh) rather than on the left. Never perform iontophoresis on the chest, especially in a child, because the current can induce cardiac arrest.

■ To prevent electric shock, use battery-powered equipment, if possible.

■ Make sure that at least 100 mg of sweat is collected in 45 minutes.

CLINICAL ALERT Stop the test immediately if the patient complains of a burning sensation, which usually indicates that the positive electrode is exposed or positioned improperly. Adjust the electrode and then continue the test.

■ Carefully seal the gauze pad or filter paper in the weighing bottle and send the bottle to the laboratory at once.

Reference values

Normal sodium values in sweat are 0 to 30 mEq/L. Normal chloride values are 10 to 35 mEq/L.

Implications of results

Abnormal sodium values are 50 to 130 mEq/L. Abnormal chloride values are 50 to 110 mEq/L. Sodium and chloride concentrations of 50 to 60 mEq/L strongly suggest cystic fibrosis. Concentrations greater than 60 mEq/L with typical clinical features confirm the diagnosis. Only a few conditions other than cystic fibrosis cause elevated sweat electrolyte levels: untreated adrenal insufficiency, type I glycogen storage disease, vasopressin-resistant diabetes insipidus, meconium ileus, and renal failure. However, cystic fibrosis is the only condition that raises sweat electrolyte levels above 80 mEq/L.

In adult females, sweat electrolyte levels fluctuate cyclically: Chloride concentrations usually peak 5 to 10 days before onset of menses, and most women retain fluid before menses. Males also show fluctuations (up to 70 mEq/L).

Posttest care

- Wash the tested area with soap and water, and dry it thoroughly.
- If the area looks red, reassure the patient that this is normal and that the redness will disappear within a few hours.
- Tell the patient that he may resume his usual activities.

Interfering factors

- Dehydration and edema, especially in the area of collection, may interfere with test results.
- Failure to obtain an adequate amount of sweat (common in neonates) prevents proper testing.
- Presence of pure salt depletion (common during hot weather) may cause false-normal test results.
- Failure to clean the skin thoroughly or to use sterile gauze pads may cause false elevations.
- Failure to seal the gauze pad or filter paper carefully may falsely elevate electrolyte levels because of evaporation.

Synovial fluid analysis

Synovial fluid is normally a viscid, colorless to pale yellow liquid found in small amounts in the diarthrodial (synovial) joints, bursae, and tendon sheaths. It's thought to be produced by the dialysis of plasma across the synovial membrane and by the secretion of hyaluronic acid, a mucopolysaccharide. Synovial fluid lubricates the joint space, nourishes the articular cartilage, and protects the cartilage from mechanical damage while stabilizing the joint.

In synovial fluid aspiration (arthrocentesis), a sterile needle is inserted into a joint space — most commonly the knee — under strict sterile conditions to obtain a fluid specimen for analysis. This procedure is indicated in patients with undiagnosed articular disease and symptomatic joint effusion (excessive accumulation of synovial fluid).

Although rare, complications associated with synovial fluid aspiration include joint infection and hemorrhage and consequent hemarthrosis (accumulation of blood in the joint).

Routine examination of synovial fluid consists of gross analysis for color, clarity, quantity, viscosity, pH, and the presence of a mucin clot as well as microscopic analysis for white blood cell (WBC) count and differential. Special examinations include microbiological analysis for formed elements (including crystals) and

SYNOVIAL FLUID FINDINGS IN VARIOUS DISORDERS

Disease	Color	Clarity	Viscosity	Mucin clot
Group I Noninflammatory				
Traumatic arthritis	Straw to bloody to yellow	Transparent to cloudy	Variable	Good to fair
Osteoarthritis	Yellow	Transparent	Variable	Good to fair
Group II Inflammatory				
Systemic lupus erythematosus	Straw	Clear to slightly cloudy	Variable	Good to fair
Rheumatic fever	Yellow	Slightly cloudy	Variable	Good to fair
Pseudogout	Yellow	Slightly cloudy (if acute)	Low (if acute)	Fair to poor
Gout	Yellow to milky	Cloudy	Low	Fair to poor
Rheumatoid arthritis	Yellow to green	Cloudy	Low	Fair to poor
Group III Septic				
Tuberculous arthritis	Yellow	Cloudy	Low	Poor
Septic arthritis	Gray or bloody	Turbid, purulent	Low	Poor

bacteria, serologic analysis, and chemical analysis for such components as glucose, protein, and enzymes.

Purpose

- To aid differential diagnosis of arthritis, particularly septic or crystal-induced arthritis (See *Synovial fluid findings in various disorders.*)
- To identify the cause or nature of joint effusion
- To relieve the pain and distention resulting from joint effusion
- To administer local drug therapy (usually corticosteroids).

WBC count; % neutrophils	Cartilage debris	Crystals	Characteristic cells	Bacteria
1,000; 25%	None	None	None	None
700; 15%	Usually present	None	None	None
2,000; 30%	None	None	Lupus erythema-tosus (LE) cells	None
14,000; 50%	None	None	Possibly LE cells	None
15,000; 70%	Usually present	Calcium pyro-phosphate	None	None
20,000; 70%	None	Urate	None	None
20,000; 70%	None	Occasionally, cholesterol	Rheumatoid arthritis cells usually present	None
20,000; 60%	None	None	None	Usually present
90,000; 90%	None	None	None	Usually present

Patient preparation

Describe the procedure to the patient, and answer any questions he may have. Explain that this test helps determine the cause of joint inflammation and swelling and helps relieve the associated pain. If glucose testing of synovial fluid is ordered, instruct him to fast for 6 to 12 hours before the test; otherwise, he needn't restrict food or fluids before the test. Tell him who will perform the test and where. Warn him that, although he'll receive a local anesthetic, he may still feel transient pain when the needle penetrates the joint capsule. (Sometimes a sedative is ordered for a young child.)

Make sure the patient or a responsible family member has signed a consent form. Check the patient's history

for hypersensitivity to iodine compounds (such as povidone-iodine), procaine, lidocaine, and other local anesthetics. Administer a sedative, as ordered.

Equipment

Surgical detergent ■ skin antiseptic (usually tincture of
povidone-iodine) ■ alcohol sponges ■ local anesthetic
(procaine or lidocaine, 1% or 2%) ■ sterile, disposable
1½" 25G needle ■ sterile, disposable 1½" to 2" 20G needle ■ sterile 5-ml syringe for injecting anesthetic ■ sterile 20-ml syringe for aspiration ■ 3-ml syringe for administering sedative ■ sterile 2" x 2" gauze pads ■ sterile
dressings ■ sterile drapes ■ elastic bandage ■ tubes for
culture, cytologic, clot, and glucose analysis ■ anticoagulants (heparin, EDTA, and potassium oxalate) ■ venipuncture equipment, if ordered.

For corticosteroid administration: ■ corticosteroid
suspension such as hydrocortisone ■ 2-ml and 5-ml
syringes (or one 10-ml syringe if procaine and steroid are
to be injected simultaneously).

Procedure

■ Position the patient as ordered, and explain that he'll
need to maintain this position throughout the procedure. Clean the skin over the puncture site with surgical
detergent and alcohol. Paint the site with tincture of
povidone-iodine, and allow it to air-dry for 2 minutes.
After the local anesthetic is administered, the aspirating
needle is quickly inserted through the skin, subcutaneous tissue, and synovial membrane into the joint
space. As much fluid as possible is aspirated into the syringe, preferably at least 15 ml. The joint (except for the
area around the puncture site) may be wrapped with an
elastic bandage to compress the free fluid into this portion of the sac, ensuring maximal collection of fluid.
■ If a corticosteroid is being injected, prepare the dose as
ordered. For instillation, the syringe is detached, leaving
the needle in the joint, and the syringe containing the
steroid is attached to the needle. After the steroid is injected and the needle withdrawn, wipe the puncture site
with alcohol. Apply pressure to the puncture site for
about 2 minutes to prevent bleeding; then apply a sterile
dressing.
■ If synovial fluid glucose is being measured, perform
venipuncture to obtain a specimen for blood glucose
analysis.
■ Apply ice or cold packs to the affected joint for 24 to
36 hours after aspiration to decrease pain and swelling.
Use pillows for support. If a large quantity of fluid was
aspirated, apply an elastic bandage to prevent fluid reaccumulation.

■ If the patient's condition permits, tell him that he may resume normal activities immediately after the procedure. However, warn him to avoid excessive use of the joint for a few days after the test, even if pain and swelling have subsided. Excessive use may cause transient pain, swelling, and stiffness.

■ Watch for increased pain and fever, which may indicate joint infection.

■ Use standard precautions in handling the dressings and linens of patients with drainage from the joint space, especially if septic arthritis is confirmed or suspected.

■ Advise the patient that he may resume his usual diet.

Precautions

■ Wear gloves when handling all specimens.

■ Don't perform this test in areas of skin or wound infections.

■ Use strict sterile technique throughout aspiration to prevent contamination of the joint space or the synovial fluid specimen.

■ Add anticoagulants to the specimen, according to the laboratory tests requested. Gently invert the tube several times to mix the specimen and anticoagulant adequately. For cultures, obtain 2 to 5 ml of synovial fluid and, if possible, inoculate the medium immediately. Otherwise, add 1 or 2 drops of heparin to the specimen. For cytologic analysis, add 5 mg of EDTA or 1 or 2 drops of heparin to 2 to 5 ml of synovial fluid. For glucose analysis, add potassium oxalate, as specified by the laboratory, to 3 to 5 ml of fluid. For crystal examination, add heparin if specified by the laboratory. For other studies, such as general appearance and clot evaluation, obtain 2 to 5 ml of synovial fluid, but don't add an anticoagulant.

■ Send the properly labeled specimens to the laboratory immediately — gonococci are particularly labile. If a WBC count is being performed, clearly label the specimen "Synovial Fluid" and "Caution — Don't use acid diluents."

Normal findings

See *Normal findings in synovial fluid*, page 564.

Implications of results

Examination of synovial fluid may reveal various joint diseases, including noninflammatory disease (traumatic arthritis and osteoarthritis), inflammatory disease (systemic lupus erythematosus, rheumatic fever, gout, pseudogout, and rheumatoid arthritis), and septic disease (tuberculous and septic arthritis). (See *Synovial fluid findings in various disorders*, pages 560 and 561.)

NORMAL FINDINGS IN SYNOVIAL FLUID	
Feature	**Results**
Gross	
Color	Colorless to pale yellow
Clarity	Clear
Quantity (in knee)	0.3 to 3.5 ml
Viscosity	5.7 to 1,160
pH	7.2 to 7.4
Mucin clot	Good
Microscopic	
White blood cell (WBC) count	0 to 200/μl
WBC differential:	
■ Lymphocytes	■ 0 to 78/μl
■ Monocytes	■ 0 to 71/μl
■ Plasma cells	■ 0 to 26/μl
■ Polymorphonuclear leukocytes	■ 0 to 25/μl
■ Other phagocytes	■ 0 to 21/μl
■ Synovial lining cells	■ 0 to 12/μl
Microbiological	
Formed elements	Absence of crystals and cartilage debris
Bacteria	None
Serologic	
Complement:	3.7 to 33.7 U/ml
■ 10 mg protein/dl	7.7 to 37.7 U/ml
■ 20 mg protein/dl	None
Rheumatoid arthritis cells	None
Lupus erythematosus cells	
Chemical	
Total protein	10.7 to 21.3 mg/dl
Fibrinogen	None
Glucose	70 to 100 mg/dl
Uric acid	2 to 8 mg/dl (men), 2 to 6 mg/dl (women)
Hyaluronate	0.3 to 0.4 g/dl
$Paco_2$	40 to 60 mm Hg
Pao_2	40 to 80 mm Hg

Interfering factors

■ Patient failure to adhere to dietary restrictions can affect glucose levels.

■ Acid diluents added to the specimen for WBC count alter the cell count.

■ Failure to mix the specimen and the anticoagulant adequately or to send the specimen to the laboratory immediately may cause inaccurate test results.

■ Contamination of the specimen can invalidate test results.

Synovial membrane biopsy

Biopsy of the synovial membrane is the needle excision of a tissue specimen for histologic examination of the thin epithelial layer lining the diarthrodial joint capsules. In a large joint, such as the knee, preliminary arthroscopy can aid selection of the biopsy site. Synovial membrane biopsy is performed when analysis of synovial fluid—a viscous, lubricating fluid contained within the synovial membrane—proves nondiagnostic or when the fluid itself is absent.

Purpose

■ To diagnose gout, pseudogout, bacterial infections and lesions, and granulomatous infections
■ To aid diagnosis of rheumatoid arthritis, systemic lupus erythematosus (SLE), or Reiter's syndrome
■ To monitor joint pathology.

Patient preparation

Describe the procedure to the patient, and ask if he has any questions. Explain that this test helps to diagnose certain joint disorders. Inform him that he needn't restrict food or fluids. Tell him who will perform the procedure and where, that the procedure takes about 30 minutes, and that test results are usually available in 1 or 2 days. Advise him that he'll receive a local anesthetic to minimize discomfort but will experience transient pain when the needle enters the joint. Tell him that complications are rare but may include infection and bleeding into the joint.

Make sure the patient has signed a consent form. Check the patient history for hypersensitivity to the local anesthetic.

Inform the patient which site—knee (most common), elbow, wrist, ankle, or shoulder—has been chosen for the biopsy (usually, the most symptomatic joint is selected). Administer a sedative, if ordered, to help him relax.

Procedure

■ Place the patient in the proper position, clean the biopsy site, and drape the area. After the local anesthetic is injected into the joint space, the trocar is forcefully thrust into the joint space, away from the site of anesthetic infiltration, to minimize the possibility of artifacts. The biopsy needle is inserted through the trocar. The hooked notch side of the biopsy needle is positioned against the synovium, and suction is applied with a 50-ml luer-lock syringe.
■ While the trocar is held stationary, the biopsy needle is twisted to cut off a tissue segment. Then the needle is withdrawn, and the specimen is placed in a properly labeled sterile container or a specimen bottle containing heparin or absolute ethyl alcohol. By changing the angle

of the biopsy needle, several specimens can be obtained without reinserting the trocar. The trocar is then removed, the biopsy site cleaned, and a pressure bandage is applied.

Precautions

Send the container with absolute ethyl alcohol to the histology laboratory immediately. Send the sterile container to the microbiology laboratory.

Normal findings

The synovial membrane contains cells that are identical to those found in other connective tissue. The membrane surface is relatively smooth, except for villi, folds, and fat pads that project into the joint cavity. The membrane tissue produces synovial fluid and contains a capillary network, lymphatic vessels, and a few nerve fibers. Pathology of the synovial membrane also affects the cellular composition of the synovial fluid.

Implications of results

Histologic examination of synovial tissue can diagnose coccidioidomycosis, gout, pseudogout, hemochromatosis, tuberculosis, sarcoidosis, amyloidosis, pigmented villonodular synovitis, or synovial tumors. Such examination can also aid diagnosis of rheumatoid arthritis, SLE, and Reiter's syndrome.

Posttest care

■ Wash the tested area with soap and water, and dry it thoroughly.
■ If the area looks red, reassure the patient that this is normal and that the redness will disappear within a few hours.
■ Tell the patient that he may resume his usual activities.

Interfering factors

Failure to obtain several biopsy specimens, to obtain the specimens away from the infiltration site of the anesthetic, to store the specimens in the appropriate solution, or to send them to the laboratory immediately may alter test results.

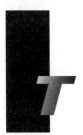

T- and B-lymphocyte assays

Lymphocytes—key cells in the immune system—recognize antigens through special receptors on their surface. The two primary kinds of lymphocytes, T and B cells, originate in the bone marrow. T cells mature under the influence of the thymus gland; B cells, without thymic influence.

Cell separation is used to isolate lymphocytes from other cellular blood elements. In this method, a whole blood sample is layered on Ficoll-Hypaque in a narrow tube, which is then centrifuged. Granulocytes and red blood cells (RBCs) form a sediment at the bottom of the tube, and lymphocytes, monocytes, and platelets form a distinct band at the Ficoll-Hypaque–plasma interface.

This procedure recovers approximately 80% of the lymphocytes but doesn't differentiate between T and B cells. The percentage of T and B cells is determined by attaching a label or marker and using different identification techniques. The E-rosette test identifies T cells, which tend to form unstable clusterlike shapes (or rosettes) after exposure to sheep RBCs at 39.2° F (4° C). Direct immunofluorescence detects B cells, which have monoclonal surface immunoglobulins; unlike T cells, B cells have receptors for complement and Fc portions of immunoglobulin.

Null cells, the remainder of the lymphocytes, have Fc receptors but no other detectable surface markers and have no diagnostic significance. Null cells are usually determined by subtracting the sum of T and B cells from total lymphocytes.

Purpose

- To aid diagnosis of primary and secondary immunodeficiency diseases
- To distinguish benign from malignant lymphocytic proliferative diseases
- To monitor response to therapy.

Patient preparation

Explain to the patient that this test measures certain white blood cells. Tell him that this test requires a blood sample, who will perform the venipuncture and when, and that he may experience transient discomfort from the needle puncture and the pressure of the tourniquet.

Procedure

Perform a venipuncture and collect the sample in a 7-ml heparinized tube.

Precautions

- Fill the collection tube completely and invert it gently several times to mix the sample and anticoagulant adequately.
- Send the sample to the laboratory immediately to make sure lymphocytes remain viable. Transport the sample at room temperature.
- If antilymphocyte antibodies are suspected, as in autoimmune disease, notify the laboratory.

Reference values

T-cell and B-cell values may differ from one laboratory to another, depending on test technique. Generally, T cells constitute 68% to 75% of total lymphocytes; B cells, 10% to 20%; and null cells, 5% to 20%. The normal total lymphocyte count is 1,500 to 3,000/µl; the T-cell count, 1,400 to 2,700/µl; and the B-cell count, 270 to 640/µl. All lymphocyte counts are higher in children than in adults.

Implications of results

An abnormal T-cell or B-cell count suggests but doesn't confirm specific diseases. The B-cell count is elevated in chronic lymphocytic leukemia (thought to be a B-cell malignancy), multiple myeloma, Waldenström's macroglobulinemia, and DiGeorge's syndrome (a congenital T-cell deficiency). The B-cell count falls in acute lymphocytic leukemia and in certain congenital or acquired immunoglobulin deficiency diseases. In other immunoglobulin deficiency diseases, especially if only one immunoglobulin class is deficient, the B-cell count remains normal.

The T-cell count rises occasionally in infectious mononucleosis and more frequently in multiple myeloma and acute lymphocytic leukemia. The T-cell count falls in congenital T-cell deficiency diseases, such as DiGeorge's, Nezelof, and Wiskott-Aldrich syndromes, and in certain B-cell proliferative disorders, such as chronic lymphocytic leukemia, Waldenström's macroglobulinemia, and acquired immunodeficiency syndrome.

Normal T-cell and B-cell counts don't necessarily reflect a competent immune system. In autoimmune diseases, such as systemic lupus erythematosus and rheumatoid arthritis, T and B cells may be present in normal numbers but may not be functionally competent.

Posttest care

■ Because many patients with T- and B-cell changes have a compromised immune system, keep the venipuncture site clean and dry.
■ If a hematoma develops at the venipuncture site, apply warm soaks.

Interfering factors

■ Failure to use the proper collection tube, to mix the sample and anticoagulant adequately, or to send the sample to the laboratory immediately can interfere with accurate testing.
■ Transporting the sample at temperature extremes (too warm or too cold) can alter results.
■ T- and B-cell counts can change rapidly with changes in health status, from the effects of stress, or after surgery, chemotherapy, steroid or immunosuppressive therapy, and radiography.
■ The presence of immunoglobulins, such as autologous antilymphocyte antibodies that sometimes occur in autoimmune disease, can alter test results.

T_3 uptake test

The triiodothyronine (T_3) uptake test indirectly measures free thyroxine (FT_4) levels by demonstrating the availability of serum thyroxine-binding globulin (TBG). The results of T_3 uptake are frequently combined with a T_4 radioimmunoassay or T_4 (D) (competitive protein-binding) test to determine the FT_4 index, a mathematical calculation that is thought to reflect FT_4 by correcting for TBG abnormalities.

The T_3 uptake test has become less popular recently because rapid tests for T_3, T_4, and thyroid-stimulating hormone are readily available.

Purpose

■ To aid diagnosis of hypothyroidism and hyperthyroidism when TBG is normal
■ To aid diagnosis of primary disorders of TBG.

Patient preparation

Explain to the patient that this test helps evaluate thyroid function. Tell him that a blood sample is needed and that the procedure, which takes a few minutes, may cause some discomfort. Inform him who will perform the venipuncture and when. Tell him the laboratory requires several days to complete the analysis. Withhold medications, such as estrogens, androgens, phenytoin, salicylates, and thyroid preparations, that may interfere with test results. If they must be continued, note this on the laboratory request.

Procedure

Perform a venipuncture and collect the sample in a 7-ml clot-activator tube.

Precautions

Handle the sample gently to prevent hemolysis.

Reference values

Normal T_3 uptake values are 25% to 35%.

Implications of results

A high T_3 uptake percentage in the presence of elevated T_4 levels indicates hyperthyroidism (implying few free TBG binding sites and high FT_4 levels). A low uptake percentage, together with low T_4 levels, indicates hypothyroidism (implying more free TBG binding sites and low FT_4 levels). Thus, in primary thyroid disease, T_4 and T_3 uptake vary in the same direction; availability of binding sites varies inversely.

Discordant variance in T_4 and T_3 uptake suggests a TBG abnormality. For example, a high T_3 uptake percentage and a low or normal FT_4 level suggest low free TBG. Low TBG may result from protein loss (as in nephritic syndrome), decreased production (due to androgen excess or genetic or idiopathic causes), or competition for T4 binding sites by certain drugs (salicylates, phenylbutazone, and phenytoin). Conversely, a low T_3 uptake percentage and a high or normal FT_4 level suggest high TBG. High TBG may reflect exogenous or endogenous estrogen (pregnancy) or idiopathic causes.

Posttest care

■ If a hematoma develops at the venipuncture site, apply warm soaks.
■ As ordered, resume administration of medications discontinued before the test.

Interfering factors

■ Radioisotope scans performed before sample collection may alter results.
■ Anabolic steroids, heparin, phenytoin, salicylates (high dose), thyroid preparations, and warfarin may produce increases in TBG and thyroxine-binding protein electrophoresis, altering results.

■ Antithyroid agents, clofibrate, estrogen, oral contraceptives, and thiazide diuretics may decrease uptake, altering results.

Terminal deoxynucleotidyl transferase test

Using indirect immunofluorescence, this test measures levels of terminal deoxynucleotidyl transferase (TdT), an intranuclear enzyme found in certain primitive lymphocytes in the normal thymus and bone marrow. Because TdT acts as a biochemical marker for these lymphocytes, it can help classify the origin of a particular tissue. Thus, the TdT test is useful in differentiating acute lymphocytic leukemia (ALL) from acute nonlymphocytic leukemia and lymphoblastic from malignant lymphoma; ALL and lymphoblastic lymphoma are marked by primitive cells that can't be identified by histology alone. Measurement of TdT in patients with these diseases may also help determine prognosis and early diagnosis of a relapse.

Purpose

■ To help differentiate acute ALL from acute nonlymphocytic leukemia
■ To help differentiate lymphoblastic lymphomas from malignant lymphomas
■ To monitor response to therapy.

Patient preparation

Explain to the patient that this test detects an enzyme that can help classify tissue origin and that it may require either a blood or bone marrow sample. If the patient is scheduled for a blood test, tell him to fast for 12 to 14 hours before the test. Tell him the test requires a blood sample, who will perform the venipuncture and when, and that he may experience transient discomfort from the needle puncture and the pressure of the tourniquet.

If the patient is scheduled for a bone marrow aspiration, describe the procedure to him and answer any questions. Inform him that he needn't restrict food or fluids before the test. Tell him who will perform the biopsy and where and that it usually takes only 5 to 10 minutes to perform. Make sure the patient or a responsible family member has signed a consent form.

Check the patient's history for hypersensitivity to the local anesthetic. After checking with the doctor, tell the patient which bone will be the biopsy site. Inform him that he'll receive a local anesthetic but will feel pressure on insertion of the biopsy needle and a brief, pulling pain when the marrow is withdrawn. As ordered, administer a mild sedative 1 hour before the test.

Procedure

■ If a blood test is scheduled, perform a venipuncture and collect samples in one 10-ml heparinized blood tube and one EDTA tube. Send the samples to the laboratory immediately.

■ If you're assisting with a bone marrow aspiration, inject 1 ml of bone marrow into a 7-ml heparinized tube and dilute it with 5 ml of sterile saline solution or submit four air-dried marrow smears. Send the sample to the laboratory immediately.

■ Because patients with leukemia may bleed excessively, apply pressure to the venipuncture site until bleeding stops completely.

Precautions

■ Contact the laboratory before performing the venipuncture to verify that they're able to process the sample and to find out how much blood to draw.

■ Because patients with leukemia are more susceptible to infection, clean the skin thoroughly before performing the venipuncture.

■ Send the samples to the laboratory immediately.

Reference values

Normally, TdT is present in less than 2% of marrow cells and is undetectable in peripheral blood.

Implications of results

Positive cells are present in more than 90% of patients with ALL, in one-third of patients with chronic myelogenous leukemia in blast crisis, and in 5% of patients with nonlymphocytic leukemias. TdT-positive cells are absent in patients with ALL who are in remission.

Posttest care

■ If a hematoma develops at the venipuncture site, apply warm soaks.

■ Check the bone marrow aspiration site for bleeding and inflammation, and observe the patient for signs of hemorrhage and infection.

Interfering factors

■ Failure to obtain a representative sample may affect the accuracy of bone marrow aspiration results.

■ Performing a bone marrow aspiration on a child may produce false-positive results because TdT is normally present in bone marrow during proliferation of prelymphocytes.

■ Bone marrow regeneration, idiopathic thrombocy-topenic purpura, and neuroblastoma may produce false-positive bone marrow aspiration results because these conditions cause TdT-positive bone marrow.

Testosterone test

The principal androgen secreted by the interstitial cells of the testes (Leydig's cells), testosterone induces puberty in the male and maintains male secondary sex characteristics. Prepubertal levels of testosterone are low. Increased testosterone secretion during puberty stimulates growth of the seminiferous tubules and the production of sperm; it also contributes to the enlargement of external genitalia, accessory sex organs (such as the prostate gland), and voluntary muscles as well as to the growth of facial, pubic, and axillary hair.

Testosterone production begins to increase at the onset of puberty, under the influence of luteinizing hormone (LH) from the anterior pituitary, and continues to rise during adulthood. Testosterone inhibits gonadotropin secretion by a negative feedback mechanism similar to that of ovarian hormones in females. Production begins to taper off at about age 40, eventually dropping to approximately one-fifth the peak level by age 80. In females, the adrenal glands and the ovaries secrete small amounts of testosterone.

This competitive protein-binding test measures plasma or serum testosterone levels. When combined with plasma gonadotropin (follicle-stimulating hormone and LH) levels, it reliably aids evaluation of gonadal dysfunction in males and females.

Purpose

■ To evaluate male infertility or other sexual dysfunction
■ To facilitate differential diagnosis of male sexual precocity (before age 10). True precocious puberty must be distinguished from pseudoprecocious puberty.
■ To aid differential diagnosis of hypogonadism. Primary hypogonadism must be distinguished from secondary hypogonadism.
■ To evaluate hirsutism and virilization in females.

Patient preparation

Explain to the patient that this test helps determine if male sex hormone production is adequate. Inform him that he needn't restrict food or fluids. Tell him this test requires a blood sample, who will perform the venipuncture and when, and that he may experience some discomfort from the needle puncture.

Procedure

■ Perform a venipuncture and collect the sample in a 7-ml clot-activator tube. Use a heparinized tube if plasma is to be collected.
■ Indicate the patient's age, sex, and history of hormone therapy on the laboratory request.

Precautions

Handle the sample gently to prevent hemolysis, and send it to the laboratory. The sample is stable and requires no refrigeration or preservative for up to 1 week. Frozen samples are stable for at least 6 months.

Reference values

Normal levels of testosterone are as follows (interlaboratory values vary slightly):
■ Males: 300 to 1,200 ng/dl
■ Females: 30 to 95 ng/dl
■ Prepubertal children: in boys, less than 100 ng/dl; in girls, less than 40 ng/dl.

Implications of results

Elevated testosterone levels in prepubertal males may indicate true sexual precocity caused by excessive gonadotropin secretion or pseudoprecocious puberty caused by male hormone production by a testicular tumor. They also suggest congenital adrenal hyperplasia, which causes precocious puberty in males (from ages 2 to 3) and pseudohermaphroditism or milder virilization of females. A benign or malignant adrenal tumor, hyperthyroidism, or incipient puberty can also increase testosterone levels. High testosterone levels in females with ovarian tumors or polycystic ovarian syndrome cause hirsutism.

Depressed testosterone levels suggest primary hypogonadism (as in Klinefelter's syndrome) or secondary hypogonadism (hypogonadotropic eunuchoidism) from hypothalamic-pituitary dysfunction. Depressed testosterone levels can also follow orchiectomy, testicular or prostatic cancer, delayed male puberty, estrogen therapy, or cirrhosis.

Posttest care

If a hematoma develops at the venipuncture site, apply warm soaks.

Interfering factors

Exogenous sources of estrogens or androgens, thyroid and growth hormones, and other pituitary hormones may interfere with test results. Estrogens decrease free testosterone levels by increasing sex hormone-binding

SEX HORMONE-BINDING GLOBULIN

This immunoassay measures levels of sex hormone–binding globulin (SHBG), also known as testosterone-binding globulin. It helps evaluate conditions related to sex hormone levels and requires no special procedure. Note the patient's sex on the laboratory request.

Normal SHBG values are 8 to 49 mmol/L for males and 20 to 106 mmol/L for females. Androgenizing or adrenal disorders can cause low SHBG values. Levels are high in women with hyperthyroidism and in those receiving estrogen.

globulin, which binds testosterone; androgens can elevate these levels. (See *Sex hormone-binding globulin.*)

Hemolysis may affect test results.

Throat culture

A throat culture is used primarily to isolate and identify group A beta-hemolytic streptococci *(Streptococcus pyogenes)*, thus allowing early treatment of pharyngitis and prevention of sequelae, such as rheumatic heart disease and glomerulonephritis. It's also used to screen for carriers of *Neisseria meningitidis*. In rare instances, a throat culture may be used to identify *Corynebacterium diphtheriae, Bordetella pertussis, Staphylococcus aureus, Streptococcus pneumoniae*, or *Haemophilus influenzae*. A throat culture may also be used to identify *Candida albicans*.

A throat culture requires swabbing the throat, streaking a culture plate, and allowing the organisms to grow for isolation and identification of pathogens. A Gram-stained smear may provide preliminary identification, which may guide clinical management and determine the need for further tests. Culture results must be interpreted in light of clinical status, recent antimicrobial therapy, and amount of normal flora.

Purpose

■ To isolate and identify pathogens, particularly group A beta-hemolytic streptococci

■ To screen asymptomatic carriers of pathogens, especially *N. meningitidis.*

Patient preparation

Explain to the patient that this test helps identify the microorganisms that could be causing his symptoms or a carrier state. Inform him that he needn't restrict food or fluids before the test. Tell him who will perform the procedure and when. Reassure him that the test takes less than 30 seconds and that test results should be available in 2 or 3 days.

Describe the procedure, and warn him that he may gag during the swabbing. Check the patient history for recent antimicrobial therapy. Determine immunization history if it's pertinent to the preliminary diagnosis. Procure the throat specimen before beginning any antimicrobial therapy.

Equipment

Gloves ■ sterile swab and culture tube with transport medium, or commercial collection and transport system.

Procedure

■ Tell the patient to tilt his head back and close his eyes. With the throat well illuminated, check for inflamed areas, using a tongue blade.

■ Swab the tonsillar areas from side to side; include any inflamed or purulent sites. Don't touch the tongue, cheeks, or teeth with the swab.

■ Immediately place the swab in the culture tube. If a commercial sterile collection and transport system is used, crush the ampule and force the swab into the medium to keep it moist.

■ Note recent antimicrobial therapy on the laboratory request. Label the specimen with the patient's name, doctor's name, date and time of collection, and origin of the specimen. Also indicate the suspected organism, especially *Corynebacterium diphtheriae* (requires two swabs and a special growth medium), and *N. meningitidis* (requires enriched selective media).

■ Rapid nonculture antigen testing methods can detect group A streptococcal antigen in as little as 5 minutes. Cultures should be performed on all negative specimens.

Precautions

■ Use gloves when performing the procedure and handling specimens.

■ Send the specimen to the laboratory immediately. Unless a commercial sterile collection and transport system is used, keep the container upright during transport. Specimens shouldn't be refrigerated in transit.

Normal findings

Throat flora normally include nonhemolytic and alpha-hemolytic streptococci, *Neisseria* species, staphylococci, diphtheroids, some *Haemophilus* species, pneumococci, yeasts, enteric gram-negative organisms, spirochetes, *Veillonella* species, and *Micrococcus* species.

Implications of results

Possible pathogens cultured include group A beta-hemolytic streptococci (*S. pyogenes*), which can cause scarlet fever or pharyngitis; *Candida albicans*, which can cause thrush; *Corynebacterium diphtheriae*, which can cause diphtheria; and *B. pertussis*, which can cause whooping cough. Other cultured bacteria include *Legionella* species and *Mycoplasma pneumoniae*. Fungi include *Histoplasma capsulatum*, *Coccidioides immitis*, and *Blastomyces dermatitidis*. Viruses include adenovirus, enterovirus, herpesvirus, rhinovirus, influenza virus, and parainfluenza virus. The laboratory report should indicate the prevalent organisms and the quantity of pathogens cultured.

Interfering factors

■ Failure to report recent or current antimicrobial therapy on the laboratory request may cause false-negative results.

■ Failure to use the proper transport media may affect the accuracy of results.

■ A delay of more than 15 minutes in sending the specimen to the laboratory may yield inaccurate results unless the specimen is in transport medium.

Thrombin time test, plasma

The plasma thrombin time test measures how quickly a clot forms when a standard amount of bovine thrombin is added to a platelet-poor plasma sample from the patient and to a normal plasma control sample. After thrombin is added, the clotting time for each sample is compared and recorded. Because thrombin rapidly converts fibrinogen to a fibrin clot, this test (also known as the thrombin clotting time test) allows a quick but imprecise estimation of plasma fibrinogen levels, which are a function of clotting time. (See *Antithrombin III test*, page 578, for information about another test that helps determine the cause of coagulation disorders.)

Purpose

■ To detect a fibrinogen deficiency or defect
■ To aid diagnosis of disseminated intravascular coagulation (DIC) and hepatic disease
■ To monitor the effectiveness of treatment with heparin or thrombolytic agents.

Patient preparation

Explain to the patient that this test helps determine if his blood clots normally. Inform him that he needn't restrict food or fluids. Tell him that the test requires a

ANTITHROMBIN III TEST

Antithrombin III (AT III) is a protein that inactivates thrombin and inhibits coagulation. AT III levels suggest the cause of abnormal coagulation, especially hypercoagulation. Normally, a balance exists between AT III and thrombin; an AT III deficiency increases coagulation.

AT III may be evaluated by a functional clotting assay or by synthetic substrates. Exogenous heparin is added to a fresh, citrated blood sample to accelerate AT III activity. Then excess thrombin (factor Xa) is added to the plasma. The amount of factor Xa not activated by AT III is quantitated by clotting time or spectrophotometrically and is compared to a normal control. Reference values may vary for each laboratory but they normally lie between 80% and 120% of normal activity.

Low AT III levels suggest disseminated intravascular coagulation or thromboembolic, hypercoagulation, or hepatic disorders. Slightly decreased levels can result from use of oral contraceptives. Elevated levels can result from kidney transplantation and use of oral anticoagulants or anabolic steroids.

blood sample, who will perform the venipuncture and when, and that he may experience discomfort from the needle puncture and the pressure of the tourniquet.

If possible, withhold heparin therapy before the test, as ordered. If heparin must be continued, note this on the laboratory request.

Procedure

Perform a venipuncture and collect the sample in a 7-ml siliconized tube.

Precautions

- To prevent hemolysis, avoid excessive probing during venipuncture and rough handling of the sample.
- Completely fill the collection tube, and invert it gently several times to mix the sample and anticoagulant adequately. If the tube isn't filled to the correct volume, an excess of citrate appears in the sample.
- Send the sample to the laboratory immediately.

Reference values

Normal thrombin times range from 10 to 15 seconds and should be within 2 seconds of the control. Test results are usually reported with a normal control value.

Implications of results

A prolonged thrombin time may indicate heparin therapy, hepatic disease, DIC, hypofibrinogenemia, or dysfibrinogenemia. Patients with prolonged thrombin times may require quantitation of fibrinogen levels; in suspected DIC, the test for fibrin split products is also necessary.

Posttest care

■ Make sure that bleeding has stopped before removing pressure.

■ If a hematoma develops at the venipuncture site, apply warm soaks.

■ If the hematoma is large, monitor pulses distal to the phlebotomy site.

Interfering factors

■ The presence of inhibitory substances such as heparin, fibrinogen, or fibrin degradation products may prolong clotting time.

■ Hemolysis caused by excessive probing during venipuncture or rough handling of the sample may affect the accuracy of test results.

■ Failure to use the proper anticoagulant in the collection tube, to mix the sample and the anticoagulant adequately, or to send the sample to the laboratory immediately may affect the accuracy of test results.

Thyroid biopsy

Thyroid biopsy is the excision of a thyroid tissue specimen for histologic examination. This procedure is indicated for patients with thyroid enlargement or nodules (even if serum triiodothyronine [T_3] and thyroxine [T_4] levels are normal), breathing and swallowing difficulties, vocal cord paralysis, weight loss, hemoptysis, or a sensation of fullness in the neck. It's commonly performed when noninvasive tests, such as thyroid ultrasonography and scans, are abnormal or inconclusive.

A thyroid tissue specimen may be obtained with a hollow needle under local anesthesia or during open (surgical) biopsy under general anesthesia. Fine-needle aspiration with a cytologic smear examination can aid in diagnosis and replace an open biopsy. Open biopsy, performed in the operating room, is more complex and provides more direct information than needle biopsy. In open biopsy, the surgeon obtains a tissue specimen from the exposed thyroid and sends it to the histology laboratory for rapid analysis. This method also permits immediate excision of suspicious thyroid tissue.

Coagulation studies should always precede thyroid biopsy.

Purpose

■ To differentiate between benign and malignant thyroid disease

■ To help diagnose Hashimoto's disease, hyperthyroidism, and nontoxic nodular goiter.

Patient preparation

Describe the procedure to the patient and answer any questions he may have. Explain that this test permits microscopic examination of a thyroid tissue specimen. Inform the patient that he needn't restrict food or fluids (unless he'll receive a general anesthetic). Tell him who will perform the biopsy and where, that it takes 15 to 30 minutes, and that results should be available in a day. Make sure the patient has signed a consent form. Check for hypersensitivity to anesthetics or analgesics.

Tell the patient he'll receive a local anesthetic to minimize pain during the procedure but may experience some pressure when the tissue specimen is procured. Advise him that he may have a sore throat the day after the test. Administer a sedative to the patient 15 minutes before the biopsy, as ordered.

Procedure

■ For needle biopsy, place the patient in the supine position, with a pillow under his shoulder blades. (This position pushes the trachea and thyroid forward and allows the neck veins to fall backward.)
■ Prepare the skin over the biopsy site. As the examiner prepares to inject the local anesthetic, warn the patient not to swallow.
■ After the anesthetic is injected, the carotid artery is palpated, and the biopsy needle is inserted parallel to and about 1″ (2.5 cm) from the thyroid cartilage to prevent damage to the deep structures and the larynx. When the specimen is obtained, the needle is removed, and the specimen is immediately placed in formalin.

Precautions

■ Thyroid biopsy should be used cautiously in patients with coagulation defects, as reflected by abnormal prothrombin time (PT) or activated partial thromboplastin time (APTT).
■ Because cell breakdown in the tissue specimen begins immediately after excision, the specimen must be placed in formalin solution immediately.

Normal findings

Histologic examination of normal tissue shows fibrous networks dividing the gland into pseudolobules that consist of follicles and capillaries. Cuboidal epithelium lines the follicle walls and contains the protein thyroglobulin, which stores T_4 and T_3.

Implications of results

Malignant tumors appear as well-encapsulated, solitary nodules of uniform but abnormal structure. Papillary carcinoma is the most common type of thyroid cancer. Follicular carcinoma, a less common form, strongly resembles normal cells.

Benign conditions such as nontoxic nodular goiter show characteristic hypertrophy, hyperplasia, and hypervascularity. Distinctive histologic patterns characterize subacute granulomatous thyroiditis, Hashimoto's disease, and hyperthyroidism.

Because many malignant thyroid tumors are multicentric and small, a negative histologic report doesn't necessarily rule out cancer.

Posttest care

■ Apply pressure to the biopsy site to stop bleeding. If bleeding continues for more than a few minutes, press on the site for up to 15 minutes more. Apply an adhesive bandage. Bleeding may persist in a patient who has abnormal PT or APTT or a large, vascular thyroid and distended veins.

■ To make the patient more comfortable, place him in semi-Fowler's position. Tell him he may avoid undue strain on the biopsy site by putting both hands behind his neck when he sits up.

CLINICAL ALERT Watch for signs of bleeding, tenderness, or redness at the biopsy site. Observe for difficulty in breathing associated with edema or hematoma, with resultant tracheal collapse. Also check the back of the neck and the patient's pillow for bleeding every hour for 8 hours. Report bleeding immediately.

■ Keep the biopsy site clean and dry.

Interfering factors

Failure to obtain a representative tissue specimen or to place the specimen in formalin solution immediately may affect the accuracy of test results.

Thyroid-stimulating hormone test

Thyroid-stimulating hormone (TSH) is a glycoprotein secreted by the anterior pituitary after stimulation by thyrotropin-releasing hormone (TRH) from the hypothalamus. TSH stimulates an increase in the size, number, and secretory activity of thyroid cells; heightens "iodine pump activity," often raising the ratio of intracellular to extracellular iodine to as much as 350:1; and stimulates the release of triiodothyronine (T_3) and thyroxine (T_4). These hormones affect total body metabo-

---

TRH CHALLENGE TEST

This test, which evaluates thyroid function and is the first direct test of pituitary reserve, is a reliable tool for diagnosing thyrotoxicosis (Graves' disease). The challenge test requires an injection of thyrotropin-releasing hormone (TRH).

One commonly accepted procedure is the following: After a venipuncture is performed to obtain a baseline thyroid-stimulating hormone (TSH) reading, synthetic TRH (protirelin) is administered by I.V. bolus in a dose of 200 to 500 mcg. As many as five samples (5 ml each) are then drawn at 5-, 10-, 15-, 20-, and 60-minute intervals to assess thyroid response. To facilitate blood collection, an indwelling catheter can be used to obtain the required samples.

A sudden spike above the baseline TSH reading indicates a normally functioning pituitary but suggests hypothalamic dysfunction. If the TSH level fails to rise or remains undetectable, pituitary failure is likely. In thyrotoxicosis or thyroiditis, TSH levels fail to rise when challenged by TRH.

---

lism and are essential for normal growth and development.

This test (also known as the serum thyrotropin test) measures serum TSH levels by immunoassay. It can detect primary hypothyroidism and can determine whether it results from thyroid gland failure or from pituitary or hypothalamic dysfunction. Normal serum TSH levels rule out primary hypothyroidism. This test may not distinguish between low-normal and subnormal levels, especially in secondary hypothyroidism.

The TRH challenge test evaluates thyroid function and can be performed after a baseline TSH reading has been obtained. (See *TRH challenge test*.)

Purpose

■ To confirm or rule out primary hypothyroidism and distinguish it from secondary hypothyroidism
■ To monitor drug therapy in patients with primary hypothyroidism.

Patient preparation

Explain to the patient that this test helps assess thyroid gland function. Tell him that the test requires a blood sample, who will perform the venipuncture and when, and that he may feel discomfort from the needle puncture. Advise him that the laboratory requires up to 2 days to complete the analysis. As ordered, withhold steroids, thyroid hormones, aspirin, and other drugs that may influence test results. If these medications must be continued, note this on the laboratory request. Keep the patient relaxed and recumbent for 30 minutes before the test.

Procedure

Between 6 a.m. and 8 a.m., perform a venipuncture. Collect the sample in a 5-ml clot-activator tube.

Precautions

Handle the sample gently to prevent hemolysis.

Reference values

Normal values for adults and children range from undetectable to 15 μIU/ml.

Implications of results

TSH levels that exceed 20 μIU/ml suggest primary hypothyroidism or, possibly, an endemic goiter (associated with dietary iodine deficiency). TSH levels may be slightly elevated in euthyroid patients with thyroid cancer.

Low or undetectable TSH levels may be normal but may occasionally reflect secondary hypothyroidism (with inadequate secretion of TSH or TRH). Low TSH levels may also result from hyperthyroidism (Graves' disease) or thyroiditis; both are marked by hypersecretion of thyroid hormones, which suppresses TSH release. Provocative testing with TRH is necessary to confirm the diagnosis.

Posttest care

■ If a hematoma develops at the venipuncture site, apply warm soaks.
■ As ordered, resume administration of drugs discontinued before the test.

Interfering factors

■ Failure to observe restrictions of medications may cause spurious test results.
■ Hemolysis caused by rough handling of the sample may affect test results.

Thyroid-stimulating hormone test, neonatal

This immunoassay (also known as the neonatal thyrotropin test) confirms congenital hypothyroidism after an initial screening test has detected low thyroxine (T_4) levels. Normally, thyroid-stimulating hormone (TSH) levels surge after birth, triggering a rise in thyroid hormone levels that's essential for neurologic development. In primary congenital hypothyroidism, the thyroid gland doesn't respond to TSH stimulation; the result is low thyroid hormone and high TSH levels. Early detection and treatment of congenital hypothyroidism are critical to prevent mental retardation and cretinism.

Purpose

To confirm a diagnosis of congenital hypothyroidism.

Patient preparation

Explain to the infant's parents that this test helps confirm a diagnosis of congenital hypothyroidism. Emphasize the test's importance in detecting the disorder early so that prompt therapy can prevent irreversible brain damage.

Equipment

For a filter paper sample: ■ alcohol or povidone-iodine swabs ■ sterile lancet ■ specially marked filter paper ■ sterile 2″ x 2″ gauze pads ■ adhesive bandage ■ labels ■ gloves.

For a serum sample: ■ venipuncture equipment.

Procedure

■ For a filter paper sample: Assemble the necessary equipment, wash your hands thoroughly, and put on gloves. Wipe the infant's heel with an alcohol or povidone-iodine swab; then dry it thoroughly with a gauze pad. Perform a heelstick. Squeezing the infant's heel gently, fill the circles on the filter paper with blood. Make sure the blood saturates the paper. Gently apply pressure with a gauze pad to ensure hemostasis at the puncture site. Allow the filter paper to dry, label it appropriately, and send it to the laboratory.

■ For a serum sample: Perform a venipuncture and collect the sample in a 3-ml clot-activator tube. Label the sample and send it to the laboratory immediately.

Precautions

Handle the samples carefully.

Reference values

The normal TSH level is 25 to 30 µIU/ml at age 2 to 3 months and less than 25 µIU/ml thereafter.

Implications of results

Neonatal TSH must be interpreted in light of T_4 concentrations. High TSH and low T_4 reflects primary congenital hypothyroidism (thyroid gland dysfunction). TSH and T_4 may be low in patients with secondary congenital hypothyroidism (pituitary or hypothalamic dysfunction). Normal TSH and low T_4 suggest hypothyroidism caused by a congenital defect in thyroxine-binding globulin or transient congenital hypothyroidism caused by prematurity or prenatal hypoxia. A complete thyroid workup must be done to confirm the cause of hypothyroidism before treatment can begin.

Posttest care

If a hematoma develops at the venipuncture site, apply warm soaks. Heelsticks require no special care.

Interfering factors

- Corticosteroids, T_3, and T_4 cause low TSH levels.
- Lithium carbonate, potassium iodide, excessive topical resorcinol, and TSH injection raise TSH levels.
- Failure to let a filter paper sample dry completely may alter test results.
- Rough handling of a serum sample may cause hemolysis and may interfere with accurate testing.

Thyroid-stimulating immunoglobulin test

Thyroid-stimulating immunoglobulin (TSI), formerly called long-acting thyroid stimulator, appears in the blood of most patients with Graves' disease. This autoantibody reacts with the cell-surface receptors that usually bind thyroid-stimulating hormone (TSH). TSI binding by these receptors activates intracellular enzymes and promotes epithelial cell activity that functions outside the normal feedback regulation mechanism for TSH. It stimulates the thyroid gland to produce and excrete excessive amounts of thyroid hormones.

About 50% to 90% of people with thyrotoxicosis have elevated TSI levels. Positive test results strongly suggest Graves' disease but don't always correlate with overt signs of hyperthyroidism.

Purpose

- To aid evaluation of suspected thyroid disease
- To aid diagnosis of suspected thyrotoxicosis, especially in patients with exophthalmos
- To monitor treatment of thyrotoxicosis.

Patient preparation

Explain to the patient that this test evaluates thyroid function. Inform him that it requires a blood sample, who will perform the venipuncture and when, and that he may experience transient discomfort from the needle puncture and the pressure of the tourniquet.

Procedure

Perform a venipuncture and collect the sample in a 5-ml clot-activator tube.

Precautions

- Handle the sample gently to prevent hemolysis.
- Send it to the laboratory promptly.
- Note on the laboratory request if the patient had a radioactive iodine scan within 48 hours of the test.

Normal findings

TSI doesn't normally appear in serum. However, it may be present in 5% of people without hyperthyroidism or exophthalmos.

Implications of results

Increased TSI levels are associated with exophthalmos, Graves' disease (thyrotoxicosis), and recurrence of hyperthyroidism.

Posttest care

If a hematoma develops at the venipuncture site, apply warm soaks to ease discomfort.

Interfering factors

- Administration of radioactive iodine within 48 hours of the test may affect the accuracy of test results.
- Hemolysis caused by excessive agitation of the sample may alter test results.

Thyroxine test

Thyroxine (T_4) is secreted by the thyroid gland in response to thyroid-stimulating hormone (TSH) from the pituitary and, indirectly, to thyrotropin-releasing hormone (TRH) from the hypothalamus. The rate of secretion is normally regulated by a complex system of negative and positive feedback involving the thyroid, anterior pituitary, and hypothalamus. The suspected precursor, or prohormone, of triiodothyronine (T_3), T_4 is believed to convert to T_3 by removing one iodine atom, which occurs mainly in the liver and kidneys.

Only a fraction of T_4 (about 0.3%) circulates freely in the blood; the rest binds strongly to plasma proteins, primarily to thyroxine-binding globulin (TBG). The minute free fraction is responsible for the clinical effects of thyroid hormone. TBG binds so tenaciously that T_4 survives in the plasma for a relatively long time; its half-life is about 6 days. This immunoassay, one of the most common thyroid diagnostic tools, measures the total circulating T_4 level when TBG is normal. An alternative test is the Murphy-Pattee or T_4 (D) test, based on competitive protein binding.

Purpose

- To evaluate thyroid function
- To aid diagnosis of hyperthyroidism and hypothyroidism
- To monitor response to antithyroid medication in hyperthyroidism or to thyroid replacement therapy in hypothyroidism (confirmation of hypothyroidism requires TSH estimates).

Patient preparation

Explain that this test helps evaluate thyroid gland function. Inform the patient that he needn't fast or restrict physical activity. Tell him a blood sample is needed, who will perform the venipuncture and when, and that he may feel some discomfort from the needle puncture.

As ordered, withhold any medications that may interfere with test results. If these medications must be continued, note this on the laboratory request. (If this test is being performed to monitor thyroid therapy, the patient continues to receive daily thyroid supplements.)

Procedure

Perform a venipuncture and collect the sample in a 7-ml clot-activator tube. Send the sample to the laboratory immediately so the serum can be separated.

Precautions

Handle the sample gently to prevent hemolysis.

Reference values

The normal range of total T_4 is 5 to 13.5 µg/dl.

Implications of results

Abnormally elevated levels of T_4 are consistent with primary and secondary hyperthyroidism, including excessive T_4 (levothyroxine) replacement therapy (factitious or iatrogenic hyperthyroidism). Subnormal levels of T_4 suggest primary or secondary hypothyroidism or T_4 suppression by normal, elevated, or replacement levels of T_3. In doubtful cases of hypothyroidism, the TSH or TRH test may be indicated. Normal T_4 levels don't guarantee euthyroidism; for example, levels are within the normal range in patients with T_3 thyrotoxicosis. Overt signs of hyperthyroidism require further testing.

Posttest care

- If a hematoma develops at the venipuncture site, apply warm soaks.
- As ordered, resume administration of medications discontinued before the test.

Interfering factors

- Estrogens, progestins, levothyroxine, and methadone increase T_4 levels.
- Free fatty acids, heparin, iodides, liothyronine sodium, lithium, methylthiouracil, phenylbutazone, phenytoin, propylthiouracil, salicylates (high doses), steroids, sulfonamides, and sulfonylureas all decrease T_4.
- Clofibrate can either increase or decrease T_4 levels.
- Hemolysis may alter test results.
- Hereditary factors and hepatic disease can change TBG concentration; protein-wasting disease (nephrotic syndrome) and androgens may reduce TBG.

Thyroxine-binding globulin test

This test measures the serum level of thyroxine-binding globulin (TBG), the predominant protein carrier for circulating thyroxine (T_4) and triiodothyronine (T_3). TBG values may be identified by adding to the sample more than enough radioactive T_4 to saturate all the available receptors on TBG, subjecting the sample to electrophoresis, and quantitating the amount of TBG by the amount of radioactive T_4 bound or by radioimmunoassay.

Any condition that affects TBG levels and subsequent binding capacity also affects the amount of free T_4 (FT_4) and free T_3 (FT_3) in circulation. This can be clinically significant because only FT_4 and FT_3 are metabolically active. An underlying TBG abnormality renders tests for total T_3 and T_4 inaccurate but doesn't alter tests for FT_3 and FT_4.

Purpose

- To evaluate abnormal thyrometabolic states that don't correlate with thyroid hormone (T_3 or T_4) values (for example, a patient with overt signs of hypothyroidism and a low FT_4 level with a high total T_4 level caused by a marked increase of TBG secondary to use of oral contraceptives)
- To identify TBG abnormalities.

Patient preparation

Explain to the patient that this test helps evaluate thyroid function. Tell him the test requires a blood sample, who will perform the venipuncture and when, and that he may feel transient discomfort from the needle puncture.

As ordered, withhold medications that may interfere with accurate testing, such as estrogens, anabolic steroids, phenytoin, salicylates, and thyroid preparations. If these medications must be continued, note this on the laboratory request. (They may be continued to determine if prescribed drugs are affecting TBG levels.)

Procedure

Draw venous blood into a 7-ml clot-activator tube.

Precautions

Be sure to handle the sample gently because excessive agitation may cause hemolysis.

Reference values

Normal values for serum TBG by electrophoresis are 10 to 26 µg T_4 (binding capacity) per deciliter. Normal values by immunoassay are 12 to 25 mg/L in males and 14 to 30 mg/L in females.

Implications of results

Elevated TBG levels may suggest hypothyroidism, congenital (genetic) excess of TBG, some forms of hepatic disease, or acute intermittent porphyria. TBG levels normally rise during pregnancy and are high in neonates. Low levels suggest hyperthyroidism or congenital deficiency and may be present in patients with active acromegaly, nephrotic syndrome, malnutrition with hypoproteinemia, acute illness, or surgical stress.

Patients with TBG abnormalities require additional testing, such as the serum FT_3 and serum FT_4 tests, to evaluate thyroid function more precisely.

Posttest care

■ If a hematoma develops at the venipuncture site, apply warm soaks.
■ As ordered, resume administration of medications that were discontinued before the test.

Interfering factors

■ Estrogens (including oral contraceptives) and phenothiazines (perphenazine) elevate TBG levels.
■ Androgens, prednisone, phenytoin, and high doses of salicylates depress TBG levels.
■ Hemolysis caused by rough handling of the sample may interfere with accurate determination of test results.

TORCH test

This test is performed on pregnant women to detect exposure to pathogens that commonly cause congenital and neonatal infections. TORCH is an acronym for *t*oxoplasmosis, *o*ther agents, *r*ubella, *c*ytomegalovirus, and *h*erpes simplex. These infections may not be clinically apparent and may cause severe central nervous system impairment. This test confirms such infection serologically by detecting specific immunoglobulin M-associated antibodies in infant blood.

Purpose

To aid diagnosis of acute, congenital, and intrapartum infections.

Patient preparation

As appropriate, explain the purpose of the test and mention that the test requires a blood sample. Tell the patient who will perform the venipuncture and when and that she may experience transient discomfort from the needle puncture and the pressure of the tourniquet.

Procedure

Obtain a 3-ml sample of venous or cord blood. Send it to the laboratory promptly for serologic testing.

Precautions

- Send the sample to the laboratory immediately.
- Don't freeze the sample.
- Handle the sample gently to prevent hemolysis.

Normal findings

Test results should be negative for TORCH agents.

Implications of results

Toxoplasmosis is diagnosed by sequential examination that shows rising antibody titers, changing titers, and serologic conversion from negative to positive; a titer of 1:256 suggests recent infection. Approximately two-thirds of infected infants are asymptomatic at birth; one-third show signs of cerebral calcification and chorio-retinitis.

In infants less than 6 months old, rubella infection is associated with a marked and persistent rise in complement-fixing antibody titer over time. Persistence of rubella antibody in an infant after age 6 months strongly suggests congenital infection. Congenital rubella is associated with cardiac anomalies, neurosensory deafness, growth retardation, and encephalitic symptoms.

Detection of herpes antibodies in cerebrospinal fluid with signs of herpetic encephalitis and persistent herpes simplex virus type 2 antibody levels confirm herpes simplex infection in a neonate without obvious herpetic lesions.

Posttest care

If a hematoma develops at the venipuncture site, apply warm soaks.

Interfering factors

Hemolysis caused by excessive agitation of the sample may affect the accuracy of test results.

Transferrin test

This test uses radial immunodiffusion or nephelometry to measure serum transferrin levels, which reflect the status of iron metabolism. Transferrin (also known as siderophilin), a glycoprotein formed in the liver, transports circulating iron obtained from dietary sources and from the breakdown of red blood cells by reticuloendothelial cells. Most of this iron is transported to bone marrow for use in hemoglobin synthesis; some is converted to hemosiderin and ferritin and stored in the liver, spleen, and bone marrow. Inadequate transferrin levels may therefore lead to impaired hemoglobin synthesis and, possibly, anemia. Transferrin is normally about 30% saturated with iron. Serum iron levels are usually obtained simultaneously.

Purpose

■ To determine the iron-transporting capacity of the blood
■ To evaluate iron metabolism in iron deficiency anemia.

Patient preparation

Explain to the patient that this test helps determine the cause of anemia. Inform him that he needn't restrict food or fluids. Tell him the test requires a blood sample, who will perform the venipuncture and when, and that he may feel some discomfort from the needle puncture and the pressure of the tourniquet. Check his medication history for drugs that may affect transferrin levels.

Procedure

Perform a venipuncture and collect the sample in a 7-ml clot-activator tube.

Precautions

Handle the sample gently and send it to the laboratory immediately.

Reference values

The normal range of serum transferrin values is 200 to 400 mg/dl, of which 65 to 170 mg/dl are usually bound to iron.

Implications of results

Depressed serum transferrin levels suggest inadequate production caused by hepatic damage or excessive protein loss from renal disease. They may also result from acute or chronic infection or from cancer. Elevated serum transferrin levels may indicate severe iron deficiency.

Posttest care

If a hematoma develops at the venipuncture site, apply warm soaks.

Interfering factors

■ Late pregnancy or the use of oral contraceptives may raise transferrin levels.

■ Hemolysis caused by rough handling of the sample may affect test results.

Triglyceride test

Triglycerides, the most prevalent form of fat in the human diet, can be produced by metabolism of carbohydrates, animal fats, or vegetable oil. The body's major source of direct and stored energy, they efficiently transport energy for direct use by the cells. Stored in the form of body fat, they provide energy reserves and insulation.

This test provides quantitative analysis of triglycerides, the main storage form of lipids, which constitute about 95% of fatty tissue. Although not in itself diagnostic, serum triglyceride analysis permits early identification of hyperlipidemia (characteristic in nephrotic syndrome and other conditions), and high levels are a risk factor for coronary artery disease (CAD).

The triglyceride molecule consists of three molecules of fatty acids (usually some combination of stearic, oleic, and palmitic) bound to one molecule of glycerol. The metabolism of triglyceride leads directly to the production of fatty acid. Carbohydrates and triglycerides furnish energy for metabolism. Serum triglycerides are associated with lipid aggregates, primarily chylomicrons, whose major function is transport. Serum that contains excessive chylomicrons appears milky, which interferes with many laboratory tests. Very-low-density lipoproteins are also rich in triglycerides, though less so than chylomicrons. When present in excessive amounts, they may cause plasma to become turbid, which also interferes with many laboratory tests.

Purpose

■ To screen for hyperlipidemias and association with possible relationship to atherosclerosis

■ To help identify nephrotic syndrome and poorly controlled type 1 and type 2 diabetes mellitus

■ To determine the risk of CAD

■ To provide a basis for calculating the low-density lipoprotein cholesterol level
■ To screen for pancreatitis
■ To monitor triglyceride levels in a patient who is receiving hyperalimentation or fat emulsions.

Patient preparation

Explain triglycerides to the patient, and tell him that
this test helps detect disorders of fat metabolism. Triglycerides are highly affected by a fat-containing meal,
with levels rising then reaching a peak 4 hours after ingesting a meal. Advise the patient to abstain from food
for 10 to 14 hours before the test and from alcohol for
24 hours, but tell him that he may drink water. Ensure
that the patient is in a steady metabolic state. If the patient has an acute illness, infection, fever, or other acute
problem, inform the doctor because this can possibly interfere with the laboratory result.

Inform the patient that the test requires a blood sample, who will perform the venipuncture and when, and
that he may experience transient discomfort from the
needle puncture and the pressure of the tourniquet.

As ordered, withhold medications that may interfere
with the accuracy of test results. These include antilipemics, corticosteroids, estrogen, and some diuretics,
which can raise or lower triglyceride levels.

Procedure

■ Have the patient sit still for 5 minutes before drawing
the blood.
■ Perform a venipuncture and collect a serum or plasma
sample in a 7-ml EDTA tube.

Precautions

■ Avoid prolonged venous occlusion. Remove the
tourniquet within 1 minute of application.
■ Send the sample to the laboratory immediately.
■ In hospitalized patients receiving I.V. hyperalimentation or fat emulsions, draw blood for the test 18 hours
after the lipid infusion is completed.

Reference values

Triglyceride values are age- and sex-related. Although
some controversy exists over the most appropriate normal ranges, 40 to 160 mg/dl in adult men and 35 to 135
mg/dl in adult women are widely accepted.

Implications of results

Increased or decreased serum triglyceride levels merely
suggest a clinical abnormality; definitive diagnosis requires additional tests. For example, cholesterol testing

may also be necessary because cholesterol and triglyceride levels vary independently. High levels of triglyceride and cholesterol reflect an increased risk of CAD.

A mild to moderate increase in serum triglyceride levels may suggest biliary obstruction, diabetes, nephrotic syndrome, endocrinopathy, or excessive consumption of alcohol. Markedly increased levels without an identifiable cause reflect congenital hyperlipoproteinemia and necessitate lipoprotein phenotyping to confirm the diagnosis. Severe elevations (greater than 1,000 mg/dl) have a significant association with abdominal pain and pancreatitis. Patients with hypertriglyceridemia may exhibit clinical manifestations such as eruptive xanthomas, corneal arcus, xanthelasma, and lipemia retinalis.

Low serum levels are rare, occurring mainly in malnutrition or abetalipoproteinemia. In the latter, serum is virtually devoid of beta-lipoproteins and the body lacks the capacity to transport preformed triglycerides from the epithelial cells of the intestinal mucosa or from the liver.

Posttest care

■ If a hematoma develops at the venipuncture site, apply warm soaks.
■ As ordered, resume medications and diet discontinued before the test.

Interfering factors

■ Failure to comply with dietary restrictions may alter test results.
■ Ingestion of alcohol within 24 hours of the test may cause elevated triglyceride levels. Excessive consumption of alcohol is a common cause of high triglyceride levels because alcohol is heavily hydrogenated, and most of the hydrogen released during alcohol metabolism ultimately ends up in triglycerides. Fatty liver is an early manifestation of this metabolic phenomenon.
■ All antilipemics lower serum lipid concentration in the bloodstream, although their mechanisms of action may differ. Some, such as cholestyramine and colestipol, raise or have no effect on triglyceride levels.
■ Long-term use of corticosteroids raises triglyceride levels, as does use of oral contraceptives, estrogen, ethyl alcohol, furosemide, or miconazole.
■ Use of glycol-lubricated collection tubes may alter test results.
■ Clofibrate, dextrothyroxine, gemfibrozil, and niacin lower cholesterol and triglyceride levels.
■ Certain drugs have a variable effect: Probucol inhibits transport of cholesterol from the intestine and may also

affect cholesterol synthesis; it lowers cholesterol and has a variable effect on triglycerides.

Triiodothyronine test

This highly specific immunoassay measures total (bound and free) serum content of triiodothyronine (T_3) to investigate clinical indications of thyroid dysfunction. T_3, the more potent thyroid hormone, is derived primarily from thyroxine (T_4) by removal of one iodine atom. At least 50% and as much as 90% of T_3 may be derived from T_4 as a result of this pivotal transformation. The remaining 10% or more is secreted directly by the thyroid gland.

Like T_4 secretion, T_3 secretion occurs in response to thyroid-stimulating hormone (TSH) released by the pituitary and, secondarily, to thyrotropin-releasing hormone from the hypothalamus through a complex negative feedback mechanism.

Although T_3 is present in the bloodstream in minute quantities and it's metabolically active for only a short time, its impact on body metabolism exceeds that of T_4. Another significant difference between the two major thyroid hormones is that T_3 binds less firmly to thyroxine-binding globulin (TBG). Consequently, T_3 persists in the bloodstream for a short time; half of it disappears in about 1 day, whereas half of T_4 disappears in 6 days.

Purpose

- To aid diagnosis of T_3 toxicosis
- To aid diagnosis of hypothyroidism or hyperthyroidism
- To monitor clinical response to thyroid replacement therapy in hypothyroidism.

Patient preparation

Explain to the patient that this test helps to evaluate thyroid gland function and to determine the cause of his symptoms. Tell him that the test requires a blood sample, who will perform the venipuncture and when, and that he may experience some transient discomfort from the needle puncture.

As ordered, withhold medications that may influence thyroid function, such as steroids, propranolol, and cholestyramine. If such medications must be continued, record this information on the laboratory request.

Procedure

- Perform a venipuncture and collect the sample in a 7-ml clot-activator tube.

■ Send the sample to the laboratory as soon as possible to avoid stasis and to allow early separation of serum from the clotted blood.

Precautions

Handle the sample gently to prevent hemolysis. If a patient must receive thyroid preparations containing T_3 (liothyronine), note the time of drug administration on the laboratory request.

Reference values

The normal range of serum T_3 levels is 90 to 230 ng/dl. These values may vary among laboratories performing this test.

Implications of results

Serum T_3 and T_4 levels usually rise and fall in tandem. However, in T_3 toxicosis, only T_3 levels rise, whereas total and free T_4 levels remain normal. T_3 toxicosis occurs in patients with Graves' disease, toxic adenoma, or toxic nodular goiter. T_3 also exceeds T_4 in patients receiving thyroid replacement containing more T_3 than T_4. In iodine-deficient areas, the thyroid may produce a greater amount of the more metabolically active T_3 than of T_4 in an effort to maintain the euthyroid state.

Generally, T_3 levels seem to reflect the presence of hyperthyroidism more accurately than T_4 levels do. Although hyperthyroidism increases both T_3 and T_4 levels in about 90% of patients, it causes a disproportionate increase in T_3. In some patients with hypothyroidism, T_3 levels may be normal and may not be diagnostically significant.

A rise in serum T_3 levels normally occurs during pregnancy. Levels may be low in euthyroid patients with systemic illness (especially hepatic or renal disease), during severe acute illness, or after trauma or major surgery. However, in such patients, TSH levels are normal. Malnourished euthyroid patients may have low T_3 levels.

Posttest care

■ If a hematoma develops at the venipuncture site, apply warm soaks.
■ As ordered, resume administration of drugs discontinued before the test.

Interfering factors

■ Failure to take into account medications that affect T_3 levels, such as steroids, clofibrate, and propranolol, may influence test results. (See *Drugs that interfere with T_3 tests.*)

DRUGS THAT INTERFERE WITH T$_3$ TESTS	
Increased T$_3$	
Clofibrate	Methadone
Estrogen	Progestins
Liothyronine sodium (T$_3$)	
Decreased T$_3$	
Clofibrate	Phenylbutazone
Ethionamide	Phenytoin
Free fatty acids	Propranolol
Heparin	Propylthiouracil
Iodides	Reserpine
Lithium	Salicylates (high doses)
Methimazole	Steroids
Methylthiouracil	Sulfonamides

■ Markedly high or low TBG levels, regardless of cause, may affect the accuracy of test results.
■ Hemolysis caused by rough handling of the sample may influence test results.

Troponin I and cardiac troponin T tests

Troponin I (cTn I) and cardiac troponin T (cTn T) are proteins in striated muscle cells; they are part of the calcium-binding complex of the thin myofilaments of myocardial tissue. Troponins are specific markers of cardiac damage. Injury to myocardial tissue releases them into the bloodstream, and blood levels rise from normally undetectable to more than 50 g/ml. Troponin levels rise within 1 hour of myocardial infarction (MI) and persist for a week or longer.

Purpose
■ To detect and diagnose acute MI and reinfarction
■ To evaluate possible causes of chest pain.

Patient preparation
Explain to the patient that this test helps assess myocardial injury and that many samples may be drawn to detect fluctuations in serum levels. Inform him that he needn't restrict foods or fluids before the test. Tell him who will perform the venipuncture and when and that he may feel some discomfort from the needle puncture and the pressure of the tourniquet.

Procedure
Perform a venipuncture and collect the specimen in a 7-ml clot-activator tube.

Precautions

Obtain each specimen on schedule and note the date and collection time on each.

Reference values

Results may vary among laboratories; some call a test positive if it shows any detectable levels and others give a normal range.

Normally, the cTn I level is less than 0.4 g/ml and the cTn T level is less than 0.1 g/ml. A cTn I level below 0.4 g/ml doesn't suggest cardiac injury, 0.5 to 1.9 g/ml is indeterminate, and greater than 2.0 g/ml is suggestive of cardiac injury. A qualitative cTn T rapid immunoassay result greater than 0.2 g/ml is considered positive for cardiac injury. In quantitative serum assays for cTn T, the upper limit for normal is 0.1 g/ml.

Implications of results

Troponin levels rise rapidly and are detectable within 1 hour of myocardial cell injury. As long as tissue injury continues, troponin levels will remain high. Troponin I levels aren't detectable in people without cardiac injury.

Posttest care

If a hematoma develops at the venipuncture site, apply warm soaks.

Interfering factors

■ Sustained vigorous exercise may increase troponin T levels in the absence of significant cardiac damage; these elevations reflect release of noncardiac-specific troponin T from skeletal muscles.
■ Cardiotoxic drugs such as doxorubicin (Adriamycin) can raise troponin levels.
Troponin T may rise in the presence of renal disease and after certain surgical procedures. Elevated troponin I levels have only been associated with myocardial injury. No other factors are known to increase these levels.

Tuberculin skin tests

These skin tests are used to screen patients for previous infection by the tubercle bacillus. They are routinely performed in children, young adults, and people with radiographic findings that suggest this infection.

In both the old tuberculin (OT) and the purified protein derivative (PPD) tests, intradermal injection of the tuberculin antigen causes a delayed hypersensitivity reaction in patients with active or dormant tuberculosis; sensitized lymphocytes gather at the injection site, causing erythema, vesiculation, and induration that peaks within 24 to 48 hours and persists for at least 72 hours.

The most accurate tuberculin test method, the Mantoux test, uses a single-needle intradermal injection of PPD, which permits precise measurement of dosage. Multipuncture tests, such as the tine test, Mono-Vacc test, and Aplitest, involve intradermal injections with tines impregnated with OT or PPD. Because multipuncture tests require less skill and are more rapidly administered than the Mantoux test, they're generally used for screening. However, a positive multipuncture test usually requires a Mantoux test for confirmation.

Purpose

■ To distinguish tuberculosis from blastomycosis, coccidioidomycosis, and histoplasmosis
■ To identify persons who need diagnostic investigation for tuberculosis because of possible exposure.

Patient preparation

Explain to the patient that this test helps detect tuberculosis. Tell him the test requires an injection into the skin, which may cause him transient discomfort.

CLINICAL ALERT Check the patient's history for active tuberculosis, the results of previous skin tests, and hypersensitivities. If the patient has had tuberculosis, don't perform a skin test; if he's had a positive reaction to previous skin tests, consult the doctor or follow your facility's policy; if he's had an allergic reaction to acacia, don't perform an OT test because this product contains acacia.

If you're performing a tuberculin test on an outpatient, instruct him to return at the specified time so that test results can be read. Inform him that a positive reaction to a skin test appears as a red, hard, raised area at the injection site. Although the area may itch, instruct him not to scratch it. Stress that a positive reaction doesn't always indicate active tuberculosis.

Equipment

Alcohol swabs ■ vial of PPD (intermediate strength)— 5 tuberculin units (TU) per 0.1 ml and 1-ml tuberculin syringe with ½" or ⅝" 25G or 26G needle for the Mantoux test ■ commercially available device (tine, Mono-Vacc, or Aplitest) for multipuncture tests ■ epinephrine (1:1,000) and 3-ml syringe (to treat anaphylactic or acute hypersensitivity reactions).

Procedure

■ Have the patient sit with his arm extended and supported on a flat surface. Clean the volar surface of the upper forearm with alcohol, and let the area dry completely.

READING TUBERCULIN TEST RESULTS

You should read the Mantoux, tine, and Aplitest skin tests 48 to 72 hours after injection; the Mono-Vacc test, 48 to 96 hours afterward.

In a well-lighted room, flex the patient's forearm slightly. Observe the injection site for erythema and vesiculation and then gently rub your finger over the site to detect induration. If induration is present, measure the diameter in millimeters, preferably with a plastic ruler marked in concentric circles of specific diameter.

In multipuncture tests, you may find separate areas of induration around individual punctures or induration involving more than one puncture site. If so, measure the diameter of the largest single area of induration or coalesced induration.

■ For the Mantoux test: Perform an intradermal injection.
■ For multipuncture tests: Remove the protective cap on the injection device to expose the four tines. Hold the patient's forearm in one hand, stretching the skin of the forearm tightly. Then, with your other hand, firmly depress the device into the patient's skin (without twisting it). Hold the device in place for at least 1 second before removing it. If you've applied sufficient pressure, you'll see four puncture sites and a circular depression made by the device on the patient's skin.
■ Record where the test was given, the date and time, and when it's to be read. Tuberculin skin tests are generally read 48 to 72 hours after injection; however, the Mono-Vacc test can be read 48 to 96 hours after the test. (See *Reading tuberculin test results.*)

Precautions
■ Tuberculin skin tests are contraindicated in patients with active tuberculosis, a current reaction to smallpox vaccinations, any type of rash, or a skin disorder.
■ Don't perform a skin test in areas with excessive hair, acne, or insufficient subcutaneous tissue, such as over a tendon or bone. If the patient is known to be hypersensitive to skin tests, use a first-strength dose in the Mantoux test to avoid necrosis at the puncture site.
■ Have epinephrine available to treat an anaphylactic or acute hypersensitivity reactions.

Normal findings
■ Mantoux test: induration less than 5 mm in diameter or no induration
■ Tine test and Aplitest: no vesiculation; no induration or induration less than 2 mm in diameter
■ Mono-Vacc test: no induration

Implications of results

A positive tuberculin reaction indicates previous infection by tubercle bacilli. It doesn't distinguish between an active and dormant infection, nor does it provide a definitive diagnosis. A positive reaction mandates a sputum smear and culture and chest X-rays.

In the Mantoux test, induration of 5 to 9 mm in diameter indicates a borderline reaction; larger induration, a positive reaction. Because patients infected with atypical mycobacteria other than tubercle bacilli may have borderline reactions, repeat testing is necessary.

In the tine test or Aplitest, vesiculation indicates a positive reaction; induration of 2 mm in diameter without vesiculation requires confirmation by the Mantoux test. Any induration in the Mono-Vacc test indicates a positive reaction but requires confirmation by the Mantoux test.

Posttest care

If ulceration or necrosis develops at the injection site, apply cold soaks or a topical steroid, as ordered.

Interfering factors

■ Corticosteroids, other immunosuppressants, or live virus vaccines (measles, mumps, rubella, or polio) given within the past 4 to 6 weeks may suppress skin reactions.

■ Subcutaneous injection, usually indicated by erythema greater than 10 mm in diameter without induration, invalidates the test.

■ Elderly people and patients with viral infection, malnutrition, febrile illness, uremia, immunosuppressive disorders, or miliary tuberculosis may have suppressed skin reactions.

■ If fewer than 10 weeks have elapsed since infection with tuberculosis, the skin reaction may be suppressed.

■ Improper dilution, dosage, or storage of the tuberculin interferes with accurate testing.

Tubular reabsorption of phosphate test

Because tubular reabsorption of phosphate is tightly regulated by parathyroid hormone (PTH), measuring urine and plasma phosphate, with creatinine clearance, is an indirect method of evaluating parathyroid function. PTH helps maintain optimum blood levels of ionized calcium and controls renal excretion of calcium and phosphate. Specifically, PTH stimulates reabsorption of calcium and inhibits reabsorption of phosphate from the glomerular filtrate. A regulatory feedback mechanism results in diminished PTH secretion as ionized calcium levels return to normal. In primary hyperparathyroidism, excessive secretion of PTH disrupts this calcium-phosphate balance.

This test is indicated to detect hyperparathyroidism in persons with clinical signs of this disorder and borderline or normal levels of serum calcium, phosphate, and alkaline phosphatase.

Purpose

- To evaluate parathyroid function
- To aid diagnosis of primary hyperparathyroidism
- To aid differential diagnosis of hypercalcemia.

Patient preparation

Explain to the patient that this test evaluates the function of the parathyroid glands and that it requires a blood sample and a 24-hour urine collection. Tell him who will perform the venipuncture and when and that he may experience transient discomfort from the needle puncture and the pressure of the tourniquet.

Instruct the patient to maintain a normal phosphate diet for 3 days before the test because low phosphate intake (less than 500 mg/day) may stimulate tubular reabsorption and a high intake (3,000 mg/day or more) may inhibit it. Common dietary sources of phosphorus include legumes, nuts, milk, egg yolks, meat, poultry, fish, cereals, and cheese; the patient should eat moderate amounts of these foods. Instruct the patient to fast after midnight the night before the test.

As ordered, withhold drugs that are known to influence test results, such as amphotericin B, thiazide diuretics, furosemide, and gentamicin. If these medications must be continued throughout the test period, note this on the laboratory request.

Procedure

First, perform a venipuncture and collect the sample in a 10-ml clot-activator tube. Then instruct the patient to empty his bladder and discard the urine; record this as time zero. Collect a 24-hour urine specimen. (Occasionally, a 4-hour collection is ordered instead.)

Precautions

- Handle the collection tube gently to prevent hemolysis and send it to the laboratory immediately.
- Keep the urine specimen container refrigerated or on ice during the collection period. Tell the patient to avoid contaminating the specimen with toilet paper or stool.
- At the end of the collection period, label the specimen and send it to the laboratory immediately.

Normal findings

Renal tubules normally reabsorb 80% or more of phosphate.

Implications of results

Reabsorption of less than 74% of phosphate strongly suggests primary hyperparathyroidism, but additional studies are needed to confirm this diagnosis as the cause of hypercalcemia. Chest and bone X-rays and bone scans should be performed because bone metastasis is the most common cause of hypercalcemia. Depressed reabsorption occurs in a small number of patients with renal calculi but without parathyroid tumor. However, reabsorption is normal in roughly 20% of patients with parathyroid tumor. Increased phosphate reabsorption may result from uremia, renal tubular disease, osteomalacia, sarcoidosis, or myeloma.

Posttest care

- After the venipuncture, allow the patient to eat and encourage fluid intake to maintain adequate urine flow.
- If a hematoma develops at the venipuncture site, apply warm soaks.
- As ordered, resume the patient's regular diet and administration of any medications that were discontinued before the test.

Interfering factors

- The patient's failure to follow guidelines for diet restrictions and phosphate intake may alter test results.
- Amphotericin B and thiazide diuretics may diminish reabsorption.
- Furosemide and gentamicin may enhance reabsorption.
- Hemolysis caused by rough handling of the sample may alter test results.
- Failure to collect all urine during the test period may affect the accuracy of test results.

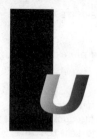

Urea clearance test

The urea clearance test is a quantitative analysis of urine urea, the main nitrogenous component in urine and the end product of protein metabolism. (See *How urea is formed.*) After filtration by the glomeruli, roughly 40% of the urea is reabsorbed by the renal tubules. Because of this reabsorption, urea clearance was once considered a precise fraction (60%) of the glomerular filtration rate (GFR). However, because the reabsorption rate of urea varies with the amount of water reabsorbed, this test actually assesses overall renal function; the creatinine clearance test reflects the GFR more accurately.

In urea clearance, blood urea content and the total amount of urea excreted in the urine are proportional only when the rate of urine flow is 2 ml/minute or higher (maximal clearance). At lower flow rates, the test's accuracy decreases.

Purpose

To assess overall renal function.

Patient preparation

Explain to the patient that this test evaluates kidney function. Instruct him to fast from midnight before the test and to abstain from exercise before and during the test. Tell him the test requires two timed urine specimens and one blood sample. Tell him how the urine specimens will be collected, who will perform the venipuncture and when, and that he may experience transient discomfort from the needle puncture.

Check the patient's medication history for drugs that may affect urea clearance. Review your findings with the laboratory, and then notify the doctor, who may want to restrict these medications before the test.

Procedure

■ Instruct the patient to empty his bladder and discard the urine. Then give him water to drink to ensure adequate urine output.

■ Collect two specimens 1 hour apart, and mark the collection time on the laboratory request. Perform a

---

HOW UREA IS FORMED

Urea, the main nitrogenous component in urine, is the final product of protein metabolism. Amino acids absorbed by the intestinal villi pass from the portal vein into the liver. The liver stores only small amounts of amino acids, which it later returns to the blood for use in the synthesis of enzymes, hormones, or new protoplasm; the excess is converted into other substances, such as glucose, glycogen, and fat.

Before this conversion, the amino acids are deaminated — that is, they lose their nitrogenous amino groups, which are converted to ammonia. Because ammonia is toxic, especially to the brain, it must be removed as quickly as it's formed. Serious liver disease raises elevated blood ammonia levels and eventually leads to hepatic coma.

In the liver, ammonia combines with carbon dioxide to form urea, which is released into the blood and ultimately secreted in urine.

---

venipuncture anytime during the collection period and collect the sample in a 7-ml clot-activator tube.

Precautions

■ Because this is a clearance test, make sure the patient empties his bladder completely and that the total amount of urine is collected from each hour's specimen.
■ Send each specimen to the laboratory as soon as it is collected.
■ If the patient is catheterized, empty the drainage bag before beginning the specimen collection.
■ Handle the blood sample gently to prevent hemolysis and send it to the laboratory immediately.

Reference values

Normally, urea clearance is 64 to 99 ml/minute with maximal clearance. If the flow rate is less than 2 ml/minute, normal clearance is 41 to 68 ml/minute. (If the urine flow rate is less than 1 ml/minute, this test should not be performed.)

Implications of results

Low urea clearance values suggest decreased renal blood flow (caused by shock or renal artery obstruction), acute or chronic glomerulonephritis, advanced bilateral chronic pyelonephritis, acute tubular necrosis, or nephrosclerosis. Low clearance may also result from advanced bilateral renal lesions (as in polycystic kidney disease, renal tuberculosis, or cancer), bilateral ureteral obstruction, heart failure, or dehydration.

High urea clearance rates are usually not diagnostically significant.

Posttest care

- If a hematoma develops at the venipuncture site, apply warm soaks.
- As ordered, resume administration of medications that were withheld before the test.
- Tell the patient that he may resume his usual diet and activities.

Interfering factors

- Caffeine and milk increase urea clearance.
- Small doses of epinephrine increase urea clearance.
- Antidiuretic hormone and large doses of epinephrine decrease urea clearance.
- Corticosteroids, amphotericin B, thiazide diuretics, and streptomycin may affect test results.
- The patient's failure to observe pretest restrictions or to empty his bladder completely, the most common error in this test, will alter test results.
- Hemolysis caused by rough handling of the blood sample may affect test results.

Uric acid test, serum

Used primarily to detect gout, this test measures serum levels of uric acid, the major end metabolite of purine. Large amounts of purines are present in nucleic acids and derive from dietary and endogenous sources. Uric acid clears the body by glomerular filtration and tubular secretion. However, uric acid isn't very soluble at a pH of 7.4 or lower. Disorders of purine metabolism, rapid destruction of nucleic acids, and conditions marked by impaired renal excretion characteristically raise serum uric acid levels.

Purpose

- To confirm diagnosis of gout
- To help detect kidney dysfunction.

Patient preparation

Explain to the patient that this test helps detect gout or kidney dysfunction. Inform him that he must fast for 8 hours before the test. Tell him that the test requires a blood sample, who will perform the venipuncture and when, and that he may feel some discomfort from the needle puncture and the pressure of the tourniquet. Check the patient's medication history for any drugs that may influence uric acid levels.

Procedure

Perform a venipuncture and collect the sample in a 7-ml clot-activator tube.

Precautions

Handle the sample gently to prevent hemolysis.

Reference values

The normal range of uric acid concentrations in men is 4.3 to 8.0 mg/dl; in women, 2.3 to 6.0 mg/dl.

Implications of results

Increased serum uric acid levels suggest gout or impaired renal function (levels don't correlate with severity of disease). Levels may also rise in heart failure, glycogen storage disease (type I, von Gierke's disease), infections, hemolytic or sickle cell anemia, polycythemia, neoplasms, or psoriasis.

Depressed uric acid levels may indicate defective tubular absorption (as in Fanconi's syndrome or Wilson's disease) or acute hepatic atrophy.

Posttest care

If a hematoma develops at the venipuncture site, apply warm soaks.

Interfering factors

■ Starvation, a high-purine diet, stress, and abuse of alcohol may raise uric acid levels.
■ Loop diuretics, ethambutol, vincristine, pyrazinamide, thiazides, and low doses of aspirin may raise uric acid levels.
■ In colorimetric assays, false elevations may be caused by acetaminophen, ascorbic acid, levodopa, and phenacetin.
■ Aspirin in high doses may decrease uric acid levels.

Uric acid test, urine

A quantitative analysis of urine uric acid levels, this test supplements serum uric acid testing for identifying disorders that alter production or excretion of uric acid (such as leukemia, gout, and renal dysfunction). Derived from dietary purines in organ meats (liver, kidney, and sweetbreads) and from endogenous nucleoproteins, uric acid (as urate) is found normally in the blood and in other tissues in amounts totaling about 1 g. Its primary site of formation is the liver, although the intestinal mucosa is also involved in urate production.

As the chief end product of purine catabolism, urate passes from the liver through the bloodstream to the kidneys, where roughly 50% is excreted daily in the urine. Renal urate metabolism is complex, involving glomerular filtration, tubular secretion, and a second reabsorption by the renal tubules.

The most specific laboratory method of detecting uric acid is spectrophotometric absorption after the specimen is treated with the enzyme uricase.

Purpose
■ To detect enzyme deficiencies and metabolic disturbances that affect uric acid production
■ To help measure the efficiency of renal clearance.

Patient preparation
Explain to the patient that this test measures the body's production and excretion of a waste product known as uric acid. Inform him he needn't restrict food or fluids before the test. Tell him the test requires a 24-hour urine specimen, and teach him the proper collection technique.

Check the patient's medication history for recent use of drugs that may influence uric acid levels. If these medications must be continued, note this on the laboratory request.

Procedure
Collect a 24-hour urine specimen.

Precautions
■ Refrigerate the specimen or put it on ice during the collection period.
■ Send the specimen to the laboratory as soon as the collection period is over.

Reference values
Normal urine uric acid values vary with diet, but generally the range is 250 to 750 mg/24 hours.

Implications of results
Elevated urine uric acid levels may result from chronic myeloid leukemia, polycythemia vera, multiple myeloma, early remission of pernicious anemia, radiation therapy of lymphosarcoma or lymphatic leukemia, or tubular reabsorption defects, such as Fanconi's syndrome and hepatolenticular degeneration (Wilson's disease).

Patients with gout have low urine uric acid levels (reflecting normal uric acid production but inadequate excretion) as do patients with severe renal damage, as occurs in chronic glomerulonephritis, diabetic glomerulosclerosis, and collagen disorders.

Posttest care
As ordered, resume administration of medications withheld before the test.

Interfering factors

■ Urine uric acid concentrations rise with a high-purine diet and fall with a low-purine diet.

■ Drugs that decrease urine uric acid excretion include pyrazinamide and diuretics, such as benzthiazide, furosemide, and ethacrynic acid.

■ Low doses of salicylates, phenylbutazone, and probenecid lower uric acid levels; high doses of these drugs cause levels to rise above normal.

■ Allopurinol, a drug used to treat gout, increases uric acid excretion.

■ Failure to observe drug restrictions or to collect all urine during the test period may alter test results.

Urinalysis, routine

Routine urinalysis is important in screening for urinary and systemic disorders. These tests evaluate color, odor, and opacity (odor, though not usually documented on laboratory reports, may be noted under specimen comments); determine specific gravity and pH; detect and measure protein, glucose, and ketone bodies; and examine sediment for blood cells, casts, and crystals.

Diagnostic laboratory methods include visual examination, reagent strip screening, refractometry for specific gravity, and microscopic inspection of centrifuged sediment.

Purpose

■ To screen urine for renal or urinary tract disease (See *Urine cytology*, page 610.)

■ To help detect metabolic or systemic disease unrelated to renal disorders.

Patient preparation

Explain that this test, which requires a urine specimen, aids diagnosis of renal or urinary tract disease and helps the clinician evaluate overall body function. Tell the patient he needn't restrict food or fluids but should avoid strenuous exercise before the test. Check the medication history for drugs that may affect test results.

Procedure

Collect a random urine specimen of at least 15 ml. If possible, obtain a first-voided morning specimen.

Precautions

■ If the patient is being evaluated for kidney stones, strain the specimen to catch stones or stone fragments. Place an unfolded 4″ x 4″ gauze pad or a fine-mesh sieve over the specimen container, and carefully pour the urine through it.

URINE CYTOLOGY

Epithelial cells line the urinary tract and exfoliate into the urine, so that a simple cytologic examination of these cells can aid diagnosis of urinary tract disease. Although urine cytology isn't performed routinely, it's useful for detecting cancer and inflammatory diseases of the renal pelvis, ureters, bladder, and urethra. It's especially useful for detecting bladder cancer in high-risk groups, such as smokers, people who work with aniline dyes (such as leather workers), and patients who have already received treatment for bladder cancer. Urine cytology can also determine whether bladder lesions that appear on X-rays are benign or malignant. This test can also detect cytomegalovirus infection and other viral diseases.

To perform the test, the patient must collect a 100- to 300-ml clean-catch urine specimen 3 hours after his last voiding. He shouldn't use the first-voided specimen of the morning. The urine specimen is sent to the cytology laboratory immediately so that it can be examined before the cells begin to degenerate.

Preparing the specimen

The specimen is prepared in one of the following ways and stained with Papanicolaou's stain:

■ *Centrifuge:* After the urine is spun down, the sediment is smeared on a glass slide and stained for examination.
■ *Filter:* Urine is poured through a filter, which traps the cells so that they can be stained and examined directly.
■ *Cytocentrifuge:* After the urine is centrifuged, the sediment is resuspended and placed on slides, which are spun in a cytocentrifuge and stained for examination.

Implications of results

Normal urine is relatively free of cellular debris but should have some epithelial and squamous cells that appear normal under a microscope. Identification of malignant cells or any other signs of malignancy may indicate cancer of the kidney, renal pelvis, ureters, bladder, or urethra. It could also indicate a metastatic tumor.

An overgrowth of epithelial cells, an excess of red blood cells, or the presence of white blood cells or atypical cells may indicate a lower urinary tract inflammation, which can result from prostatic hyperplasia, urinary calculi, bladder diverticula, strictures, or malformation.

Large intranuclear inclusions may indicate a cytomegalovirus infection, which usually affects the renal tubular epithelium. This type of viral infection commonly occurs in cancer patients undergoing chemotherapy and in transplant patients receiving immunosuppressant drugs. Cytoplasmic inclusion bodies may also indicate measles and may precede the characteristic Koplik's spots.

■ Send the specimen to the laboratory immediately, or refrigerate it if analysis will be delayed longer than 1 hour.

Normal findings

See *Normal findings in routine urinalysis.*

NORMAL FINDINGS IN ROUTINE URINALYSIS

Element	Findings
Macroscopic	
Color	Straw to dark yellow
Odor	Slightly aromatic
Appearance	Clear
Specific gravity	1.005 to 1.035
pH	4.5 to 8.0
Protein	None
Glucose	None
Ketones	None
Bilirubin	None
Urobilinogen	Normal
Hemoglobin	None
Red blood cells	None
Nitrite (bacteria)	None
White blood cells	None
Microscopic	
Red blood cells	0 to 2/high-power field
White blood cells	0 to 5/high-power field
Epithelial cells	0 to 5/high-power field
Casts	None, except 1 to 2 hyaline casts/low-power field
Crystals	Present
Bacteria	None
Yeast cells	None
Parasites	None

Implications of results

Nonpathologic variations in normal values may result from diet, use of certain drugs, nonpathologic conditions, specimen collection time, and other factors. (See *Drugs that influence routine urinalysis results*, pages 612 and 613.) For example, specific gravity influences urine color and odor: as specific gravity increases, urine becomes darker and its odor becomes stronger.

Urine pH is greatly affected by diet and medications; it influences the appearance of urine and the composition of crystals. An alkaline pH (above 7.0)—characteristic of a vegetarian diet—causes turbidity and formation of phosphate, carbonate, and amorphous crystals. Alkaline urine may also be caused by ammonia-splitting bacteria, sodium bicarbonate and acetazolamide intake, excess intake of carbonated beverages, and conditions

DRUGS THAT INFLUENCE ROUTINE URINALYSIS RESULTS

Change of urine color
Amitriptyline (blue-green)
Antraquinone laxatives (reddish brown)
Chloroquine (rusty yellow)
Chlorzoxazone (orange to purple-red)
Deferoxamine mesylate (red)
Fluorescein sodium I.V. (yellow-orange)
Furazolidone (brown)
Iron salts (black)
Levodopa (dark)
Methylene blue (blue-green)
Metronidazole (dark)
Nitrofurantoin (brown)
Oral anticoagulants, indanedione derivatives (orange)
Phenazopyridine (orange, red, or orange-brown)
Phenolphthalein (red to purple-red)
Phenolsulfonphthalein (pink or red)
Phenothiazines (dark)
Phenytoin (red to reddish brown or pink)
Quinacrine (deep yellow)
Riboflavin (yellow)
Rifabutin (red-orange)
Rifampin (red-orange)
Sulfasalazine (orange-yellow)
Sulfobromophthalein (red)
Triamterene (blue-green)

Urine odor
Antibiotics
Paraldehyde
Vitamins

Increased specific gravity
Albumin
Dextran
Glucose
Radiopaque contrast media

Acidic pH
Ammonium chloride
Ascorbic acid
Diazoxide
Methenamine compounds
Metolazone

Alkaline pH
Acetazolamide
Amphotericin B
Carbonic anhydrase inhibitors
Mafenide
Potassium citrate
Sodium bicarbonate

False-positive for protein
Acetazolamide (Combistix)
Aminosalicylic acid (sulfosalicylic acid or Exton's method)
Captopril
Cephalothin in large doses (sulfosalicylic acid method)
Dichlorphenamide
Fenoprofen
Methazolamide
Nafcillin (sulfosalicylic acid method)
d-Penicillamine
Sodium bicarbonate
Tolbutamide (sulfosalicylic acid method)
Tolmetin (sulfosalicylic acid method)

True proteinuria
Aminoglycosides
Amphotericin B
Bacitracin
Cephalosporins
Cisplatin
Etretinate
Gold preparations
Isotretinoin
Nonsteroidal anti-inflammatory drugs
Phenylbutazone
Polymyxin B
Sulfonamides
Trimethadione

Either true proteinuria or false-positive for protein
Penicillin in large doses (except with Ames reagent strips); some penicillins cause true proteinuria
Sulfonamides (sulfosalicylic acid method)

False-positive for glucose
Aminosalicylic acid (Benedict's test)
Ascorbic acid (Clinistix, Diastix, Tes-Tape)
Ascorbic acid in large doses (Clinitest tablets)
Cephalosporins (Clinitest tablets)
Chloral hydrate (Benedict's test)
Chloramphenicol (Clinitest tablets)
Isoniazid (Benedict's test)
Levodopa (Clinistix, Diastix, Tes-Tape)
Levodopa in large doses (Clinitest tablets)
Methyldopa (Tes-Tape)
Nalidixic acid (Benedict's test or Clinitest tablets)
Nitrofurantoin (Benedict's test)

DRUGS THAT INFLUENCE ROUTINE URINALYSIS RESULTS

(continued)

False-positive for glucose

(continued)

Penicillin G in large doses (Benedict's test)

Phenazopyridine (Clinistix, Diastix, Tes-Tape)

Probenecid (Benedict's test, Clinitest tablets)

Salicylates in large doses (Clinitest tablets, Clinistix, Diastix, Tes-Tape)

Streptomycin (Benedict's test)

Tetracycline (Clinistix, Diastix, Tes-Tape)

Tetracyclines, due to ascorbic acid buffer (Benedict's test, Clinitest tablets)

Unasyn (ampicillin/sulbactam)

True glycosuria

Ammonium chloride

Asparaginase

Carbamazepine

Corticosteroids

Dextrothyroxine

Estrogens

Lithium carbonate

Nicotinic acid (large doses)

Phenothiazines (long-term)

Phenytoin

Thiazide diuretics

False-positive for ketones

Sulfobromophthalein

Isoniazid

Isopropanol

Levodopa (Ketostix, Labstix)

Phenazopyridine (Ketostix or Gerhardt's reagent strip shows atypical color)

Phenolsulfonphthalein (Rothera's test)

Phenothiazines (Gerhardt's reagent strip shows atypical color)

Salicylates (Gerhardt's reagent strip shows reddish color)

Sulfobromophthalein (Bili-Labstix)

True ketonuria

Ether (anesthesia)

Insulin (excessive doses)

Isoniazid (intoxication)

Isopropyl alcohol (intoxication)

Increased white blood cell count

Allopurinol

Ampicillin

Aspirin (toxicity)

Kanamycin

Methicillin

Hematuria

Aspirin

Bacitracin

Caffeine

Amphotericin B

Coumarin derivatives

Gold

Indomethacin

Methenamine in large doses

Methicillin

Para-aminosalicylic acid

Phenylbutazone

Sulfonamides

Casts

Amphotericin B

Aspirin (toxicity)

Bacitracin

Ethacrynic acid

Furosemide

Gentamicin

Griseofulvin

Isoniazid

Kanamycin

Neomycin

Penicillin

Radiographic agents

Streptomycin

Sulfonamides

Crystals in acidic urine

Acetazolamide

Aminosalicylic acid

Ascorbic acid

Nitrofurantoin

Theophylline

Thiazide diuretics

causing metabolic alkalosis. An acidic pH (below 7.0)—typical of a high-protein diet—causes turbidity and formation of oxalate, cystine, leucine, tyrosine, amorphous urate, and uric acid crystals.

Protein is normally absent from urine, but it may be present in a benign condition known as orthostatic (postural) proteinuria. Most common in patients age 10 to 20, it appears after prolonged standing and disappears after recumbency. Transient benign proteinuria can also accompany fever, exposure to cold, emotional stress, or strenuous exercise. Systemic diseases that may cause proteinuria include lymphoma, hepatitis, diabetes mellitus, toxemia, hypertension, lupus erythematosus, and febrile illnesses.

Sugars are usually absent from urine but may be present under normal conditions. The most common sugar in urine is glucose. Transient, nonpathologic glycosuria may result from emotional stress or pregnancy and may follow ingestion of a high-carbohydrate meal.

Centrifuged urine sediment contains cells, casts, crystals, bacteria, yeasts, and parasites. Red blood cells (RBCs) don't usually appear in urine without pathologic significance, but hard exercise can cause hematuria.

The following abnormal findings generally suggest pathologic conditions.

■ Color: Color change can result from diet, drugs, and many diseases.

■ Odor: In diabetes mellitus, starvation, and dehydration, a fruity odor indicates the presence of ketones. In urinary tract infections, a common fetid odor suggests *Escherichia coli*. Maple syrup urine disease and phenylketonuria also cause distinctive odors.

■ Turbidity: Turbid urine may contain RBCs or white blood cells (WBCs), bacteria, fat, or chyle; it may reflect renal infection.

■ Specific gravity: Low specific gravity (<1.005) is characteristic of diabetes insipidus, acute tubular necrosis, and pyelonephritis. Fixed specific gravity, in which values remain 1.010 regardless of fluid intake, occurs in chronic glomerulonephritis with severe renal damage. High specific gravity (>1.035) occurs in nephrotic syndrome, dehydration, acute glomerulonephritis, heart failure, liver failure, and shock.

■ pH: Alkaline urine may result from Fanconi's syndrome, urinary tract infection, or metabolic or respiratory alkalosis. Acidic urine is associated with renal tuberculosis, pyrexia, phenylketonuria, alkaptonuria, or acidosis.

■ Protein: Proteinuria may result from renal failure or disease (including nephrosis, glomerulosclerosis, glomerulonephritis, nephrolithiasis, and polycystic kidney disease) or, possibly, multiple myeloma.

■ Sugars: Glycosuria usually indicates diabetes mellitus but may result from pheochromocytoma, Cushing's syndrome, impaired tubular reabsorption, advanced renal disease, or increased intracranial pressure. I.V. solutions containing glucose and total parenteral nutrition containing from 10% to 50% glucose can cause glucose to spill over the renal threshold, leading to glycosuria. Lactosuria is a normal finding during pregnancy and lactation. Fructosuria, galactosuria, or pentosuria generally suggests a rare hereditary metabolic disorder, but pentosuria and fructosuria may follow excessive ingestion of pentose or fructose.

■ Ketones: Ketonuria occurs in diabetes mellitus when cellular energy needs exceed available cellular glucose. In the absence of glucose, cells metabolize fat for energy. Ketones—the end products of incomplete fat metabolism—accumulate in plasma and are excreted in the urine. Ketonuria may also occur during starvation, pregnancy, or lactation or after diarrhea or vomiting.

■ Bilirubin: Bilirubin in urine suggests obstructive jaundice, hepatotoxicity from drugs or toxins, or fibrosis of the biliary canaliculi (as in cirrhosis). Chlorpromazine can cause a false-positive result.

■ Urobilinogen: Bacteria in the duodenum metabolize bilirubin to urobilinogen, which the liver reprocesses into bile. Excessive urobilinogen in the urine suggests liver damage, hemolytic disease, or severe infection. Low levels suggest biliary obstruction, inflammatory disease, antimicrobial therapy, severe diarrhea, or renal insufficiency.

■ Cells: Hematuria indicates bleeding in the genitourinary tract, and it may be the only symptom of renal carcinoma. Other common causes of hematuria include infection, obstruction, inflammation, and a long list of other conditions. Strenuous exercise or exposure to toxic chemicals may also cause hematuria.

WBCs and white cell casts in urine suggest renal infection or inflammatory disease. A very high number of WBCs in urine usually implies urinary tract inflammation, especially cystitis or pyelonephritis. Numerous epithelial cells suggest renal tubular degeneration, which occurs in heavy metal poisoning, eclampsia, or kidney transplant rejection.

■ Casts: These plugs of high-molecular-weight mucoprotein form in the renal tubules and collecting ducts by agglutination of protein cells or cellular debris and are flushed loose by urine flow. Excessive casts indicate renal disease.

–Hyaline casts are associated with renal parenchymal disease, inflammation, and trauma to the glomerular capillary membrane

–epithelial casts, with renal tubular damage, nephrosis, eclampsia, amyloidosis, and heavy metal poisoning

–coarse and fine granular casts, with acute or chronic renal failure, pyelonephritis, and chronic lead intoxication

–fatty and waxy casts, with nephrotic syndrome, chronic renal disease, and diabetes mellitus

–RBC casts, with renal parenchymal disease (especially glomerulonephritis), renal infarction, subacute bacterial endocarditis, vascular disorders, sickle cell anemia, scurvy, blood dyscrasias, malignant hypertension, collagen disease, and acute inflammation

–WBC casts, with acute pyelonephritis and glomerulonephritis, nephrotic syndrome, pyogenic infection, and lupus nephritis.

■ Crystals: Some crystals are normally present

–numerous calcium oxalate crystals suggest hypercalcemia

–calcium carbonate, calcium phosphate, and magnesium phosphate crystals often form in alkaline urine

–xanthine, uric acid, urate, and cystine crystals are often present in acidic urine

–cystine crystals (cystinuria) reflect an inborn error of metabolism.

■ Other components: Bacteria, yeast cells, and parasites in urinary sediment reflect genitourinary tract infection or contamination of external genitalia. Yeast cells, which may be mistaken for RBCs, are identifiable by their ovoid shape, lack of color, variable size, and, frequently, signs of budding. The most common parasite in urinary sediment is *Trichomonas vaginalis*, which causes vaginitis, urethritis, and prostatovesiculitis.

Interfering factors

■ Strenuous exercise before routine urinalysis may cause transient myoglobulinuria, resulting in inaccurate test results.

■ Povidone-iodine washed into the urine will give a false-negative result for occult blood.

■ Many drugs influence the results of urinalysis.

■ Failure to follow the proper collection procedure, to send the specimen to the laboratory immediately, or to refrigerate the specimen may affect the accuracy of test results.

Urinary calculi test

Urinary calculi (commonly known as urinary stones) are insoluble substances that range in size from microscopic to several centimeters and may form anywhere in the urinary tract. Most calculi have well-defined nuclei — made of bacteria, fibrin, blood clots, or epithelial cells — enclosed in a protein matrix. Mineral salts accumulate around this core in layers.

Calculi commonly form in the kidney, pass into the ureter, and are excreted in the urine. Because not all calculi pass spontaneously, they may require surgical extraction. Calculi don't always cause symptoms, but when they do, hematuria is most common. If calculi obstruct the ureter, they may cause severe flank pain, dysuria, urine retention, urinary frequency, and urinary urgency.

Purpose

To detect and identify calculi in the urine.

Patient preparation

Explain to the patient that the test detects urinary stones and that, if such stones are found, laboratory analysis will reveal their composition. Tell him the test requires that all of his urine be collected and strained. Advise him that he needn't restrict food or fluids before the test. Reassure him that symptoms will subside immediately after any stones are excreted. Administer medication to control pain, as ordered.

Equipment

Strainer (unfolded 4″ x 4″ dressing or fine-mesh sieve) ■ specimen container.

Procedure

■ After the patient voids into the strainer, inspect the strainer carefully because calculi may be minute. Calculi may look like gravel or sand. Document the appearance of the calculi and the number, if possible. Then place the calculi in a properly labeled container and send the container to the laboratory immediately for prompt analysis.

■ Observe for severe flank pain, dysuria, urine retention, urinary frequency, or urinary urgency. Hematuria should subside after passage of the stone.

Precautions

If the patient has received analgesics, be sure to keep the strainer and urinal or bedpan within his reach because he may be drowsy and unable to get out of bed to void.

Normal findings

Calculi aren't normally present in the urine.

TYPES AND CAUSES OF CALCULI

A
Calcium oxalate calculi usually result from idiopathic hypercalciuria, a condition that reflects absorption of calcium from the bowel.

B
Calcium phosphate calculi usually result from primary hyperparathyroidism, which causes excessive resorption of calcium from bone.

C
Cystine calculi result from primary cystinuria, an inborn error of metabolism that prevents renal tubular reabsorption of cystine.

D
Urate calculi result from gout, dehydration (causing elevated uric acid levels), acidic urine, or hepatic dysfunction.

E
Magnesium ammonium phosphate calculi result from the presence of urea-splitting organisms, such as *Proteus*, which raises ammonia concentration and makes urine alkaline.

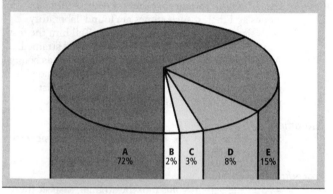

Implications of results

More than half of all calculi in urine are of mixed composition, containing two or more mineral salts; calcium oxalate is the most common component. Determining the composition of calculi helps identify various metabolic disorders. (See *Types and causes of calculi.*)

Posttest care

- Inform the patient of dietary restrictions intended to prevent formation of calculi.
- Teach the patient that increasing mobility, if allowed, may help decrease the incidence of calculi.
- Teach the importance of increasing fluid intake to 3,000 to 4,000 ml per day, unless contraindicated.
- Teach the importance of continuing medications such as allopurinol for gout.
- Teach the patient how to monitor urine pH.

Interfering factors

None reported.

Urine 17-hydroxycorticosteroid test

This test measures urine levels of 17-hydroxycortico-steroids (17-OHCS)—metabolites of the hormones that regulate glyconeogenesis. More than 80% of all urinary 17-OHCS are metabolites of cortisol, the primary adrenocortical steroid. Test findings thus reflect cortisol secretion and, indirectly, adrenocortical function.

Because cortisol secretion varies diurnally and in response to stress and many other factors, urine 17-OHCS levels are most accurately determined from a 24-hour specimen. Plasma cortisol, urine free cortisol, and urine 17-ketosteroids may be measured, and the corticotropin stimulation and suppression test may confirm the results of this test.

Purpose

To assess adrenocortical function.

Patient preparation

Explain to the patient that this test evaluates how his adrenal glands are functioning. Inform him that he needn't restrict food or fluids but should avoid excessive physical exercise and stressful situations during the testing period. Tell him the test requires collection of a 24-hour urine specimen, and teach him the proper collection technique.

Check the patient's medication history for drugs that may affect 17-OHCS levels. Review your findings with the laboratory and notify the doctor, who may restrict medications before the test.

Procedure

Collect a 24-hour urine specimen in a bottle containing a preservative to prevent deterioration of the specimen.

Precautions

Refrigerate the specimen or place it on ice during the collection period.

Reference values

- Males: 4.5 to 12 mg/24 hours
- Females: 2.5 to 10 mg/24 hours
- Children age 8 to 12: 4.5 mg/24 hours
- Children under age 8: 1.5 mg/24 hours

Levels normally rise slightly during the first trimester of pregnancy. Patients who are obese or very muscular may excrete slightly higher amounts of 17-OHCS because of increased cortisol catabolism.

Implications of results

Elevated urine 17-OHCS levels suggest Cushing's syndrome, adrenal carcinoma or adenoma, or pituitary tumor. Values may also be high in patients with virilism, hyperthyroidism, or severe hypertension. Extreme stress induced by such conditions as acute pancreatitis and eclampsia also increases urine 17-OHCS levels.

Low urine 17-OHCS levels suggest Addison's disease, hypopituitarism, or myxedema.

Posttest care

■ Tell the patient that he may resume activities restricted during the test.

■ As ordered, resume administration of any medications withheld before the test.

Interfering factors

■ The following drugs may elevate urine 17-OHCS levels: meprobamate, phenothiazines, spironolactone, ascorbic acid, chloral hydrate, colchicine, erythromycin, paraldehyde, glutethimide, chlordiazepoxide, penicillin G, hydroxyzine, quinidine, quinine, iodides, and methenamine.

■ The following drugs may suppress urine 17-OHCS levels: estrogens, oral contraceptives, phenothiazines, hydralazine, phenytoin, thiazide diuretics, nalidixic acid, and reserpine.

■ Failure to follow drug restrictions, to collect all urine during the test period, or to store the specimen properly may interfere with test results.

Urine 17-ketogenic steroid test

This test measures urine levels of 17-ketogenic steroids (17-KGS), which consist of the 17-hydroxycorticosteroids—such as cortisol and its metabolites—and other adrenocortical steroids, such as pregnanetriol, that can be oxidized in the laboratory to 17-ketosteroids.

Because 17-KGS represent such a large group of steroids, this test provides an excellent overall assessment of adrenocortical function. For accurate diagnosis of specific disease, abnormal 17-KGS must be evaluated in the context of other test results, including plasma corticotropin, plasma cortisol, corticotropin stimulation, single-dose metyrapone, and dexamethasone suppression.

Purpose

■ To evaluate adrenocortical function

■ To aid diagnosis of Cushing's syndrome and Addison's disease.

Patient preparation

Explain to the patient that this test evaluates adrenal function. Inform him that he needn't restrict food or fluids before the test but should avoid excessive physical exercise and stressful situations during the collection period. Tell him the test requires 24-hour urine collection, and teach him how to collect the specimen correctly.

Check the medication history for drugs that may affect 17-KGS levels. Review your findings with the laboratory, and notify the doctor, who may want to withhold such medications before the test.

Procedure

Collect a 24-hour urine specimen in a bottle containing a preservative to keep the specimen at a pH of 4.0 to 4.5.

Precautions

Refrigerate the specimen or keep it on ice during the collection period. Send the specimen to the laboratory as soon as the collection is completed.

Reference values

- Men: 4 to 14 mg/24 hours
- Women: 2 to 12 mg/24 hours
- Children age 11 to 14: 2 to 9 mg/24 hours
- Younger children and infants: 0.1 to 4.0 mg/24 hours

Implications of results

Elevated 17-KGS levels reflect hyperadrenalism, as in Cushing's syndrome; some cases of adrenogenital syndrome (congenital adrenal hyperplasia); and adrenal carcinoma or adenoma. Levels also rise with severe physical or emotional stress.

Low levels may reflect hypoadrenalism, as in Addison's disease, as well as panhypopituitarism, cretinism, and general wasting.

Posttest care

- Tell the patient that he may resume activities restricted before the test.
- As ordered, resume administration of drugs withheld before the test.

Interfering factors

- Urine 17-KGS levels may be elevated by corticotropin therapy and by such drugs as meprobamate, phenothiazines, spironolactone, penicillin, oleandomycin, and hydralazine.

17-KS FRACTIONATION VALUES

Through gas-liquid chromatography, the 17-ketosteroid (17-KS) fractionation test shows which specific steroids in the 17-KS group are elevated or suppressed and thus aids differential diagnosis of conditions characterized by abnormal 17-KS levels. All values in the chart below are expressed in number of milligrams per 24 hours.

Steroid	Adult males	Adult females
Androsterone	2.2 to 5.0	0.5 to 2.4
Dehydroepiandrosterone	0 to 2.3	0 to 1.2
Etiocholanolone	1.9 to 4.7	1.1 to 3.0
11-Hydroxyandrosterone	0.5 to 1.3	0.2 to 0.6
11-Hydroxyetiocholanolone	0.3 to 0.7	0.2 to 0.6
11-Ketoandrosterone	0 to 0.1	0 to 0.2
11-Ketoetiocholanolone	0.2 to 0.7	0.2 to 0.6
Pregnanediol	0.6 to 1.6	0.2 to 2.4
Pregnanetriol	0.6 to 1.3	0.1 to 1.0
5-Pregnanetriol	0 to 0.3	0 to 0.3
11-Ketopregnanetriol	0 to 0.2	0 to 0.4

■ Levels may be suppressed by estrogens, quinine, reserpine, thiazide diuretics, and long-term corticosteroid therapy.
■ Nalidixic acid and dexamethasone may elevate or suppress urine 17-KGS levels.
■ Failure to observe drug restrictions, to collect all urine, or to store the specimen properly may alter test results.

Urine 17-ketosteroid test

This test measure urine levels of 17-ketosteroids (17-KS). These steroids and their metabolites are characterized by a ketone group on carbon 17 in the steroid nucleus. They originate primarily in the adrenal glands but also in the testes (which produce one-third of 17-KS in males) and the ovaries (which produce a minimal amount of 17-KS in females).

Although not all 17-KS are androgens, all cause androgenic effects. For example, excessive secretion of 17-KS may cause hirsutism and increased clitoral or phallic size; in utero, elevated 17-KS levels may cause a female fetus to develop a male urogenital tract.

Because 17-KS don't include all the androgens (such as testosterone, the most potent androgen), this test provides only a rough estimate of androgenic activity. To provide more information about androgen secretion,

Males age 10 to 15	Females age 10 to 15	Both sexes age 0 to 9
0.2 to 2.0	0.2 to 2.5	≤1
<0.4	<0.4	<0.2
0.1 to 1.6	0.7 to 3.1	≤1
0.1 to 1.1	0.2 to 1.0	≤1
<0.3	0.1 to 0.5	≤0.5
<0.1	<0.1	<0.1
0.2 to 0.6	0.1 to 0.6	≤0.7
0.1 to 0.7	0.1 to 1.2	<0.5
0.2 to 0.6	0.1 to 0.6	<0.3
<0.3	<0.3	<0.2
<0.3	<0.2	<0.2

plasma testosterone and 17-KS fractionation tests may be performed. (See *17-KS fractionation values.*)

Purpose

■ To aid diagnosis of adrenal and gonadal dysfunction
■ To aid diagnosis of adrenogenital syndrome (congenital adrenal hyperplasia)
■ To monitor cortisol therapy in the treatment of adrenogenital syndrome.

Patient preparation

Explain to the patient that this test evaluates hormonal balance. Inform him that he needn't restrict food or fluids before the test but should avoid excessive physical exercise and stressful situations during the collection period. Tell him the test requires 24-hour urine collection, and instruct him in the proper collection technique.

If the female patient is menstruating, urine collection may have to be postponed because blood in the specimen interferes with test findings.

Check the patient's medication history for drugs that may affect test results. Review your findings with the laboratory and notify the doctor, who may want to restrict such drugs before the test.

Procedure

Collect a 24-hour urine specimen in a bottle containing a preservative to keep the specimen at a pH of 4.0 to 4.5.

Precautions

Refrigerate the specimen or place it on ice during the collection period. Send the specimen to the laboratory as soon as the collection is completed.

Reference values

- Men: 6 to 21 mg/24 hours
- Women: 4 to 17 mg/24 hours
- Children age 11 to 14: 2 to 7 mg/24 hours
- Younger children and infants: 0.1 to 3 mg/24 hours

Implications of results

Elevated urine 17-KS levels may result from adrenal hyperplasia, carcinoma or adenoma, or adrenogenital syndrome. In women, elevated levels may also indicate ovarian dysfunction (such as polycystic ovarian disease [Stein-Leventhal syndrome] or lutein cell tumor of the ovary) or androgenic arrhenoblastoma. In men, elevated 17-KS levels may indicate interstitial cell tumor of the testis. Characteristically, 17-KS levels also rise during pregnancy, severe stress, chronic illness, or debilitating disease.

Depressed urine 17-KS levels may result from Addison's disease, panhypopituitarism, eunuchoidism, or castration and may occur in cretinism, myxedema, and nephrosis. When this test is used to monitor cortisol therapy for adrenogenital syndrome, 17-KS levels typically return to normal with adequate therapy.

Posttest care

- Tell the patient that he may resume activities restricted during the test.
- As ordered, resume administration of medications withheld before the test.

Interfering factors

- Meprobamate, phenothiazines, spironolactone, spironolactone, and oleandomycin may elevate urine 17-KS levels. Corticotropin, antibiotics, and dexamethasone may also elevate levels.
- Estrogens, penicillin, ethacrynic acid, and phenytoin may suppress 17-KS levels.
- Nalidixic acid and quinine may elevate or suppress 17-KS levels.
- Failure to observe drug restrictions, to collect all urine, or to store the specimen properly may affect test results.

Urine 5-hydroxyindoleacetic acid test

This test measures urine levels of 5-hydroxyindoleacetic acid (5-HIAA) and is used mainly to screen for carcinoid tumors (argentaffinomas). Urine 5-HIAA levels reflect plasma concentrations of serotonin (5-hydroxytryptamine). This powerful vasopressor is produced by argentaffin cells, primarily in the intestinal mucosa, and is metabolized to 5-HIAA.

Carcinoid tumors, found generally in the intestine or appendix, secrete an excessive amount of serotonin, which is reflected by high 5-HIAA levels. A 24-hour urine specimen can detect small or intermittently secreting carcinoid tumors.

Purpose

To aid diagnosis of carcinoid tumors.

Patient preparation

Explain to the patient what serotonin is and why this test is important. Instruct him not to eat foods containing serotonin, such as bananas, plums, pineapples, avocados, eggplants, tomatoes, and walnuts, for 4 days before the test. Tell him the test requires collection of a 24-hour urine specimen, and teach him the proper collection technique.

Check the patient's medication history for recent use of drugs that may affect test results. Review your findings with the laboratory, and notify the doctor, who may want to withhold these drugs before the test.

Procedure

Collect a 24-hour urine specimen in a bottle containing a preservative to keep the specimen at a pH of 2.0 to 4.0.

Precautions

Refrigerate the specimen or keep it on ice during the collection period. Send the specimen to the laboratory as soon as the collection is completed.

Reference values

The normal urine 5-HIAA value is less than 6 mg/24 hours.

Implications of results

Markedly elevated urine 5-HIAA levels, possibly as high as 200 to 600 mg/24 hours, are diagnostic of a carcinoid tumor. However, because these tumors vary in their capacity to store and secrete serotonin, some patients with carcinoid syndrome (metastatic carcinoid tumors) may not have elevated levels. Repeated testing is often necessary.

Posttest care

- As ordered, resume administration of medications withheld before the test.
- Tell the patient that he may resume his normal diet.

Interfering factors

- Melphalan, reserpine, fluorouracil, and methamphetamine raise urine 5-HIAA levels.
- Ethanol, tricyclic antidepressants, monoamine oxidase inhibitors, methyldopa, and isoniazid usually lower urine 5-HIAA levels.
- Methenamine compounds, phenothiazines, salicylates, guaifenesin, methamphetamine, methocarbamol, and acetaminophen may raise or lower 5-HIAA levels.
- Failure to observe drug and dietary restrictions, to collect all urine during the test period, or to store the specimen properly may affect test results.
- Severe GI disturbance or diarrhea may affect test results.

Urine culture

Laboratory examination and culture of urine are necessary to evaluate urinary tract infections (UTIs) — most commonly bladder infections. Although urine in the kidneys and bladder is normally sterile, a small number of bacteria are usually present in the urethra and, consequently, may pass into the urine. Nevertheless, bacteriuria generally results from prevalence of a single type of bacteria. Indeed, the presence of more than two distinct bacterial species in a urine specimen strongly suggests contamination during collection. However, a single negative culture doesn't always rule out infection, as in chronic, low-grade pyelonephritis. Urine cultures also identify pathogenic fungi, such as *Coccidioides immitis*. (See *Culture sites for common pathogenic fungi.*)

Many laboratories perform a quick and easy screen on urine submitted for culture. A common screening test used is the leukocyte esterase-nitrate dipstick. The purpose of the screen is to determine if bacteria or white blood cell (WBC) counts are high. Only the urine with bacteria or WBCs is processed for culture; urine that doesn't contain either of these is classified as negative by urine screen.

Significant results of urine culture are possible only after quantitative examination. To distinguish between true bacteriuria and contamination, it's necessary to know the number of organisms in a milliliter of urine,

CULTURE SITES FOR COMMON PATHOGENIC FUNGI

Organism	Culture sites
Aspergillus species*	Skin, respiratory secretions, nasal sinuses, ear, gastric washings
*Blastomyces dermatitidis**	Respiratory secretions, skin, oropharyngeal ulcer, bone, prostate
Candida species*	Mucous membranes, skin, gastric washings, blood, stool, sputum, body fluids, bone
Cladosporium species*	Respiratory exudates, skin, nails, nose, cornea
*Coccidioides immitis**	Sputum, skin, cerebrospinal fluid (CSF), joint fluid, urine
*Cryptococcus neoformans**	Respiratory tract, CSF, blood, urine, cornea, ocular orbit, vitreous humor
Epidermophyton floccosum	Skin, nails
*Histoplasma capsulatum**	Sputum, blood, CSF, pleural fluid, vaginal secretions, larynx
Microsporum species	Skin, hair
Mucor species	Wound specimens, sputum, ear, cornea, vitreous humor, stool
Paracoccidioides brasiliensis	Mucous membrane lesions, including those of the nose, gingiva and, less commonly, conjunctiva
Penicillium species	Bronchial washings, skin, ear, cornea, urine
Pseudallescheria boydii	Sputum, skin, cornea, gastric washings
*Sporothrix schenckii**	Sputum, skin, joint fluid, CSF, ear, conjunctiva, maxillary sinuses
Trichophyton species	Skin, hair, nails
Zygomycetes species (not *Mucor*)	Nasal mucosa, palate, sinuses, lung fluid, GI tract

* Serum tests are available for these fungi.

estimated by a culture technique known as a "colony count." In addition, a quick centrifugation test can determine where a UTI originates. (See *Quick centrifugation test*, page 628.)

Clean-catch specimen collection, rather than suprapubic aspiration or catheterization, is now the method of choice for obtaining a urine specimen.

Purpose

■ To diagnose UTI
■ To monitor microorganism colonization after urinary catheter insertion.

QUICK CENTRIFUGATION TEST

This test can determine whether the source of a urinary tract infection (UTI) is in the lower tract (bladder) or the upper tract (kidneys). The test involves centrifugation of urine in a test tube, followed by staining of the sediment with fluorescein. If at least one-fourth of the bacteria fluoresce when viewed under a fluorescent microscope, an upper tract UTI is present; if bacteria don't fluoresce, a lower tract UTI is present.

Patient preparation

Explain to the patient that this test helps detect UTI. Advise him that it requires a urine specimen and that he needn't restrict food or fluids. Teach him how to collect a clean-catch specimen, and emphasize the importance of cleaning the external genitalia thoroughly. Or, if appropriate, explain catheterization or suprapubic aspiration to the patient, and inform him that he may experience some discomfort during specimen collection.

Tell the patient with suspected urogenital tuberculosis that specimen collection may be required on three consecutive mornings. Check the patient history for current use of antimicrobial drugs.

Equipment

Gloves ■ sterile specimen cup ■ premoistened, antiseptic towelettes. Commercial clean-catch urine kits are available; many include instructions in several languages.

Procedure

■ Collect a urine specimen as ordered. Record the suspected diagnosis, the collection time and method, current antimicrobial therapy, and fluid- or drug-induced diuresis on the laboratory request.
■ No specific post-test care is necessary.

Precautions

■ Use gloves when performing the procedure and handling specimens.
■ Collect at least 3 ml of urine, but don't fill the specimen cup more than halfway.
■ Seal the cup with a sterile lid and send it to the laboratory at once. If transport is delayed for more than 30 minutes, store the specimen at 39.2° F (4° C) or place it on ice, unless a urine transport tube containing preservative is used.

Normal findings

Culture results of sterile urine are normally reported as "no growth," which usually indicates the absence of UTI.

Implications of results

Bacterial counts of 100,000 or more organisms of a single microbe species per milliliter indicate probable UTI. Counts under 100,000/ml may be significant, depending on the patient's age, sex, history, and other individual factors; however, they usually suggest contamination, except in symptomatic patients or those with urologic disorders. All growths from catheterized urine or suprapubic aspirations are considered significant and mandate susceptibility tests to identify the causative organism. A special test for acid-fast bacteria can isolate *Mycobacterium tuberculosis*, thus diagnosing tuberculosis of the urinary tract.

Isolation of more than two species of organisms or of vaginal or skin organisms usually suggests contamination and requires a repeat culture. Prolonged catheterization or urinary diversion may cause polymicrobial infection.

Posttest care

As ordered, resume administration of medications withheld before the test.

Interfering factors

■ Fluid- or drug-induced diuresis and antimicrobial therapy may lower bacterial counts.
■ Improper collection technique may contaminate the specimen.
■ Improper preservation or delays in sending the specimen to the laboratory may lead to inaccurate counts.

Urobilinogen test, fecal

Urobilinogen, the end product of bilirubin metabolism, is a brown pigment formed by bacterial enzymes in the small intestine. It's excreted in feces or reabsorbed into portal blood, where it's returned to the liver and re-excreted in bile; a small amount of urobilinogen is excreted in urine. Because bilirubin metabolism depends on a properly functioning hepatobiliary system and a normal erythrocyte life span, measurement of fecal urobilinogen is a useful indicator of hepatobiliary and hemolytic disorders. However, this test is rarely performed because serum bilirubin and urine urobilinogen can be measured more easily.

Purpose

To aid diagnosis of hepatobiliary and hemolytic disorders.

Patient preparation

Explain to the patient that this test evaluates the function of the liver and bile ducts or detects red blood cell disorders. Inform him that he needn't restrict food or fluids before the test. Tell him the test requires collection of a random stool specimen.

Withhold broad-spectrum antibiotics, sulfonamides, and salicylates for 2 weeks before the test, as ordered. If these medications must be continued, note this on the laboratory request.

Procedure

Collect a random stool specimen.

Precautions

- Tell the patient not to contaminate the stool specimen with toilet tissue or urine.
- Use a light-resistant collection container because urobilinogen breaks down to urobilin on exposure to light.
- Send the specimen to the laboratory immediately. If transport or testing is delayed more than 30 minutes, refrigerate the specimen; if testing is being performed by an outside laboratory, freeze the specimen.

Reference values

Normally, fecal urobilinogen values range from 50 to 300 mg/24 hours.

Implications of results

Low levels or absence of urobilinogen in the feces indicates obstructed bile flow, which may result from intrahepatic disorders (such as hepatocellular jaundice caused by cirrhosis or hepatitis), extrahepatic disorders (such as tumor of the head of the pancreas, the ampulla of Vater, or the bile duct), or choledocholithiasis. Low fecal urobilinogen levels are also characteristic of depressed erythropoiesis, as occurs in aplastic anemia.

Posttest care

Resume administration of medications withheld before the test, as ordered.

Interfering factors

- Broad-spectrum antibiotics can depress fecal urobilinogen levels by inhibiting bacterial growth in the colon.
- Sulfonamides, which react with the reagent used by the laboratory in this test, and large doses of salicylates can raise fecal urobilinogen levels.

■ Failure to use a light-resistant collection container or contamination of the specimen will affect the accuracy of test results.

Urobilinogen test, urine

This test detects impaired liver function by measuring urine levels of urobilinogen, the colorless, water-soluble product that results from the reduction of bilirubin by intestinal bacteria. Up to 50% of intestinal urobilinogen returns to the liver, where some of it is resecreted into bile and, eventually, into the intestine through enterohepatic circulation. Small amounts of the reabsorbed urobilinogen also enter the general circulation and are ultimately excreted in the urine (urobilinogenuria).

Purpose

■ To aid diagnosis of extrahepatic obstruction, such as blockage of the common bile duct
■ To aid differential diagnosis of hepatic and hematologic disorders.

Patient preparation

Explain to the patient that this test helps assess liver and biliary tract function. Inform him that he needn't restrict food or fluids, except for bananas, which he should avoid for 48 hours before the test. Tell him that the test may require a random specimen or a 2-hour urine specimen, and teach him how to collect the specimen.

Check the patient's history for drugs that may affect urine urobilinogen levels. Review your findings with the laboratory and the doctor, who may restrict such drugs before the test.

Procedure

■ Most laboratories request a random urine specimen; others prefer a 2-hour specimen, usually during the afternoon (ideally, between 1 p.m. and 3 p.m.), when urobilinogen levels peak. (See *Random specimen test for urobilinogen*, page 632.)
■ As ordered, resume administration of drugs restricted before the test.
■ Tell the patient he may resume his usual diet.

Precautions

Send the specimen to the laboratory immediately. This test must be performed within 30 minutes of collection because urobilinogen quickly oxidizes to an orange compound called urobilin.

RANDOM SPECIMEN TEST FOR UROBILINOGEN

Quantitative tests for urinary urobilinogen excretion can be performed with reagent strips, such as Bili-Labstix or N-Multistix (dip-and-read test).

To perform such tests, collect a clean-catch urine specimen in a clean, dry container—preferably in the afternoon, when urine urobilinogen levels peak—and test the specimen immediately. A fresh urine specimen is essential for reliable results because urobilinogen is unstable when exposed to room temperature and light.

Dip the strip into the urine, and as you remove it, start timing the reaction. Carefully remove excess urine by tapping the edge of the strip against the container or a clean, dry surface to prevent color changes along the edge of the test area. When using N-Multistix (or a similar product for multiple testing), hold the strip in a horizontal position to prevent mixing of chemicals from adjacent reagent areas. Place the strip near the color block on the bottle and carefully compare the colors. Read the results at 45 seconds. The color results correspond to the number of Ehrlich units per deciliter of urine, as shown below.

Normally, a random specimen contains a small amount of urobilinogen. This test cannot establish the absence of urobilinogen in the specimen being tested.

Para-aminosalicylic acid may cause unreliable results with this reagent strip test. Drugs containing azo dyes, such as Azo Gantrisin (sulfisoxazole/phenazopyridine), mask test results by causing a golden color.

Color	Value (Ehrlich units/dl)
Yellow-green to yellow (normal)	0.1 to 1
Yellow-orange (positive)	2
Medium yellow-orange (positive)	4
Light brown-orange (positive)	8
Brown-orange (positive)	12

Reference values

Normal urine urobilinogen values in women: 0.1 to 1.1 Ehrlich units/2 hours; in men: 0.3 to 2.1 Ehrlich units/2 hours.

Implications of results

Absence of urine urobilinogen may reflect complete obstructive jaundice or treatment with broad-spectrum antibiotics, which destroy the intestinal flora. Low levels may reflect congenital enzymatic jaundice (hyperbilirubinemia syndromes) or treatment with drugs that acidify urine, such as ammonium chloride or ascorbic acid.

Elevated levels may indicate hemolytic jaundice, hepatitis, or cirrhosis.

Posttest care

Resume administration of medications withheld before the test, as ordered.

Interfering factors

■ Bananas eaten up to 48 hours before the test may raise urobilinogen levels.

■ The following drugs affect the test reagent and may affect the accuracy of test results: para-aminosalicylic acid, phenazopyridine, procaine, mandelate, phenothiazines, and sulfonamides.

■ Highly alkaline urine, which may be caused by acetazolamide or sodium bicarbonate, may elevate urobilinogen levels.

Urogenital secretions test for trichomonads

Microscopic examination of urine or vaginal, urethral, or prostatic secretions can detect urogenital infection by *Trichomonas vaginalis* — a parasitic, flagellate protozoan that's usually transmitted sexually. This test is performed more often on females than on males because more females exhibit symptoms. Males with trichomoniasis may have symptoms of urethritis or prostatitis.

Purpose

To confirm trichomoniasis.

Patient preparation

Explain that this test can identify the cause of urogenital infection. Tell the female patient that it requires a specimen of vaginal secretion or urethral discharge and that she shouldn't douche before the test. Tell the male patient that a specimen of urethral or prostatic secretion is required. Inform the patient who will perform the procedure and when.

Equipment

Gloves ■ cotton swab ■ test tube containing a small amount of normal saline solution (.9% normal saline solution) ■ vaginal speculum ■ specimen cup (for urine specimen).

Procedure

■ Vaginal secretion: With the patient in the lithotomy position, insert an unlubricated vaginal speculum and collect the discharge with a cotton swab. Then place the swab in the tube containing normal saline solution, and remove the speculum. Another method is to smear the specimen on a glass slide, allow it to air dry, and then transport it to the laboratory.

■ Prostatic material: After prostatic massage, collect secretions with a cotton swab, and place the swab in normal saline solution.

■ Urethral discharge: Collect the discharge with a cotton swab, and place the swab in normal saline solution.
■ Urine: Include the first portion of a voided random specimen (not midstream).
■ Label the specimen appropriately, including the date and time of collection.
■ Provide perineal care.

Precautions

■ Remember to use gloves when performing procedures and handling specimens.
■ If possible, obtain the urogenital specimen before treatment with a trichomonacide begins.
■ Send the specimen to the laboratory immediately because trichomonads can be identified only while still motile.

Normal findings

Trichomonads are normally absent from the urogenital tract. In approximately 25% of females and most infected males, trichomonads may be present without associated pathology.

Implications of results

The presence of trichomonads confirms trichomoniasis.

Interfering factors

■ Collection of the specimen after trichomonacide therapy begins decreases the number of parasites in the specimen.
■ Failure to send the specimen to the laboratory immediately causes trichomonads to lose their motility.
■ Improper collection technique may interfere with detection.

Uroporphyrinogen I synthase test

This test measures blood levels of uroporphyrinogen I synthase, an enzyme that converts porphobilinogen to uroporphyrinogen during heme biosynthesis. This enzyme (also known as uroporphyrinogen I synthetase and porphobilinogen deaminase) is normally present in erythrocytes, fibroblasts, lymphocytes, liver cells, and amniotic fluid cells. However, a hereditary deficiency can reduce uroporphyrinogen I synthase levels by 50% or more, resulting in acute intermittent porphyria (AIP). An autosomal dominant disorder of heme biosynthesis, AIP can be latent indefinitely, until certain factors (some sex hormones and drugs, a low-carbohydrate diet, or an infection) precipitate active disease.

An improvement over traditional urine tests, which can detect AIP only during an acute episode, the uroporphyrinogen I synthase test can detect AIP even during its latent phase. Thus, it can identify affected persons before their first acute episode. Because it's specific for AIP, this test can also differentiate AIP from other types of porphyria.

Purpose

To aid diagnosis of latent or active AIP.

Patient preparation

Explain to the patient that this test helps detect a red blood cell disorder. Inform him that he'll need to fast for 12 to 14 hours before the test and to abstain from alcohol for 24 hours, but that he may drink water. Tell him that the test requires a blood sample, who will perform the venipuncture and when, and that he may experience slight discomfort from the needle puncture and the pressure of the tourniquet.

If the patient's hematocrit is available, record this on the laboratory request. Check the patient's history for any medications that may decrease enzyme levels, and withhold them as ordered. If they must be continued, note this on the laboratory request.

Procedure

Perform a venipuncture and collect the sample in a 10-ml heparinized tube.

Precautions

- Handle the sample gently.
- Send the specimen, on ice, to the laboratory immediately.

Reference values

Normal values for this enzyme are greater than or equal to 7 nmol/sec/L.

Implications of results

Low levels usually indicate latent or active AIP; symptoms differentiate these phases. Levels below 6 nmol/sec/L confirm AIP; levels from 6 to 6.9 nmol/sec/L are indeterminate. When levels are indeterminate, urine and stool tests for the porphyrin precursors ALA and porphobilinogen may be ordered.

Posttest care

- If a hematoma develops at the venipuncture site, apply warm soaks.
- As ordered, instruct the patient to resume his usual diet and medications.

Interfering factors

■ Failure to fast before the test may increase enzyme levels.

■ Hemolytic and hepatic diseases may elevate uroporphyrinogen I synthase levels.

■ Hemolysis caused by rough handling of the sample may alter test results.

■ Failure to freeze the sample will cause false-positive results.

■ A low-carbohydrate diet, alcohol, infection, and use of the certain drugs (such as steroid hormones, estrogens, barbiturates, sulfonamides, phenytoin, griseofulvin, chlordiazepoxide, meprobamate, glutethimide, and ergot) may decrease enzyme levels.

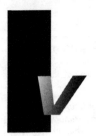

Vanillylmandelic acid test, urine

This test measures urine levels of vanillylmandelic acid (VMA), the most prevalent catecholamine metabolite in the urine. It is the product of hepatic conversion of epinephrine and norepinephrine; urine VMA levels reflect endogenous production of these major catecholamines.

Like the test for urine total catecholamines, this test helps detect catecholamine-secreting tumors — especially pheochromocytoma — and helps evaluate the function of the adrenal medulla, the primary site of catecholamine production. A 24-hour urine specimen is preferred over a random specimen to overcome the effects of diurnal variations in catecholamine secretion. Other catecholamine metabolites — metanephrine, normetanephrine, and homovanillic acid (HVA) — may be measured at the same time. (See *Urinary metabolite values in pheochromocytoma*, page 638.)

Purpose

■ To help detect pheochromocytoma, neuroblastoma, and ganglioneuroma
■ To evaluate the function of the adrenal medulla.

Patient preparation

Explain to the patient that this test evaluates hormone secretion. Instruct him to restrict foods and beverages containing phenolic acid, such as coffee, tea, colas, bananas, citrus fruits, chocolate, and vanilla, for 3 days before the test and to avoid stressful situations and strenuous physical activity during the urine collection period. Tell him the test requires collection of a 24-hour urine specimen, and teach him the proper collection technique.

Check the patient's medication history for drugs that may affect test results. Review your findings with the laboratory, and notify the doctor, who may want to restrict these drugs before the test.

Procedure

Collect a 24-hour urine specimen in a bottle containing a preservative to keep the specimen at a pH of 3.0.

URINARY METABOLITE VALUES IN PHEOCHROMOCYTOMA

Metabolite levels in urine increase in patients with pheochromocytoma, as shown below.

Metabolite	Normal excretion rate (mg/24 hours)	Usual range in pheochromocytoma (mg/24 hours)
Free catecholamines	<0.1	0.2 to 4
Metanephrine and normetanephrine	<1.3	2.5 to 40
Vanillylmandelic acid	<6.8	10 to 250

Precautions

Refrigerate the specimen or keep it on ice during the collection period. Send the specimen to the laboratory as soon as the collection is completed.

Reference values

Normal urine VMA values are 0.7 to 6.8 mg/24 hours.

Implications of results

Elevated urine VMA levels may result from a catecholamine-secreting tumor. Further testing, such as measurement of urine HVA levels to rule out pheochromocytoma, is necessary for a precise diagnosis. (See *Diagnosing catecholamine-secreting tumors*.) If a pheochromocytoma is confirmed, the patient may be tested for multiple endocrine neoplasia, an inherited condition commonly associated with pheochromocytoma. (Family members of a patient with confirmed pheochromocytoma should also be carefully evaluated for multiple endocrine neoplasia.)

Posttest care

■ As ordered, resume administration of medications withheld before the test.
■ Tell the patient that he may resume his normal diet and activities.

Interfering factors

■ Excessive physical exercise or emotional stress may raise VMA levels.
■ Epinephrine, norepinephrine, lithium carbonate, and methocarbamol may raise urine VMA levels. Chlorpromazine, guanethidine, reserpine, monoamine oxidase inhibitors, and clonidine may lower VMA levels. Levodopa and salicylates may raise or lower them.

DIAGNOSING CATECHOLAMINE-SECRETING TUMORS

Although a pheochromocytoma is a catecholamine-producing tumor of the adrenal medulla, not every patient with this disorder has elevated urine catecholamine (epinephrine and norepinephrine) levels. Moreover, hypertension, a prime clue in this condition, is sometimes absent. Thus, an analysis of one or more catecholamine metabolites is helpful in confirming the diagnosis.

When catecholamine levels remain normal in the presence of hypertension, elevated vanillylmandelic acid (VMA) levels may signal a tumor. Or, metanephrine may be high when VMA and catecholamines are essentially unchanged. VMA assay is also an alternative method when catecholamine analysis has been compromised by interfering food or drugs. Increased excretion of homovanillic acid (HVA) typically indicates malignant pheochromocytoma, although the incidence of malignancy is very low.

Measurement of urine VMA is also useful for diagnosing two neurogenic tumors—neuroblastoma, a common soft-tissue tumor that's a leading cause of death in infants and young children, and ganglioneuroma, a well-defined tumor of the sympathetic nervous system that occurs in older children and young adults. Both tumors primarily produce dopamine and thus show the expected high readings of dopamine's metabolite, HVA, especially in their malignant forms. But both tumors also show abnormal increases in urine VMA levels.

■ Failure to observe drug and dietary restrictions, to collect all urine during the test period, or to store the specimen properly may affect test results.

Venereal Disease Research Laboratory test

This flocculation test, commonly known as the VDRL test, is widely used to screen for primary and secondary syphilis. The test demonstrates the presence of reagin—an antibody relatively specific for *Treponema pallidum*, the spirochete that causes syphilis—in serial dilutions of a serum sample. The last dilution to reveal flocculation is taken as the titer.

Unfortunately, transient or permanent biologic false-positive reactions can make accurate interpretation difficult. A biologic false-positive reaction can result from viral or bacterial infection, chronic systemic illness, or nonsyphilitic treponemal disease.

The VDRL test may be performed on cerebrospinal fluid to test for tertiary syphilis, but it is less sensitive than the fluorescent treponemal antibody absorption test. (See *Serodiagnostic tests for syphilis*, page 640.) The rapid plasma reagin test can also be used to diagnose syphilis. (See *Rapid plasma reagin test*, page 641.)

SERODIAGNOSTIC TESTS FOR SYPHILIS

The fluorescent treponemal antibody absorption (FTA-ABS) test — which uses a strain of the *Treponema pallidum* antigen itself as a reagent — is more sensitive than the Venereal Disease Research Laboratory (VDRL) test or the rapid plasma reagin (RPR) test in detecting all stages of untreated syphilis (as shown in the graph below). However, the test's complexity and the incidence of false-positive results make it an impractical screening tool. The VDRL and RPR tests are preferred for wide-scale screening and when primary- or secondary-stage disease is suspected. In advanced syphilis, when more than one-third of infected people may have a negative VDRL, the FTA-ABS test is preferred for sensitivity.

The VDRL test also can be used to monitor response to treatment. Untreated syphilis produces titers that are low in the primary stage (<1:32), elevated in the secondary stage (>1:32), and variable in the tertiary stage. Successful therapy markedly reduces titers, with two-thirds of patients reverting to a negative VDRL, especially during the first two stages of the disease. Third-stage therapy seldom produces a nonreactive VDRL, but maintenance of low-reactive values during the 6- to 12-month posttherapy period indicates success. A subsequent rise signals reinfection. By comparison, FTA-ABS test results usually remain positive after treatment.

A significant number of patients with infectious diseases show temporary false-positive VDRL test results. Chronic false-positive VDRL and FTA-ABS results are associated with immune complex diseases.

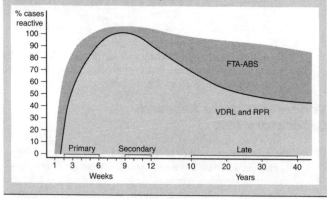

Purpose
- To screen for primary and secondary syphilis
- To confirm primary or secondary syphilis in the presence of syphilitic lesions
- To monitor response to treatment.

Patient preparation
Explain to the patient that this test detects syphilis. Tell him that he needn't restrict food, fluids, or medications but should abstain from alcohol for 24 hours before the test. Advise him that the test requires a blood sample,

---

RAPID PLASMA REAGIN TEST

This rapid, macroscopic serologic test is an acceptable substitute for the Venereal Disease Research Laboratory (VDRL) test in diagnosing syphilis. The rapid plasma reagin (RPR) test, available as a kit, uses a cardiolipin antigen to detect reagin, the antibody relatively specific for *Treponema pallidum*, the causative agent of syphilis.

In the RPR test, the patient's serum is mixed with cardiolipin on a plastic-coated card, rotated mechanically, and then examined with the unaided eye. If flocculation occurs, the test sample is diluted until no visible reaction occurs. The last dilution to show visible flocculation is the titer of the reagin antibody.

In the RPR test, like the VDRL test, normal serum shows no flocculation.

---

who will perform the venipuncture and when, and that he may experience transient discomfort from the needle puncture and the pressure of the tourniquet.

Procedure

Perform a venipuncture and collect the sample in a 7-ml clot-activator tube.

Precautions

■ Handle the specimen carefully to prevent hemolysis.
■ If a hematoma develops at the venipuncture site, apply warm soaks.

Normal findings

Absence of flocculation is reported as a nonreactive test.

Implications of results

Definite flocculation is reported as reactive; slight flocculation as weakly reactive. The VDRL is reactive in about 50% of patients with primary syphilis and in nearly all patients with secondary syphilis. A reactive VDRL test is diagnostic in the presence of syphilitic lesions; if no lesions are evident, a reactive VDRL test necessitates retesting and consideration of known causes of biologic false-positive reactions, such as infectious mononucleosis, malaria, leprosy, hepatitis, systemic lupus erythematosus, rheumatoid arthritis, or nonsyphilitic treponemal diseases, such as pinta or yaws.

A nonreactive test doesn't rule out syphilis because *T. pallidum* causes no detectable immunologic changes in the serum for 14 to 21 days after infection. However, dark-field microscopic examination of exudate from suspicious lesions can provide early diagnosis by identifying the causative spirochetes.

Interfering factors

- Ingestion of alcohol within 24 hours of the test can produce transient, nonreactive results.
- Immune system dysfunction can cause nonreactive results.
- Hemolysis of the sample can interfere with test results.

Vitamin A and carotene test, serum

This test measures serum levels of vitamin A (retinol) and its precursor, carotene. A fat-soluble vitamin normally supplied by diet, vitamin A is important for reproduction, vision (especially night vision), and epithelial tissue and bone growth. It also maintains cellular and subcellular membranes and synthesis of mucopolysaccharides (the ground substance of collagenous tissue).

The body absorbs vitamin A from the intestines as a fatty acid ester; chylomicrons in the lymphatic system then transport it to the liver, where nearly 90% is stored. Absorption of vitamin A requires the presence of adequate amounts of dietary fat and bile salts. Thus, impaired fat absorption or biliary obstruction inhibits vitamin A absorption, causing a deficiency of this vitamin. Serum levels of vitamin A can remain normal as long as the liver retains even a low reserve of vitamin A.

In this serum test, the color reactions produced by vitamin A and related compounds with various reagents provide both quantitative and qualitative determinations.

Purpose

- To investigate suspected vitamin A deficiency or toxicity
- To aid diagnosis of visual disturbances, especially night blindness and xerophthalmia
- To aid diagnosis of skin diseases, such as keratosis follicularis or ichthyosis
- To screen for malabsorption.

Patient preparation

Explain to the patient that this test measures the level of vitamin A in the blood. Instruct him to fast overnight, but advise him that he need not restrict water before the test. Tell him the test requires a blood sample, who will perform the venipuncture and when, and that he may feel some discomfort from the needle puncture and the pressure of the tourniquet.

Procedure

Perform a venipuncture and collect the sample in a chilled, 7-ml siliconized tube.

Precautions

■ Protect the sample from light because vitamin A characteristically absorbs light.

■ Handle the sample gently and send it to the laboratory immediately.

■ Keep the specimen on ice.

Reference values

Normal carotene levels are 50 to 300 µg/dl in adults and 40 to 130 µg/dl in children. Normal vitamin A values differ according to age and gender. The normal range in adults is 30 to 95 µg/dl, with values for men usually 20% higher than for women. In children ages 1 to 6, the range is 20 to 43 µg/dl; at ages 7 to 12, 26 to 50 µg/dl; and at ages 13 to 19, 26 to 72 µg/dl.

Implications of results

Low serum levels of vitamin A (hypovitaminosis A) suggest impaired fat absorption, as in celiac disease, infectious hepatitis, cystic fibrosis of the pancreas, or obstructive jaundice. Low levels are also associated with protein-calorie malnutrition (marasmic kwashiorkor), a rare condition in the United States but a major nutritional disorder worldwide, especially among children. Low vitamin A levels may also result when chronic nephritis causes excessive loss of vitamin A in urine.

Elevated vitamin A levels (hypervitaminosis A) usually reflect chronic excessive intake of vitamin A supplements or of foods high in vitamin A. Associated disorders include hyperlipemia and hypercholesterolemia associated with uncontrolled diabetes mellitus.

Low serum carotene levels suggest impaired fat absorption or, rarely, insufficient dietary intake of carotene. Carotene levels may also fall during pregnancy as the body's metabolic demand for carotene rises. Elevated carotene levels indicate grossly excessive dietary intake.

Interfering factors

■ Patient failure to observe overnight fast may influence test results.

■ Ingestion of mineral oil, neomycin, or cholestyramine may suppress vitamin A and carotene levels. Glucocorticoids and oral contraceptives may increase levels.

■ Hemolysis caused by rough handling of the sample may alter test results.

Vitamin B₁ test, urine

This test is used to detect a deficiency of vitamin B_1 (thiamine). This water-soluble vitamin helps metabolize carbohydrates, fats, and proteins and requires folic acid (folate) for effective uptake. It is absorbed in the duodenum and excreted in the urine. Urine levels of vitamin B_1 reflect dietary intake and metabolic storage of thiamine.

Rare in the United States, vitamin B_1 deficiency (also called beriberi) is most common in Asia, where the subsistence diet is polished rice. Vitamin B_1 deficiency may result from inadequate dietary intake, usually associated with alcoholism; impaired absorption, malabsorption syndrome; impaired utilization, as in hepatic disease; or conditions that increase the metabolic demand, such as pregnancy, lactation, fever, exercise, hyperthyroidism, surgery, or high carbohydrate intake.

Purpose

To help confirm vitamin B_1 deficiency and to distinguish it from other causes of polyneuritis.

Patient preparation

Explain to the patient that this test evaluates the body's stores of vitamin B_1. Tell him the test requires a 24-hour urine specimen. Check his diet history to rule out a deficiency associated with inadequate intake. If the patient is to collect the specimen, teach him the proper technique.

Procedure

Collect a 24-hour urine specimen.

Precautions

- Tell the patient not to contaminate the urine specimen with toilet tissue or stool.
- Refrigerate the specimen or place it on ice during the collection period.

Reference values

The normal range of urinary excretion is 100 to 200 µg/24 hours.

Implications of results

Deficient urine levels of vitamin B_1 can result from inadequate dietary intake, hyperthyroidism, alcoholism, severe hepatic disease, chronic diarrhea, or prolonged diuretic therapy. Negative results indicate neuritis unrelated to vitamin B_1 deficiency.

Interfering factors

Failure to collect all urine during the test period or to store the specimen properly may alter test results.

Vitamin B$_2$ test, serum

This test evaluates the nutritive status and metabolism of vitamin B$_2$ (riboflavin) and thus helps to detect vitamin B$_2$ deficiency. Absorbed from the intestinal tract and excreted in urine, vitamin B$_2$ is essential for growth and tissue function. In the tissues, it combines with phosphate to produce the coenzymes flavin mononucleotide and flavin adenine dinucleotide (FAD); these coenzymes then participate in oxidation-reduction reactions with oxidative enzymes, such as glutathione reductase.

In this test, glutathione reductase activity is measured before and after administration of exogenous FAD. Normally, glutathione reductase binds with FAD. If vitamin B$_2$ supply is inadequate, glutathione reductase activity and the degree of FAD unsaturation are increased, inversely proportional to vitamin B$_2$ concentration.

This serum test is considered more reliable than the urine vitamin B$_2$ test, which can produce artificially high values in patients after surgery or prolonged fasting.

Purpose

To detect vitamin B$_2$ deficiency.

Patient preparation

Explain to the patient that this test evaluates vitamin B$_2$ levels. Instruct him to maintain a normal diet before the test. Inform him that the test requires a blood sample, who will perform the venipuncture and when, and that he may experience some discomfort from the needle puncture and the pressure of the tourniquet.

Procedure

Perform a venipuncture and collect the sample in a 7-ml siliconized tube.

Precautions

- Handle the sample gently to prevent hemolysis.
- Send the sample to the laboratory immediately.
- Don't refrigerate or freeze the sample.

Reference values

Normally, glutathione reductase has an activity index of 0.9 to 1.3.

Implications of results

An index of 1.4 or greater reflects vitamin B$_2$ deficiency.

Posttest care

If a hematoma develops at the venipuncture site, ease discomfort by applying warm soaks.

Interfering factors

Hemolysis caused by rough handling of the sample may alter test results.

Vitamin B$_6$ test, serum

Vitamin B$_6$ consists of four enzymes—pyridoxol (pyridoxine), pyridoxal, pyridoxal phosphate, and pyridoxic acid—that participate in many biochemical reactions. This test uses high-pressure liquid chromatography to evaluate the serum levels and metabolism.

Purpose

To detect vitamin B$_6$ deficiency.

Patient preparation

Explain to the patient that this test determines the body stores of vitamin B$_6$ by measurement in serum. Instruct him to maintain a normal diet before the test. Inform him that the test requires a blood sample, who will perform the venipuncture and when, and that he may experience some discomfort from the needle puncture and the pressure of the tourniquet.

Procedure

Perform a venipuncture and collect the sample in a 7-ml clot-activator tube.

Precautions

- Handle the sample gently to prevent hemolysis.
- Send the sample to the laboratory immediately.

Reference values

- Pyridoxol: normal, 0.2 to 2.5 µg/L; marginally low, 0.1 to 0.2 µg/L.
- Pyridoxal: normal, 2 to 30 µg/L; marginally low, 1 to 2 µg/L.
- Pyridoxal phosphate: normal, 5 to 50 µg/L; marginally low, 3 to 5 µg/L.
- Pyridoxic acid: normal, 3 to 30 µg/L; marginally low, 1 to 3 µg/L.

Implications of results

Pyridoxol levels less than 0.1 µg/L, pyridoxal levels less than 1 µg/L, pyridoxal phosphate levels less than 3 µg/L, and pyridoxic acid levels less than 1 µg/L indicate vitamin B$_6$ deficiency.

Posttest care

If a hematoma develops at the venipuncture site, ease discomfort by applying warm soaks.

Interfering factors

Hemolysis caused by rough handling of the sample may alter test results.

Vitamin B$_{12}$ test, serum

Vitamin B$_{12}$ is also known as cyanocobalamin, antipernicious anemia factor, and extrinsic factor. This test is usually performed concurrently with measurement of serum folic acid levels because deficiencies of vitamin B$_{12}$ and folic acid are the two most common causes of megaloblastic anemia.

A water-soluble vitamin containing cobalt, vitamin B$_{12}$ is essential to hematopoiesis, synthesis and growth of deoxyribonucleic acid, and myelin synthesis and nervous system integrity. (See *Cobalt: Critical trace element*, page 648.) Ingested almost exclusively in animal products, such as meat, shellfish, milk, and eggs, vitamin B$_{12}$ is absorbed from the ileum after forming a complex with intrinsic factor and is stored in the liver.

A clinical dietary vitamin B$_{12}$ deficiency takes years to develop because almost total conservation is provided by a cyclic pathway (enterohepatic circulation) that reabsorbs vitamin B$_{12}$ from bile. Deficiency of intrinsic factor causes malabsorption of vitamin B$_{12}$ and may cause pernicious anemia.

Purpose

■ To aid differential diagnosis of megaloblastic anemia, which may be associated with a deficiency of vitamin B$_{12}$ or folic acid
■ To aid differential diagnosis of central nervous system (CNS) disorders affecting peripheral and spinal myelinated nerves.

Patient preparation

Explain that this test determines the amount of vitamin B$_{12}$ and folic acid. Instruct the patient to observe an overnight fast before the test. Tell him this test requires a blood sample, who will perform the venipuncture and when, and that he may feel some discomfort from the needle puncture and pressure of the tourniquet.

Procedure

Perform the venipuncture and collect the sample in a 7-ml siliconized tube.

COBALT: CRITICAL TRACE ELEMENT

A trace element found mainly in the liver, cobalt is an essential component of vitamin B$_{12}$ and therefore is a critical factor in hematopoiesis.

A balanced diet supplies sufficient cobalt to maintain hematopoiesis. However, excessive ingestion of cobalt may have toxic effects. For example, people who consumed large quantities of dietary supplements containing cobalt as a stabilizer suffered toxicity, resulting in heart failure from cardiomyopathy.

Because quantitative analysis of cobalt alone is difficult because so little is present in the body, cobalt is often measured by bioassay along with vitamin B$_{12}$ tests. The normal cobalt concentration in human plasma is about 60 to 80 pg/ml.

Precautions

Handle the sample gently to prevent hemolysis and send it to the laboratory immediately.

Reference values

Normal ranges of serum vitamin B$_{12}$ values are 200 to 900 pg/ml in adults and 160 to 1,200 pg/ml in newborns.

Implications of results

Low serum levels suggest inadequate dietary intake of vitamin B$_{12}$, especially if the patient is a strict vegetarian; malabsorption syndromes such as celiac disease; isolated malabsorption of vitamin B$_{12}$ from previous ileal or gastric surgery; hypermetabolic states such as hyperthyroidism; pregnancy; or CNS damage, such as posterolateral sclerosis or funicular degeneration.

High serum levels suggest excessive dietary intake; hepatic disease, such as cirrhosis or acute or chronic hepatitis; or myeloproliferative disorders such as myelocytic leukemia. These conditions raise levels of serum vitamin B$_{12}$-binding proteins, causing high serum levels of vitamin B$_{12}$.

Posttest care

- If a hematoma develops at the venipuncture site, apply warm soaks.
- As ordered, have the patient resume his normal diet.

Interfering factors

- Drugs such as neomycin, metformin, anticonvulsants, oral contraceptives, and ethanol may decrease vitamin B$_{12}$ levels.
- Failure to fast overnight and administration of substances that decrease absorption of vitamin B$_{12}$ may alter test results.

Vitamin C test, plasma

This chemical assay measures plasma levels of vitamin C, also known as ascorbic acid, a water-soluble vitamin required for collagen synthesis and cartilage and bone maintenance. It also promotes iron absorption, influences folic acid metabolism, and may be necessary for withstanding the stresses of injury and infection.

After vitamin C is absorbed from the small intestine, it's transported in the blood to the kidneys and oxidized to dehydroascorbic acid. Then it's stored in the adrenal and salivary glands, pancreas, spleen, testes, and brain. Because the adrenal glands contain high concentrations of vitamin C, stimulation of these glands by corticotropin may deplete stores of vitamin C.

This vitamin is present in generous amounts in citrus fruits, berries, tomatoes, raw cabbage, green peppers, and green leafy vegetables. Severe vitamin C deficiency, or scurvy, causes capillary fragility, joint abnormalities, and numerous systemic symptoms.

Purpose

To aid diagnosis of scurvy, scurvy-like conditions, and metabolic disorders, such as malnutrition and malabsorption syndromes.

Patient preparation

Explain to the patient that this test detects the amount of vitamin C in the blood. Instruct him to observe an overnight fast before the test. Tell him that this test requires a blood sample, who will perform the venipuncture and when, and that he may feel some discomfort from the needle puncture and the pressure of the tourniquet.

Procedure

Perform the venipuncture and collect the sample in a 7-ml heparinized tube.

Precautions

■ Avoid rough handling or excessive agitation of the sample to prevent hemolysis.
■ Send the sample to the laboratory immediately.

Reference values

Plasma vitamin C values of 0.3 mg/dl or more are considered acceptable.

Implications of results

Vitamin C values of 0.2 to 0.29 mg/dl are considered borderline; values under 0.2 mg/dl indicate deficiency. Vitamin C levels diminish during pregnancy and reach a

RISKS OF INGESTING HIGH-DOSE VITAMIN C

In the early 1970s, Nobel Laureate Linus Pauling sparked interest in vitamin C when he suggested that megadoses of this vitamin might increase resistance to viral and bacterial infection, increase resistance to cancer, and decrease serum cholesterol levels. Pauling recommended daily doses of vitamin C at two to five times the recommended dietary allowance (60 mg daily for adults) and much higher doses during times of stress or illness. In particular, he advocated very high doses to treat cancer and to relieve common cold symptoms.

To date, clinical studies haven't supported Pauling's theories. In fact, some studies proved definitively that high-dose vitamin C is no more effective than a placebo in the treatment of cancer. Other studies have shown that high-dose vitamin C has little or no effect on the severity of colds. However, despite this, many people supplement their diets with high doses of vitamin C. In addition to delaying proper treatment, such high doses can cause severe adverse effects.

The most common adverse effects of vitamin C are diarrhea and vomiting. However, in some people, high-dose vitamin C promotes formation of uric acid crystals, which may trigger or intensify gout, and causes oxalic acid accumulation in the kidneys, which may lead to formation of calculi. Vitamin C also promotes iron absorption, which may lead to iron toxicity.

Additional risks include interference with drug metabolism and diagnostic tests. For example, high-dose vitamin C impairs the effectiveness of warfarin and other anticoagulants and can cause rapid excretion of other drugs by acidifying urine pH. Also, it interferes with fecal occult blood testing and produces false-positive test results for glycosuria.

---

low point immediately postpartum. Depressed levels accompany infection, fever, anemia, and burns. Severe deficiencies result in scurvy.

High plasma levels can reflect excessive intake of the vitamin. Excess vitamin C is converted to oxalate, which is excreted in the urine. Excessive oxalate can produce urinary calculi. (See *Risks of ingesting high-dose vitamin C.*)

Posttest care
■ If a hematoma develops at the venipuncture site, apply warm soaks.
■ As ordered, resume diet that was discontinued before the test.

Interfering factors
■ Failure to follow dietary restrictions or to transport the sample to the laboratory promptly may alter test results.

■ Hemolysis caused by rough handling of the sample may affect test results.

Vitamin D₃ test, serum

Vitamin D_3 (cholecalciferol) is produced in the skin by the sun's ultraviolet rays and occurs naturally in fish oils, egg yolks, liver, and butter. Like other fat-soluble vitamins, vitamin D_3 is absorbed from the intestine in the presence of bile salts and is stored in the liver. To become active, this vitamin must undergo conversion to 25-hydroxycholecalciferol, its circulating metabolite, and then to 1,25-dihydroxycholecalciferol, a hormone that controls bone mineralization.

The hormonal function of vitamin D_3 closely parallels that of parathyroid hormone in maintaining calcium and phosphorus homeostasis. Low serum calcium and phosphorus levels stimulate production of parathyroid hormone, which then stimulates renal secretion of 1,25-dihydroxycholecalciferol to promote intestinal absorption of calcium and phosphate. Together the two hormones stimulate renal absorption of calcium and mobilization of calcium from bone.

This test, a competitive protein-binding assay, determines serum levels of 25-hydroxycholecalciferol after chromatography has separated it from other vitamin D metabolites and contaminants. Clinically useful in evaluating nutritional status and the biological activity of vitamin D_3, this test is commonly combined with measurement of serum calcium and alkaline phosphatase levels.

Purpose

■ To evaluate skeletal diseases, such as rickets and osteomalacia
■ To aid diagnosis of hypercalcemia
■ To detect vitamin D toxicity
■ To monitor therapy with vitamin D_3.

Patient preparation

Explain to the patient that this test measures vitamin D in the body. Tell him that he shouldn't eat or drink anything for 8 to 12 hours before the test, that the test requires a blood sample, who will perform the venipuncture and when, and that he may feel discomfort from the needle puncture and the tourniquet. Check for drugs that may alter test results, such as corticosteroids and anticonvulsants. If these drugs must be continued, note this on the laboratory request.

Procedure

Perform a venipuncture and collect the sample in a 7-ml siliconized tube.

Precautions

Handle the sample carefully to prevent hemolysis.

Reference values

The normal range of serum vitamin D_3 levels is 10 to 55 ng/ml; values are typically higher in summer.

Implications of results

Low or undetectable levels suggest vitamin D deficiency, which can cause rickets or osteomalacia. Such deficiency may stem from poor diet, decreased exposure to the sun, or impaired absorption of vitamin D (secondary to hepatobiliary disease, pancreatitis, celiac disease, cystic fibrosis, or gastric or small-bowel resection). Low levels may also be related to various hepatic diseases that directly affect vitamin D metabolism.

Elevated levels (over 100 ng/ml) suggest toxicity caused by excessive self-medication or prolonged therapy. Elevated levels associated with hypercalcemia suggest hypersensitivity to vitamin D, as in sarcoidosis.

Posttest care

■ If a hematoma develops at the venipuncture site, apply warm soaks.
■ Tell the patient that he may resume his normal diet.

Interfering factors

■ Drugs that may decrease vitamin D_3 levels include anticonvulsants, isoniazid, mineral oil, glucocorticoids, aluminum hydroxide, cholestyramine, and colestipol.
■ Anticonvulsants and corticosteroids may lower serum levels by inhibiting formation of vitamin D_3 metabolites.
■ Hemolysis may alter test results.

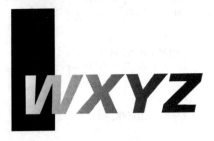

White blood cell count

Part of the complete blood count, the white blood cell (WBC), or leukocyte, count reports the number of WBCs found in a microliter (cubic millimeter) of whole blood. The counting process uses a hemacytometer or an electronic device, such as the Coulter counter.

On any given day, WBC counts may vary by as much as 2,000 cells/μl. Such variation can be the result of strenuous exercise, stress, or digestion. The WBC count may rise or fall significantly in certain diseases but is diagnostically useful only when interpreted in light of the WBC differential and the patient's current clinical status.

Purpose
- To determine infection or inflammation
- To determine the need for further tests, such as the WBC differential or bone marrow biopsy
- To monitor response to chemotherapy or radiation therapy.

Patient preparation
Explain to the patient that this test helps detect an infection or inflammation. Inform him that he needn't restrict food or fluids but should avoid strenuous exercise for 24 hours before the test. Also tell him that he should avoid ingesting a heavy meal before the test. Explain to him that the test requires a blood sample, who will perform the venipuncture and when, and that he may experience transient discomfort from the needle puncture and the pressure of the tourniquet.

If the patient is being treated for an infection, advise him that this test will be repeated to monitor his progress. Review his drug history for medications that may alter test results. Note the use of such medications on the laboratory request.

Procedure
Perform a venipuncture and collect the sample in a 7-ml EDTA tube.

Precautions

Completely fill the sample collection tube, and invert it gently several times to adequately mix the sample and the anticoagulant.

Reference values

The normal range is 4,000 to 10,000/μL.

Implications of results

An elevated WBC count (leukocytosis) commonly signals infection, such as an abscess, meningitis, appendicitis, or tonsillitis. Other causes include leukemia, tissue necrosis caused by burns, myocardial infarction, or gangrene.

A low WBC count (leukopenia) may reflect bone marrow depression caused by viral infections or reactions to drugs or other toxins. Leukopenia characteristically accompanies influenza, typhoid fever, measles, infectious hepatitis, mononucleosis, and rubella.

Posttest care

■ If a hematoma develops at the venipuncture site, ease discomfort by applying warm soaks.
■ As ordered, advise the patient that he may resume normal activities that he discontinued before the test.

Interfering factors

■ Exercise, stress, or digestion raises the WBC count.
■ Some drugs, including most antineoplastic agents; anti-infectives, such as metronidazole and flucytosine; anticonvulsants, such as phenytoin derivatives; thyroid hormone antagonists; and nonsteroidal anti-inflammatory drugs such as indomethacin lower the WBC count.
■ Hemolysis caused by rough handling of the sample may affect test results.

White blood cell differential test

The white blood cell (WBC) differential evaluates the distribution and morphology of white cells, and therefore it provides specific information about a patient's immune status. The laboratory classifies 100 or more white cells in a stained film of peripheral blood into the five major types of leukocytes—neutrophils, eosinophils, basophils, lymphocytes, and monocytes—and reports the percentage of each type.

The differential count is the relative number of each type of white cell in the blood. Multiplying the percentage value of each type by the total WBC count yields the absolute number of each type of white cell. Abnormally high values are associated with various allergic reactions and parasitic infections. When high levels are reported,

LAP STAIN

Levels of leukocyte alkaline phosphatase (LAP), an enzyme found in neutrophils, may be altered by infection, stress, chronic inflammatory diseases, Hodgkin's disease, and hematologic disorders. Most of these conditions elevate LAP levels; only a few, notably chronic myelogenous leukemia (CML), depress them. Thus, this test is most often used to differentiate CML from other disorders that produce an elevated white blood cell count.

Procedure

To perform this test, obtain a blood sample by venipuncture or fingerstick. Collect a venous blood sample in a 7-ml EDTA tube and transport it immediately to the laboratory, where a blood smear is prepared. The peripheral blood sample is smeared on a 3″ glass slide and fixed in cold formalin-methanol. The blood smear is then stained to show the amount of LAP present in the cytoplasm of the neutrophils. One hundred neutrophils are counted and assessed; each is assigned a score of 0 to 4, according to the degree of LAP staining. Normally, values for LAP range from 40 to 100, depending on the laboratory's standard.

Implications of results

Depressed LAP values typically indicate CML; however, values may also be low in paroxysmal nocturnal hemoglobinuria, aplastic anemia, or infectious mononucleosis. Elevated levels suggest Hodgkin's disease, polycythemia vera, or a neutrophilic leukemoid reaction—a response to such conditions as infection, chronic inflammation, or pregnancy.

After a diagnosis of CML, the LAP stain may also be used to help detect onset of the blastic phase of the disease, when LAP levels typically rise. However, since LAP levels also increase in response to therapy, test results must be correlated with the patient's condition.

an eosinophil count is sometimes ordered as a follow-up to the white cell differential. The eosinophil count is also appropriate if the differential WBC count shows a depressed eosinophil level.

Purpose

■ To evaluate the body's capacity to resist and overcome infection
■ To detect and identify various types of leukemia (See *LAP stain*, for information on another test used to identify leukemia.)
■ To determine the stage and severity of an infection
■ To detect allergic reactions and parasitic infections and assess their severity (eosinophil count)
■ To distinguish viral from bacterial infection.

Patient preparation

Explain to the patient that this test evaluates how well his immune system is functioning. Inform him that he needn't restrict food or fluids but should refrain from

DRUGS THAT INFLUENCE EOSINOPHIL COUNT		
Many drugs can affect the accuracy of the eosinophil count, as shown in the chart below.		
Increase or decrease count	Decrease count	Increase count by provoking an allergic reaction
methysergide desipramine	indomethacin procainamide	anticonvulsants capreomycin d-penicillamine gold compounds isoniazid nalidixic acid novobiocin para-aminosalicylic acid paromomycin penicillins phenothiazines rifampin streptomycin sulfonamides tetracyclines

strenuous exercise for 24 hours before the test. Tell him the test requires a blood sample, who will perform the venipuncture and when, and that he may experience transient discomfort from the needle puncture and the pressure of the tourniquet.

Review the patient's history for use of medications that may interfere with test results. (See *Drugs that influence eosinophil count.*)

Procedure

Perform a venipuncture and collect the sample in a 7-ml EDTA tube.

Precautions

Completely fill the collection tube, and invert it gently several times to mix the sample and the anticoagulant adequately. Handle the tube gently to prevent hemolysis.

Reference values

For normal values for neutrophils, eosinophils, basophils, lymphocytes, and monocytes in adults and children, see *Interpreting WBC differential values.* However, keep in mind that, for an accurate diagnosis, differential test results must always be interpreted in relation to the total WBC count.

Implications of results

Abnormal differential patterns suggest a wide range of disease states and other conditions. (See *How disease affects differential values*, pages 658 and 659.)

INTERPRETING WBC DIFFERENTIAL VALUES

The differential count measures the types of white blood cells (WBCs) as a percentage of the total WBC count (the relative value). The absolute value is obtained by multiplying the relative value of each cell type by the total WBC count. Both the relative and absolute values must be considered to obtain an accurate diagnosis.

For example, consider a patient whose WBC count is 6,000/μL and whose differential shows 30% neutrophils and 70% lymphocytes. His relative lymphocyte count seems to be quite high (lymphocytosis), but when this figure is multiplied by his WBC count (6,000 × 70% = 4,200 lymphocytes/μL), it is well within the normal range.

This patient's neutrophil count is low (30%); when this figure is multiplied by the WBC count (6000 x 30% = 1,800 neutrophils/μL), the result is a low absolute number, which suggests depressed bone marrow function.

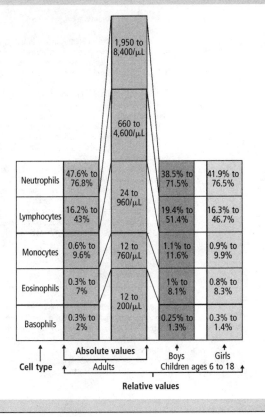

Cell type	Adults		Boys	Girls
Neutrophils	47.6% to 76.8%	1,950 to 8,400/μL	38.5% to 71.5%	41.9% to 76.5%
Lymphocytes	16.2% to 43%	660 to 4,600/μL	19.4% to 51.4%	16.3% to 46.7%
Monocytes	0.6% to 9.6%	24 to 960/μL	1.1% to 11.6%	0.9% to 9.9%
Eosinophils	0.3% to 7%	12 to 760/μL	1% to 8.1%	0.8% to 8.3%
Basophils	0.3% to 2%	12 to 200/μL	0.25% to 1.3%	0.3% to 1.4%

Absolute values
Adults — Children ages 6 to 18
Relative values

CLINICAL ALERT An absolute neutrophil count of 1,000 μL or less mandates the need for neutropenic precautions, including protective isolation.

HOW DISEASE AFFECTS DIFFERENTIAL VALUES

Cell type	How affected
Neutrophils	**Increased by:** ■ Infections: osteomyelitis, otitis media, salpingitis, septicemia, gonorrhea, endocarditis, smallpox, chickenpox, herpes, Rocky Mountain spotted fever ■ Ischemic necrosis caused by myocardial infarction, burns, cancer ■ Metabolic disorders: diabetic acidosis, eclampsia, uremia, thyrotoxicosis ■ Stress response associated with acute hemorrhage, surgery, excessive exercise, emotional distress, third trimester of pregnancy, childbirth ■ Inflammatory diseases: rheumatic fever, rheumatoid arthritis, acute gout, vasculitis, myositis **Decreased by:** ■ Bone marrow depression caused by radiation or cytotoxic drugs ■ Infections: typhoid, tularemia, brucellosis, hepatitis, influenza, measles, mumps, rubella, infectious mononucleosis ■ Hypersplenism: hepatic disease and storage diseases ■ Collagen vascular diseases, such as systemic lupus erythematosus ■ Deficiency of folic acid or vitamin B_{12}
Eosinophils 	**Increased by:** ■ Allergic disorders: asthma, hay fever, food or drug sensitivity, serum sickness, angioneurotic edema ■ Parasitic infections: trichinosis, hookworm, roundworm, amebiasis ■ Skin diseases: eczema, pemphigus, psoriasis, dermatitis, herpes simplex ■ Neoplastic diseases: chronic myelocytic leukemia, Hodgkin's disease, metastasis and necrosis of solid tumors ■ Collagen vascular disease, adrenocortical hypofunction, ulcerative colitis, polyarteritis nodosa, scarlet fever, pernicious anemia, excessive exercise, splenectomy **Decreased by:** ■ Stress response associated with trauma, shock, burns, surgery, mental distress ■ Cushing's syndrome
Basophils 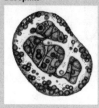	**Increased by:** ■ Chronic myelocytic leukemia, polycythemia vera, some chronic hemolytic anemias, Hodgkin's disease, systemic mastocytosis, myxedema, ulcerative colitis, chronic hypersensitivity states, nephrosis **Decreased by:** ■ Hyperthyroidism, ovulation, pregnancy, stress

Posttest care

If a hematoma develops at the venipuncture site, ease discomfort by applying warm soaks.

HOW DISEASE AFFECTS DIFFERENTIAL VALUES (continued)

Cell type	How affected
Lymphocytes 	**Increased by:** ■ Infections: pertussis, brucellosis, syphilis, tuberculosis, hepatitis, infectious mononucleosis, mumps, rubella, cytomegalovirus ■ Thyrotoxicosis, hypoadrenalism, ulcerative colitis, immune diseases, lymphocytic leukemia **Decreased by:** ■ Severe debilitating illnesses, such as congestive heart failure, renal failure, advanced tuberculosis ■ Defective lymphatic circulation, high levels of adrenal corticosteroids, immunodeficiency caused by immunosuppressive therapy
Monocytes 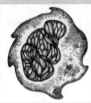	**Increased by:** ■ Infections: subacute bacterial endocarditis, tuberculosis, hepatitis, malaria, Rocky Mountain spotted fever ■ Collagen vascular diseases: systemic lupus erythematosus, rheumatoid arthritis, polyarteritis nodosa ■ Carcinomas, monocytic leukemia, lymphomas

Interfering factors

■ Hemolysis caused by rough handling of the sample may affect the accuracy of test results.

■ Failure to use the proper anticoagulant, to completely fill the collection tube, or to mix the sample and anticoagulant adequately may affect the accuracy of test results.

Wound culture

A wound culture consists of growing a specimen from a lesion under specific circumstances and microscopic analysis to confirm infection. Wound cultures may be aerobic (for detection of organisms that usually require oxygen to grow and typically appear in a superficial wound) or anaerobic (for organisms that need little or no oxygen and appear in areas of poor tissue perfusion, such as postoperative wounds, ulcers, or compound fractures). Indications for wound culture include fever as well as inflammation and drainage in damaged tissue.

Purpose

To identify an infectious microbe in a wound.

Patient preparation

Explain to the patient that this test identifies infectious microbes. Advise him that a drainage specimen from the wound will be withdrawn by a syringe or removed on cotton swabs. Tell him who will perform the procedure and when.

Equipment

■ Sterile cotton swabs and sterile culture tube, or commercial sterile collection and transport system (for aerobic culture) ■ sterile cotton swabs or sterile 10-ml syringe with 21G needle, and special culture tube containing carbon dioxide or nitrogen (for anaerobic culture) ■ sterile gloves ■ alcohol wipes ■ sterile gauze and povidone-iodine solution.

Procedure

Using gloves, prepare a sterile field and clean the area around the wound with antiseptic solution.

For aerobic culture: Express the wound and swab as much exudate as possible, or insert the swab deep into the wound and gently rotate. Immediately place the swab in the aerobic culture tube.

For anaerobic culture: Insert the swab deep into the wound, gently rotate it, and immediately place it in the anaerobic culture tube; or insert the needle into the wound, aspirate 1 to 5 ml of exudate into the syringe, and immediately inject the exudate into the anaerobic culture tube. If the needle is covered with a rubber stopper, the aspirate may be sent to the laboratory in the syringe.

Record on the laboratory request recent antimicrobial therapy, the source of the specimen, and the suspected organism. Also, label the specimen container appropriately with the patient's name, the doctor's name, the hospital number, and the wound site and time of specimen collection.

Dress the wound as necessary.

Precautions

■ Clean the area around the wound thoroughly to limit contamination of the culture by normal skin flora, such as diphtheroids, *Staphylococcus epidermidis*, and alphahemolytic streptococci. However, don't clean the area around a perineal wound.
■ Make sure no antiseptic enters the wound.
■ Obtain exudate from the entire wound, using more than one swab.
■ Because some anaerobes die in the presence of even a small amount of oxygen, place the specimen in the cul-

ture tube quickly, take care that no air enters the tube, and check that double stoppers are secure.
■ Keep the specimen container upright and send it to the laboratory within 15 minutes to prevent growth or deterioration of microbes.
■ Use gloves during the procedure and when handling the specimen, and take necessary isolation precautions when sending the specimen to the laboratory.

Normal findings

No pathogenic organisms should be present in a clean wound.

Implications of results

The most common aerobic pathogens in wounds are *S. aureus*, group A beta-hemolytic streptococci, *Proteus* species, *Escherichia coli* and other Enterobacteriaceae, and some *Pseudomonas* species; the most common anaerobic pathogens are some *Clostridium*, *Bacteroides*, *Peptococcus*, and *Streptococcus* species.

Interfering factors

■ Failure to report recent or current antimicrobial therapy may cause false-negative results.
■ Poor collection technique (for example, exposing some specimens to oxygen) may contaminate or invalidate the specimen.
■ Failure to use the proper transport media may cause the specimen to dry up and the bacteria to die, affecting the accuracy of test results.

APPENDICES

APPENDIX A: GUIDE TO ABBREVIATIONS

<	less than
>	greater than
17-KS	17-ketosteroid
ABG	arterial blood gas
ACTH	adrenocorticotropic hormone
ADH	antidiuretic hormone
AFP	alpha-fetoprotein
ALT	alanine aminotransferase
ANA	antinuclear antibodies
APTT	activated partial thromboplastin time
ASO	antistreptolysin-O
AST	aspartate aminotransferase
BUN	blood urea nitrogen
C_3	third component of complement
Ca	calcium
CBC	complete blood count
CEA	carcinoembryonic antigen
CK	creatine kinase
Cl	chloride
cm^3	cubic centimeter
CO_2	carbon dioxide
CSF	cerebrospinal fluid
CT	computed tomography
CXR	chest X-ray
D&C	dilatation and curettage
DNA	deoxyribonucleic acid
dl	deciliter
EBV	Epstein-Barr virus
ECG	electrocardiogram
EEG	electroencephalogram
ELISA	enzyme-linked immunosorbent assay
EMG	electromyography
ESR	erythrocyte sedimentation rate
FEV_1	forced expiratory volume in 1 second
FSH	follicle-stimulating hormone

FSP	fibrin split products
FVC	forced vital capacity
g	gram
GFR	glomerular filtration rate
GH	growth hormone
Hb	hemoglobin
hCG	human chorionic gonadotropin
HCO_3^-	bicarbonate
Hct, HCT	hematocrit
HDL	high-density lipoprotein
hGH	human growth hormone
HIV	human immunodeficiency virus
HLA	human leukocyte antigen
^{131}I	radioiodine 131
Ig	immunoglobulin
IU	international unit
K	potassium
kg	kilogram
KUB	kidney-ureter-bladder
L	liter
LD	lactate dehydrogenase
LDL	low-density lipoprotein
LH	luteinizing hormone
m^2	square meter
mcg, μg	microgram
mEq	milliequivalent
Mg	magnesium
mg	milligram
MHC	major histocompatibility complex
mIU	milli-international unit
ml	milliliter
mm	millimeter
mm^3	cubic millimeter
mm Hg	millimeter of mercury
mmol	millimole
mOsm	milliosmole
MRI	magnetic resonance imaging
mμ	millimicron
mU	milliunit
μ	micron
μg	microgram
μIU	micro-international unit

μl	microliter
μmol	micromole
μU	microunit
ng	nanogram
nmol	nanomole
Pa_{CO_2}	partial pressure of arterial carbon dioxide
Pa_{O_2}	partial pressure of arterial oxygen
Pap	Papanicolaou
PAWP	pulmonary artery wedge pressure
PET	positron emission tomography
PFT	pulmonary function test
pg	picogram
PT	prothrombin time
PTH	parathyroid hormone
PTT	partial thromboplastin time
RAST	radioallergosorbent test
RBC	red blood cell
RF	rheumatoid factor
RPR	rapid plasma reagin (test)
sec	second
SI	Système International d'Unités (units)
T_3	triiodothyronine
T_4	thyroxine
TBG	thyroxine-binding globulin
TSH	thyroid-stimulating hormone
U	unit
VDRL	Venereal Disease Research Laboratory (test)
VLDL	very-low-density lipoprotein
WBC	white blood cell

APPENDIX B: ILLUSTRATED GUIDE TO HOME TESTS

In recent years, the number of diagnostic tests that people can perform themselves at home has greatly increased. The teaching aids on the following pages describe how to accurately perform many of the newest and most common home tests, including tests for blood cholesterol levels, pacemaker function, and the presence of human immunodeficiency virus.

When you review one of these tests with your patient, be sure to:
- stress the need to follow the manufacturer's instructions precisely
- explain unfamiliar terms
- review any special forms that the patient must complete, such as the diary needed when using a Holter monitor
- discuss how to follow up on test results.

TESTING YOUR BLOOD CHOLESTEROL LEVEL

Dear Patient:
Testing your blood cholesterol level can tell you whether you're at risk for heart disease. If you are on a low-cholesterol diet or are taking cholesterol-lowering medication, testing your blood cholesterol level will help you determine whether your cholesterol is under control. If you have any questions about your test results or the risk factors associated with heart disease, always consult your doctor.

Follow these steps to learn how to obtain a blood sample and how to perform the test. Remember, because cholesterol levels can change from day to day and can be affected by stress, weight loss, illness, or pregnancy, one cholesterol reading may not be final.

Getting ready
1. Begin by assembling the necessary equipment included in the packet: the test device, the cholesterol test result chart, and a lancet.
2. Read the instructions thoroughly before you stick your finger.

Obtaining blood
1. Wash your hands thoroughly and dry them. Choose a site on the end or side of any fingertip. To enhance blood flow, hold your finger under warm water for a minute or two.
2. Hold your hand below your heart and milk the blood toward the fingertip you plan to pierce. Squeeze that fingertip with the thumb of the same hand. Place your fingertip (with your thumb still pressed against it) on a firm surface such as a table.
3. Twist off the lancet's protective cap. Then grasp the lancet and quickly pierce your fingertip just to the side of the finger pad, where you have more blood vessels and fewer nerve endings.

4. Remove your thumb from your fingertip to permit blood flow. Then milk your finger gently until you get a large, hanging drop of blood.
5. Point your finger down directly over the blood well, and place the hanging drop of blood into the blood well, making sure that you fill the black circle completely. Then wait at least 2 but no more than 4 minutes.

Reading the results
When the display windows indicate that the test is finished, read the results. Use the chart included in the packet to identify the exact reading on the test device (as shown). Then compare this reading with the chart to identify your cholesterol level. Remember to inform your doctor about the results.

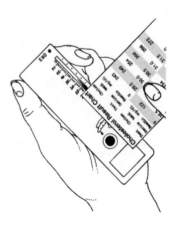

TESTING YOUR BLOOD GLUCOSE LEVEL

Dear Patient:
Testing your blood glucose level daily will tell you whether your diabetes is under control. Follow these steps to learn how to obtain blood for testing and how to perform the test.

Getting ready

1. Begin by assembling the necessary equipment: your glucose meter, a lancet, and a vial with reagent strips.
2. Remove a reagent strip from the vial. Then replace the cap, making sure it's tight.
3. Turn on the glucose meter and insert the reagent strip according to the manufacturer's instructions. Wait for the display window to show that the meter is ready for the blood sample.

Obtaining blood

1. Wash your hands thoroughly and dry them. Choose a site on the end or side of any fingertip. To enhance blood flow, hold your finger under warm water for a minute or two.
2. Hold your hand below your heart, and milk the blood toward the fingertip you plan to pierce. Squeeze that fingertip with the thumb of the same hand. Then place your fingertip (with your thumb still pressed against it) on a firm surface such as a table.
3. Twist off the lancet's cap. Then grasp the lancet and quickly pierce your fingertip just to the side of the finger pad, where you have more blood vessels and fewer nerve endings (as shown below).

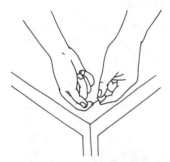

4. Remove your thumb from your fingertip to permit blood flow. Then milk your finger gently until you get a large, hanging drop of blood (as shown below).

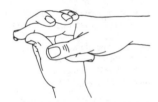

Testing blood

1. When the display window indicates that the meter is ready, touch the drop of blood to the reagent strip at the indicated spot. The drop of blood will automatically start the meter's timer.
2. After the meter has finished the test, you can read the results from the display window. The meter will automatically store the date, time, and results of the test.

PERFORMING A HOME OVULATION TEST

Dear Patient:

A home ovulation test helps you determine the best time to try to become pregnant. It works by monitoring the amount of luteinizing hormone (LH) that is found in your urine.

Normally, during each menstrual cycle, levels of this hormone rise suddenly (LH surge), causing an egg to be released from the ovary 24 to 36 hours later. The release of the egg is known as ovulation. Ovulation normally occurs once a month, about 2 weeks before your period, and lasts about 24 hours. This is your most fertile period — the only time each month that you can become pregnant.

Follow these directions to test your urine for the presence of LH and to determine when you are most likely to become pregnant. To know when to begin testing, you'll need to know the length of your menstrual cycle. Count from the beginning of one period to the beginning of the next period. (Count the first day of bleeding as day 1.) Use the chart below to determine when to begin testing.

Length of cycle	Start test this many days after your last period begins	Length of cycle	Start test this many days after your last period begins
21	5	31	14
22	5	32	15
23	6	33	16
24	7	34	17
25	8	35	18
26	9	36	19
27	10	37	20
28	11	38	21
29	12	39	22
30	13	40	23

Getting ready

1. Read the instructions thoroughly before you perform the test. This test can be performed any time of the day or night but should be performed at the same time each day.

Note: Don't urinate for at least 4 hours before taking this test, and don't drink a lot of liquids for several hours before testing.

2. Remove the test stick from the package and remove the cap.

Performing the test

1. Sit on the toilet. Direct the absorbent end of the test stick downward and directly into your urine stream for at least 5 seconds or until it's thoroughly wet. *Don't urinate on the windows of the stick.* You can also urinate into a clean dry cup and dip the test stick (absorbent tip only) into the urine for at least 5 seconds.

2. Lay the test stick on a clean, dry, flat surface.

Reading the results

1. Wait at least 5 minutes to read the results. When the test is finished, a line will appear in the small window (control window).

2. *If there is no line in the large rectangular window* (test window) *or if the line is lighter than the line in the small rectangular window,* you haven't begun your LH surge. You should continue with daily testing.

3. *If you see one line in the large window that is similar to or darker than the line in the small window* (as shown at the right), you've detected an LH surge. This means that you should ovulate within the next 24 to 36 hours. Once you've determined that you're about to ovulate, you know you're at the start of the most fertile time of your cycle.

PERFORMING A HOME PREGNANCY TEST

Dear Patient:

A home pregnancy test will detect a hormone in your urine that your body produces only if you are pregnant. The test can detect this hormone — human chorionic gonadotropin, or hCG — as early as 1 day after you miss your period. If you have been pregnant or had a miscarriage within the past 8 weeks, or if you are taking a medication that contains hCG or that's used in combination with hCG, the test may produce a false-positive result. In any case, always consult your doctor before and after taking this test.

Follow these steps to learn how to perform the test.

Getting ready

1. Read the instructions thoroughly before you perform the test. This test can be performed any time of the day or night — it doesn't need to be done first thing in the morning. However, the concentration of hCG is greatest in the first voided specimen, so doing it first thing decreases the chance of a false-negative result.

2. Remove the test stick from the package and slide the clear splash guard back to expose the absorbent tip.

Performing the test

1. Sit on the toilet and hold the test stick by the thumb grip.

2. Direct the absorbent tip downward and directly into your urine stream for at least 5 seconds or until it is thoroughly wet (as shown above). Do not urinate on the windows.

3. You can also urinate into a clean, dry cup or container and dip the test stick (absorbent tip only) into the urine for at least 5 seconds.

4. Lay the test stick on a clean, dry, flat surface.

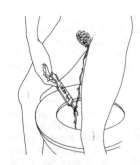

Reading the results

1. Wait at least 3 minutes to read the results. When the test is finished, a line will appear in the small rectangular window.

2. *If you see one line in the round and rectangular windows* (as shown below), the test has indicated that you are pregnant. You should consult your doctor as soon as possible to discuss your pregnancy.

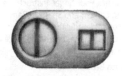

3. *If the only visible line is in the control* (rectangular window), the test has indicated that you aren't pregnant. You can perform a repeat test with a new test kit if your period doesn't start within a week.

Note: If results appear in the round window but not in the rectangular control window, don't read the results because they may be inaccurate. Call the toll-free number located on the test box or package insert.

PERFORMING A HOME HIV TEST

Dear Patient:

Human immunodeficiency virus (HIV) is a virus that attacks your immune system and causes acquired immunodeficiency syndrome (AIDS). By testing your blood, you can determine if you've been infected with HIV. Remember that, even if you've been exposed to HIV, it may not become evident in your blood for 6 months. If you have any questions about your test results or the risk factors associated with HIV, always consult a doctor. Follow these steps to learn how to obtain a blood sample and how to perform the test.

Getting ready

1. Begin by assembling the necessary equipment included in the packet: a lancet, a test card with your personal identification number (to receive the confidential and anonymous test results), and the envelope in which to send the test card to the laboratory.

2. Read the instructions thoroughly before you stick your finger. Instructions appear in English and Spanish. Remove the personal identification card from the bottom of the test card and place it in a safe place.

Obtaining blood

1. Wash your hands thoroughly and dry them. Choose a site on the end or side of any fingertip. To enhance blood flow, hold your finger under warm water for a minute or two.

2. Hold your hand below your heart, and milk the blood toward the fingertip you plan to pierce. Squeeze that fingertip with the thumb of the same hand. Place your fingertip, with your thumb still pressed against it, on a firm surface such as a table.

3. Twist off the lancet's protective cap. Then grasp the lancet and quickly pierce your fingertip just to the side of the finger pad, where you have more blood vessels and fewer nerve endings.

4. Remove your thumb from your fingertip to permit blood flow. Then milk your finger gently until you get a large, hanging drop of blood.

5. Point your finger down directly over the three circles on the test card. Completely fill each circle with blood.

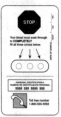

6. Place any used lancets in the containers attached to the mailing card. Slip the test card in the postage-paid mailer, seal the mailer, and send it to the address printed on the front. Save the part of the card that lists the toll-free phone number to call for results.

Obtaining the results

In about 1 week, call the toll-free number on the identification card. Give the person who answers your identification number and wait for the results. If your test is positive for HIV, a specially trained counselor will advise you what to do next and will tell you about HIV and AIDS organizations nationwide. If your test results are negative for HIV, the trained counselor will advise you how to maintain your negative HIV status.

Remember, a negative test result doesn't necessarily mean you're free from HIV infection. It may simply mean that the antibodies are not yet present in your blood. To be certain, repeat the test in 6 months.

TESTING FOR BLOOD IN YOUR STOOL

Dear Patient:
A home fecal occult blood test is an easy, inexpensive way to detect blood in your stool. For accurate results, follow the directions given by the nurse or doctor, read the instructions included with the test kit, and review these guidelines.

How to get ready
Don't eat red meat or raw fruits and vegetables for 3 days before you take the test and during the test period. Avoid diet supplements containing iron or vitamin C and painkillers containing aspirin or ibuprofen (such as Advil and Nuprin) for the same time period. All of these substances can affect test results.

Increase your intake of high-fiber foods, such as whole grain breads and cereals. Your doctor may also ask you to eat popcorn or nuts.

How to perform the test
1. Make sure all your supplies are in one place. They may include your test cards (or slides), a chemical developer, a wooden applicator, and a watch with a second hand.
2. Obtain a stool sample from the toilet bowl. Use the applicator to smear a thin film of the sample onto the slot marked "A" on the front of the test card. Smear a thin film of a second sample from a different area of the same stool onto the slot marked "B" on the same side of the card.
3. *If the doctor or a lab will be analyzing the test samples,* close slots A and B. Put your name and the date on the test kit and return the card (or slide) to the doctor or lab as soon as possible.

If you're doing the test yourself, turn the card over and open the back window. Apply two drops of the chemical developer to the paper covering each

A   B

1. Collect small stool specimen on applicator. Apply thin smear in box A.
2. Reuse applicator to obtain another sample from a different part of the stool. Apply thin smear in box B.
3. Close cover. Place slide away from heat and light. Return slide to doctor.

sample. Wait 1 minute; then read the results.

If either slot has a bluish tint, the test results are positive for blood in the stool. If neither slot looks blue, the test results are normal. Write down the results.

4. Repeat the test on your next two bowel movements. Report the results of all the tests to the doctor. Even if only one of the six test results is positive, the doctor may recommend other tests.

Discard any unused supplies when you've completed all tests.

Dear Patient:

Your doctor wants you to have your urine tested. A urine test can tell whether you have a infection or whether you have too much or too little of certain substances in your body. To make sure that the test results are accurate, your urine shouldn't contain germs from your hands or your penis.

Follow these directions carefully. Read them through to the end before collecting the specimen.

Note: Don't drink a lot of water before the test. This could affect the accuracy of test results.

1. Wash your hands thoroughly. Open the package of disposable wipes that the nurse gave you and place it on a clean, dry surface nearby.

2. Remove the lid from the specimen cup and place it flat side down. Do not touch the inside of the cup or lid.

3. Prepare to urinate. If you're uncircumcised, first pull back your foreskin. Using a disposable wipe, clean the head of your penis from the urethral opening toward you, as shown. Then discard the used wipe.

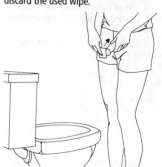

4. Urinate a small amount into the toilet. After 1 or 2 seconds, catch about 1 ounce (30 milliliters) of urine in the specimen cup.

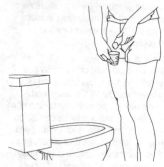

The nurse will tell you how far to fill the cup. As a rule, you'll fill it about one-fourth or more full.

Don't allow the cup to touch your penis at any time. When you're done, place the lid on the cup and return it to the nurse.

COLLECTING A URINE SPECIMEN: FOR FEMALES

Dear Patient:

Your doctor has asked you to provide a urine specimen for testing. The specimen can tell whether you have an infection or whether you have too much or too little of certain substances in your body.

To make sure that the test results are accurate, your urine shouldn't contain germs from your hands, labia, or urethral opening.

Follow the instructions below carefully. Read them through to the end before collecting your specimen.

Note: Don't drink a lot of water before the test. This could affect the accuracy of test results.

1. Wash your hands thoroughly. Open the package of disposable wipes that the nurse gave you and place it on a clean, dry, surface nearby.

2. Remove the lid from the specimen cup and place it flat side down. Do not touch the inside of the cup or lid.

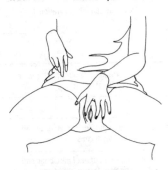

3. Sit as far back on the toilet as possible. Spread your labia apart with one hand, keeping the folds separated for the rest of the procedure.

4. Using the disposable wipes, clean the area between the labia and around the urethra thoroughly from front to back. Use a new wipe for each stroke.

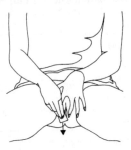

5. Urinate a small amount into the toilet. After 1 or 2 seconds, hold the specimen cup below your urine stream and catch about 1 ounce (30 milliliters) of urine in the cup. Don't allow the cup to touch your skin at any time.

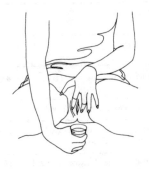

6. Place the lid on the cup and return it to the nurse.

APPENDIX C: CRITICAL LABORATORY VALUES

The abnormal laboratory test values listed below have immediate life-and-death significance to the patient. Report such values to the patient's doctor immediately.

Test	Low value	Common causes and effects
Ammonia	< 15 µg/dl	Renal failure
Calcium, serum	< 7 mg/dl	Vitamin D or parathyroid hormone deficiency: tetany, seizures
Carbon dioxide and bicarbonate, blood	< 10 mEq/L	Complex pattern of metabolic and respiratory factors
Creatine kinase isoenzymes (CK-MB)		
Creatinine, serum		
D-dimer, serum or cerebrospinal fluid (CSF)		
Glucose, blood	< 40 mg/dl	Excess insulin administration: brain damage
Gram stain, CSF		
Hemoglobin	< 8 g/dl	Hemorrhage, vitamin B_{12} or iron deficiency: heart failure
International Normalized Ratio (INR)		
Partial pressure of carbon dioxide in arterial blood ($Paco_2$)	< 20 mm Hg	Complex pattern of metabolic and respiratory factors
Partial pressure of oxygen in arterial blood (Pao_2)	< 50 mm Hg	Complex pattern of metabolic and respiratory factors
Partial thromboplastin time (PTT)		
pH, arterial blood	< 7.2	Complex pattern of metabolic and respiratory factors
Platelet count	< 50,000/µl	Bone marrow suppression: hemorrhage

High value	Common causes and effects
> 50 µg/dl	Severe hepatic disease leading to hepatic coma, Reye's syndrome, GI hemorrhage, heart failure
> 12 mg/dl	Hyperparathyroidism: coma
> 40 mEq/L	Complex pattern of metabolic and respiratory factors
> 5%	Acute myocardial infarction (MI)
> 4 mg/dl	Renal failure: coma
> 250 µg/ml	Disseminated intravascular coagulation (DIC), pulmonary embolism, arterial or venous thrombosis, subarachnoid hemorrhage (CSF only), secondary fibrinolysis
> 300 mg/dl (with ketonemia and electrolyte imbalance)	Diabetes: diabetic coma
Gram positive or gram negative	Bacterial meningitis
>18 g/dl	Chronic obstructive pulmonary disease: thrombosis, polycythemia vera
> 3.0	DIC, uncontrolled oral anticoagulation
> 70 mm Hg	Complex pattern of metabolic and respiratory factors
> 40 sec (> 70 sec for patient on heparin)	Anticoagulation factor deficiency: hemorrhage
> 7.6	Complex pattern of metabolic and respiratory factors
> 500,000/µl	Leukemia, reaction to acute bleeding: hemorrhage

(continued)

Test	Low value	Common causes and effects
Potassium, serum	< 3 mEq/L	Vomiting and diarrhea, diuretic therapy: cardiotoxicity, arrhythmia, cardiac arrest
Prothrombin time (PT)		
Sodium, serum	< 120 mEq/L	Diuretic therapy: cardiac failure
Troponin I		
White blood cell (WBC) count	< 2,000/µl	Bone marrow suppression: infection
WBC count, CSF		

High value	Common causes and effects
> 6 mEq/L	Renal disease, diuretic therapy: cardiotoxicity, arrhythmia
> 14 sec (> 20 sec for patient on warfarin)	Anticoagulant therapy, anticoagulation factor deficiency: hemorrhage
> 160 mEq/L	Dehydration: vascular collapse
> 2 µg/ml	Acute MI
> 20,000/µl	Leukemia: infection
> 10/µl	Meningitis, encephalitis: infection

SELECTED READINGS

Bausch, D.G., et al. "Diagnosis and Clinical Virology of Lassa Fever as Evaluated by Enzyme-Linked Immunosorbent Assay, Indirect Fluorescent-Antibody Test, and Virus Isolation," *Journal of Clinical Microbiology* 38(7):2670-2677, July 2000.

Carithers, R.L., Jr, et al. "Diagnostic testing for hepatitis C," *Seminars in Liver Disease,* 20(2):159-171, 2000.

Cavanaugh, B.M. *Nurse's Manual of Laboratory and Diagnostic Tests,* 3rd ed. Philadelphia: F.A. Davis Co., 1999.

Cohen, D.E., et al. "Diagnostic tests for type IV or delayed hypersensitivity reactions," *Clinical Allergy and Immunology,* 15:287-305, 2000.

Diagnostics: An A-to-Z Nursing Guide to Laboratory Tests and Diagnostic Procedures. Springhouse, Pa.: Springhouse Corp., 2001.

Ernst, D.J. "Collecting Blood Culture Specimens," *Nursing99* 29(7):56-58, July 1999.

Fauci, A.S., et al., eds. *Harrison's Principles of Internal Medicine,* 14th ed. New York: McGraw-Hill Book Co., 1998.

Fischbach, F.T.. *A Manual of Laboratory and Diagnostic Tests,* 6th ed. Philadelphia: Lippincott-Raven Pubs., 2000.

Handbook of Diagnostic Tests, 2nd ed. Springhouse, Pa.: Springhouse Corp., 1999.

Heifets, L. "Dilemmas and realities of rapid diagnostic tests for tuberculosis," *Chest,*118(1):4-5, July 2000.

Yu, M., et al. "Screening tests of disseminated intravascular coagulation: guidelines for rapid and specific laboratory diagnosis," *Critical Care Medicine,* 28(6):1777-1780, June 2000.

Yunginger, J.W., et al. "Quantitative IgE antibody assays in allergic diseases," *Journal of Allergy and Clinical Immunology,* 105(6PtI):1077-1084, June 2000.

INDEX